Ethnic Considerations in Facial Plastic Surgery

gy

c Surgery

neiro

Executive Editor: Timothy Hiscock
Managing Editor: J. Owen Zurhellen IV
Editorial Assistant: Kate Barron
Director, Editorial Services: Mary Jo Casey
Production Editor: Kenneth L. Chumbley
International Production Director: Andreas Schabert
Vice President, Editorial and E-Product Development: Vera Spillner
International Marketing Director: Fiona Henderson
International Sales Director: Louisa Turrell
Director of Sales, North America: Mike Roseman
Senior Vice President and Chief Operating Officer: Sarah Vanderbilt
President: Brian D. Scanlan

Medical Illustrators: Emily Ciosek and Thomson Digital
Front Cover Illustration: Emily Ciosek

Library of Congress Cataloging-in-Publication Data
Ethnic considerations in facial plastic surgery / [edited by] Roxana Cobo.
p. ; cm.
Includes bibliographical references.
ISBN 978-1-62623-023-1 (alk. paper)—ISBN 978-1-62623-024-8 (eBook)
I. Cobo, Roxana, editor.
[DNLM: 1. Face—surgery. 2. Reconstructive Surgical Procedures. 3. Cultural Competency. 4. Culturally Competent Care. 5. Surgery, Plastic—methods. WE 705]
RD119.5.F33
617.5'20592—dc23
2015026381

Thieme Publishers New York
333 Seventh Avenue, New York, NY 10001 USA
+1 800 782 3488, customerservice@thieme.com

Thieme Publishers Stuttgart
Rüdigerstrasse 14, 70469 Stuttgart, Germany
+49 [0]711 8931 421, customerservice@thieme.de

Thieme Publishers Delhi
A-12, Second Floor, Sector-2, Noida-201301
Uttar Pradesh, India
+91 120 45 566 00, customerservice@thieme.in

Thieme Publishers Rio de Janeiro, Thieme Publicações Ltda.
Edifício Rodolpho de Paoli, 25º andar
Av. Nilo Peçanha, 50 – Sala 2508
Rio de Janeiro 20020-906, Brasil
+55 21 3172 2297

Cover design: Thieme Publishing Group
Typesetting by Prairie Papers

Printed in India by Replika Press Pvt. Ltd. 5 4 3 2 1

ISBN 978-1-62623-023-1

Also available as an e-book:
eISBN 978-1-62623-024-8

Dedicated to the men in my life: to my dad for showing me the value of quality, perseverance, and persistence;
to Giuliano, for his patience and understanding after all these months of hard work;
and to my boys, Aulo and Carlo, who know that when things are done with determination,
dedication, and passion the sky is the limit to what can be achieved.

Contents

Section IV The Asian Perspective

Section V The Mediterranean and Middle Eastern Perspective

Section VI Special Topics

Menu of Accompanying Videos

Foreword

In spite of the many different textbooks on facial plastic surgery that are available today, there is not one as unique as Roxana Cobo's *Ethnic Considerations in Facial Plastic Surgery*. Only when you open the cover of this book will you realize how much you needed it and what a valuable resource it will be in your management of the ethnic patient. Although our specialty has always recognized the differences in anatomy, surgery, and management of the ethnic patient, it is only in the last decade that we have begun to seriously study these patients, learn from them, and share our experiences with each other. This is a corollary to our globalization and increasing understanding of the impact of race and culture on our perception of attractiveness and beauty. These ubiquitous forces, especially as propagated by the Internet, have made it imperative that every surgeon, no matter where he or she practices, be aware of the special needs of the ethnic patient. Further, in all cultures the traditional aesthetic goals are evolving due to these very same forces.

Ethnic Considerations in Facial Plastic Surgery begins with a section on general considerations. It reviews the essence of beauty, both physically and psychologically, and leads us to better comprehend the aesthetic goals we should aspire to for our patients. Chapters on racial anatomical differences, especially regarding the nose, are followed by an important chapter on the consultation process.

Dr. Cobo then has internationally renowned experts from their respective regions deliver comprehensive, yet succinct, information on surgery within their ethnic groups. This includes all of the world's major ethnicities: Latin American/Mestizo, African, Asian, Mediterranean, and Middle Eastern. Each section begins with a chapter on aesthetic, ethnic, and cultural considerations. These chapters provide a fountain of fascinating and useful background information to enhance understanding of the treatment challenges ahead. In addition, current aesthetic trends are reviewed and put into perspective. Cultural, ethnic, and religious factors affecting the ethnic patient are explored in an insightful, reasoned, and wise manner. Even the philosophy of ancient Chinese-face reading is included! The reader not only learns but is left to reflect upon his or her own views and practices.

With this background, each section has subsequent chapters revealing in detail both surgical and nonsurgical aesthetic management of the ethnic face. It is appropriate that rhinoplasty—being the most challenging procedure and arguably having the most differences ethnically—receives prime attention. Additionally, there are chapters covering ethnic blepharoplasty, face and neck lifting, and noninvasive procedures. The final section of the book covers important subjects, such as fat grafting, management of scars and keloids, and skin tightening devices for the ethnic patient.

This book benefits from a beautiful layout with subsections in each chapter. There are exceptional patient illustrations, intraoperative photographs, graphics, and tables to illustrate the concepts presented and to enhance learning. Each chapter has a reliable and extensive list of references for the reader seeking more explicit inquiry into the topic at hand. The layout is simple and attractive, and the font is comfortable to read.

In creating *Ethnic Considerations in Facial Plastic Surgery*, Dr. Cobo has drawn on her personal wealth of experience and knowledge as a renowned surgeon and respected teacher in the international community. Her carefully chosen and internationally esteemed contributing authors similarly reveal their mastery of their topics and their ability to impart their wisdom.

This book (with its accompanying videos) is a new and exciting literary addition to our specialty. It provides well-organized, comprehensive, and valuable information about the care of the ethnic patient. It is a highly desirable book for all practicing facial plastic surgeons and a mandatory book for all those planning to treat ethnic patients.

Read, learn, enjoy.

Peter A. Adamson, MD, FRCSC, FACS
Professor and Head
Division of Facial Plastic and Reconstructive Surgery
Department of Otolaryngology–Head and Neck Surgery
University of Toronto
Toronto, Ontario, Canada
President, International Board for Certification in Facial Plastic and Reconstructive Surgery
Senior Advisor, American Board of Facial Plastic and Reconstructive Surgery
Past President, American Academy of Facial Plastic and Reconstructive Surgery
Past President, Canadian Academy of Facial Plastic and Reconstructive Surgery

Preface

The world has become globalized. Migration patterns have increased and changed dramatically over time, leading to vivid changes in all populations. The constant blending of races has resulted in more mixed cultures and ethnic groups. Nevertheless, human beings continue to cherish and pursue a feeling of attractiveness that defines social behavior regardless of ethnicity or race. Developments in communications, such as social networks and web searching, have increased the availability of information across populations. This data explosion brings with it a greater awareness of appearances, as well as a more globalized idea of beauty on the whole. In addition, cosmetic procedures cease to be a privilege of the wealthy and have become available to patients regardless of their economic status. This is why, in the last few decades, there has been an exponential increase in cosmetic procedures globally.

Facial plastic surgery is no exception. Advances in technology and surgical techniques have made this specialty a rapidly changing one. Patients that come to our offices are diverse. As a result, we need to have a broader understanding of the different cultural, ethnic, racial, and anatomic differences in the populations we are treating. It then becomes our responsibility to understand and deal with continuously changing global concepts of beauty.

When I started my practice of facial plastic surgery over 20 years ago, I soon realized that I was dealing with patients that did not fit the prototype within the literature. Over time and after teaching all around the world, I was amazed to find that my perception was shared by many friends and colleagues. It was interesting to see and learn new particular techniques and concepts. These have nurtured and formed my own unique approach to the multiethnic patients I face on a daily basis.

Most of today's publications focus on specific topics in facial plastic surgery. Some deal with the specialty as a whole, but to date, we do not have a comprehensive source focusing on the many considerations that should be taken into account when dealing with patients of multiethnic backgrounds. This book was written to address that dearth of information.

The contributors to this book are experts in the field from different regions of the world. There is a bank of information deposited in these pages that reflects the different authors' views on how they approach different ethnic groups, and what different types of procedures can be offered. The distribution of the book is relatively straightforward. It starts with a section on general concepts where topics we have to deal with on a daily basis are presented: today's definition of beauty, knowledge of important anatomical differences, ethnic reflections with emphasis on the nose (rhinoplasty is the most frequently performed facial plastic procedure globally), and recommendations for a successful consultation with the facial plastic patient.

The book is then divided into four important ethnic sections: the Latin American/Mestizo patient, the African patient, the Asian patient, and the Mediterranean and Middle Eastern patient. Each section starts with a very important chapter where aesthetic, ethnic, and cultural considerations of each group are presented and discussed, as well as current cosmetic trends respective to each. It is fascinating to see how interests and requests vary depending on where the patient comes from. Each section also features special topics, depending on which are the most important surgical and nonsurgical procedures performed.

The final section of the book includes some special topics, which are either independent of any specific ethnic group, or have become very important procedures performed by all facial plastic surgeons. With this type of distribution my intention is to orient the reader to focus either on specific ethnic groups or in areas of interest. All chapters contain valuable illustrations and photographs of surgical techniques and of pre- and postoperative cases, offering readers a greater, more comprehensive educational experience.

Through the content of this book, it is my goal to provide a broader perspective when dealing with ethnic patients. Everything we do will have an impact on the patient's overall well-being. Needs and desires of patients can change but it is our duty to try to accomplish an end result that not only will be aesthetically pleasing but will also be safe and reliable, and accompanied by patient satisfaction.

Roxana Cobo, MD

Acknowledgments

This book is a dream come true and the result of great teamwork. None of it would have been accomplished without the support from Thieme Medical Publishers Inc. To Timothy Hiscock who believed this project could be accomplished, to J. Owen Zurhellen for his infinite patience, and to Kate Barron, Kenny Chumbley, and the rest of the team at Thieme for their hard work and perseverance that has made this project possible.

Thank you to all of the authors from all around the globe, who took time off their busy agendas to put in writing their amazing knowledge in the field of facial plastic surgery. For many of them, English is not their first language, so the effort was even greater.

I would not be what I am today without the mentorship of Dr. Pedro Blanco, chief of the Department of Otolaryngology in Cali, Colombia, and without the ongoing support, guidance, and friendship of Ted Cook and Gilbert Nolst Trenité, amazing facial plastic surgeons, teachers, and teammates of incredible academic projects.

Contributors

Tareq Alotaibi, MD
Department of Otolaryngology–Head and Neck Surgery
Facial Plastic Division
College of Medicine
King Saud University
Riyadh, Kingdom of Saudi Arabia

Fazil Apaydin, MD
Professor of Otorhinolaryngology
Department of Otorhinolaryngology
Ege University
Bornova-Izmir, Turkey

Scott A. Asher, MD
Director, The Facial Plastic and Reconstructive Center
Tallahassee Ear, Nose, and Throat–Head and Neck Surgery
Clinical Assistant Professor
Florida State University College of Medicine
Tallahassee, Florida

Babak Azizzadeh, MD, FACS
Director of the Center for Advanced Facial Plastic Surgery
Associate Clinical Professor
Department of Head and Neck Surgery
David Geffen School of Medicine
University of California–Los Angeles
Beverly Hills, California

Sameer Ali Bafaqeeh, MD
Senior Consultant and Professor
Department of Otolaryngology–Head and Neck Surgery
Chairman, Facial Plastic Division
College of Medicine
King Saud University
Riyadh, Kingdom of Saudi Arabia

Scott Bevans, MD
MAJ, United States Army
Department of Facial Plastic and Reconstructive Surgery
Head and Neck Oncology and Microvascular Surgery
University of Washington
Seattle, Washington

Chiara Botti, MD
Plastic Surgeon
Director, Villa Bella Clinic
Salò, Italy

Giovanni Botti, MD
Clinical Professor of Plastic Surgery
University of Verona
ISAPS Traveling Professor
Villa Bella Clinic
Salò, Italy

Tara E. Brennan, MD
Assistant Professor, Facial Plastic and Reconstructive Surgery
Department of Surgery
Division of Otolaryngology–Head and Neck Surgery
University of New Mexico
Albuquerque, New Mexico

Roxana Cobo, MD
Head, Department of Otolaryngology
Centro Médico Imbanaco
Cali, Colombia
Ad-Honorem Professor, Facial Plastic Surgery
Department of Otolaryngology
Nueva Granada Military Hospital
Nueva Granada Military University
Bogotá, Colombia

Christian P. Conderman, MD
Assistant Professor
Division of Facial Plastic Surgery
Department of Otorhinolaryngology–Head and Neck Surgery
University of Texas Health Science Center at Houston
Houston, Texas

Tara Davison, BS
Director of Operations
Campbell Facial Plastics
Sheboygan, Wisconsin

Steven H. Dayan, MD, FACS
Clinical Assistant Professor
Division of Facial Plastic Surgery
Department of Otolaryngology–Head and Neck Surgery
University of Illinois–Chicago
Chicago, Illinois

Tatiana K. Dixon, MD
Assistant Professor, Facial Plastic and Reconstructive Surgery
Department of Otolaryngology–Head and Neck Surgery
University of Illinois–Chicago
Chicago, Illinois

Rafael Espinosa Delgado, MD
ENT and Facial Plastic Surgeon
CEO, San Jose Laser Spa
Department of Otolaryngology and Facial Plastic Surgery
Hospital San Jose de Hermosillo
Hermosillo, Mexico

Jaime Fandiño Izundegui, MD
Chairman
Department of Otolaryngology–Head and Neck Surgery
Department of Facial Plastic Surgery
Hospital Español de Mexico
Mexico City, Mexico

Hossam M. T. Foda, MD
Professor and Head
Facial Plastic Surgery Division
Faculty of Medicine
Alexandria Medical School
Alexandria University
Alexandria, Egypt

Néstor Ricardo González Marín, MD
Otolaryngologist and Epidemiologist
Department of Otolaryngology
Nueva Granada Military University
Bogotá, Colombia

Monte Oyd Harris, MD, FACS
Founder, Center for Aesthetic Modernism
Chevy Chase, Maryland
Clinical Assistant Professor
Department of Otolaryngology–Head and Neck Surgery
Georgetown University Medical Center
Washington, DC

Rolando Hidalgo Moiron, MD
Facial Plastic Surgeon
Private Practice
Professor
Department of Otolaryngology–Head and Neck Surgery
Lluvenis Medical Center and Spa
Ciudad Satélite, Mexico

Melissa Hu, MD
Department of Otolaryngology–Head and Neck Surgery
Louisiana State University Health
Shreveport, Louisiana

Yong Ju Jang, MD, PhD
Professor
Department of Otolaryngology
Asan Medical Center
University of Ulsan College of Medicine
Seoul, South Korea

Iman Khodaei, MD, FRCSI, FRCS (ORL–HNS)
Locum Consultant, Ear, Nose, and Throat Surgeon
Department of Ear, Nose, and Throat
Leighton Hospital
Cheshire, United Kingdom

Min Joo Kim, MD
Department of Otolaryngology
Asan Medical Center
University of Ulsan College of Medicine
Seoul, Republic of Korea

Russell W. H. Kridel, MD, FACS
Clinical Professor and Director
Division of Facial Plastic Surgery
Department of Otorhinolaryngology–Head and Neck Surgery
University of Texas Health Science Center at Houston
Private Practice
Facial Plastic Surgery Associates
Houston, Texas

Samuel M. Lam, MD, FACS
Private Practice
Willow Bend Wellness Center
Plano, Texas

Wayne F. Larrabee Jr., MD, FACS
Director, Larrabee Center for Plastic Surgery
Clinical Professor, Facial Plastic Surgery
Department of Otolaryngology–Head and Neck Surgery
University of Washington
Seattle, Washington

Hyoung Jin Moon, MD
President, Dr. Moon's Aesthetic Surgery Clinic
Clinical Professor
Department of Otolaryngology–Head and Neck Surgery
The Yonsei University Medical College
Seoul, South Korea

Xiongzheng Mu, MD
Professor
Department of Plastic Surgery
Huashan Hospital
Fudan University
Shanghai, China

Gilbert J. Nolst Trenité, MD, PhD
Professor
Departments of Ear, Nose, Throat and Facial Plastic Surgery
Amsterdam, The Netherlands

Pietro Palma, MD
Private Practice
The Face Clinic
Milan, Italy
Clinical Professor
Department of Otolaryngology–Head and Neck Surgery
University of Insubria
Varese, Italy

José Roberto Parisi Jurado, MD, DDS
Facial Plastic Surgeon
Department of Otolaryngology
University of São Paulo
São Paulo, Brazil

Jose Antonio Patrocinio, MD
Chairman and Full Professor
Department of Otolaryngology
Federal University of Uberlândia
Uberlândia, Brazil

Lucas G. Patrocinio, MD, PhD
Assistant Professor
Department of Otorhinolaryngology and Facial Plastic Surgery
Federal University of Uberlândia
Uberlândia, Brazil

Tomas G. Patrocinio, MD
Assistant Professor
Division of Facial Plastic Surgery
Department of Otolaryngology
Federal University of Uberlândia
Uberlândia, Brazil

Santdeep Paun, MBBS, FRCS
Consultant Facial Plastic Surgeon
Department of Otolaryngology–Head and Neck Surgery
St Bartholomew's and The Royal London Hospitals
London, United Kingdom

Fernando Pedroza Campo, MD
Facial Plastic Surgeon and General Director
La Font Ltda./CES University
Facial Plastic Surgery Specialization
Bogotá, Colombia

Luis Fernando Pedroza, MD
Facial Plastic Surgeon and Medical Director
La Font Ltda.
Plastic Surgery Clinic
Bogotá, Colombia

Leila Freire Rêgo Lima, MD
Otolaryngologist/Facial Plastic Surgeon
Academic Member of the Post-Graduate Course in Facial Plastic Surgery–Instituto Jurado
São Paulo, Brazil

Thomas Romo III, MD, FACS
Director, Facial Plastic and Reconstructive Surgery
Lenox Hill Hospital
Manhattan Eye, Ear, and Throat Hospital
The New York Head and Neck Institute
New York, New York

Frank Rosengaus Leizgold, MD
Facial Plastic Surgeon
Medical Director
Ultimate Medica
Mexico City, Mexico

Hangyan Shi, MD
Department of Plastic and Reconstructive Surgery
Zhejiang Provincial People's Hospital
Hangzhou, China

Choladhis Sinrachtanant, MD
Head of Facial Plastic Division
Department of Otolaryngology
Faculty of Medicine, Siriraj Hospital, Mahidol University
Founding President
Facial Plastic and Reconstructive Surgery Association of Thailand
Bangkok, Thailand

Gordon M. S. Soo, MD
Clinical Associate Professor (hon.)
Chief of Facial Plastic Surgery
Department of Otorhinolaryngology–Head and Neck Surgery
The Chinese University of Hong Kong
Hong Kong

Fred J. Stucker, MD, FACS
Jack W. Pou Professor and Chairman
Department of Otolaryngology–Head and Neck Surgery
Louisiana State University Health
Shreveport, Louisiana

Valerie Tay, MBBS, MRCS, MMed, FAMS
Medical Director
Singapore Medical Group ENT Centre
Visiting Consultant
Department of Otolaryngology
Tan Tock Seng Hospital
Singapore

J. Regan Thomas, MD, FACS
Mansueto Professor and Chairman
Department of Otolaryngology–Head and Neck Surgery
University of Illinois–Chicago
Chicago, Illinois

Dean M. Toriumi, MD
Professor
Department of Otolaryngology–Head and Neck Surgery
College of Medicine
University of Illinois–Chicago
Chicago, Illinois

Miriam de la Torre Campos, MD
ENT and Facial Plastic Surgeon
Medical Director, San Jose Laser Spa
Department of Otolaryngology and Facial Plastic Surgery
Hospital San Jose de Hermosillo
Hermosillo, Mexico

Satyen Undavia, MD
Private Practice
Head and Neck Associates
Wynnewood, Pennsylvania

Ignacio Viza-Puiggros, MD
International Fellow
European Academy of Facial Plastic and Reconstructive Surgery
Department of Otolaryngology–Head and Neck Surgery
Lenox Hill Hospital
New York, New York
Hospital Plato
Barcelona, Spain

Frederick T. C. Wong, MD
Clinical Assistant Professor (hon.)
Division of Facial Plastic Surgery
Department of Otorhinolaryngology–Head and Neck Surgery
The Chinese University of Hong Kong
Hong Kong

Sufan Wu, MD, PhD
Professor and Head
Department of Plastic and Reconstructive Surgery
Zhejiang Provincial People's Hospital
Hangzhou, China

Yingzhi Wu, MD
Department of Plastic Surgery
Huashan Hospital
Fudan University
Shanghai, China

Eduardo C. Yap, MD, FPSO-HNS
Department of Facial Plastic Surgery
Belo Medical Group
Manila, Philippines

Ian Loh Chi Yuan, MBBS, MRCS, FAMS
Director
Facial Plastic and Reconstruction Service
Consultant
Department of Otorhinolaryngology–Head and Neck Surgery
Changi General Hospital
Singapore

Section I

General Considerations

1 The New Definition of Beauty

Tara Davison and Steven H. Dayan

1.1 Introduction

Throughout time, the meaning of beauty has been defined and redefined by everyone from ancient philosophers to today's fashion magazine editors. Scientists tend to appreciate a more Darwinian approach to beauty: beauty serves a utilitarian purpose, namely for survival of one's genes. Hence, beauty is a universal signal that one is healthy and viable, and, over time, certain physical characteristics have remained associated with beauty. Symmetry, averageness, and youthfulness are all associated with beauty.

From an evolutionary perspective, beauty exists as a form of subliminal communication facilitating the projection of our genes onto and into the next generation. But beauty is raw and primary, and humans rely on much more before deciding if someone or something is beautiful or attractive to them. The context within which that beauty is identified and perceived is as influential as the absolute beauty. Additionally, other factors, such as posture, adornments, fashion, and expression, all affect the perceived degree of beauty projected. We label the perceived beauty that takes into account all of these factors as attraction. Therefore, the value of beauty is best appreciated within the context of attraction. The same way that a karaoke version of a hit song may sound awful, a beautiful person has the ability to appear highly unattractive in certain contexts. While studies have shown that being beautiful may get one further in life, beauty is more advantageous if the person has the ability to communicate their beauty in an attractive way.[1] Conversely, consider a celebrity who is undeniably physically attractive, such as Mel Gibson. Regardless of his looks, when found in a compromised situation of being caught yelling vulgar profanities following a drunken driving incident, he appeared highly unattractive.

In contrast, beauty has the potential to be overlooked when not presented in an expected context. This was demonstrated in a social experiment conducted by *The Washington Post* on 12 January 2007. During morning rush hour, the famed violinist Joshua Bell played a set of classical music on a very rare violin at a Washington D.C. Metro stop. Almost no one stopped to listen: the hurrying pedestrians barely noticed that one of the world's most celebrated musicians was playing extraordinary music on a multimillion-dollar Stradivarius violin, when only two days earlier he had played a sold-out Boston amphitheater where seats cost $100 apiece. The goal of the test was to see how his music would be perceived in a different environment. After 45 minutes of his performing at the Metro stop, his violin case had a mere $27 in it.

The way in which the element of raw beauty is wrapped, delivered, and interpreted by an observer is what I refer to as the first impression. First impressions are judgments that are formed immediately from no preconceived associations. They are based on specific parameters that are rapidly evaluated and subconsciously processed. Factors that influence first impressions consist of the raw physical characteristics of beauty that we are innately prewired to recognize. Secondary factors also contribute, such as cosmetics, accessories, expression, posture, or clothing, but these also have the potential to overwhelm raw physical traits of beauty. The packaged impression that these factors portray results in a person's being considered attractive or unattractive based on their delivery. First impressions are meaningful and consequential. As a species evolving over 3.5 million years, *Homo sapiens* has developed an incredibly reliable system of first impressions. The appropriateness and accuracy of a first impression are critical for survival. But, of course, we have learned that, despite the relative accuracy of first impressions, they can be misleading. The context within which that first impression is created and perceived has significant influence on the judgment and elicited behaviors of both the subject projecting as well as the one receiving the impression.

Attractiveness is a fluid, conceptual construction formulated by the basic elements of beauty. However, being perceived as attractive is more than just encompassing individual components of beauty. Attractiveness is dynamic and exists within a framework of social and cultural norms. As an example, on the east coast of Africa among certain native tribes, a 14-cm plate placed within the lip of a young female may be seen as beautifying, increasing her attractiveness; however, those in a Western culture may find it unsightly. In contrast, the natives of the Mursi tribe of Ethiopia would probably not find over-inflated hyaluronic-plumped lips attractive. Beauty is more likely to be perceived as attractive when delivered and accepted in an expected manner. The state of mind of the observer is also fundamental to the interpretation.

Just as Joshua Bell's music may not be interpreted as attractive in a subway corridor, if a physically beautiful person passes you the day you lost your best friend, you may not recognize that person as attractive. However, at a later date, while enjoying a leisurely moment, that same person walking by in a form-fitting outfit may spark your attention. The take-home is that while one may possess the raw characteristics of what nature defines as physically beautiful, beauty is only as important as its strength of delivery and the ability for it to be received.

1.2 Female Beauty in the Raw

An evolutionary biologist would likely favor the notion that beauty has evolved as a reliable indicator of superior health and viable genes. Furthermore, it must be presumed that the ability to recognize such elements as beautiful is innate. Infants as young as three months old can recognize beautiful faces and will stare at them longer than at less beautiful faces.[2] Furthermore, research done by Jones and Hill with the Hiwi and Ache Indian tribes of Venezuela and Paraguay showed that, despite having little or no exposure to Western media, the tribal members were attracted to the same facial characteristics as observers from Brazil, the United States, and Russia.[3]

1.3 Less Is More

We have made the linear argument that the manner in which beauty is transmitted and received determines whether it is considered attractive. However, it is the authors' opinion that the transmission of this information is most successful if it remains subconsciously perceived. Once the receiver's conscious awareness is tipped off, the message loses its effectiveness as a positive indicator. This contradictory response occurs when we are required to evaluate whether something is beautiful because conscious evaluation is less pleasurable than assessing it without thinking.[4] In other words, if you have to think about whether something is beautiful, you are no longer rewarded in the same way as you would have been if merely observing it inattentively.

Consider this scenario: we are dismayed by someone trying to defy their true age when signs of cosmetic surgery become overtly apparent. We experience equal aversion to someone using too much makeup as to someone wearing indecently revealing and unflattering clothing they do not fit into properly. Although a woman may take these measures in an attempt to enhance her beauty, the message received is that the woman actually lacks the natural beauty traits that she believes she is highlighting. In fact, studies have indicated that makeup applied inappropriately or excessively triggers negative impressions.[5] The message perceived by observers is that the woman who applies makeup in excess is not vital, healthy, or a good gene holder. Men are similarly perceived if they attempt to highlight their sexually defining or sexually dimorphic character traits. A strong chin, a strong jawline, a full head of hair, and tall stature all are beauty-defining features in a male, but if he attempts a "comb-over" to cover a balding vertex or wears platform shoes in an attempt to compensate for his lack of height, these measures will be recognized subconsciously by females as physically unattractive. Any attempt to hide a genetic weakness must be covert; otherwise it loses its value. This is the reason Michael Jordan, the famed Chicago Bulls basketball star, looks better bald than he did with a receding hairline. If his hair loss isn't recognizable in contrast to his scalp, the uniformity of his head provides a more youthful appearance.

The raw tenets of beauty that pertain to the face can be categorized into the core traits of symmetry, averageness, and youthfulness.

1.4 Symmetry

The more symmetric an object is, the more favorably it is perceived. This is true across the contexts of art, nature, and humans. The explanation for this fact is linked to the brain's ability to process symmetry fluently and rapidly. The brain shows preference for what it is able to do more easily and quickly.[6] As symmetry diminishes, the brain needs more time to process an image, as it has to reconcile any unexpected glitches. Accordingly, the less symmetric that an image is, the longer it takes the brain to process it, and the longer it takes for the brain to do something, the less pleasure it receives.

Dr. Ingo Springer and colleagues demonstrated that symmetry is particularly important in regard to the midline of the face,[7] because the brain processes symmetry from the middle and works its way laterally. In their study, they showed that an asymmetric mole is often considered unattractive when near the midline of the face but is considered increasingly less unattractive when toward the outside of the face. In other words, it is the reason why Cindy Crawford's mole near her outer lip is referred to as a beauty mark, but a mole in the middle of her forehead would likely be judged less attractive.

With the location of the nose being right in the middle of the face, it is no surprise that the nose is one of the first features (after the eyes) to be noticed by observers. Subsequent to its position, the nose also plays a key role in the processing of facial symmetry. A person with an oddly shaped or sized nose is less likely to elicit an impression of supreme health and vitality. If the nose becomes too distracting, it also deters from the appearance of the eyes. For this reason, many satisfied rhinoplasty patients report that their peers tend not to comment on their altered nose, but more often comment on the beauty of their eyes.

1.5 When Being the Best Is Not Best

Years spent striving to be the best may have been time wasted—that is, in an evolutionary sense. Darwinian principles indicate that the more common something is, the more likely it is to thrive. Just like outliers in a dataset, extremes in any direction are often discarded, because they are not representative of the majority. Accordingly, beauty is most desirable when it is the average appearance of a population. This results in its being most familiar and comfortable. The reason nature selects for those beauty traits found in the middle of the pack is due to the brain's processing what it is familiar with more easily than something foreign. This ease results in the translation of something as more beautiful and pleasing. This postulation was reinforced by a study performed by Langlois and Roggman, who found that attractive faces were also the most average faces of a population.[8] They determined this using the blended composite photos of a population, which were deemed the most attractive by the study subjects. Darwinian principles would suggest that the preference is reinforced by the fact that the most blended individual would embody the most diverse gene combination, thus providing them with the best chance of survival in any environment. Thus, nature selects for averageness.

1.6 What's in the Fountain of Youth?

Nature favors youth: it has the most potential for procreation and is less likely to contract disease. Furthermore, for a female, the more infantile her features, the more attractive she is perceived to be. In a study done by Victor Johnston, computer composite photos of females were evaluated by 40 people (20 men and 20 women) ranging from 18 to 30 years of age.[9] Precise anthropometric sites were marked on the photographed faces and were used to determine the exact positions and sizes of the lips, nose, chin, eyes, and other features. The photos that the evaluators found most attractive were associated with large lips, a small chin, a high hairline, and large eyes—features strongly associated with younger women. The average age of the faces judged to be the most beautiful was calculated to be 24.9 years.

Even across cultures, youthful characteristics remain the same: high cheekbones, large eyes, a small chin, even skin tone, and plump lips. A youthful face draws attention to the eyes and positions an imaginary inverted triangle with its width spanning the cheekbones and its most narrow point occurring at the chin.

1.7 It's All in the Eyes

A youthful face is deeply rooted in the eyes. Heterosexual males selecting for a mate are attracted to large eyes in females, particularly if their pupils are enlarged. Furthermore, it was shown by a study done in Norway that women in their ovulatory phase produced a maximum dilation of up to 8%.[10] The ability to recognize the dilation is not necessarily a conscious effort; however, the subconscious picks up on the subtle changes. Furthermore, males prefer blue eyes over other colors because the lighter color renders the pupils easier to discern for the male.

Advertisers and artists have caught on to this phenomenon. A close look at popular dolls and children's books reveals that Barbies and princesses all have wide, doe-like eyes with large pupils. The editors in charge of Photoshopping magazine images also engage in altering the models' eyes to garner more attention from the audience. For women, more contrast between the color around the eyes and the surrounding skin increases attractiveness.[11] This explains why nearly 70% of women in the United States use mascara. It also goes a long way to account for the hundreds of thousands of options women have for eye shadow shades and eyeliners to accentuate their eyes with the dark, colorful framing. Cosmetic medicine has tools to further draw attention to the eyes. An intradermal injection of a small amount of neurotoxin a few millimeters inferior to the ciliary margin at the mid-pupillary line can be used to weaken the muscle as a means of opening the palpebral aperture of the eye. This results in a more open appearance of the eye and the appearance of increased friendliness. This is used in conjunction with neurotoxin injections to the corrugator supercilii, procerus, depressor supercilii, and orbicularis oculi muscles. Weakening these muscles effectively inhibits frowning, creates the appearance of eyes set further apart, and raises eyebrows. The collective benefit of such results is a more friendly and approachable appearance—which is considered beautiful **(Fig. 1.1)**.

1.8 Lips

Direct indicators of youthfulness are full, red lips defined by a distinctive white border. Lips plump slightly during the height of female fertility. In a study in which males identified the size lips they found most attractive, they chose the photos of females with lips of 19.4 mm.[9] The male's subconscious mind recognizes large lips and correlates them with youth and fertility. Beautiful lips are also marked by an upper lip that protrudes 1 to 2 mm further than the bottom lip.

Lip enhancements tend to be one of the most talked about nonsurgical procedures when it comes to celebrities. When they are done well, nobody should notice that anything was done, but when overfilled, lips are the "Scarlet Letter" of cosmetic enhancement. (Unfortunately, "duck lips" have become an everyday phrase in patients' list of concerns, but they are completely avoidable.) As women age, they tend lose their lip roll, which once provided youthful definition. Additionally, the lip body loses volume and the upper cutaneous lip elongates, both of which are tell-tale signs of aging.[12] To combat this, filler with a higher viscosity can be used in the upper and lower vermilion body and border to recreate the roll. To address the loss of volume, a hydrophilic hyaluronic acid filler can be injected into the upper and lower vermilion body to create a more plump lip.

1.9 A Youthful Glow

In cosmetics, we tend to become caught up in use of injectables for their quick way of addressing structural deficiencies. However, a person is only as beautiful as the skin

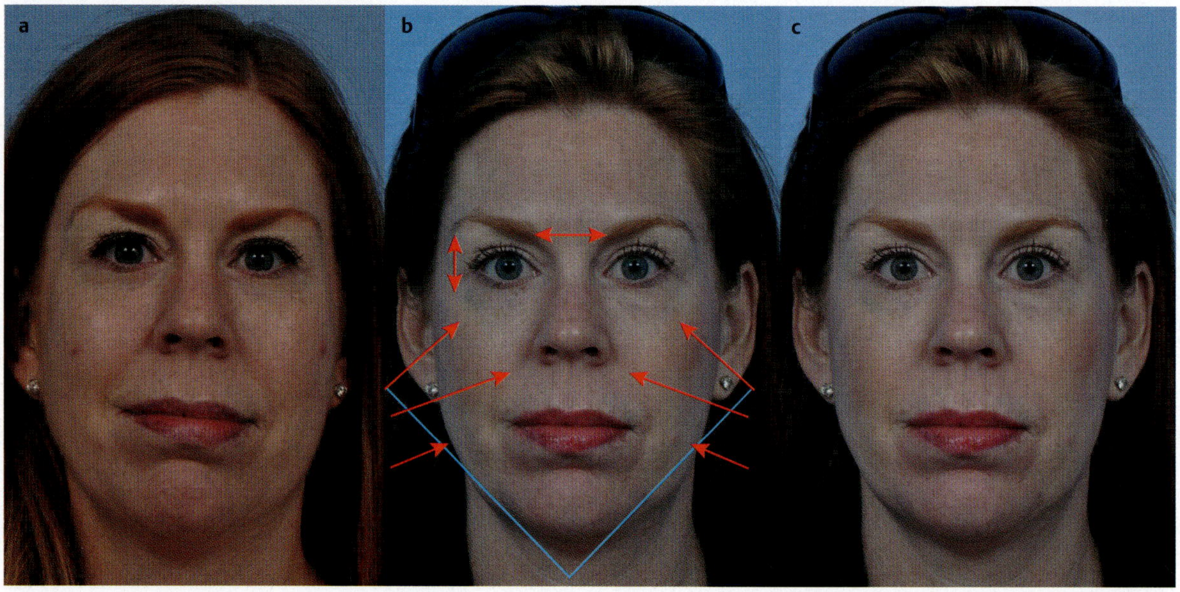

Fig. 1.1 (a–c) Non-surgical treatments, such as fillers and botulinum neuromodulators, can be utilized to make subtle changes in the face resulting in the patient projecting an improved first impression. The alterations result in a natural outcome we call "subliminal difference."

that displays their features. Historically, youthful skin has homogeneous tone and color. Health and youth correlate with translucent and clear skin. As blood is pumped to the skin, light bounces off the blood vessels, which produces the desirable pinkish tint that exudes health and viability and attracts the opposite sex. Consistently across all cultures, female beauty results from skin that is a few shades lighter than their male counterparts' skin tone. Biologically, this creates an advantage for women by allowing the absorption of more sunlight, resulting in the increased production of vitamin D, a nutrient essential for pregnancy.

As a woman ages, collagen denatures, soft tissue and fat atrophy, and skin volume is lost. This process partly results in wrinkling and creping of skin. Additionally, as a woman goes through pregnancy and beyond, her skin begins to darken and take on a more uneven appearance. Aging also results in the visibility of tiny blood vessels in the skin, known as spider veins or telangiectasia, which detracts from homogeneity and signifies the loss of youth and/or health. From an evolutionary perspective, abnormal skin coloring signals potential disease. Someone seeking a mate would likely be more inclined to spend their energy and resources on someone apparently more youthful and a better carrier for their genes.

Luckily, skin-care companies have recognized the value of science and have developed products that not only protect skin from the harmful rays of the sun, but also correct damage that has already occurred and slow the rate of collagen breakdown. The combination of nonsurgical treatments that includes filler neurotoxin to alter facial architecture coupled with chemical balancing peels and topical skin care can improve the first impression the person projects as well as the individual's self-esteem.[13] Combination ablative and nonablative lasers target pigment issues as well as work on resurfacing and retexturizing the skin. The complete and prudent cosmetic provider will incorporate a skin-care regimen into their practice to enhance both the skin and the well-being of patients.

During the aging process, the soft tissue, fat, and muscle that once created "apple-like" cheeks descend. The area around the eyes subsequently becomes hollow, and the soft tissue starts to fall over the jawline, creating jowling. This in turn makes the jawline appear squarer, a masculinizing trait that leads to a less physically beautiful female appearance. And while there are aggressive surgical procedures to treat an isolated jowl or hollowing, it is the complete face within the holistic context of the person's individual desires and goals that we must consider.

1.10 The Subliminal Creation of Beauty

Traditional plastic surgery training seems to have fixated on the physical "ideals of beauty," but too often the ideals may be taken out of the context of how they fit the individual person. As a result, surgeons aim beyond natural results to a glorified ideal that may not proportionally or emotionally match the individual patient. To improve appearance and well-being, we need to dampen radical changes in exchange for placing focus on subtle ones. It is the collective minor facial alterations, although barely detectable, that will stimulate the subconscious mind of both the individual and the unknowing observer to interpret them as beauty.

Accordingly, the authors have adopted a new philosophy, "Subliminal Difference," which allows one to factor in the evolutionary aspect of beauty along with the neuropsychiatric interpretation of how it is perceived **(Fig. 1.1)**. This has added a third dimension, the subconscious mind, to the two dimensions of form and function formerly used as guiding forces. The philosophy of Subliminal Difference embraces mostly nonsurgical facial cosmetic treatments, but it can be translated to strategic surgical procedures that serve to illuminate the eyes and deemphasize the lower third of the face. As an example, combination in-office neurotoxin and filler treatments can be a more readily available means for aging gracefully. Treating the upper one-third of the face with a neurotoxin can result in the elevation of the brow, creating a subtle separation of the medial clubs of the brow, which results in the reduction of forehead wrinkles and the opening of the eyelid aperture. This conveys a more friendly and youthful message. Eyelashes are easily enhanced, drawing attention to the eyes. The use of filler in the malar cheeks further pedestals the eyes and draws attention away from the lower third of the face. If the jaw appears too square and masculine, the lower third of the face may be deemphasized and the width of the mandible narrowed with injection of a neurotoxin into the masseters. This allows the lips to become more noticeable. If a patient has volume loss in the vermilion body or border, hyaluronic acid filler may be used to subtly redefine them. Ablative and nonablative laser treatments or chemical peeling may be used to address discoloration and texture changes that are associated with aging, and this is followed with a home skin-care regimen. The importance of a proper diet and adequate exercise is discussed during aesthetic interventions, as it is our belief diet and exercise benefit the psyche and ultimately our patients' satisfaction and outcome.

Although the approach described here was specifically developed as a way to achieve subtle results from in-office procedures with little to no downtime, the same "less is more" doctrine can and should be applied surgically. For example, if a patient requests a drastically smaller nose, the surgeon cannot look at the nose alone. Just as with a sculpture, alteration of one piece must be considered only within the context of the entire piece of art. While the patient may be underwhelmed at first with the computer imaging projecting the expected result, subsequently they are further informed that the end result is the surgeon's best effort to enhance all of the other characteristics of beauty that they possess. This includes the eyes, as well as the creation of facial balance and harmony that is most pleasing. The surgical (or nonsurgical) result is a face that conveys femininity/masculinity, youthfulness, and beauty while remaining subtle, natural, and within the context of the patient's age. Ultimately, patients feel better about themselves.

Our efforts have shown that all it takes is mild, barely perceptible alterations in facial appearance to impact the first impression the patient projects and to elevate patients' self-esteem and quality of life.[14,15,16,17] And, as our colleagues in neuropsychology and behavioral psychology have shown, regardless of physical appearance, those with elevated self-esteem stand taller, appear more extroverted, handle conflict better, and even can earn more money.[18,19] A confident disposition can, and often will, trump physical perfection. In the authors' opinion, our goal as plastic surgeons and cosmetic physicians, regardless of culture, ethnicity, or language, is not to improve the patient's appearance per se bur to use our aesthetic skills and interventions to elevate our patients' self-esteem.[20] Those who feel beautiful project a more favorable impression and are awarded all the social benefits of beauty. Ultimately, those who feel beautiful are beautiful, and that, in essence, is what we aim to achieve.

References

1. Mulford M, Orbell J, Shatto C, et al. Physical attractiveness, opportunity, and success in everyday exchange. Am J Sociol 1998;103(6):1565–1592
2. Slater A, Von der Schulenburg C, Brown E, et al. Newborn infants prefer attractive faces. Infant Behav Dev 1998;21(2):345–354
3. Jones D, Hill K. Criteria of facial attractiveness in five populations. Hum Nat 1993;4(3):271–296
4. Winston JS, O'Doherty J, Kilner JM, Perrett DI, Dolan RJ. Brain systems for assessing facial attractiveness. Neuropsychologia 2007;45(1):195–206
5. Workman JE, Johnson KK. The role of cosmetics in impression formation. Cloth Text Res J 1991;10(1):63–67
6. Reber R, Schwarz N, Winkielman P. Processing fluency and aesthetic pleasure: is beauty in the perceiver's processing experience? Pers Soc Psychol Rev 2004;8(4):364–382
7. Springer IN, Wannicke B, Warnke PH, et al. Facial attractiveness: visual impact of symmetry increases significantly towards the midline. Ann Plast Surg 2007;59(2): 156–162
8. Langlois JH, Roggman LA. Attractive faces are only average. Psychol Sci 1990;1(2):115–121
9. Johnston VS, Solomon CJ, Gibson SJ, Pallares-Bejarano A. Human facial beauty: current theories and methodologies. Arch Facial Plast Surg 2003;5(5):371–377
10. Laeng B, Falkenberg L. Women's pupillary responses to sexually significant others during the hormonal cycle. Horm Behav 2007;52(4):520–530
11. Russell R. Sex, beauty, and the relative luminance of facial features. Perception 2003;32(9):1093–1107
12. Gunn DA, Rexbye H, Griffiths CE, et al. Why some women look young for their age. PLoS ONE 2009;4(12):e8021
13. Dayan S. The focus on triple arm cosmeceutical therapy. Presentation IMCAS Feb. 2014.
14. Dayan S, Clark K, Ho AA. Altering first impressions after facial plastic surgery. Aesthet Plast Surg 2004;28(5): 301–306

15. Dayan SH, Arkins JP, Gal TJ. Blinded evaluation of the effects of hyaluronic acid filler injections on first impressions. Dermatol Surg 2010;36(Suppl 3):1866–1873

16. Dayan SH, Arkins JP, Patel AB, Gal TJA. A double-blind, randomized, placebo-controlled health-outcomes survey of the effect of botulinum toxin type A injections on quality of life and self-esteem. Dermatol Surg 2010;36(Suppl 4): 2088–2097

17. Dayan SH, Lieberman ED, Thakkar NN, Larimer KA, Anstead A. Botulinum toxin A can positively impact first impression. Dermatol Surg 2008;34(Suppl 1):S40–S47

18. Naumann LP, Vazire S, Rentfrow PJ, Gosling SD. Personality judgments based on physical appearance. Pers Soc Psychol Bull 2009;35(12):1661–1671

19. Hamermesh DS, Biddle JE. Beauty and the labor market (No. w4518). National Bureau of Economic Research; 1993

20. Dayan SH. Subliminally Exposed. New York, NY: Morgan James Publishing; 2013

2 Surgical Anatomy of the Face: Evaluating Racial Differences

Wayne F. Larrabee Jr. and Scott Bevans

2.1 Introduction

The racial and ethnic differences that we see in each other are the visible product of anatomical differences. A facial phenotype is the product of the facial skeleton, the thickness and position of overlying soft tissue layers, and skin tone, which create a literal mask—and our identity. Many of these anatomical features are predictable and have been both well studied and well described. For decades, forensic scientists have been able to analyze skulls to deduce racial origin and to create facial profiles of victims or perpetrators. Similarly, anthropologists have attempted to describe the facial features of our predecessors from centuries past. Despite these studies, and the fact that nearly 40% of the world's population live in Asia, the vast majority of facial anatomy textbooks are based on Caucasians—a worldwide minority.[1]

In this metaphorical "small world," both patient access to facial plastic surgery and patient desires have changed. Most patients who request aesthetic surgery would like a more youthful appearance or refinement of a specific bothersome feature. Some will also request that the aesthetic surgeon preserve, augment, or minimize some defining racial characteristic. This can create a surgical paradox, as exemplified by the dilemma of the patient who wants a dorsal nasal hump reduced, but still wants to "leave a little" of this family heirloom. The solution is, of course, to be aware of what facial anatomical differences may be underlying and plan appropriately. Careful attention to the ethnically diverse patients in our practices will result in both a high level of individual patient satisfaction and an excellent reputation among local ethnic enclaves.

To lay the foundation for this understanding, this chapter begins by comparing the bony foundation of the face, progressing from deep to superficial. Finally, because so much of human facial recognition is associated with the midface, we address differences in periorbital, nasal, and perioral anatomical regions.

2.2 Facial Skeleton and Facial Proportions

Measurements of bony and surface landmarks of the facial anatomy have been recorded for hundreds of years. The detailed story of anthropometrics reveals a humbling tale of racism, beginning with the Greeks, who attempted to prove racial superiority by claiming "optimal" facial aesthetics belonged to their specific set of anthropometric measurements.[2] These artistic renditions became "canons" of facial proportions for centuries, based as much (or more) on the aesthetics of the age than on rigorous comparative anatomical studies. It wasn't until the early 1900s that more specific and objective values began to appear in medical literature (**Fig. 2.1** and **Fig. 2.2**).[2]

Over the past 40 years, racial differences in the facial skeleton have been increasingly well documented. Gray's anatomy describes these major differences in craniofacial features by grouping them into four historic categories correlating with geographic areas.[3]

1. Caucasoid—Descendants of North American and European peoples, extending through the Middle East and into Northern Africa.
2. Mongoloid—Descendants of peoples from Asia, Polynesia, and Central and South America.
3. Australoid—Descendants of Pacific Islanders, Indonesians, Malaysians, and Australian Aborigines; originally including people from regions of present-day India and probably even Native Americans
4. Negroid—Descendants of peoples from Africa extending northward toward sub-Saharan Africa.

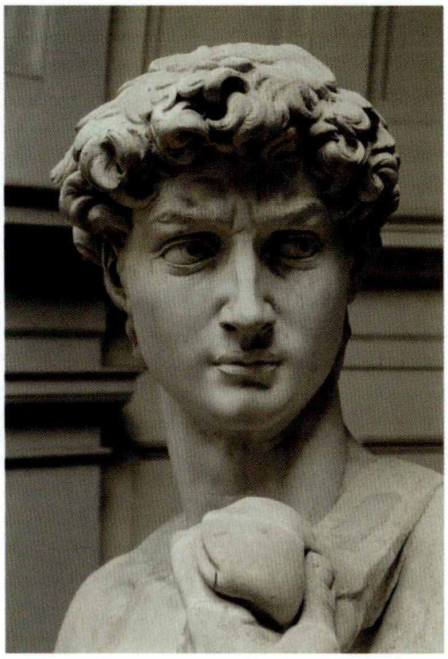

Fig. 2.1 Michelangelo's David. Artists from the Renaissance heavily influenced our historical perception of "ideal facial proportions." Michelangelo (Buonarroti, Michelangelo 1475–1564): David—detail (head from front). Florence, Accademia. © 2015. Photo Scala, Florence—courtesy of the Ministero Beni e Att. Culturali.

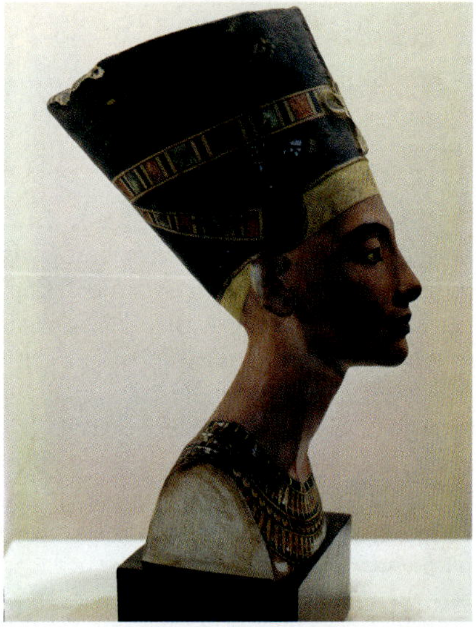

Fig. 2.2 Note the facial features of the bust of Nefertiti, one of the most famous among sculptures representing ideals of feminine facial features. The bust predates Michelangelo's David by nearly 3000 years. Egyptian art: Head of Queen Nefertiti: in profile (plaster cast). Florence, Archaeological Museum. © 2015. Photo Scala, Florence—courtesy of the Ministero Beni e Att. Culturali.

See **Table 2.1** for comparisons of the cranial skeletal differences among these groups and **Fig. 2.3** for direct comparisons.

Some authors fold the Australoid subgroup into either the Mongoloid or Negroid category because of their respective similarities. Also, note the use of the Mongoloid skull shape to describe the skull of ethnicities from Central and South American regions, which many authors refer to as "Mestizo." Because Mestizo is used more commonly as an ethnic descriptor in medical literature, the more specific anthropologic terminology for comparison of skulls or craniofacial features is used here.

Most studies compare Caucasoid, Mongoloid, and Negroid structural skull differences, which are summarized in **Table 2.1**. The defining features tend to be the shape of the piriform aperture, the width of the bi-zygomatic arch, the maxilla, the mandible, the presence of prognathism, and orbital shape.

Additional, more recent dental studies of bony facial dimensions using cross-sectional imaging and lateral cephalograms comparing Asian populations (Chinese, Korean, and Japanese most prevalently published) to

Table 2.1 Anthropomorphic differences in facial skeleton among racial groups

	Caucasoid	Mongoloid	Australoid	Negroid
Shape	Rounded to long	Rounded portrait, flat profile	Heterogeneous	Long, convex profile
Forehead	Steep, moderate supraorbital rim	Vertical/flat	Prominent supraorbital ridge (largest)	Rounded
Orbits	Narrow interorbital distance, more rectangular/rhomboid	Rounded orbits	Rounded orbits, large supraorbital arches	Widened interorbital distance, square or rectangular orbit
Zygoma	Not overly prominent	Well-developed, high, and well-projected malar eminences	Moderate	Reduced relative to Mongoloid, similar to Caucasoid
Nasal piriform	Narrowed aperture, triangular shape, prominent nasal spine, long nasal bones	Medium width, round-shaped aperture, low nasal bridge, short nasal bones, tented nasal root, short nasal spine	Broad aperture, triangular in shape	Wide, oval aperture, low nasal root with nearly reduced nasal spine, medium to small nasal bones
Maxilla	Little prognathism, narrow, long palate	Foreshortened palate	Wide palate, large teeth, somewhat prognathic	Strongly prognathic, wide palate
Mandible	Angled with prominent and relatively wide chin, tendency to mandibular retrusion	Rotated forward, widened at angles, robust	Large, heavy mandible	Reduced chin projection, moderate width

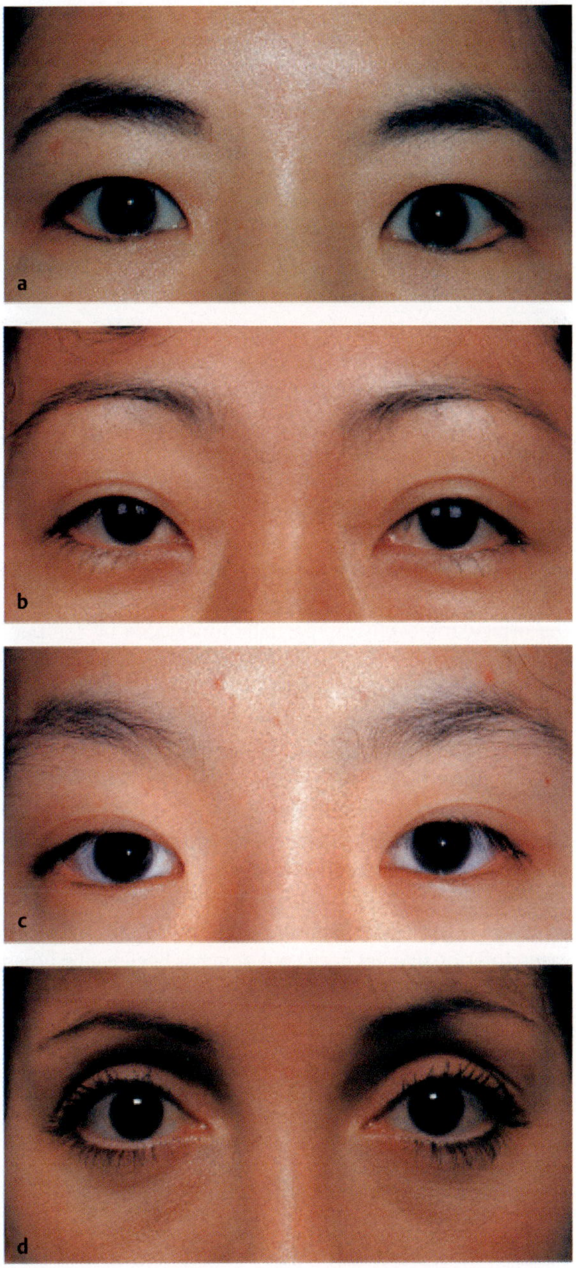

Fig. 2.3 Racial variation in upper eyelid appearance. **(a)** "Single lid" (no eyelid crease) but epicanthal fold present. **(b)** "Double lid" with supratarsal crease 3 to 5 mm from the lash line and minimal epicanthal fold. **(c)** "Inner double lid" with the epicanthal fold crossing over the supratarsal crease. **(d)** Caucasian eyelid with supratarsal crease set back 8 to 10 mm from the lash line. (Used with permission from Larrabee WF, Makielski KH, Henderson JL. Surgical Anatomy of the Face. 2nd ed. Philadelphia, PA: Lippincott Williams & Wilkins; 2004.)

Caucasians found overall smaller midfaces and a shorter mandible among the Asians. Both sexes of the Asians studied tended to have increased lower anterior facial height, with increased protrusion of the soft tissue profile of the upper and lower lips.[4] The mandibular angle and bizygomatic width increase the lateral projection, causing increased facial width. These combined factors create a more rounded facial appearance.[5,6]

Among African ethnicities, a slightly wider piriform aperture is common, averaging 26 to 27 mm, relative to 23 to 24 mm in Caucasians. This difference in bony craniofacial skeleton is not the only cause of the wider nasal appearance, however. The nasal soft tissue is also significantly wider, with an average 44 mm interalar width for African noses and 36 mm for Caucasians.[7] Nasal spine angulation and soft tissue profile comparison revealed a significantly more acute nasolabial angle (79 ± 15 degrees) relative to Caucasian populations (102 ± 8 degrees).[8,9] Data from measurements taken on hundreds of lateral cephalograms from various African ethnic groups showed less soft tissue nasal projection, more maxillary prognathism, and significantly greater soft tissue thickness of the upper lip relative to Caucasian populations.[10] The result is a less prominent nose but greater midfacial convexity and lower facial third prominence.

Mestizo ethnicities tend to have more mandibular and maxillary prognathism, resulting in greater lip protrusion relative to Caucasians.[11] Many of the remaining facial measurements (vertical thirds, horizontal fifths, lip soft tissue thickness, etc.) fell between those of the Caucasoid and Negroid features. There are several additional differences in the nasal structure and soft tissue composition specific to the Mestizo nose, which are addressed below.

Leslie Farkas has multiple comprehensive publications on the topic of craniofacial differences among ethnic groups. In analyzing nearly 1500 healthy subjects from five major regions (a total of 18 countries), he recorded significant differences in facial proportions. The measurements compared differences in superficial landmarks, incorporating differences in both bony and soft tissue composition. Most commonly, the measurements for each race included alar facial height, vertical facial thirds, alar width, monocular and binocular orbital width, mouth width, and mandibular width, which he then compared with North American Caucasians.[12] After screening for statistical significance, the Farkas team found the most defining ethnic features to be as listed below.

General facial proportions:

- Facial height greater in Iranians
- Facial height and lower one-third height smaller in Egyptians
- Face and mandible width greater in Thais, Japanese, and Chinese
- Facial width smaller in Portuguese males and females

- Croatians and Iranians have smaller foreheads
- Lower face smaller in Hungarian and Slovakian females
- Mouth width larger in Hungarian males
- Mouth width smaller in Vietnamese males
- Mandible width greater in male Turks and Iranian females
- Mandible width smaller in Portuguese males and females
- Mandible width larger in Italians and Slovaks
- Ear height 40% smaller among African males

Orbital anatomy differences:

- More widely variable within the five major ethnic groupings (both intra- and intercountry variation)
- Turkish males and females have wider eyes
- Iranians have smaller intercanthal distances
- Intercanthal width is greater in nearly all Asian ethnicities
- Chinese females and Vietnamese males have smaller eye fissures
- Bi-ocular width is increased in Indian females and Japanese

Nasal anatomy differences:

- Greater nasal height in Iranians, Turks, Greek females, and Portuguese males and females
- Shorter nasal height in Indian males and females, Hungarian females
- Nasal width increased in all Asian ethnicities and African ethnic groups
- Nasal inclination greater in Slovenian and Russian females

In Farkas' data, while many trends were consistent, there were outliers in nearly every measurement and generally greater variability among the females of each ethnicity. This heterogeneity reinforces the concept that, even as we detail anatomical differences among ethnic groups, there are broad facial differences within ethnic groups that we must remain mindful of.

2.3 Facial Soft Tissue Differences

The muscles of facial expression likely make a large contribution to our individual ethnic facial features. Just as there are consistent differences in craniofacial skull shape, differences in soft tissue thickness in the forehead, zygoma, and lips have been determined by comparing computerized tomography studies among different races (largely to assist forensic scientists in recreating soft tissue envelopes on remains).[4] These studies, however, have not been of sufficient resolution to delineate interracial differences in facial musculature. To date, there have been no anatomical studies detailing differences in position, relative strength, or size of specific facial muscle groups (e.g., zygomaticus major, orbicularis oris, orbicularis oculi, or frontalis). Similarly, although intuitively it seems that differences must exist, at the time of the writing of this chapter, we could not locate data regarding differences in fat compartment position or size.

2.4 Nerves

The course of the facial nerve, its pattern of arborization, and even the distal mimetic site of innervation between individuals of the same ethnicity may also be more highly variable than initially described in classic anatomy texts. Three recent studies of facial nerve characteristics in Japanese and Korean patients have challenged the long-held views that the temporal and zygomatic branches innervate the upper and lower portions of the orbicularis oculi and the buccal or mandibular branches innervate the respective divisions of the orbicularis oris. Cadaveric studies demonstrated that the orbicularis oculi was partially innervated by the buccal branch in more than 30% of cases. Similarly, the orbicularis oris was at least partially innervated by the zygomatic branch in up to 40% of cases.[13,14] At the time of this writing, no additional data about the terminal innervation patterns in other races/ethnicities are available. Therefore, we are unable to determine if these described differences are truly racially related anatomical variants or are correction of long-held inaccurate ideas applied across all ethnicities.

As one may have assumed based on differing skull shapes, the position of sensory nerves also differs among races. Inferior alveolar nerve position has been well studied and reported in the dental literature. The mental foramen, and therefore the inferior alveolar nerve position, can be located between the first and second premolars in most Middle Eastern and Caucasian patients, while it is located directly below the long axis of the second premolar in Asian races and inferior to slightly posterior to the second premolar in African races.[15,16]

2.5 Facial Skin

The most obvious skin difference among racial groups is that of color, which is determined by the amount of melanin within the basal keratinocytes in the epidermis; however, skin color can vary quite dramatically within ethnic groups. Multiple studies have shown that increased melanin confers greater resistance to photoaging (termed photoprotection).[17] The signs of photoaging include pigment irregularities, fine rhytids, and increased laxity, thought to be a result of protease activity in the epidermis

The overall appearance of skin, as well as its chemical and mechanical properties, however, are functions of its composition, including:

- Ceramides—waxy lipids present largely in the extracellular spaces in the stratum corneum.
- Overall moisture—linked closely to ceramide level, but also influenced by sebum secretion, rate of desquamation, etc.
- Transepidermal water loss—the amount of water vapor escaping from the skin when not sweating.
- pH—found to be inversely proportional to elasticity and likely influencing both microflora and water content.
- Pore size and sebaceous gland density.
- Skin reactivity—based on concentrations of inflammatory and mast cells.

Table 2.2 compares these differences in detail. Most important to the surgeon, however, may be the overall skin thickness and ability for adherence in the skin, as well as the skin's resistance to photoaging. For surgeons considering superficial skin regenerative procedures, it is also important to consider density of pilosebaceous units, which correlates with differences in cross-sectional hair shape.

Reports comparing the stratum corneum of African skin to that of Caucasians have varied regarding overall thickness. Berardesca and Maibach reported equivalent thickness of the stratum corneum between the groups, but they found African skin had more layers within the stratum corneum and more cohesion.[18] Rawlings' data support the finding of increased intercellular cohesion in African skin,

Table 2.2 Comparison of skin characteristics among ethnic groups

	Pigment	Stratum corneum	Ceramide level	Water content	Transepidermal water loss	Pores and sweat glands	pH	Skin reactivity/ Mast cell activity
Caucasian	Lower melanin	Moderate thickness	Low	Medium	Low	Highest number and density	Middle	Moderate reactivity
Asian	Increased melanin and carotene levels	Similar to Caucasian skin, thick subcuticular skin	Highest	Highest	Highest	Lowest number and density	Higher	Highly reactive
Mestizo	Similar to Asian skin	Moderate thickness	Medium	Higher	Middle	Moderate to high pore number, lower gland number/ size	Middle	Likely similar to Caucasian
African	High density of melanin	More cohesive, more compact, with increased desquamation rate	Lowest	Lowest	High	More pore anchors, slightly lower number than in Caucasians	Lower	Larger mast cell granules, lower reactivity

Data from:

- Rawlings AV. Ethnic skin types: are there differences in skin structure and function? Int J Cosmet Sci 2006;28(2):79–93.
- Wan DC, et al. Moisturizing different racial skin types. J Clin Aesthet Dermatol 2014;7(6):25–32.
- Wesley NO, Maibach HI. Racial (ethnic) differences in skin properties: the objective data. Am J Clin Dermatol 2003;4(12):843–860.
- Berardesca E, Maibach H. Racial differences in skin pathophysiology. J Am Acad Dermatol 1996;34(4):667–672.
- Akazawa T, Sathmåry EJE. Prehistoric Mongoloid Dispersals. New York, NY: Oxford University Press; 1996.
- Montagu A. Growing Young. Westport, CT: Greenwood Publishing Group; 1989.
- Muizzuddin N, et al. Structural and functional differences in barrier properties of African American, Caucasian and East Asian skin. J Derm Sci 2010;59(2):123–128.

making it more compact, and Rawlings suggests that this contributes to a somewhat increased barrier function.[17] The increased number of granulocytes and mast cells may also contribute to the tendency for keloid formation.

Asian skin also tends to have a thicker subcuticular component, with an abundance of carotene.[19] Sweat gland density per square inch of skin surface was 50% less than that of Caucasian skin and pore size was the smallest among the races compared.[20,21]

2.6 Midface Identity

Many have argued that, as subunits, the midface and lower face are the two most critical portions of the face for both communication and identity. Although they comprise less than 5% of total body surface area, the eyes, nose, and mouth allow us to recognize a single face from among 200,000 others.[22] For this reason and the great difficulty of reconstructing them, loss of one or both of the eyes or oral subunits is an indication for facial transplantation.[23] The differences among various racial and ethnic groups are therefore obviously critical components of our identity.

2.6.1 Eyes and Eyelids

One of the dominant racial variations in the periorbital region is variation in the upper eyelid shape and crease in Asian individuals. In most Asian populations, the supratarsal crease is lower than in Caucasian individuals or altogether absent **(Fig. 2.3)**. Recall that, in Caucasian anatomy, the supratarsal crease is created by fusion of the levator aponeurosis and orbital septum near the superior edge of the tarsal plate, with insertion of the fibers into the skin. In Asian eyelids, the fusion of the orbital septum and the levator aponeurosis occurs below the tarsal border and/or the levator aponeurosis attachment to the skin is absent.[24] These factors combined allow the pre-aponeurotic fat pad to descend and protrude. This is shown in **Fig. 2.4**. Cadaveric and MRI studies have also revealed a larger amount of pretarsal, sub-orbicularis, and subcutaneous fat in Asian specimens.[25,26] Other common eyelid features are narrowed palpebral fissure and the presence of an epicanthal fold.[27] This is nicely characterized in **Fig. 2.4**.

2.6.2 Nose

The nose is probably the most frequently studied and described feature for defining ethnic anatomy. **Table 2.3** compiles data from several studies to allow side-by-side comparison. The most telling differences in nasal features include the dorsal profile, alar width, and nasal projection. Surgically, the amount of available septal cartilage for reconstruction is highly pertinent and varies widely from Asian (very little) to Middle Eastern patients (often overgrown). The alar width and external valve support in both Asian and African populations is also relevant to surgical planning **(Fig. 2.5)**.

In addition, a recent study by Chun and colleagues assessed the anatomical cause for the differences in alar lobule structure that contribute to the appearance of "the Asian nose." The authors noted that the size of the Asian alar cartilages was similar to the size in Caucasians. Rather, the more flared Asian nostrils were secondary to the increased size of the dilator naris muscles and the increased thickness of the vestibular skin.[28]

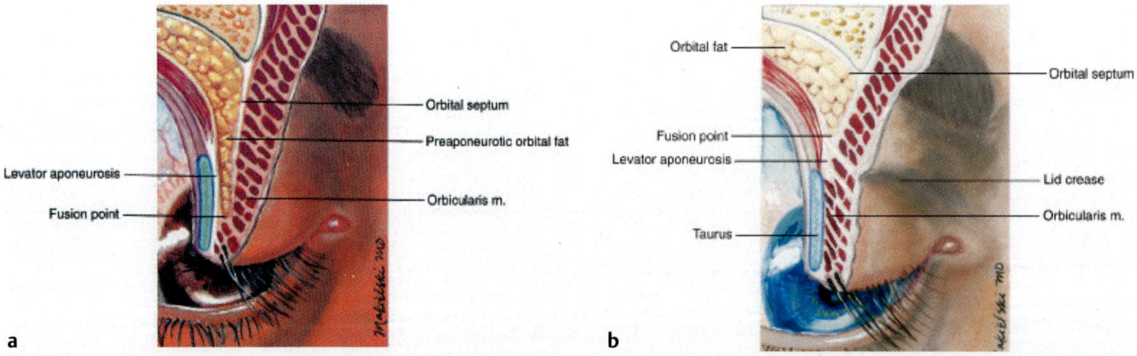

Fig. 2.4 Differences in eyelid structure contributing to presence of supratarsal crease and epicanthal fold. **(a)** Non-Asian eyelid. Notice the fusion of the levator aponeurosis with the orbital septum superior to the tarsal plate with extension directly to dermis at this level, creating the characteristic supratarsal crease. **(b)** Asian eyelid. After fusing with the tarsal crease, the dermal attachments are absent, which allow the pre-aponeurotic fat pad to extend to the lash line below the orbicularis oculi muscle. (Used with permission from Larrabee WF, Makielski KH, Henderson JL. Surgical Anatomy of the Face. 2nd ed. Philadelphia, PA: Lippincott Williams & Wilkins; 2004.)

Table 2.3 Soft tissue characteristics of ethnic nose

	African	Asian	Mestizo	Middle Eastern
Skin envelope	Thick	Moderate to thick	Moderate to thick, sebaceous	Moderate to thick
Dorsal profile	Wide, low dorsum	Shallow nasion, decreased projection	Wide, low dorsum	Full to normal radix, often with bony/ cartilaginous dorsal hump
Tip support	Weak	Weak	Weak	Moderate to weak
Tip profile	Flat, amorphous	Rounded	Underprojected	Flattened tip, bulbous
Nostril shape	Round to flat (horizontal), wide alar lobule	Wide lobule	Wide lobule, rounded to flattened	Widened, asymmetric
Nasolabial angle	Hyperacute (prognathism)	Acute	Acute	Acute
Septum	Shortened	Thin and small	Relatively small, weak caudally	Oversized, deviated
Columella	Short	Moderately retracted, short, decreased nasolabial angle	Acute nasolabial angle	Lengthened nasal platform

Data from:

- Daniel RK. Middle Eastern rhinoplasty: anatomy, aesthetics, and surgical planning. Facial Plast Surg FPS 2010;26(2):110–118.
- Nolst Trenité GJ. Considerations in ethnic rhinoplasty. Facial Plast Surg FPS 2003;19(3):239–245.
- Jang YJ, Alfanta EM. Rhinoplasty in the Asian nose. Facial Plast Surg Clin N Am 2014;22(3):357–377.
- Rohrich RJ, Bolden K. Ethnic rhinoplasty. Clin Plast Surg 2010;37(2):353–370.
- Chun KW, et al. Anatomy of the alar lobule in the Asian nose. J Plast Reconstr Aesthet Surg 2008;61(4):400–407.

2.7 Lips and Lower Face

The appearance of the lips and lower third of the face is heavily influenced by the underlying maxillary, mandibular, and dental characteristics **(Fig. 2.6)**. While the skeletal differences are often significant (as referenced above), the soft tissue visible even on lateral cephalometric studies consistently suggests further differences exist. However, surprisingly limited data are available regarding the cause of anatomical differences in soft tissue composition. Evaluations of the smile arc (that is, the arc made by both the teeth and lips during smiling) have shown statistically significant different patterns among Caucasian, Korean, and Japanese groups.[29,30] However, very few further investigations of differences in the surrounding musculature are available to date.

In one of the few studies evaluating the cause of soft tissue differences between ethnicities, McAlister et al used ultrasound to evaluate the thickness of the lip levator musculature. The group found essentially no difference between Asian and Caucasian subjects. Instead, they describe sexual dimorphism in both ethnicities, with women having more robust levator anguli oris and zygomaticus major muscle groups, as well as more mean gingival exposure (although the authors were unable to show a statistical correlation between the degree of muscle hypertrophy and gingival show).[31]

Among Mestizo populations, lateral cephalometric evaluations showed that, in addition to slightly greater prognathism and lower third projection, the soft tissue profile of the region tended to be thicker, and overall facial shape was, as a result, more convex.[11]

Regarding *desired* lip appearance and *preferred* lower facial proportions in African American and Caucasian females, a 2011 publication by Iglesias-Linares et al in the *Journal of Oral and Maxillofacial Surgery* found that similar preferences existed for cervicomental angles, lip width, and lip projection, as well as overall facial convexity.[32] They

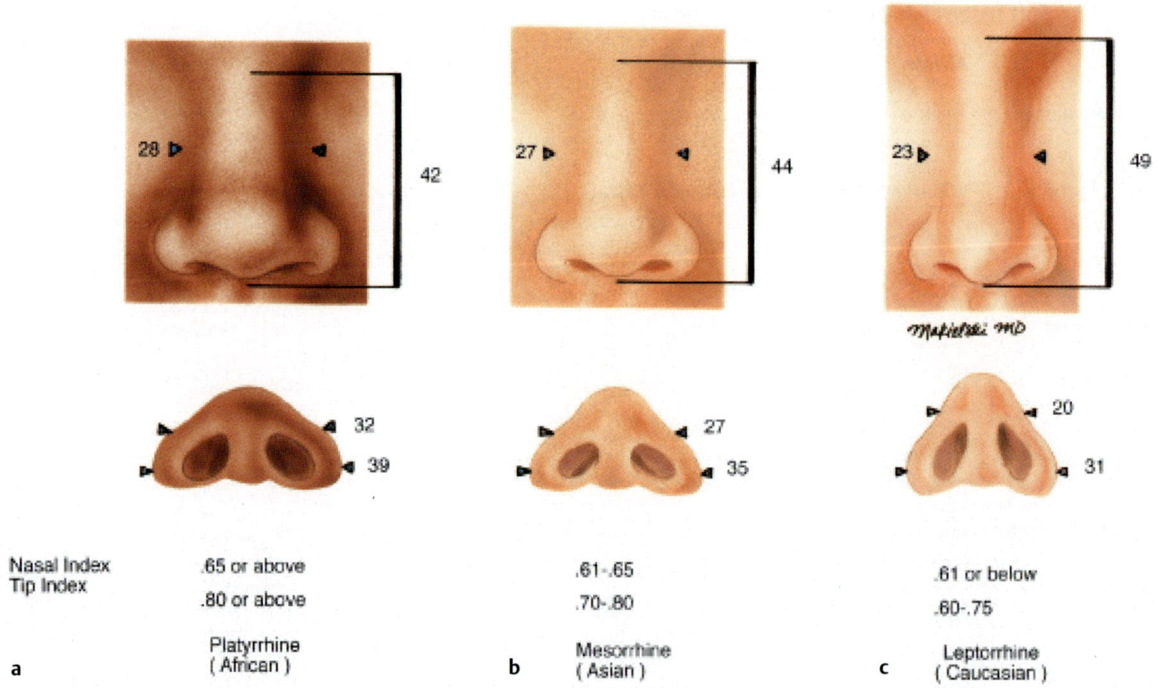

Fig. 2.5 **(a–c)** Nasal variations with race. The illustrations demonstrate the differences between nasal width, projection, and nostril shape based on race. The nasal index is a ratio of the nasal width (measured at the piriform aperture) and the nasal height. A larger nasal index therefore indicates a "shorter" and "wider" nose, with a smaller nasal index indicating a longer, more narrowed nose. The tip index is a ratio of the soft tissue width of the nose at the level of the apex of the nostril and the soft tissue width at the widest point of the ala. A larger tip index indicates more rounded, wider nostril shape. (Data ranges from the Hinderer analysis: Hinderer KH. Fundamentals of Anatomy and Surgery of the Nose. Birmingham, AL: Aesculapius Publishing; 1971:54. Used with permission from Larrabee, Makielski, Henderson. Surgical Anatomy of the Face. 2nd ed. Philadelphia, PA: Lippincott Williams & Wilkins; 2004.)

noted similarities in the preferred amount of lower lip protrusion (to be less than the upper lip) and upper lip width between African American and Caucasian celebrities. Differences existed, however, relative to historical Caucasian soft tissue profiles in the "ideal" lip volume, with more voluminous upper lips (and more projection) coming into vogue. Their discussion indicates this is a gradual shift, noted in the medical literature as early as 1990, toward a traditionally more "African aesthetic" soft tissue profile.

Khosravanifard et al, in their 2013 study on factors influencing the attractiveness of the soft tissue profile, generally agree with these tenets. Their study discusses the preference of Mestizo and Asian judges for relatively retruded lips, while Africans preferred more voluminous upper lips in particular. The authors compared their results to a handful of other studies and showed concordance, in that either a more full upper lip adjacent to a smaller nose, and/or more fullness in upper lips relative to lower lips, were considered the aesthetically most attractive combinations across ethnicities.[33]

2.8 Neck

The neck contour is heavily affected by mandibular anatomy. With varying mandibular projection, obviously the cervicomental angle and thyromental distances will be greatly influenced. No data are currently available on consistent racial differences in platysmal characteristics and in the great auricular or external jugular venous systems.

Ozgur et al make reference to differences in the position, size, and insertion of the anterior belly of the digastric, which influence the profile appearance of the neck and affect plans for surgical intervention. They found two broad patterns of insertion. The first, and more common, pattern was central diastasis. The second pattern, in which the anterior heads crossed, was less common.[34] The intuitive difference in profile and potential for central hollowing after submental procedures is noted.

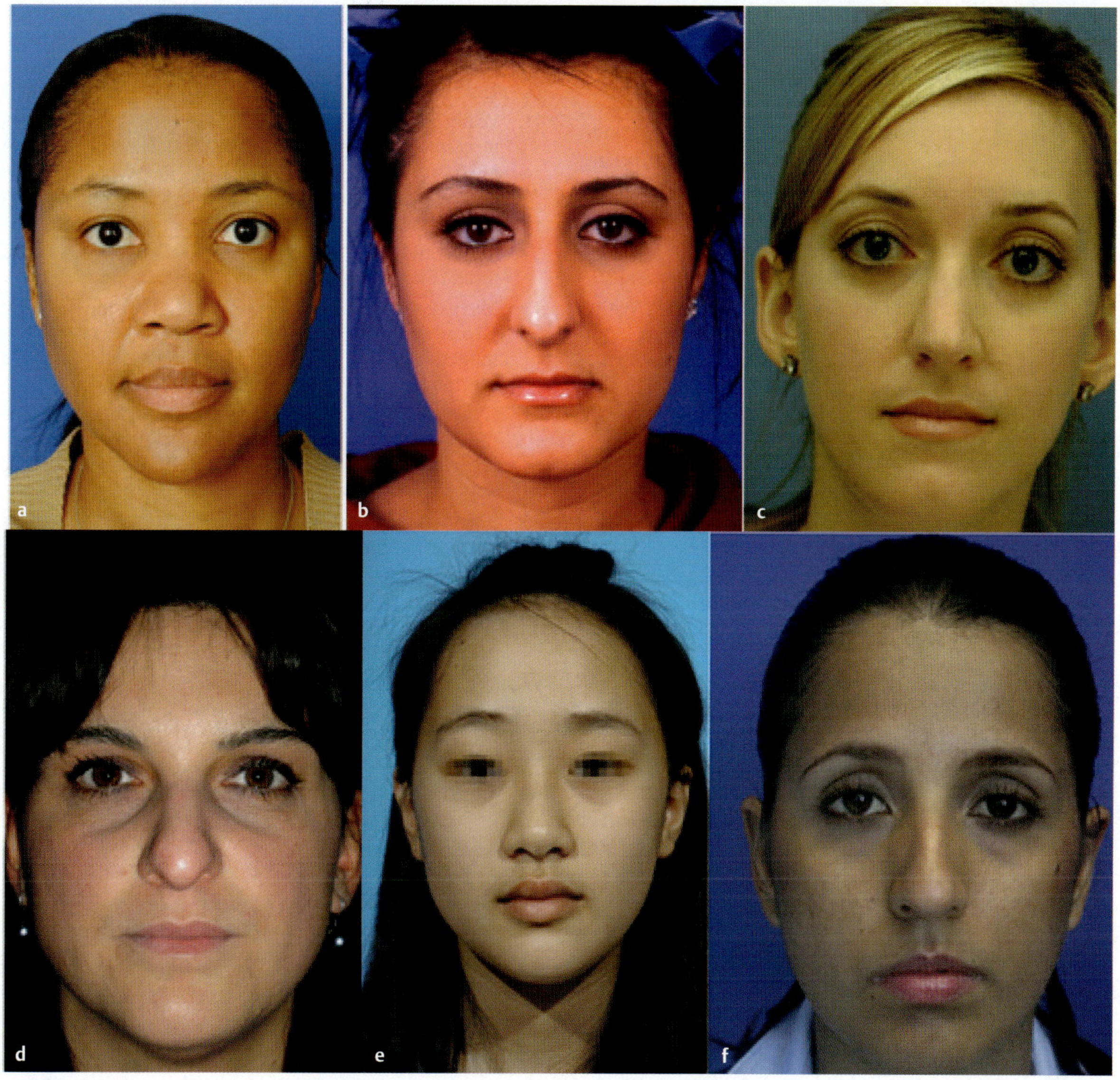

Fig. 2.6 Wide variation in middle-aged females' lip size, shape, and projection between and within various races. **(a)** African, **(b)** Mid-Eastern, **(c)** Northern European/Caucasian, **(d)** Mediterranean, **(e)** Asian, **(f)** Mestizo. (Used with permission from Sclafani AP. Rhinoplasty: The Experts' Reference. New York, NY: Thieme; 2015.)

2.9 Clinical Pearls

- Differences exist in the craniofacial skeleton among patients of different racial backgrounds and contribute to differences in overall facial shape and profile (**Table 2.1**). Understanding these skeletal differences is important in ascertaining how much modification of the soft tissue may (or may not) affect form and function.
- There are structural differences in skin thickness and composition, which result in differing susceptibilities to both aging and surgical intervention. Moisture content likely has implications for postoperative moisturizing therapy (**Table 2.2**).

- The most defining characteristics contributing to racial (and individual) appearances are those of the eyes, nasal anatomy, and perioral regions.
  - Asian eyelids are identified by the lack of supratarsal crease (caused by absent or low skin insertion of the levator aponeurosis), epicanthal fold, and narrowed palpebral fissure **(Fig. 2.4)**.
  - Nasal projection and alar width tend to be inversely related, and they are influenced by nasal aperture, cartilage strength and position, and thickness of the skin and soft tissue envelope **(Table 2.3)**.
  - Mestizo and African lips are more full than those of Asians and Caucasians.
  - Aesthetic ideals show more volume and projection of the upper lip relative to the lower lip.

References

1. United Nations, Department of Economic and Social Affairs, Population Division. 2014. World Population Prospects: The 2012 Revision, Methodology of the United Nations Population Estimates and Projections, Working Paper No. ESA/P/WP.235.
2. Vegter FMD, Hage JJ. Clinical anthropometry and canons of the face in historical perspective. Plast Reconstr Surg 2000;106(5):1090–1096
3. Standring S, et al. External skull. Gray's Anatomy. 4th ed. 2008; 409–421
4. Phillips VM, Smuts NA. Facial reconstruction: utilization of computerized tomography to measure facial tissue thickness in a mixed racial population. Forensic Sci Int 1996;83(1):51–59
5. Gu Y, McNamara JA Jr, Sigler LM, Baccetti T. Comparison of craniofacial characteristics of typical Chinese and Caucasian young adults. Eur J Orthod 2011;33(2):205–211
6. Uhm KI, Lew JM. Prominent zygoma in Orientals: classification and treatment. Ann Plast Surg 1991;26(2): 164–170
7. Hoffman BE, McConathy DA, Coward M, Saddler L. Relationship between the piriform aperture and interalar nasal widths in adult males. J Forensic Sci 1991;36(4): 1152–1161
8. Fadeju AD, Otuyemi OD, Ngom PI, Newman-Nartey M. A study of cephalometric soft tissue profile among adolescents from the three West African countries of Nigeria, Ghana and Senegal. J Orthod 2013;40(1):53–61
9. McNamara JA Jr, Brust EW, Riolo ML. Soft tissue evaluation of individuals with an ideal occlusion and a well balanced face. In: McNamara JA Jr, ed. Esthetics and treatment of facial form. Monograph 28, Craniofacial Growth Series. Ann Arbor, MI: Centre for Human Growth and Development, The University of Michigan; 1992:115–146
10. Ikenna Isiekwe G, Olatokunbo DaCosta O, Chukwudi Isiekwe M. A cephalometric investigation of horizontal lip position in adult Nigerians. J Orthod 2012;39(3): 160–169
11. Vela E, Taylor RW, Campbell PM, Buschang PH. Differences in craniofacial and dental characteristics of adolescent Mexican Americans and European Americans. Am J Orthod Dentofacial Orthop 2011;140(6):839–847
12. Farkas LG, Katic MJ, Forrest CR, et al. International anthropometric study of facial morphology in various ethnic groups/races. J Craniofac Surg 2005;16(4):615–646
13. Mitsukawa N, Moriyama H, Shiozawa K, Satoh K. Study on distribution of terminal branches of the facial nerve in mimetic muscles (orbicularis oculi muscle and orbicularis oris muscle). Ann Plast Surg 2014;72(1):71–74
14. Hwang K, Lee DK, Lee EJ, Chung IH, Lee SI. Innervation of the lower eyelid in relation to blepharoplasty and midface lift: clinical observation and cadaveric study. Ann Plast Surg 2001;47(1):1–5, discussion 5–7
15. Santini A, Alayan I. A comparative anthropometric study of the position of the mental foramen in three populations. Br Dent J 2012;212(4):E7
16. Mbajiorgu EF, Mawera G, Asala SA, Zivanovic S. Position of the mental foramen in adult black Zimbabwean mandibles: a clinical anatomical study. Cent Afr J Med 1998;44(2):24–30
17. Rawlings AV. Ethnic skin types: are there differences in skin structure and function? Int J Cosmet Sci 2006;28(2): 79–93
18. Berardesca E, Maibach H. Racial differences in skin pathophysiology. J Am Acad Dermatol 1996;34(4):667–672
19. Akazawa T, Sathmåry EJE. Prehistoric Mongoloid Dispersals. New York, NY: Oxford University Press; 1996
20. Montagu A. Growing Young. Greenwood Publishing Group; 1989
21. Sugiyama-Nakagiri Y, Sugata K, Hachiya A, Osanai O, Ohuchi A, Kitahara T. Ethnic differences in the structural properties of facial skin. J Dermatol Sci 2009;53(2): 135–139
22. Soni CV, Barker JH, Pushpakumar SB, et al. Psychosocial considerations in facial transplantation. Burns 2010; 36(7):959–964
23. Alam DS, Chi JJ. Facial transplantation for massive traumatic injuries. Otolaryngol Clin North Am 2013;46(5): 883–901
24. Kakizaki H, Selva D, Asamoto K, Nakano T, Leibovitch I. Orbital septum attachment sites on the levator aponeurosis in Asians and whites. Ophthal Plast Reconstr Surg 2010;26(4):265–268
25. Jeong S, Lemke BN, Dortzbach RK, Park YG, Kang HK. The Asian upper eyelid: an anatomical study with comparison to the Caucasian eyelid. Arch Ophthalmol 1999; 117(7):907–912
26. Koh K, Choi JW, Ishii CH. Asian facial cosmetic surgery. Section 1: Aesthetic Surgery of the Face. Plastic Surgery. Neligan, Peter C; 2013

27. Batniji RK, Perkins SW. Upper and midfacial rejuvenation in the non-Caucasian face. Facial Plast Surg Clin North Am 2010;18(1):19–33

28. Chun KW, Kang HJ, Han SK, et al. Anatomy of the alar lobule in the Asian nose. J Plast Reconstr Aesthet Surg 2008;61(4):400–407

29. Dong JK, Rashid RG, Rosenstiel SF. Smile arcs of Caucasian and Korean youth. Int J Prosthodont 2009;22(3): 290–292

30. Kopuz C, Turgut S, Yavuz S, Ilgi S. Distribution of facial nerve in parotid gland: analysis of 50 cases. Okajimas Folia Anat Jpn 1994;70(6):295–299

31. McAlister RW, Harkness EM, Nicoll JJ. An ultrasound investigation of the lip levator musculature. Eur J Orthod 1998;20(6):713–720

32. Iglesias-Linares A, Yáñez-Vico RM, Moreno-Manteca B, Moreno-Fernández AM, Mendoza-Mendoza A, Solano-Reina E. Common standards in facial esthetics: craniofacial analysis of most attractive black and white subjects according to *People* magazine during previous 10 years. J Oral Maxillofac Surg 2011;69(6):e216–e224

33. Khosravanifard B, Rakhshan V, Raeesi E. Factors influencing attractiveness of soft tissue profile. Oral Surg Oral Med Oral Pathol Oral Radiol 2013;115(1):29–37

34. Ozgur Z, Govsa F, Ozgur T. The cause of the difference in the submental region: aberrant muscle bundles of the anterior belly of the digastric muscle. J Craniofac Surg 2007;18(4):875–881

3 Ethnic Reflections Emphasizing the Nose

Gilbert J. Nolst Trenité

3.1 Introduction

In recent decades, facial plastic surgeons in Europe and North America have been confronted more frequently with patients from a specific ethnic background who seek cosmetic surgery and who have been influenced by the Caucasian standard of beauty shown in the media. Nowadays, however, as the world is becoming a melting pot of different races, the standard of beauty is less specifically Caucasian and is shifting rapidly to a more general standard of beauty in which the different facial units are in harmony. "Ethnic beauty" is a new trademark.

It is difficult to define ethnicity: the literature is rather confusing about general ethnic differences, which are determined by geographical, racial, cultural, and historical factors. Nevertheless, it is helpful to give guidelines for aesthetic surgery of the face and more specifically of the nose, to differentiate the non-Caucasian groups in five geographically defined ethnic groups: African, Asian, Latin American, Mediterranean, and Middle Eastern. Noses from these five "ethnic regions" have specific general anatomical characteristics, knowledge of which helps us to evaluate the facial characteristics and to make an adequate surgical plan.[1,2] In this chapter, the focus is on communication, specific anatomical problems, and surgical solutions to preserve ethnic facial balance, and less on general surgical procedures of the nose.

3.2 Communication/ Consultation

Communication with the patient is of utmost importance in general, and with an ethnic patient it is especially important to take ample time to find out if the patient's cosmetic desires are based purely on beauty and harmony of the face, or instead on obscuring the patient's own ethnic background.[3] If the latter, then it can be difficult to find harmony and beauty. With every patient seeking cosmetic surgery, formulating realistic expectations and excluding those with body dysmorphic disorder are important. Computer imaging, as well as standard photographs, can be helpful in discussing preservation of ethnicity. Photographs are also important as a reference during surgery, for analyzing the final outcome, and for medico-legal purposes. Possible complications, such as bleeding, hematomas, infections, and especially scar tissue formation, should be discussed. In dark-skinned patients particularly, keloid formation is a possibility; it will not happen in the nasal triangle, but it is a realistic problem when harvesting ear or rib cartilage for reconstruction of the nasal skeleton.

3.3 Physical Examination

It is important to see the face as a whole and to be aware of the fact that, in addition to the nose, there are four other major aesthetic components in the facial complex: forehead, eyes, lips, and chin. Every ethnic group has its specific ethnic conformation of facial components, which should be in harmony to create beauty. Be aware of facial asymmetries and characteristics that could be important for the final aesthetic outcome and discuss them with the patient. The nose, in the center of the face, should not distract the attention from the eyes, as it will when the nose is deformed, crooked, too big, or too small. The goal in ethnic rhinoplasty is that the long-term outcome should be in harmony with the other ethnic features of the face.

The following points are helpful in preoperative evaluation of the nose.

External inspection to evaluate:

- skin type
- width and height of the nasal bridge
- saddling or hump formation
- tip shape, supra tip fullness, infra tip lobule and projection
- nasal base width
- alar and nostril shape
- columellar show and double break
- nasolabial angle

Internal inspection to evaluate:

- septal deviations
- internal nasal valve
- mucosa and turbinates

Dynamic inspection to evaluate:

- alar insufficiency
- internal valve collapse (Cottle test)

Palpation of the nose is important to evaluate:

- skin thickness and elasticity
- length of the bony pyramid
- strength of the nasal tip cartilages
- tip support
- cartilaginous septum for harvesting purposes

3.4 General Nasal Anatomical Considerations for the Five Geographical Ethnic Groups

Although numerous variations can occur within the same ethnic group, it is helpful to categorize the most common characteristic anatomical features for each group as a checklist to help make a surgical plan.

African nasal anatomy:

- thick, sebaceous, dark skin
- low nasal dorsum
- wide nasal bridge
- underprojected, undefined tip
- flimsy alar cartilages, broad domes, and short columella
- acute nasolabial angle
- wide, flaring nasal base
- horizontal, round nostrils
- poor tip support

Asian nasal anatomy:

- moderate to thick skin (skin is thinner in the nasion and dorsum and thinner in the nasal tip area)
- low, shallow nasion
- wide nasal bridge
- underprojected, moderately undefined tip
- flimsy alar cartilages and short columella
- acute to normal nasolabial angle
- wide, flaring nasal base
- oblique-shaped nostrils
- poor tip support

Latin-American/Mestizo nasal anatomy:

- moderate to thick skin
- small to normal dorsum
- normal to wide nasal bridge
- underprojected, wide, undefined tip
- flimsy alar cartilages and short to normal columella
- normal to acute nasolabial angle
- normal to wide nasal base with thick alar side walls
- normal to horizontally shaped nostrils
- poor tip support

Mediterranean nasal anatomy:

- moderate to thick skin
- straight to convex nasal dorsum
- normal to narrow nasal bridge
- plunging tip with wide, strong cartilages
- normal to acute nasolabial angle
- normal to narrow nasal base
- vertically shaped nostrils
- normal to weak tip support

Middle Eastern nasal anatomy:

- moderate to thick skin
- high, arched nasal dorsum often extending into the glabellar region
- high nasal bridge
- underprojected tip with downward rotation
- wide alar cartilages with undefined tip
- acute nasolabial angle
- normal nasal base
- oval to vertically shaped nostrils
- normal to strong tip support

3.5 Surgical Considerations

After an accurate evaluation, keeping in mind the ethnic background and the desires of the patient, the surgeon should set up a surgical plan. The surgical approach (non-delivery, delivery, or external approach) depends on the extent of the surgical goal and on the expertise of the surgeon. The modern generation of surgeons will in most cases use an external approach, which gives more control and is easier when grafts for reconstruction are used. Often in Middle Eastern countries, patients with an Islamic background don't want a columellar scar.

The choice of implant material is often a point of discussion.[4] In Western countries, the adage "autogenous material (fascia and cartilage, no bone) is still the first choice in rhinoplasty" is still valid (**Fig. 3.1**). Yet in Asia there is a long tradition of using Silastic implants for augmentation purposes. If performed with the state-of-the-art approaches (sterile circumstances and no tension on the surrounding tissues), the success rate is high, with a low complication rate. But if a complication, such as infection of the implant, occurs, it could be a disaster if not adequately treated.

Some surgical tips:

- Surgery in the correct surgical plane diminishes perioperative bleeding, causes fewer postoperative ecchymoses, and promotes quicker healing.
- Tight pockets are helpful for dorsal side and onlay grafts, which should be smooth and not too big.
- In cases of a thin soft tissue envelope, an extra layer of fascia is helpful to disguise any dorsal irregularity.
- Using the middle part of rib cartilage prevents warping.
- Crushed cartilage is ideal for contouring and camouflage.
- To project the tip, lateral crural steal, cap grafts are appropriate for moderate augmentation, while shield grafts and a lengthened columella strut are useful for more tip projection.
- A bulbous, broad tip with thick skin asks for reconstruction instead of reduction (**Fig. 3.2**).

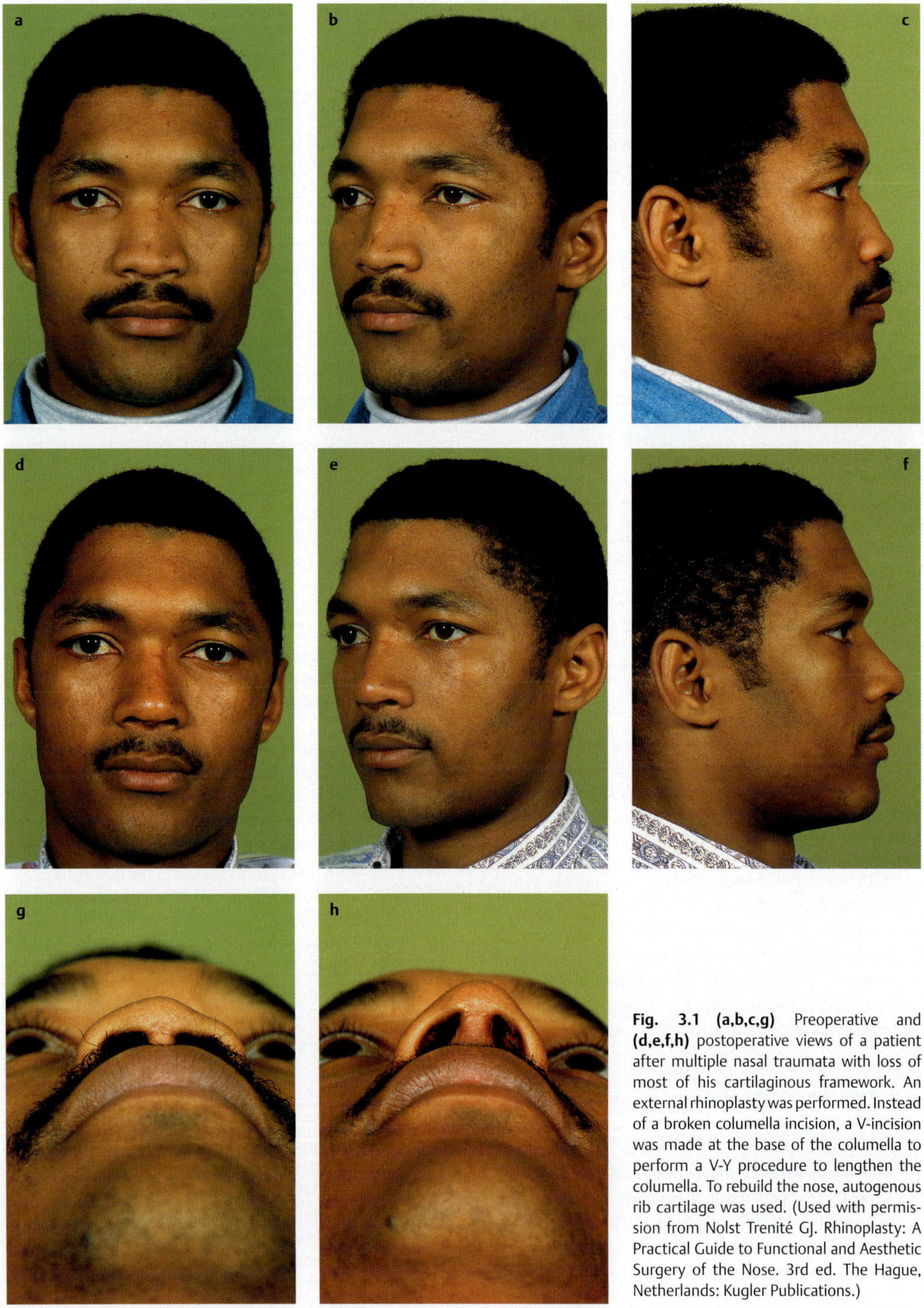

Fig. 3.1 (a,b,c,g) Preoperative and **(d,e,f,h)** postoperative views of a patient after multiple nasal traumata with loss of most of his cartilaginous framework. An external rhinoplasty was performed. Instead of a broken columella incision, a V-incision was made at the base of the columella to perform a V-Y procedure to lengthen the columella. To rebuild the nose, autogenous rib cartilage was used. (Used with permission from Nolst Trenité GJ. Rhinoplasty: A Practical Guide to Functional and Aesthetic Surgery of the Nose. 3rd ed. The Hague, Netherlands: Kugler Publications.)

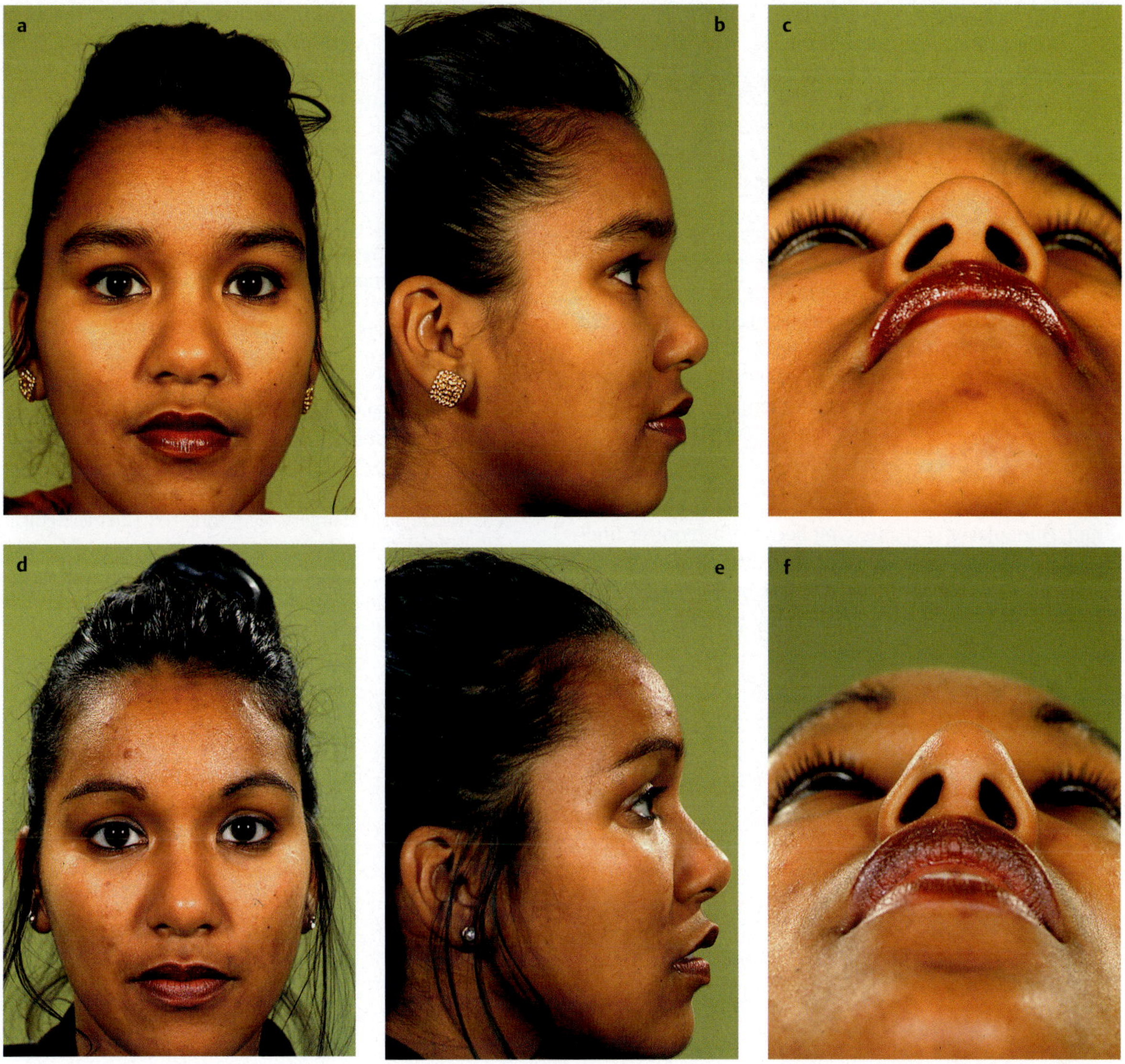

Fig. 3.2 (a–c) Preoperative and **(d–f)** postoperative views of a patient with a bulbous tip with lack of projection and low nasal bridge. An external rhinoplasty was performed for more dorsal and tip projection and more tip refinement with the use of autogenous cartilage. (Used with permission from Nolst Trenité GJ. Rhinoplasty: A Practical Guide to Functional and Aesthetic Surgery of the Nose. 3rd ed. The Hague, Netherlands: Kugler Publications.)

- In a very thick soft tissue envelope, conservative reduction of fat tissue without disturbing blood supply and innervation is an option.
- The sharp nasolabial angle more commonly seen in the African nose can be treated with plumping grafts in moderate cases, and with a caudal extension of an enlarged columella strut.
- Alar base wedge resections can be divided into three main types, to narrow nostril size, to reduce a too-broad nasal base, or to correct alar flaring. It is important to prevent over-resection and to employ adequate suturing of the wound.

3.6 Pitfalls

Apart from the common general pitfalls of rhinoplastic surgery, there are some specific pitfalls in surgery of the ethnic nose. They occur in:

- Communication about preservation of ethnicity
- Evaluation of the characteristics of the nasal skeleton, especially the thickness of the skin envelope and tip support
- Graft harvesting procedures (e.g., the risk of keloid formation and of warping of rib cartilage)

- Alar base wedge over-resection, resulting in unnatural straightening of the ala
- Suturing technique after alar base wedge resection, resulting in ugly scarring

3.7 Postoperative Care

Besides the standard packing for one day with a 2-cm cotton strip with antibiotic ointment and dressing restricted to the nose itself for a week, it is helpful in the thick-skinned ethnic patient to have prolonged taping in the supra tip area to prevent a soft tissue Polly beak. With severe, prolonged postoperative swelling, subdermal (not intradermal!) injections of Kenacort can be useful.

3.8 Conclusion

Ethnic rhinoplasty is challenging because it requires finding a balance between preserving the patient's specific ethnic features and the individual desires of the patient. The surgeon should be aware that harmony in the face creates beauty. Knowledge of the ethnic characteristics of the nose and face, meticulous evaluation, including both inspection and palpation, and use of atraumatic surgical techniques will help create satisfying results for the patient and the surgeon as well.

References

1. Cobo R, Nolst Trenité GJ. Ethnic rhinoplasty. In: Nolst Trenité GJ, ed. Rhinoplasty: A Practical Guide to Functional and Aesthetic Surgery of the Nose. 3rd ed. The Hague, Netherlands: Kugler Publications; 2005:309–321
2. Earle Matory W Jr. Definition of beauty in the ethnic patient. In: Earle Matory W Jr, ed. Ethnic Considerations in Facial Aesthetic Surgery. Philadelphia, New York: Lippincott-Raven; 1998:61–85
3. Leong SC, Eccles R. Race and ethnicity in nasal plastic surgery: a need for science. In: Kridel RWH, Rowe-Jones J, eds. Facial Plastic Surgery. New York, NY: Thieme Medical Publishers; 2010:63–69
4. Tardy ME Jr, Denneny J III, Fritsch MH. The versatile cartilage autograft in reconstruction of the nose and face. Laryngoscope 1985;95(5):523–533

4 The Consultation

Roxana Cobo and Néstor Ricardo González Marín

4.1 Introduction

A facial plastic surgeon must understand the changing concept of beauty. Today, aesthetic ideals involve facial harmony, balance, and symmetry whenever possible.[1,2] These concepts vary depending on the patients' cultural, social, religious, and ethnic backgrounds. Current aesthetic ideals are influenced by multiculturalism, which is the result of globalization, migration, and social media. Geographic and cultural barriers have started to disappear, transforming the concept of beauty into a more global one. Mixed heritage is becoming a common denominator in the world, as is already the case in many developed countries. Different people will no doubt continue to mix, and the physical features of mixed heritage will be the high point in beauty.[1,2] A single attractive individual will have physical features of different races without necessarily having the predominant features of one race.

Patients come to facial plastic surgeons because they want to look and feel more attractive, and our goal is to satisfy our patients. A successful outcome of any surgical or nonsurgical facial plastic procedure begins with the initial contact with the patient in the office. The consultation is the moment when the specialist tries to define the patient's needs, desires, and expectations. Ideally, for any type of intervention, an adequate patient–physician relationship has been established, and both specialist and patient are satisfied with the final result of whatever intervention is performed.

4.2 The Consultation

Patients' motives for undertaking a facial plastic surgery procedure vary, but most are related to the current definition of beauty, which over time has been influenced by the media and Internet. Patients' motives are also related to the instinctive drives for survival and reproductive success. Today, survival includes the capacity to obtain a better job, higher income, or better academic grades. People also want to "fit in" and "be part of a group," especially if they are from ethnic groups that differ from those among whom they are living. Fitting in increases their social acceptance and raises their self-esteem. Another very common motive in seeking facial plastic procedures is to delay the appearance or improve the changes associated with aging, as well as to improve facial harmony. People of all races, ethnic groups, and ages are interested in looking attractive.[1,2,3,4]

4.2.1 Initial Contact

Initial contact and the interview are key points for establishing a solid communication channel that allows both the surgeon and the patient to obtain essential and immediate information that will define the quality of the patient–physician relationship, and thus the level of satisfaction and success of any procedure that is performed.[5] The first impressions that our staff members and we as specialists have of the patient are very important and should always be taken into consideration. Patients should be received in an environment that is relaxing and friendly. Waiting rooms should not be overcrowded or attended by personnel who are not friendly. Appointment times should be respected and scheduling personnel should be trained so that the specialist does not feel he has to rush with the consultation because he or she has a long line of patients waiting to be seen.

The surgeon should greet the patient with a secure and friendly attitude. This will give the patient a sense of trust in the surgeon and will establish a foundation for conversation. Next, the patient should be asked about the main concerns and reasons for seeking a consultation with a facial plastic surgeon. The patient should be asked to express in their own words why they sought a consultation, what is their main complaint or facial aspect they want changed, modified, or corrected, and what specific procedure (surgical or nonsurgical) they want performed.[6] These initial questions, together with other questions regarding expectations surrounding the procedure, must be asked openly, without inducing responses from the individual, while always showing an attitude of interest and real concern regarding the problem or complaint that brings the patient to the office.

4.2.2 Defining the "Problem"

After eliciting the initial reasons for consultation, it is important to define which aspects of their facial image the patient wants to work on. Patients should be asked to point to the areas of the face they want to work on. This is easily done using a three-way mirror while keeping an active conversation between the patient and the physician.[6] In addition, we must systematically look for signs and symptoms associated with the main complaint that could be resolved at the same time. For example, with a patient consulting for a nasal deformity, ideally we should ask if there is any related functional problem, such as obstruction, snoring, allergies, or sinusitis. Once a problem has been identified, it is necessary to determine if the patient's expectations are realistic and possible to achieve.

4.2.3 Understanding Expectations

Success in facial plastic surgery is synonymous with patient satisfaction. To increase the probability of success in any facial plastic procedure, it is essential to identify unrealistic expectations and other aspects that could cause a disparity between the result obtained and the patient's desires.[7] Open questions should be formulated without leading or giving any answers to the patient. The first question that must be asked is: "What do you hope this procedure (surgical or nonsurgical) will do for you?" It is important to identify patients who expect a miracle to happen. Such answers include: "I will be beautiful and finally be confident and happy," "I expect to be more successful in my career," "I will be more loved by my mate," "I will get my spouse back," and "I am sure everything that you do will be perfect."[7,8] Additionally, it is important to identify whether the expectations are only those of the patient or if there are other people who also expect to be satisfied by the result. In this case, it is useful to ask: "Who else would be affected by your decision to have surgery?" In other words, is there a significant other who also has expectations that could later be projected to the patient? Through these questions, the surgeon establishes whether the patient's expectations are unrealistic and whether there are other motives that have not been expressed during the interview. If you receive sensible responses, you will be able to educate the patient regarding the procedure and subsequent care, thus increasing the probability of success and patient satisfaction. Sensible responses include: "I know surgery cannot make people happy" and "I am doing this for myself, and not others."[8]

4.2.4 Building Trust

The patient's feeling of trust in the physician is vitally important, and is developed through the patient–physician relationship. Strategies that can be used to build up trust include: showing an interest in the patient's problems, answering questions in a clear and unhesitant manner, showing patients what results could be obtained by using computer imaging programs, and taking the time to explain the procedure that is going to be performed.

4.2.5 Background Information

Before considering surgery and examining the patient, a complete medical history should be recorded, including physical and mental issues, so that the patient is selected correctly.[8,9] It is essential to identify conditions that can have a negative effect on the final result of the procedure, such as smoking or consumption of medicines and/or foods that must be discontinued several weeks before the procedure (**Table 4.1**). Concurrent and pre-existing illnesses must be controlled and should be properly treated before any procedure is scheduled.[9] When necessary, the patient should be cleared by their primary care physician. When surgery is going to be performed, the anesthesiologist must also evaluate the patient and define what is needed for the surgical procedure.

4.2.6 Psychiatric History and Assessment

Identifying the high-risk patient from a psychological standpoint is important to avoid negative short- and long-term outcomes. Patients with overly high and unrealistic expectations, those who are rude during the initial assessment, psychopaths, and patients with obsessive disorders present a higher risk of dissatisfaction after the surgical procedure.

Much has been published in the literature about identifying high-risk patients. For example, the acronym SIMON (single, immature, male, overly expectant or obsessive, narcissistic) can help the surgeon to assess the patient's risk level and to identify the need for preliminary assessment by a psychologist or psychiatrist. In general, if the patient's expectations are unrealistic, or if the patient is overly demanding, demands immediate surgical intervention, tends toward extreme adulation, is going through a crisis, or feels unhappy or apathetic, it is best to request a second opinion prior to the procedure.[10]

The first warning sign is if the surgeon feels an aversion to the patient or personal antipathy. Psychiatrists summarize this feeling as: "If you can't get your patient to smile, then don't operate."[10]

Body dysmorphic disorder is another warning sign for the surgeon. Its prevalence in the general population is 1% and increases from 6 to 16 times in candidates for aesthetic surgery, with a higher prevalence among adolescents. Generally, patients with this disorder worry about one or more physical defects that are not observable or that are usually not noticed by others. They tend to engage in repetitive behaviors, such as looking at the mirror frequently and anxiously, or avoiding looking at mirrors. They clean themselves excessively, scratch their skin, compare themselves to others, show dissatisfaction with their physical appearance, tend to cover up their "defects," and tend to be

Table 4.1 Medications and herbal health supplements to discontinue prior to surgery

Medication	Mechanism of action	Recommended stop date (before surgery)
NSAIDs: aspirin, ibuprofen, naproxen, meloxicam, celecoxib	Inhibit platelet synthesis Vitamin K antagonists (clotting cascade)	2 weeks
Warfarin	Inhibits platelet synthesis	1 week
Clopidogrel	Inhibits platelet aggregation	1 week
Alcohol	Inhibits platelet synthesis	1 week
Systemic steroids	Inhibit platelet aggregation	1 week
Isotretinoin	Alters wound healing	3–6 weeks
Herbal/Health supplements	**Mechanism of action**	**Recommended stop date (before surgery)**
Foods high in salicylate: Curry, cayenne pepper, ginger, paprika, thyme, cinnamon, dill, oregano, turmeric, licorice, peppermint, raisins, cherries, cranberries, oranges, prunes, grapes, strawberries, chewing gum, honey, wine, cider, vinegar	Inhibit platelet synthesis	2 weeks
Vitamin E, fish oil/omega-3 fatty acids	Vitamin K antagonists	1 week
Gingko biloba	Inhibits platelet synthesis	2 weeks

Data from Karimi K, Adamson P. Patient analysis and selection in aging face surgery. Facial Plast Surg 2011;27(1):5–15.

dissatisfied with any previous surgical procedures.[11] A simple screening questionnaire is recommended for patients suspected of having this disorder[12]:

1. Do you currently think often about your physical appearance? What features do you dislike? Do you think your appearance is ugly or unpleasant?
2. How well known do you think your features are to other people?
3. On an average day, how many hours do you spend thinking about your physical appearance?
4. Is your physical appearance an important source of worry to you?
5. How times a day do you usually check your physical appearance? (In the mirror, on a reflective surface, or with your fingers?)
6. How often you feel anxious in social encounters due to your physical appearance? Could this lead you to stay away from such social encounters?
7. Has your physical appearance affected your work, studies, or friendships?

If the surgeon suspects the presence of body dysmorphic disorder, the patient should be referred to a psychiatrist and must be completely cleared before any cosmetic procedures are performed.[12]

On the other hand, some patient traits indicate a low psychological risk. These characteristics are summarized by the acronym SYLVIA (secure, young, listens, verbal, intelligent, attractive). A brief summary of favorable and unfavorable risk factors for facial plastic surgery is shown in **Table 4.2**.

4.3 Physical Examination

In the first part of the interview, we focus on understanding what the patient wants and expects. In the physical examination part of the consultation, the objective is to establish what the patient needs. An accurate physical examination of the different anatomical structures of the face will allow the surgeon to establish efficiently the different findings of the face. In this way, a precise definition of the different problems can be established, enabling the surgeon to define the solutions that can be offered.[13]

Table 4.2 High- and low-risk patient characteristics for facial plastic surgery

High-risk characteristics	Low-risk characteristics
Obsessive traits	Secure patient
Demanding patient	Attractive patient
Unrealistic expectations	Communicative patient
Overly expectant patient	Young patient (not adolescent)
Unhappy patient	Intelligent patient
Narcissistic traits	No affective disorders
Poor relationship with the surgeon	Good relationship with the surgeon

The first step is to examine the patient as a whole and to carry out a complete analysis, identifying aspects that are affecting facial harmony. It is advised that findings not be mentioned out loud, to avoid giving opinions that the patient dislikes. Afterward, a complete inspection and palpation of the soft tissue, cartilage, and bones should be performed, while keeping in mind the patient's motive for the consultation and the functional condition of the structures involved. When we have linked the information obtained in the first part of the interview with the findings of the physical exam, it is time to begin dialog with the patient on critical points and other related findings that can be changed to obtain a better result. For example, patients with nasal deformities and microgenia could benefit from simultaneous rhinoplasty and mentoplasty.

When performing the physical examination, the face, head, and neck area should be evaluated as a whole and then divided into thirds for adequate evaluation of each subdivision. All components should be taken into consideration: the bony facial skeleton, the cartilaginous structures, the soft tissues, and the skin. If facial asymmetries are present, they should be pointed out and documented. Key points that bother the patient should be closely evaluated and registered in the clinical chart.

4.3.1 Photographic Documentation

Photographic documentation is crucial in facial plastic surgery. Pre- and postoperative photographs must be standardized and taken in a controlled setting by either the physician or a trained assistant. Analysis of the patient's pictures is essential for surgical planning. They allow the surgeon to assess problems that could have been missed in the initial physical exam; when combined with computer imaging, they are an excellent tool to show patients what the surgical result could look like. Imaging can also help identify non-ideal surgical patients. During surgery, the images help guide the surgeon. Additionally, they are useful as clinical and legal evidence, because they document the patient's preoperative state; they are useful as a reminder for patients who forget their preoperative appearance; and they serve as a reference point for assessing surgical outcomes.[13,14,15,16]

Standard photographs should be taken using the same focal length, same distance from the patient, same lighting system, and the same standard views. Ideally, patients should be photographed without makeup, jewelry, or eyeglasses. Hair should be pinned back and ears must be visible. Five standard views are used for most facial plastic procedures: anteroposterior (AP) view, right and left lateral view, and right and left oblique view (**Fig. 4.1**).

The frontal, lateral, and oblique views should all be taken in the Frankfort plane. The Frankfort plane is a horizontal line that extends from the superior tragus (superior edge of the external auditory canal) passing through the inferior orbital rim (**Fig. 4.2**). The oblique views that the authors recommend are more "three-fourths" views, where the medial canthus is aligned with the oral commissure (**Fig. 4.3**).

Depending on the type of procedure planned, additional views may be needed. In rhinoplasty, a base view to evaluate the alar–columellar complex is added. In the base view, the tip of the nose should be placed between the brows or, alternatively, as some authors prefer, the tip of the nose should be placed at the level of the glabella (**Fig. 4.4**). For blepharoplasty, close-up views with the patient looking ahead, gazing upward, and with the eyes closed are necessary (**Fig. 4.5**).

For rhytidectomy, the same five standard images are taken, but they should include the full face and neck. In otoplasty, additional images include a posterior image and close-up views of each ear (**Fig. 4.6, Table 4.3**).

4.3.2 Computer Imaging

Computer programs are useful tools that permit surgeons to assess if the patient is a good candidate for surgery, and the use of software to modify presurgical photographs is an excellent communication tool. Morphing presurgical images and showing patients approximate results often help both surgeon and patient decide if what is being discussed is a feasible option and if it fulfills the patient's expectations.

Most programs are two-dimensional, but recently three-dimensional computer imaging programs have become available, and they have an added benefit because the morphing of images allows results to be shown at different angles and positions. The great advantage of these programs is that the surgeon can show the patient in a

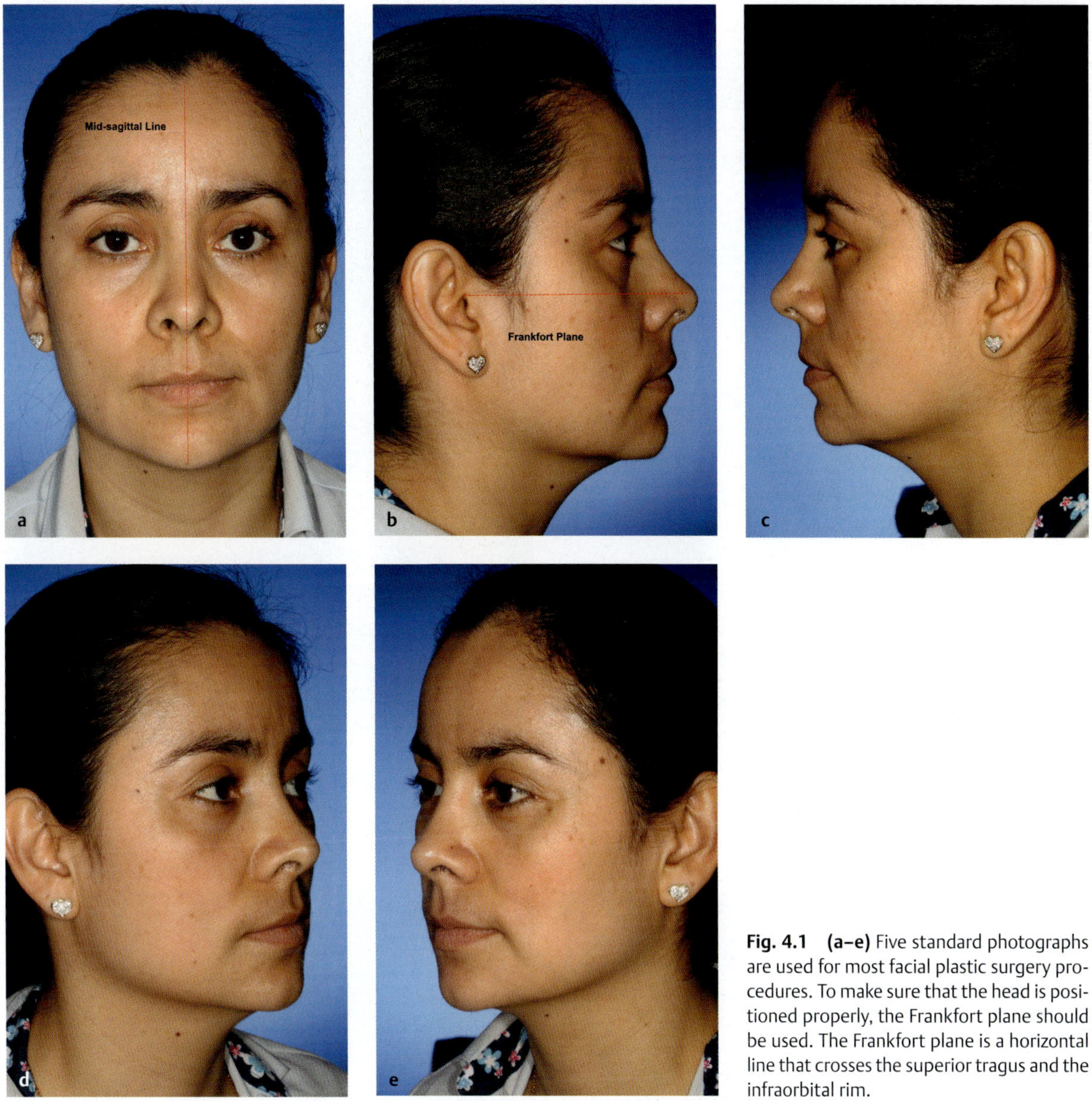

Fig. 4.1 **(a–e)** Five standard photographs are used for most facial plastic surgery procedures. To make sure that the head is positioned properly, the Frankfort plane should be used. The Frankfort plane is a horizontal line that crosses the superior tragus and the infraorbital rim.

realistic fashion how the postoperative results can look. The imaging is a simulation, but it still permits us to educate our patients, to clarify any doubts regarding the procedure, and to identify patients who have unrealistic expectations of what is going to be accomplished. From a legal standpoint, patients need to be told that computer programs are simulations and that the final result will never be exactly what was shown in the computer screen **(Fig. 4.7)**.[5] In countries that consider that photographic imaging is a contract guaranteeing results, an additional paragraph can be included in the informed consent that indicates that the patient accepts that the imaging is merely an educational tool used as an additional support during the consultation.

A disadvantage of computer imaging is when young, inexperienced surgeons become overly enthusiastic about the expected postoperative changes expected. Morphing of images must be approached conservatively, and patients should be told that imaging is simply a tool that helps them understand what can be achieved in surgery. An additional disadvantage of imaging is the increased time required for the consultation, many times involving a second or third consultation with the patient.

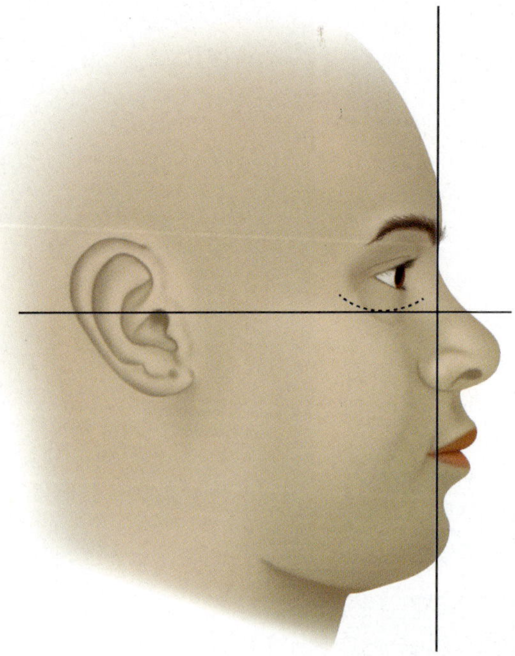

Fig. 4.2 Frankfort plane is a horizontal line that extends from the top of the tragus and passes through the infraorbital rim. The patient's head should be positioned so that the horizontal line is parallel with the floor.

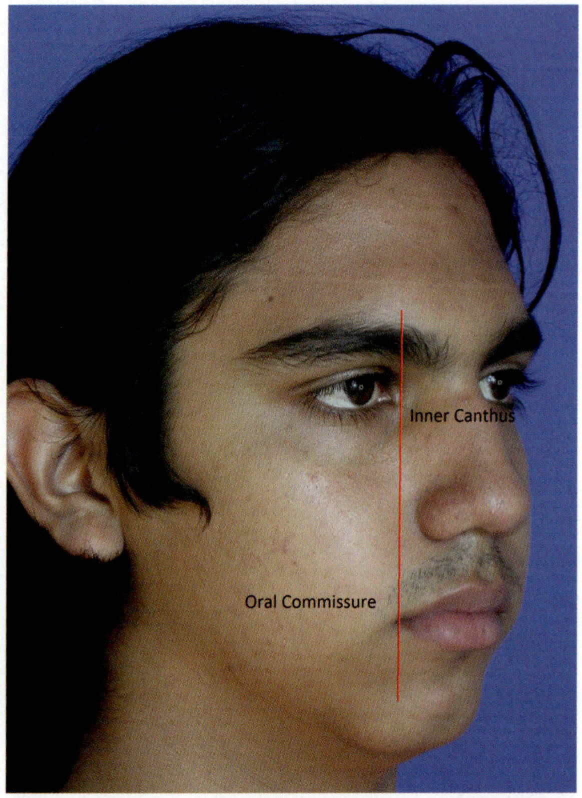

Fig. 4.3 Oblique view. The patient's ipsilateral canthus is aligned with the oral commissure.

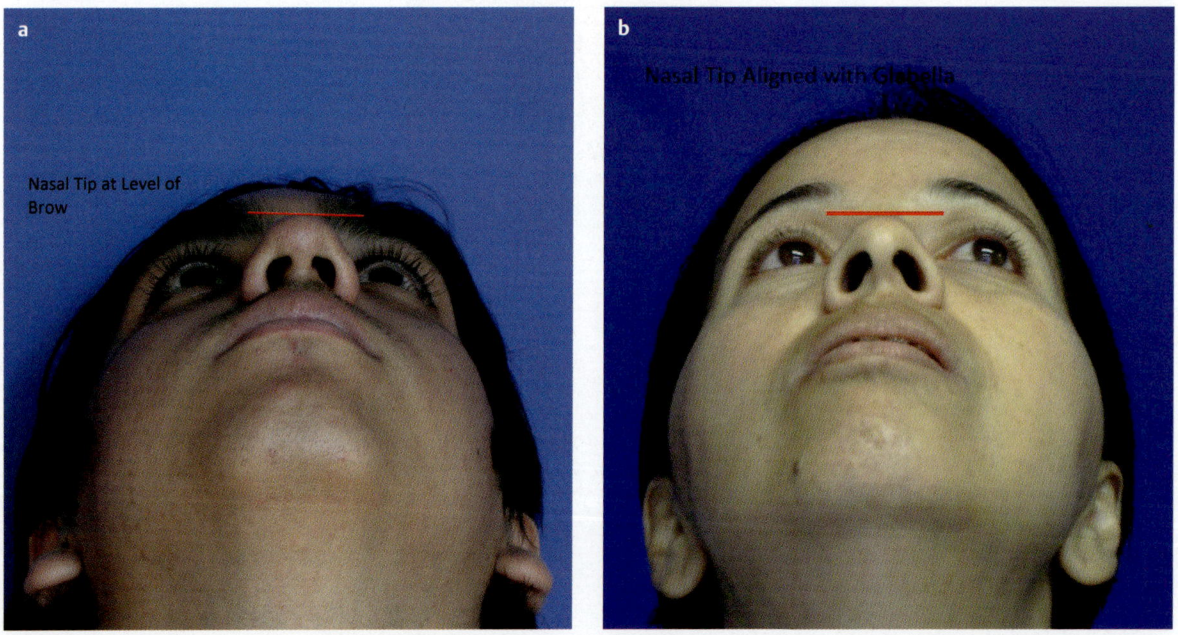

Fig. 4.4 Basal views. The basal view evaluates the alar–columella complex. **(a)** The nasal tip is positioned at the level of a horizontal line that is passed through the interbrow area. **(b)** The nasal tip is positioned at the level of a horizontal line crossing the glabella.

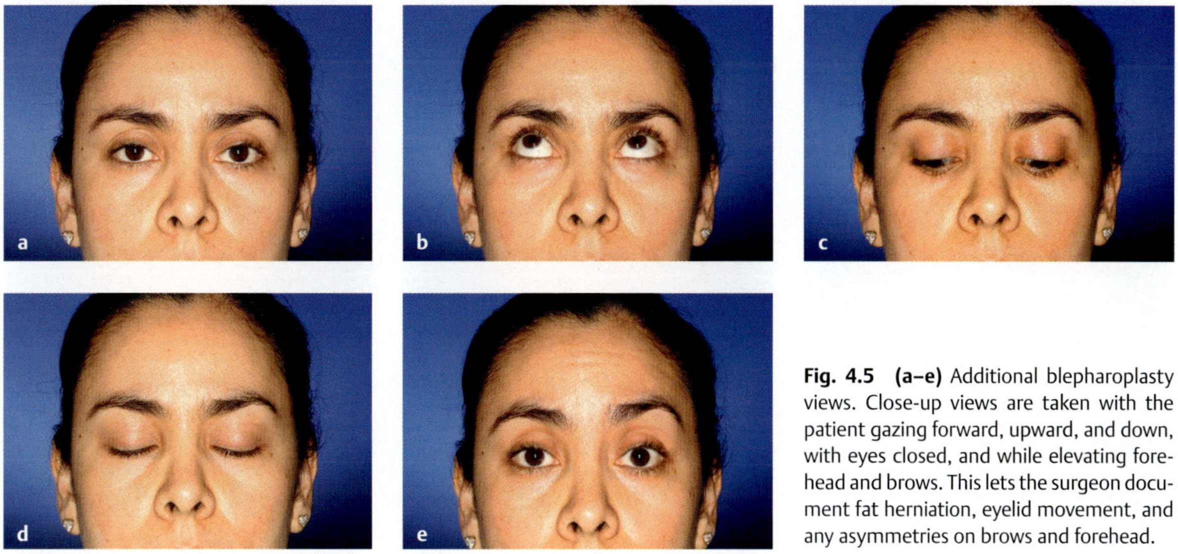

Fig. 4.5 **(a–e)** Additional blepharoplasty views. Close-up views are taken with the patient gazing forward, upward, and down, with eyes closed, and while elevating forehead and brows. This lets the surgeon document fat herniation, eyelid movement, and any asymmetries on brows and forehead.

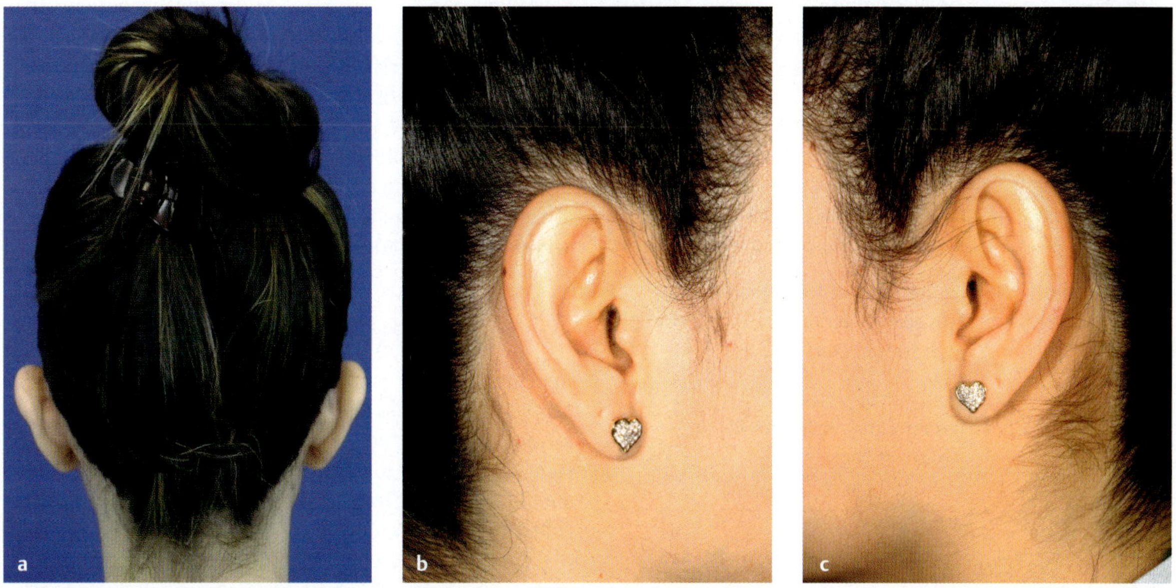

Fig. 4.6 Otoplasty views. When documenting patients for otoplasty, it is important that patients pin hair back, so that the surgeon can evaluate the auricle and its relationship with the scalp. **(a)** Posterior image of ears. **(b,c)** Additional close-up images of left and right ear.

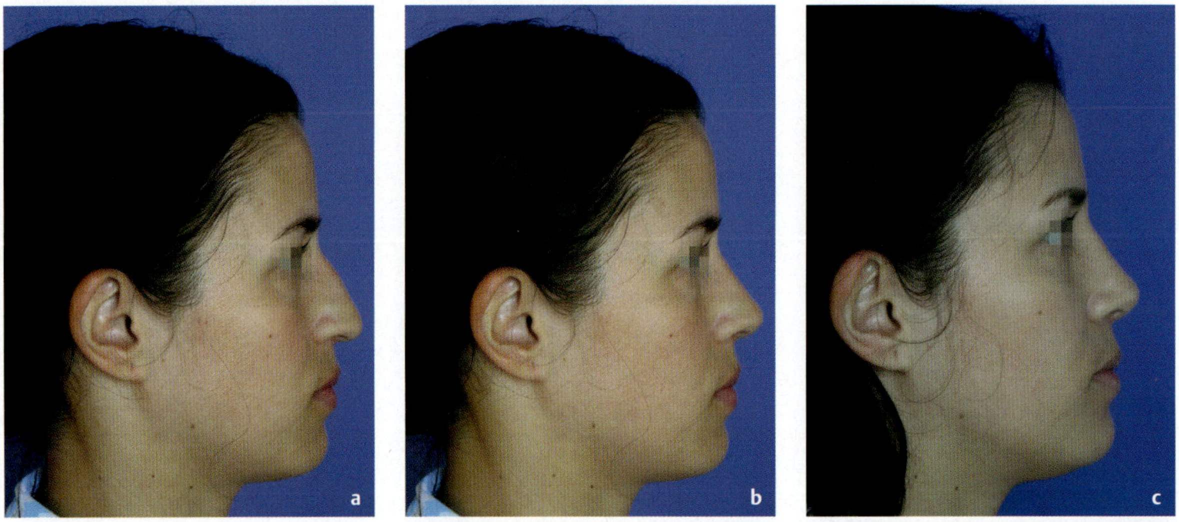

Fig. 4.7 Simulation of potential postoperative results using computer imaging. **(a)** Preoperative photography (lateral projection). **(b)** Morphed image. **(c)** Postoperative image (lateral projection).

Table 4.3 Standard photographs for facial plastic surgery

Procedure	Standard photographs
Rhinoplasty	Frontal Right/Left lateral Right/Left oblique Base
Rhytidectomy	Frontal (including neck) Right/Left lateral (including neck) Right/Left oblique (including neck)
Blepharoplasty/ Frontoplasty	Frontal (face with forehead clear) Eyes open/closed/upward gaze (close up) Right/Left lateral (close up)
Otoplasty	Frontal (hair pulled back) Posterior (hair pulled back) Right/Left lateral Right/Left lateral (close up)

4.4 Treatment Plan

Once the patient's complaints have been clearly understood, the physical exam has been completed, and the photographs have been discussed, specific treatment plans can be discussed with the patient. It is necessary to outline all surgical and nonsurgical options and to decide on what best fits the patient's needs and desires. It is important to clearly understand what the patient's expectations are and to define if they are realistic or not. Finally, all complications and limitations and unpredictable outcomes of the procedures should be explained.[3]

When deciding on a procedure with a patient, it is always important to ask ourselves if we have the proper training and expertise to perform whatever we are offering the patient. With minimally invasive treatments, it is imperative to have the proper training and to have available the appropriate devices and instruments before offering those options to our patients. Being humble and honest about what we can offer our patients will avoid unnecessary problems and dissatisfied patients.

4.5 Informed Consent

Informed consent is legally required and must be signed *before* any type of surgical or nonsurgical procedure is performed. The informed consent gives the patient the legal right to accept or to reject the proposed treatment and it should be signed freely after the patient has read all of its content.

The informed consent should describe the procedure(s) that is/are going to be performed and should include possible complications, limitations, risks, and unfavorable outcomes. The informed consent should not omit any details and the surgeon should elicit feedback from the patient to ensure that the patient understands the explanations. It is also important to obtain specific consent to take grafts from other parts of the body (e.g., ear, ribs) or to place synthetic implants.[14]

The patient must understand that no procedure is without risk or is complication free. The patient should also understand that the surgeon and his team will do everything possible to solve whatever problems arise. Patients must understand that they will need to schedule follow-up visits and that, if the result is not satisfactory or is unfavorable, additional procedures may be needed. The surgeon's policies regarding fees for additional surgeries must be clearly stipulated for the patient. Revision surgery has greater risk than the first operation, and this should be explained to the patient.

In addition, it should be made clear before the procedure how and when payment will be made; the surgeon's policies should be very strict on this matter. Patients who cannot comply with these conditions or who cause difficulties with the agreements are more likely not to be good patients after the surgery, and it is recommended that you reassess them as candidates for aesthetic facial surgery. Ideally, all patients should receive written postoperative or postprocedure recommendations. In the case of surgery, patients should have a companion (family member, friend, nurse) who can assist them during their recovery process.

4.6 Other Aspects to Be Considered

4.6.1 Internet and the Initial Consultation

Advances in information communication and technology have changed communication between individuals and health care professionals. Recent studies show that 66% of Americans with Internet access seek medical information online before meeting with a health care professional. This access can give patients the power to make well-informed decisions and allows them to talk with their doctors with greater confidence, which results in a more balanced interaction between patients and health care professionals.[17]

The Internet has become an important means for facial plastic surgeons to attract potential patients to their clinical practice. Most professionals have a Website on which patients can access information about procedures and services offered and about the professional's academic training. The American Medical Association recommends that the Website have information regarding the professional's training, the basic rate charged, and payment methods, and it recommends not showing general results but instead clarifying that results of procedures can vary between patients depending on the specific conditions of each person before the procedure.[18] These guidelines are not generally followed on most facial plastic surgery sites and information varies depending on the owner of the site.

Becker, in his article "Website for Rhinoplasty and Facial Plastic Surgery," offers some suggestions for building a new Website.[19] For example, the Website should describe the surgeon's care policy, the type of practice, and the surgeon's training. It should also provide educational material on the procedure(s) offered. Patient education helps build patients' confidence by allowing them to read the information and to resolve their doubts, and ultimately it improves patient outcomes.

The most important aspect of a Website is its content. It is a powerful marketing tool, and care should be taken to ensure that it shows the material in a way that is truthful and understandable for everyone.[20] Most people prefer sites that show a large number of photos from before and after the procedure. (All published patient material should have written consent from the patient.) It is common to find a section of frequently asked questions. Some professionals' Websites include videos in which the physician explains the procedures, video clips from television programs on which the physician appeared, or academic articles that the physician has written.

It is always important to seek advice from an attorney before building a Website. Issues regarding physician–patient communication, privacy of images, content used, and mechanisms for providing medical advice to potential patients not seen in person should all be discussed. This is especially important when information found on the Web can be used for different purposes or can be distorted by the potential patient. Electronic media can shorten distances between doctor and patient, especially if the patient lives outside the physician's immediate area, but patients who use electronic media should be selected with care. Without in-person contact, it is easier for patients to distort information, to lie about medical issues, or to omit relevant information (including psychiatric issues).

It is also important to ask patients about the sources of the information they have obtained, because generally they consult more than one Website for professional opinions and information regarding surgical alternatives.[21] It is also very common for patients to consult sites that offer misleading information. All of this can lead to confusing and even contradictory information from professionals, which creates even more confusion in the potential patient. For this reason, educating the patient on how to obtain reliable information online can be useful. The advantages and disadvantages of telecommunication in medical/surgical practice are summarized in **Table 4.4**.[22]

4.7 Conclusion

The consultation can be the most important step in performing a surgical or nonsurgical procedure on a patient. It is crucial to establish a solid patient–physician relationship, with good communication, trust, and confidence in what is going to be done.

Patient selection is important, and it is necessary to establish mechanisms for identifying the "not ideal" patient or the patient who is unstable or who has unrealistic expectations. All information and findings should be recorded in a consistent and reproducible fashion. It is always useful

Table 4.4 Advantages and disadvantages of telecommunication in medical/surgical practice

Advantages	Disadvantages
– Improves delivery of health care information to patients – Improves physician–patient communication – Gives additional information about the surgeon's training – Photographs increase the patient's confidence in the surgeon's abilities – Patients who have reviewed online information (video, explanations, and articles) can optimize consultation time by resolving any additional questions – An informed patient can become more involved in decision making and can be more objective when deciding on the type of procedure to undertake	– Misinterpretation of published information can result in inappropriate requests for surgical and nonsurgical procedures – Published photographs can generate false expectations in patients – Impossible to determine if published images are real cases or not – Patients can become overly confident and not follow surgeon's specific recommendations – Answering questions and giving clinical opinions online without knowing the patient can lead to misinformation

to be able to revise information, photographs, and procedure plans. The ideal scenario is a satisfied patient and a satisfied facial plastic surgeon. As caregivers, we have to be active listeners and acute observers who show genuine interest in our patients' welfare and satisfaction.

References

1. Sands NB, Adamson PA. Global facial beauty: approaching a unified aesthetic ideal. Facial Plast Surg 2014;30(2): 93–100
2. Weeks DM, Thomas JR. Beauty in a multicultural world. Facial Plast Surg Clin North Am 2014;22(3):337–341
3. Cobo R, García CA. Aesthetic surgery for the Mestizo/Hispanic patient: special considerations. Facial Plast Surg 2010;26(2):164–173
4. Rowe-Jones JM. Facial aesthetic surgical goals in patients of different cultures. Facial Plast Surg Clin North Am 2014;22(3):343–348
5. Palma P, Khodaei I, Tasman AJ. A guide to the assessment and analysis of the rhinoplasty patient. Facial Plast Surg 2011;27(2):146–159
6. Steiger JD. The rhinoplasty consult. Facial Plast Surg 2011; 27(5):393–396
7. Chatham DR. The difficult patient. Preface. Facial Plast Surg Clin North Am 2008;16(2):xi–xii
8. Chatham DR. Avoiding and correcting complications in facial plastic surgery: patient selection. Facial Plast Surg 2012;28(3):253–259
9. Karimi K, Adamson P. Patient analysis and selection in aging face surgery. Facial Plast Surg 2011;27(1):5–15
10. Tasman AJ. The psychological aspects of rhinoplasty. Curr Opin Otolaryngol Head Neck Surg 2010;18(4):290–294
11. American Psychiatric Association, ed. Diagnostic and Statistical Manual of Mental Disorders. 5th ed. Arlington, VA: American Psychiatric Publishing; 2013
12. Veale D. Body dysmorphic disorder. Postgrad Med J 2004; 80(940):67–71
13. Cobo R. Rhinoplasty in the Mestizo nose. Facial Plast Surg Clin North Am 2014;22(3):395–415
14. Godin M. Preparation is essential. In: Godin M, ed. Rhinoplasty Cases and Techniques. New York, NY: Thieme; 2011:1–19
15. Tardy ME. Principles of photography in facial plastic surgery. New York, NY: Thieme; 1992
16. Henderson JL, Larrabee WF Jr, Krieger BD. Photographic standards for facial plastic surgery. Arch Facial Plast Surg 2005;7(5):331–333
17. McMullan M. Patients using the Internet to obtain health information: how this affects the patient-health professional relationship. Patient Educ Couns 2006;63(1–2): 24–28
18. Winker MA, Flanagin A, Chi-Lum B, et al; American Medical Association. Guidelines for medical and health information sites on the Internet: principles governing AMA Web sites. JAMA 2000;283(12):1600–1606
19. Becker DG. Website for rhinoplasty and facial plastic surgery. Facial Plast Surg 2006;22(1):70–74
20. Carroll J. Legal examination of physician advertising on the Internet. Facial Plast Surg 2006;22(1):75–79
21. Patrick K. How patients use the Web for second opinions. West J Med 1999;170(6):332–333
22. Wald HS, Dube CE, Anthony DC. Untangling the Web—the impact of Internet use on health care and the physician-patient relationship. Patient Educ Couns 2007;68(3): 218–224

Section II

The Latin American/Mestizo Perspective

5 Aesthetic, Ethnic, and Cultural Considerations and Current Cosmetic Trends in Mestizo Patients in Latin America

Roxana Cobo

5.1 Introduction

Access to the Internet and the different social networks has increased exponentially the awareness of cosmetic procedures worldwide. Latin America is no exception. Initially, Brazil became known as a big place for plastic surgery procedures and Ivo Pitanguy was the plastic surgery icon of the 1960s. Venezuela is known for having the highest number of Miss Universe beauty queens, especially in the past 10 years. Colombia and Mexico have quickly become referral centers for facial plastic surgery procedures and Argentina is known for its cosmetic procedures. Many Latin American countries receive visitors looking for cheaper surgical options than they can find in their home countries. Medical tourism is a growing business in Latin America, and cosmetic procedures comprise a good percentage of this business.

Aesthetic trends have changed over the years and are dominated by what is dictated in the media, social networks, and fashion magazines. Patients want to "blend in" and want to be part of what they see globally. Although facial characteristics can vary from place to place, cosmetic tendencies tend to follow a "fashion trend" that is usually imposed by actors, singers, and different countries' popular idols. To be able to understand what our patients want, it is necessary to understand where they come from and what factors are important in defining their cosmetic ideals.

5.2 Geographic Composition and Migration Patterns

Latin America comprises a vast territory covering a geographic area that starts in Mexico (southern border of United States) and goes all the way down to the tip of Argentina, as well as including the Caribbean. Spanish is the main language in most countries except Brazil, where Portuguese is spoken, and some Caribbean islands, where French is the main language.

The early permanent settlements in Latin America were the local Indian tribes. The most advanced civilizations were the Mayas, who settled in Mexico, Guatemala, Belize, and El Salvador; the Aztecs, who settled in the Valley of Mexico; and the Incas, who settled in Cuzco, Peru. With the European invasion in the 1400s, all of the indigenous tribes were finally taken over by the Spanish invaders in the west side of South America and the Portuguese in the east side, which is Brazil today. The Roman Catholic Church became the most important political and economic power and Catholicism the most important religion in the entire region.

Africans were brought over as slaves to work in the mines and the plantations in the sixteenth century. Additional migrations were the Chinese to Peru and the Japanese, mainly into Brazil but also into Peru and Mexico. During World War I and World War II, Europeans migrated to different Latin American countries, mainly Argentina, Chile, Paraguay, Uruguay, and Brazil. Middle Eastern people also migrated during this period, settling down in the different Latin American countries.[1,2,3]

Today, migration patterns have changed due to political happenings, insecurity, and job opportunities. There is a steady migration of inhabitants of the different Latin American countries to more developed countries, like the United States, Canada, and Europe. In the United States, the Latin American population has become the biggest ethnic or racial minority group.[4]

Because of the great variety of races that have settled in Latin America, today it is considered one of the most diverse regions of the globe. Intermixing between Indigenous people and the different racial groups that settled over the years has been common. The different "ethnic" groups that can be found in Latin America are:

1. Indigenous or Indian groups—They were dramatically reduced during the colonization period. Today, they are a majority in Bolivia, Guatemala, and Peru. In Ecuador and Mexico, they are an important minority group.[5]
2. Asians—The majority of Asians in Latin America settled in Peru and Brazil. Brazil has the largest Japanese community outside Japan and Peru has the largest Chinese community outside China. The Japanese are also an important Asian group in Peru.[6]
3. Blacks—Africans were brought over as slaves in the sixteenth century. They were sent mainly to the Caribbean islands and Brazil, but important settlements are also found in Cuba, Colombia, Venezuela, and Dominican Republic.

4. Whites—Europeans colonized America in the fifteenth century. Brazil was colonized by Portugal and the rest of the continent was colonized by Spain. Additional migrations were seen during the different world wars.
5. Mestizo—*Mestizo* is a term used originally in Spain and in Latin America to describe a person of mixed European and Indian descent. The intermixing began during the colonial period in Latin America and has been extensive. Mestizos are present in all countries of Latin America and make up the majority of the population in most countries.
6. Mulatto—*Mulatto* is a term used to define a person of mixed European and African descent. Brazil has the largest Mulatto population in Latin America. Mulattos are also majority in Dominican Republic. Cuba, Colombia, Panama, and Costa Rica have important Mulatto populations. Mulattos are present in most countries of Latin America where Africans were brought over as slaves.
7. Zambo—A Zambo is a person of mixed African and Indigenous heritage. Zambos are found mainly in Brazil, Colombia, Venezuela, and Ecuador, although they can be present in any country where Africans and Indigenous groups lived.

Today, it is common to see intermixing of more than one ethnic group. The term *Mestizo* today is commonly used to define a person of mixed race. In the United States and some European nations, patients from Latin America are usually known as *Hispanics* or *Latinos*. For this reason, it is more appropriate to refer to the "mixed race" patient **(Fig. 5.1)**.

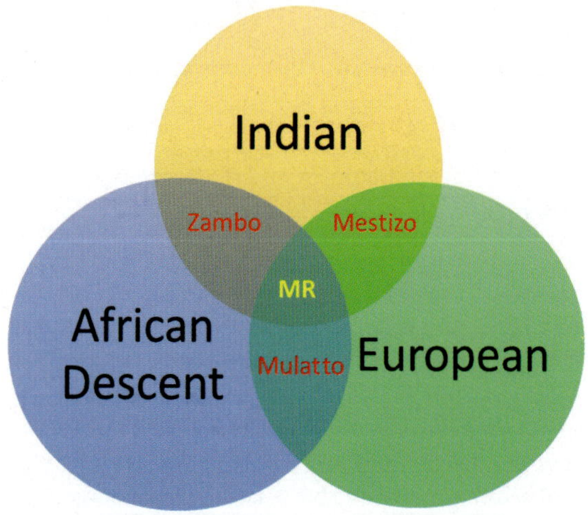

Fig. 5.1 Racial and ethnic composition in Latin America. Racial and ethnic composition in Latin America is of mixed race. Mestizos are the result of intermixing of Indians and Europeans. Mulattos are the result of intermixing of Europeans and Africans. Zambos are the result of intermixing of Indians and Africans. Today, the mixture of all these different groups is considered the new Mestizo generation in Latin America, which is a mixed-race population.

5.3 Facial Features and Aesthetic Considerations

Mestizos are present in all Latin American countries and make up the majority of the population in most of these countries.

Mestizo patients have faces that tend to be broad with a skin–soft tissue envelope (S-STE) that is thicker and heavier and has less elasticity than that of Caucasian patients. Malar eminences tend to be more prominent in Mestizos, but their faces look rounder. Their chins have a tendency to be slightly retrusive. Upper eyelids have a tendency for hooding. Their noses tend to look wide, lacking definition and projection. The skin color varies from white to black, being mostly a mixture of tonalities **(Fig. 5.2, Table 5.1)**.[7,8]

With the aging process, Mestizo facial features become more prominent. The thicker S-STE has a tendency to sag more, making nasolabial folds and the jowl area more prominent. Hooding of eyelids tends to be more pronounced, and there is a tendency for eyebrows to droop because of the loss of support. Redundant skin in the neck will appear not only loose but also heavy **(Fig. 5.3)**.

5.4 Current Cosmetic Trends/ Cultural and Religious Considerations

Most of the population in Latin America is Roman Catholic. Although religion plays an important role in patients' family structure, it is not the predominant feature and usually does not affect cosmetic trends. All countries in Latin America have a strong Occidental influence, mainly from the United States and to a lesser degree from Europe (mainly Spain). The younger generations want to look like their idols or the people they see as their role models. These usually include movie actors and actresses, singers, and athletes. Today, there is a strong trend to cultivate the body, to look fit and athletic, and to have a face with more defined features. Patients don't want to have an "operated" look, but they do want to improve the areas that they think need improving. Symmetry is very important for achieving harmony, and, although ethnicity is also important, today patients simply want to look a bit more like their role models and to blend in better with what they consider ideal.

What, then, do our patients want? Women want more defined noses with tips that are slightly upturned (not

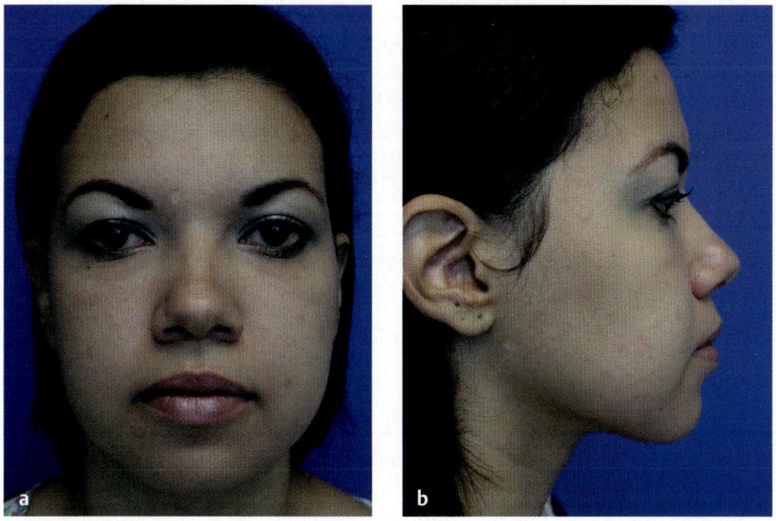

Fig. 5.2 (a,b) Facial characteristics of Mestizo patients. Mestizo faces have a tendency to be broad and to appear rounder. The S-STE can be thick and inelastic. There can be hooding in the lateral brow area and noses can look bulbous and undefined, with a lack of projection and rotation.

Table 5.1 Mestizo facial characteristics

Facial area	Characteristic
Skin	Normal–thick/sebaceous
Skin–soft tissue envelope (S-STE)	Thick
Shape of face	Round
Eyelids	Heavy skin with upper lateral eyelid hooding
Malar eminence	Normal to prominent
Chin	Normal to slightly retrusive
Nasal dorsum	Normal–low radix Wide nasal bridge
Nasal bones	Short
Lower third of nose/nasal tip	Flimsy/unsupported/bulbous

completely straight). Eyelids should not be hooded and the tail of the eyebrows should be arched and slightly slanted upward laterally. Ideally, cheekbones are slightly prominent and well defined, with a slight hint of cheek hollow. Faces should have some definition and not look round. Lips should be slightly full. With aging, the main complaints from women are about the presence of bags under their eyes, prominent nasolabial folds, jowls, and neck skin laxity.

Men, on the other hand, want noses that are more defined but not small. They prefer a straight profile. What tends to bother them the most is to have a wide nasal bridge and a wide base. None of them want an upturned nose because this is considered feminine. Faces should have defined, markedly angled features with strong bony structures. Chins should be strong without adiposity in the neck. With aging, the main complaint from men involves the eyes. Even though loose skin in the neck and jowls can bother them, they are more cautious before having any extensive rejuvenation procedures done. For men, it is very important not to have the stigma of surgery or any telltale scars around the ear.

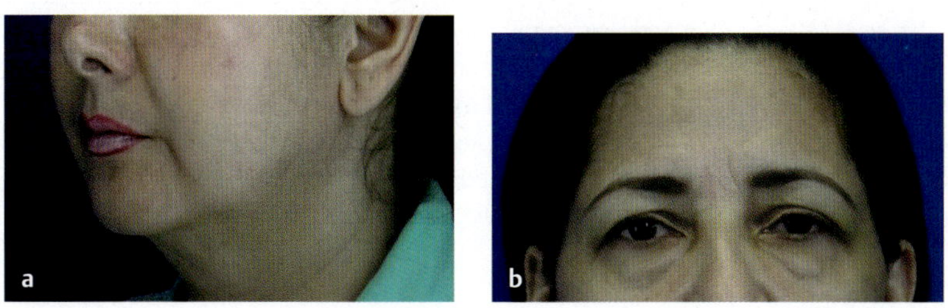

Fig. 5.3 (a,b) Aging process in Mestizo patients. In the upper third of the face, it is common to find upper eyelid hooding, with descent of the tail of the brows. Lower eyelids can look puffy, with bags under the eyes. The nasojugal fold can be more prominent.

Latin America is a continent where people are frequently having cosmetic procedures performed. Looks play an important role in people's lives. With the boom in minimally invasive procedures and the wide variety of options that exist today, most patients at some point will use one of these as an adjunct to improve their appearance. Costs, time taken off work or school, and complications are limiting factors and could be the reason why many times a minimally invasive procedure is chosen over a surgical procedure. This is especially true with facial rejuvenation surgeries like face-lifts, forehead lifts, midface lifts, etc. Interestingly, surgeries like rhinoplasty are still consistently in demand by younger people, especially teenage girls. Again, wanting to avoid the "operated look" is crucial for patients.

Procedures can be divided into the nonsurgical and the surgical.

5.5 Nonsurgical Procedures

Nonsurgical procedures have become extremely popular in Latin America. Unfortunately, many of them are not completely regulated and it is not uncommon to have them performed by personnel who do not have adequate knowledge or training. The great advantages that nonsurgical procedures offer patients are that there is very little or no time off work or school, complications are minimal, and nonsurgical approaches are less expensive than a surgical procedure. They are also an excellent option for patients who are not ready for rejuvenation surgery but who still want their faces to look "young and fresh."

The most commonly performed nonsurgical procedures are[9]:

5.5.1 Neurotoxin Injections

Neurotoxin injection is the most popular nonsurgical procedure. Many patients use it on a regular basis and as a complement to other rejuvenation surgeries. The toxins available in Latin America are: Botox (onabotulinumtoxin A), Dysport (abobotulinumtoxin A), Xeomin (incobotulinumtoxin A), Siax (onabotulinumtoxin A), and Lantox (onabotulinumtoxin A). Siax and Lantox do not have FDA approval in the United States.

5.5.2 Injection of Filler Agents

Filler agents are frequently used to fill in, augment, and contour. Depending on the composition of the filler, it can be considered short term (6–12 months), long term, semi-permanent (12–24 months), or permanent. The filler most frequently used is hyaluronic acid (HA), a short-term filler. HA comes in a gel form of different sizes depending on what its clinical application is going to be. The semi-permanent fillers available are hydroxylapatite and poly-L-lactic acid, and permanent fillers are polymethylmethacrylate and pure liquid silicone. Filler agents available outside the United States are not necessarily FDA approved. It is the responsibility of the professional injecting the material to make sure he is using a substance that will not result in complications that later can be very hard to correct.

5.5.3 Skin Tightening

Skin-tightening procedures are becoming extremely popular among patients. The complication rate is low, there is no lay-off time, and skin tightening is cheaper than surgery. The downside to all of these procedures is that many times the results are not long lasting, the machines are expensive, and most procedures use disposable devices, which in many countries can become a problem and can increase costs for physicians and patients. Newer devices like Ulthera (Ulthera, Inc., Mesa, Arizona) and Thermi RF (ThermiAesthetics, Irving, Texas) give better long-term results although they are slightly more invasive than the previous skin-tightening devices.

5.5.4 Fractional Carbon Dioxide (CO_2) Laser

The CO_2 laser is used for skin rejuvenation, resurfacing, and tightening procedures. The downside is possible postinflammatory hyperpigmentation in patients with darker skin pigmentation (Fitzpatrick skin type IV–VI). Patients need to have adequate skin preparation before the procedure and should follow strict recommendations after the procedure has been performed.[10]

5.6 Surgical Procedures

Facial plastic surgery is performed mainly by general plastic surgeons, facial plastic surgeons, and otolaryngologists. Otolaryngologists and facial plastic surgeons tend to do mainly rhinoplasties and chin augmentations, while general plastic surgeons perform more facial rejuvenation procedures. As training programs in facial plastic surgery have evolved in Latin American countries, the trend is changing and facial plastic surgeons are being more widely recognized as the "face experts." The most common facial plastic surgery procedure performed in Latin America is rhinoplasty, followed by otoplasty, chin augmentation, and blepharoplasty. Facial rejuvenation procedures like rhytidectomies, midface lifts, and frontoplasty are performed less frequently.[9]

5.6.1 Gender

Facial plastic surgery procedures are still a female domain. Women in Latin America are very keen on anything new related to cosmetic procedures and actively seek out and share information in this regard. Looks are very important and procedures are discussed openly at social events, in schools, and in universities.

Even though the number of male patients seeking cosmetic procedures is increasing, it is not a topic that is openly discussed in social circles. If men have procedures done, they want to be discreet about it and do not want to have results that are too obvious or that will give them away. Many times the excuse for doing something cosmetic is disguised as a functional surgery, such as a septoplasty or turbinate surgery to conceal rhinoplasty, or performing a blepharoplasty with the excuse that excess skin is going to be resected from sagging upper eyelids. Whatever is done, incisions must be well placed so that the final scar will be well hidden and results will not be too obvious.

5.6.2 Age

In Latin America, when girls reach age 15 it is a very important social event. Many times the birthday gift is a rhinoplasty, which frequently is done at least 6 months before the girl's fifteenth birthday so that the swelling will have gone down before the birthday pictures. Not all girls are good candidates for surgery at this age. Patients must be chosen carefully, and the surgical techniques used must be as conservative as possible.

5.6.3 Common Facial Plastic Surgery Procedures

Rhinoplasty

As mentioned above, rhinoplasty is the surgery that is more frequently performed in both men and women all over Latin America independent of the age group.[9] Most rhinoplasties in Latin America are done using endonasal approaches, although open techniques have grown increasingly popular. Reductive techniques with resection of important support structures of the nose have slowly been replaced by techniques where grafts and sutures are used to give additional support to the existing nasal structures (**Fig. 5.4**).

Facial Rejuvenation Procedures

Rejuvenation of the Upper Third of the Face

Today, endoscopic approaches are still used to treat the frontal region, but many techniques are now done using direct vision and illuminated retractors. Brow lifting is a minor surgical procedure that is frequently done in all age groups.

Midface Lift

The midface lift is popular because it can be used to correct jowls and to reposition malar fat that has descended with the aging process. Additionally, the approach does not necessarily require an endoscope; the incisions that are used are usually not very big and are placed within the hair in the temporal area. Depending on the technique used, suspension sutures can be placed transcutaneously, through the temporal incision, or by a combination approach using a Caldwell-Luc incision intraorally.

Blepharoplasty

Blepharoplasty techniques include approaches where fat is preserved or repositioned and the hollow eye is filled in using either fillers or fat. It is not uncommon for upper eyelid surgery to be combined with a midface lift or brow elevation.

Rhytidectomy and Neck Lifting Procedures

Many different techniques have been described for facelifting. Our patients always worry about the scar, because many have darker skin types that can be thick and oily, making scars more visible. For this reason, patients are always looking for techniques that use shorter scars or that do not involve a preauricular scar. Edema is always a problem, and swelling and inflammation can take longer to resolve. Adjunctive measures like lymphatic drainage can help patients in the postoperative period.

Micro Fat Grafting

Fat grafting is a nice complement to facial rejuvenation procedures. When done as a single procedure it can be an excellent option for rejuvenation in patients who are not ready for a facelift. The time required is very short, the cost is less, and the complication rate is low. Care must be taken to inject with the proper cannulas, and not to over-inject, especially around the inferior orbital rim (**Fig. 5.5**).

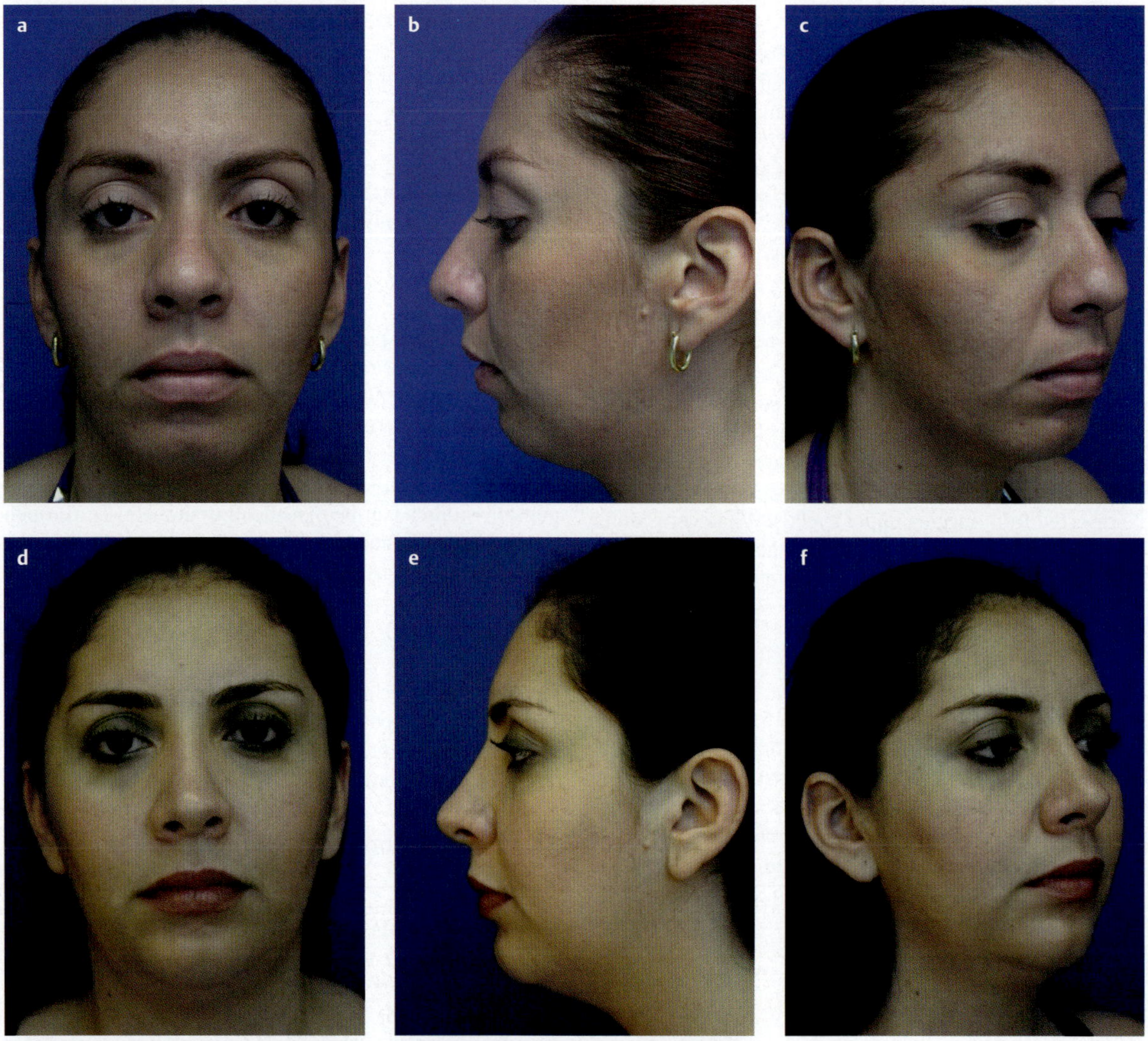

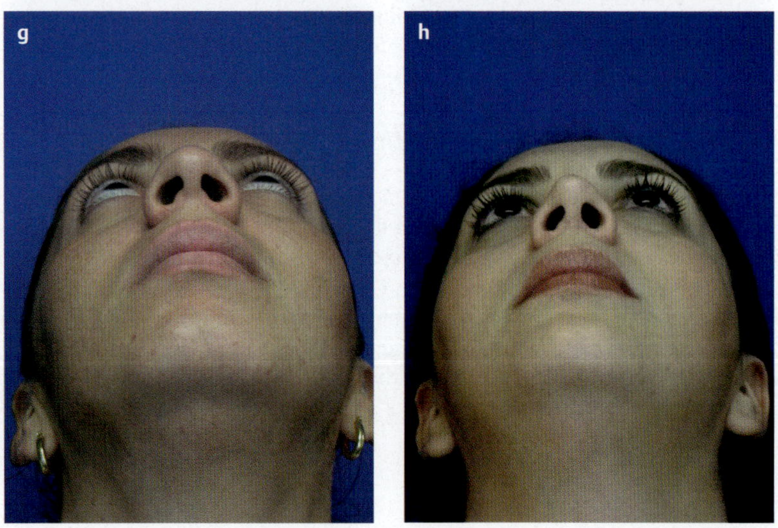

Fig. 5.4 **(a,b,c,g)** Before rhinoplasty and **(d,e,f,h)** 5-year postsurgical result in a Mestizo patient. A structural approach was used. Conservative rasping was done on the dorsum, and medial and lateral osteotomies were performed, with placement of spreader grafts in the middle third of the nose. Tip definition was achieved with dome-defining sutures, placement of a shield graft, alar rim grafts, and morcelized cartilage over the nasal tip. Alar wedge resection was performed and an intraoral chin implant was placed.

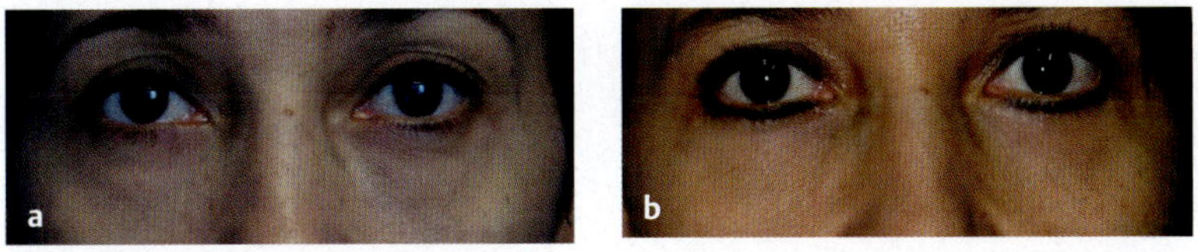

Fig. 5.5 Micro fat grafting in the inferior orbital rim. **(a)** Presurgical image of the eyes showing pseudoherniation of fat and dark circles under the eyes. **(b)** One year after surgery, the image shows important correction of dark circles and fat pseudoherniation. There are no visible irregularities in the infraorbital rim.

5.7 Conclusion

Before doing any type of facial plastic surgery procedure, it is necessary to understand what our patients want. Today, patients are constantly exposed to information on the Web, social networks, TV, etc. Beauty ideals have changed and patients want to follow the fashion and beauty trends set by their idols (beauty queens, actors, etc.). Even though society has become more global, there can be marked differences among patients depending on where they are coming from. As surgeons, we need to be informed so that we can offer our patients the best options possible.

5.8 Pearls

- Have a clear understanding of current beauty ideals and what patients are looking for.
- Patients in Latin America are a mixture of mainly white, black, and Indian races.
- Try to define where the patient is coming from and what facial characteristics are found in the physical exam. This will aid correct surgical planning.
- Rhinoplasty is still the most common facial plastic surgery procedure. Most patients want more defined, smaller-looking noses.
- With the increasing number of nonsurgical and minimally invasive procedures available, we need to be able to offer our patients new technologies safely.

References

1. Ethnic Groups. The World Factbook 2013–14. Washington, DC: Central Intelligence Agency, 2013. Available at: https://www.cia.gov/library/publications/the-world-factbook/index.html
2. Halperin Donghi T. Historia Contemporánea de America Latina. Madrid, Spain: Alianza Editorial; 2013
3. Fox A. Latinoamérica: Presente y Pasado. 3rd ed. Prentice Hall; 2006
4. Hispanic Heritage Month 2014. Release Number: CB14-FF.22 Sept 2014. At: www.census.gov
5. Fernández FL. Composición Étnica de las Tres Áreas Culturales del Continente Americano al Comienzo del Siglo XXI. Convergencia. Rev Cienc Soc 2005;12(38):185–232
6. Rodriguez H. Herederos del Dragón: Historia de la Comunidad China en el Perú. Fondo Editorial del Congreso del Perú. 2000
7. Cobo R, García CA. Aesthetic surgery for the Mestizo/Hispanic patient: special considerations. Facial Plast Surg 2010;26(2):164–173
8. Cobo R. Facial aesthetic surgery with emphasis on rhinoplasty in the Hispanic patient. Curr Opin Otolaryngol Head Neck Surg 2008;16(4):369–375
9. Cobo R. Trends in facial plastic surgery in Latin America. Facial Plast Surg 2013;29(3):149–153
10. Delgado RE, Torre MdeL. Use of fractional laser in mixed-race patients. Facial Plast Surg 2013;29(3):161–166

6 Mestizo Rhinoplasty Using a Structural Open Approach

Roxana Cobo

6.1 Introduction

No matter where they come from or what ethnic group they belong to, people have always had an interest in looking attractive. Thus, it is necessary for the facial plastic surgeon to understand patients' needs and to have a clear understanding of what is considered beautiful today.

The world today is very different from what was true in the past. Political happenings, conquests, and religious crusades have changed regions around the globe, and Latin America is no exception. Ethnic groups have become more mixed and less distinct. Concepts of beauty are constantly changing. With globalization and the broad access to information, patients today want to imitate their favorite people, who tend to be the actors, beauty queens, sports celebrities, and models they see in glossy magazines or on the Internet. Patients want their noses to have more rounded tips, a wider nasal base, and in general a softer look. This can be explained because most people who are considered beautiful today are of mixed race. But then the question is, why do we consider them beautiful? One reason is because, even though they are of mixed race, their faces and noses are symmetrical, and they may have one or two distinctive features that make them stand out among the crowd.

Rhinoplasty is the most frequently performed facial plastic surgery in men and women of all age groups in all Latin American countries.[1] The surgery for rhinoplasty has changed: Reductive surgeries were performed all over Latin America for many years, but the approach has been slowly changing. This chapter describes a structural approach, in which support structures are reinforced or built, and how, using this approach, consistent, satisfactory, functional, and cosmetic long-term results can be achieved in Latin American mixed-race patients.

6.2 The Mestizo Nose

Mestizo patients are of mixed race. In Latin America, *mixed race* today means the intermixing of Indians (local Indian tribes) or Negroes (Africans brought over as slaves) with Europeans (see Chapter 5).[2,3] Migration patterns have changed, and in the past 50 years many people have migrated from Latin America to developed regions like the United States and Europe (mainly Spain) to look for better opportunities or for political reasons. In the United States, the biggest minority ethnic group is the Latin group, who are commonly referred to as Hispanics and Latinos instead of Mestizos.[4]

Nasal characteristics in Mestizo patients are, therefore, those of a mixed-race patient. It is often impossible to define a predominant racial characteristic in a particular patient in our office. In general, the Mestizo nose has a thicker skin–soft tissue envelope (S-STE) and a weak underlying bony and cartilaginous framework. Bones tend to be small and cartilages thin, with poor support. The result is a nose that has a bulbous, undefined nasal tip, skin that can be normal to thick, a wide alar base, and a dorsum that is a bit low, sometimes with a small hump or pseudohump (**Fig. 6.1, Table 6.1**).[5]

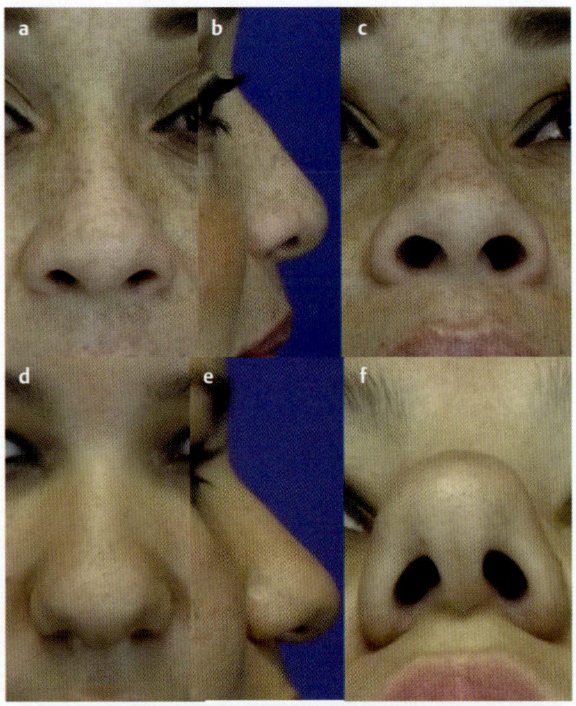

Fig. 6.1 Mestizo noses. Mestizo noses frequently have a skin–soft tissue envelope that has a tendency to be thick and a weak bony and cartilaginous structure. **(a,d)** On the frontal view, bones appear small, wide, and slightly flattened. Tips are wide and bulbous, with poor definition. **(b,e)** On the lateral view, the radix can be low and it is not uncommon to find a pseudohump. Tip recoil is poor and nasolabial angles are acute. **(c,f)** On the base view, the columella can be normal to short, with a nasal base that can be wide, with flaring ala.

Table 6.1 Mestizo nasal characteristics

Nasal Bones
Small and slightly wide
Low nasion
Small dorsal hump or pseudohump
Upper Lateral Cartilages
Thin with a tendency to be narrow in the middle third
Can be wide and flattened
Alar Cartilages
Bulbous
Undefined
Thin and flimsy
Wide
Nasal Spine
Normal to short
Can result in acute nasolabial angle
Columella
Normal to short
Nostrils
Horizontal shape
Flaring
Nasal Base
Tendency to be slightly wide

Used with permission from Cobo R. Structural rhinoplasty in Latin American patients. Facial Plast Surg 2013;29:171–183.

6.3 The Consultation

The consultation is probably the most important step when planning a rhinoplasty. It is very important to establish a solid relationship with the patient. The surgeon needs to understand what patients want, to define their needs, and to evaluate if they are good candidates for cosmetic surgery (see Chapter 4). In summary, the key points that should be covered are:

- Definition of the problem
- The patient's desires
- The patient's expectations
- Important previous clinical history/previous surgeries/medications

6.4 The Physical Examination

A complete facial and nasal examination should be performed and registered in an adequate and reproducible fashion. The nose is inspected internally with a nasal speculum and, when needed, with a rigid or flexible scope to define any functional problems. Septal deviations, turbinate hypertrophies, presence of synechiae, and internal or external nasal valve insufficiencies are properly documented. Availability of septal cartilage is crucial when planning a rhinoplasty, especially in mixed-race patients, for whom support is an important consideration.

Externally, the nose is evaluated by inspecting the S-STE. Size, shape, and asymmetries in bony and cartilaginous structures are documented (including depressions, irregularities, and deviations). Tip recoil is evaluated and measurements are recorded.

6.5 Photographic Documentation

All photographs should be taken in a controlled setting with adequate lighting, using the same standards for all photographs. Six standard rhinoplasty views are used: front, base, left lateral, left oblique, right lateral, and right oblique. Occasionally, a helicopter view (image taken from above the patient's nose) and a lateral view with the patient smiling can also be taken to complement the standard pictures (**Fig. 6.2**).

Digital imaging and morphing programs have changed dramatically the way surgeons interact with patients. Digital images are morphed to show patients what can be achieved with surgery, and it is the surgeon's responsibility to show patients realistic changes. Patients are usually very impressed with the changes shown in the lateral views, but the frontal image is the view where morphing has to be done carefully so patients can perceive how they may look after surgery. New digital software now uses 3D images, which can be very useful, especially for frontal views.

Preoperative images are used not only during the consultation, but also in surgery, and in postoperative visits to show patients the progress of their surgical results. Photographs are a very important part of patients' records. A new set of photographs is routinely taken 6 months and 1 year after surgery. If possible, photographs should be taken on a yearly basis thereafter to evaluate long-term results. Images are a very important tool for surgeons to evaluate their own surgical techniques, and they are very useful in the unfortunate event of a lawsuit or any legal problem that might arise.

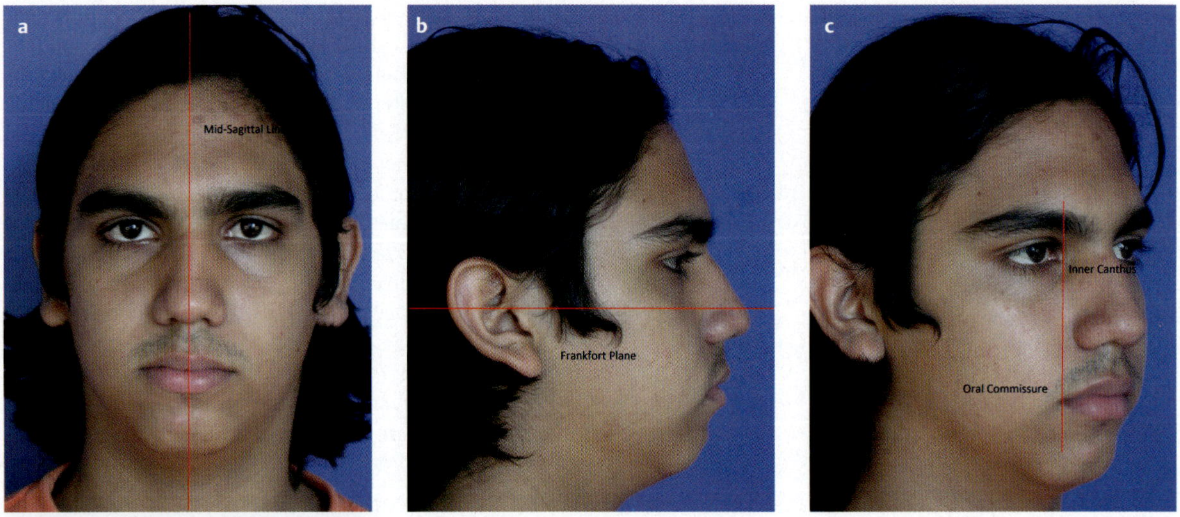

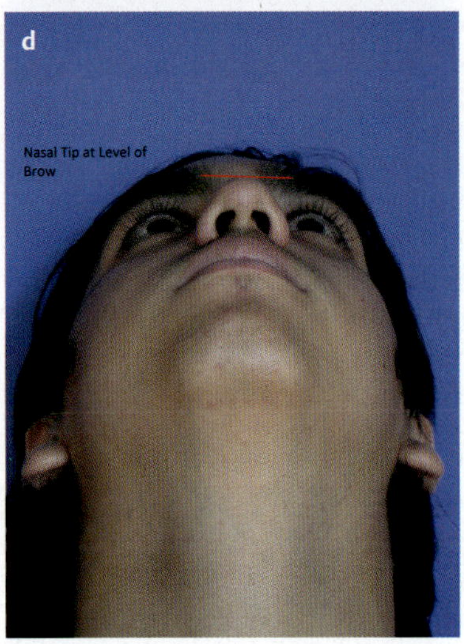

Fig. 6.2 (a–d) Standard rhinoplasty photographs should be taken using the Frankfort plane (an imaginary horizontal line that is drawn from the top of the tragus to the infraorbital bony rim) as a reference to position patients in a standard reproducible manner. Photographs are taken in the front plane (using a midsagittal vertical line), in left and right lateral views, in left and right oblique views, and in a base view, where the nasal tip should be positioned either between the eyebrows or at the level of the glabella.

6.6 Discussing Surgical Options

It is important to clearly understand patients' desires, what bothers them, and what they want changed. This information should be evaluated in light of the patient's physical findings. An adequate anatomical diagnosis is required to determine if there are surgical options that can satisfy the patient's needs and desires. Limitations and complications of the procedure must be clearly understood by the patient. Consent forms should be discussed and signed before surgery. Ideally, the final result is a happy patient with a happy surgeon.

As mentioned earlier, Mestizo patients are of mixed race. Trying to define a predominant ethnic or racial background many times is impossible. What is important is to make adequate anatomical diagnoses so that real surgical solutions can be offered. Our patients want noses that have more definition and projection (see Chapter 5). As surgeons, our challenge is to create noses that have a strong underlying structural framework with greater definition but without looking big or over-projected. This requires the use of sutures and grafts to obtain these results.

6.7 Structural Approach to the Mestizo Nose

For more than 20 years, the author has used a structural approach that is tailored to the patient's needs. The philosophy behind this approach is:

- Conservative tissue excision
- Preservation and, when necessary, reinforcement of support structures of the nose

- Structural grafting to reinforce and improve the strength of existing anatomical structures
- Definition of nasal tip structures using grafts and sutures

To help organize surgery efficiently, the nose is divided into anatomical thirds:

- Upper third of the nose (bony dorsum)
- Middle third of the nose (cartilaginous dorsum)
- Lower third of the nose (nasal tip)

Specific techniques are planned for each area and cartilage grafting is planned depending on the needs of each individual patient.

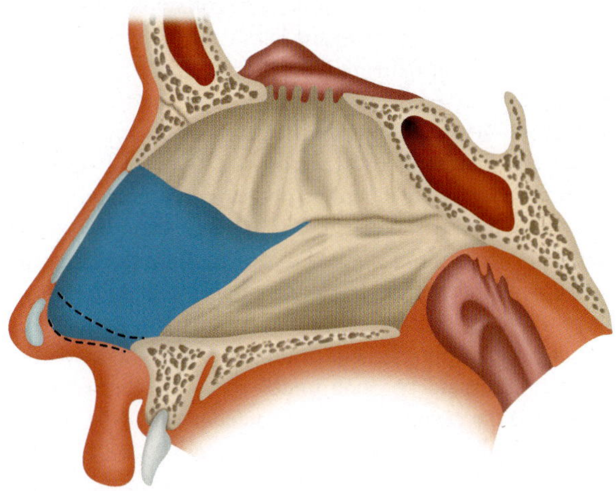

Fig. 6.3 Septal incisions: the caudal incision is placed at the edge of the nasal septum and the Killian incision is made a few mm behind the caudal incision.

6.8 Surgical Technique

All surgeries are done under general anesthesia. The nose is infiltrated using 1 to 2% lidocaine (Xylocaine) + epinephrine 1:100,000.

6.9 Harvesting of Cartilage

The septum is usually managed before opening the nose. Depending on the anatomical findings, a Killian incision or an incision at the caudal edge of the septum is performed **(Fig. 6.3)**. Septal cartilage is the first and best choice for cartilage grafting. Mestizo patients tend to have noses with a mesorrhine configuration, and the quadrangular cartilage is usually not very big and tends to be thin (2–3 mm). When harvesting the septal cartilage, it is important to take the cartilage out as a complete block, leaving an inverted L strip of at least 1.0 to 1.5 cm dorsally and caudally. This inverted L will become a very important support to the nose postoperatively. Before closing the septum, any deviations should be corrected and, if necessary, caudal fixation to the nasal spine should be reinforced. Septal mucosa is closed using absorbable 5–0 mattress sutures. Usually no packing is left inside the nose **(Fig. 6.4)**.

6.10 The Open Approach

Using a no. 15 blade, an inverted V incision is done at the midcolumellar region immediately above the feet of the medial crura. The incision extends laterally 2 mm behind

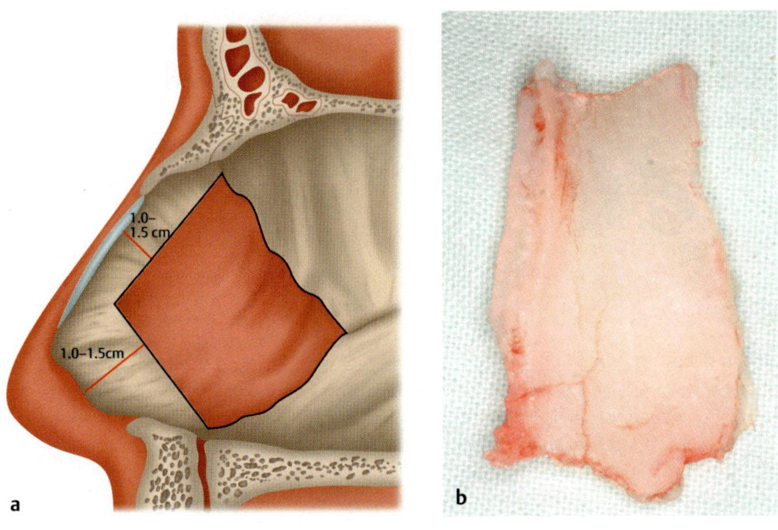

Fig. 6.4 The septum is approached using a Killian or caudal incision. **(a)** When harvesting septal cartilage, it is important to leave an inverted L-shaped strip of at least 1.0 to 1.5 cm. **(b)** Image of harvested piece of septum. Notice there are no breaks in the cartilage.

the crura and is extended superiorly following the caudal margin of the intermediate and lateral crura of the alar cartilages. All cuts on skin are done perpendicularly. Elevation of the flap is done using converse scissors and two-prong retractors, keeping the plane of dissection immediately above the cartilaginous structures of the nasal tip. This provides a relatively bloodless dissection plane and makes dissection a lot easier. Once skin has been elevated off the nasal tip, dissection is moved to the midline, elevating the S-STE over the middle third and upper third of the nose. Over the cartilaginous dorsum, the dissection plane is directly above the perichondrium, and over the bone, the dissection should be done under the periosteum all the way up to the nasofrontal angle if needed (**Fig. 6.5**).

6.11 The Upper Third of the Nose (Bony Dorsum)

Nasal bones tend to be short and somewhat flattened, and the bony dorsum can be slightly wide.

6.11.1 Anatomical Findings: Wide Nasal Dorsum without Hump/ Adequate Dorsal Height

Surgical Technique: Medial and Lateral Osteotomies

Osteotomies can help narrow a wide dorsum without making important changes in dorsal height. Medial osteotomies should be done first, using a 3 to 4 mm curved osteotome. The osteotome is engaged between the dorsal edge of the septum and the caudal edge of the bony dorsum. It is angled 20 to 30 degrees off the midline in the direction of the medial canthus. The thick frontal bone is avoided. Lateral osteotomies are done with a 2.2 guarded osteotome and using a high-low-high technique that starts in the lateral nasal mucosa perpendicular to the head of the inferior turbinate (**Fig. 6.6**).

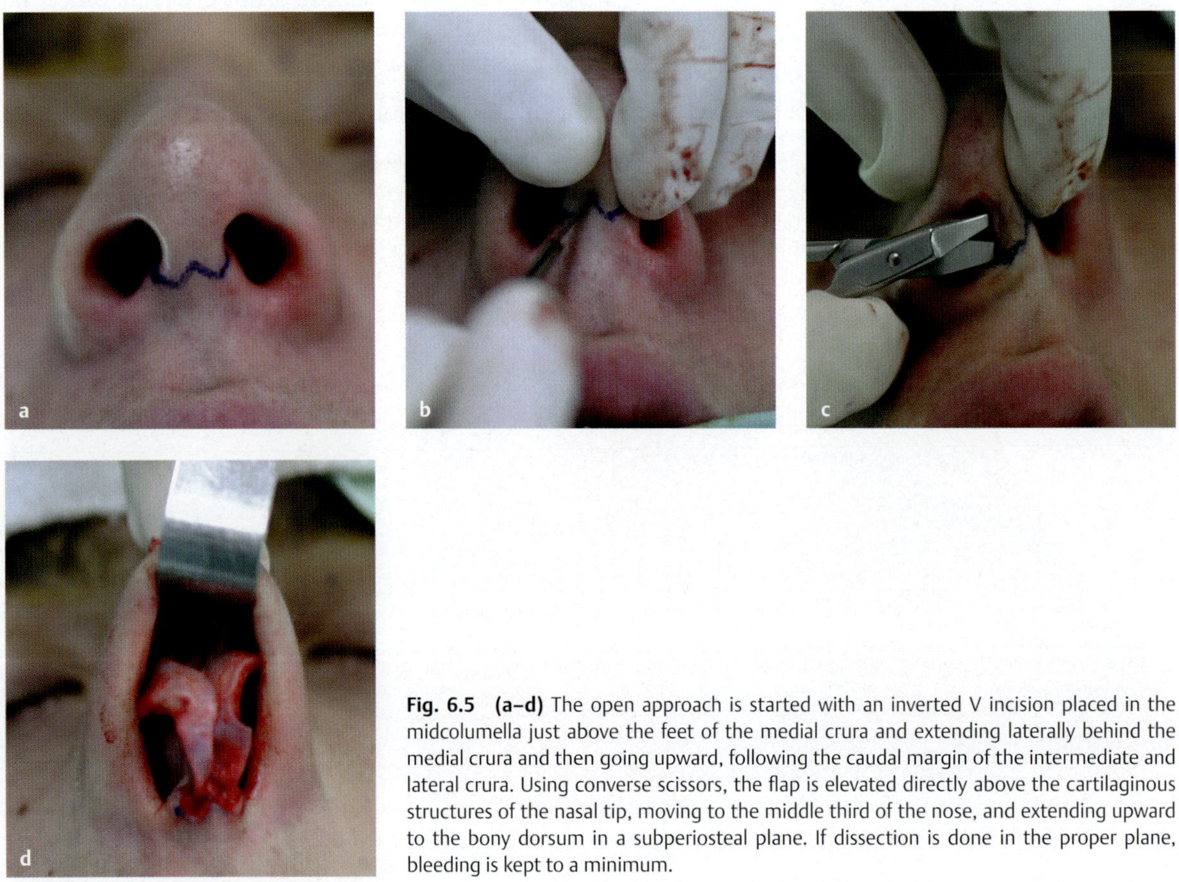

Fig. 6.5 (a–d) The open approach is started with an inverted V incision placed in the midcolumella just above the feet of the medial crura and extending laterally behind the medial crura and then going upward, following the caudal margin of the intermediate and lateral crura. Using converse scissors, the flap is elevated directly above the cartilaginous structures of the nasal tip, moving to the middle third of the nose, and extending upward to the bony dorsum in a subperiosteal plane. If dissection is done in the proper plane, bleeding is kept to a minimum.

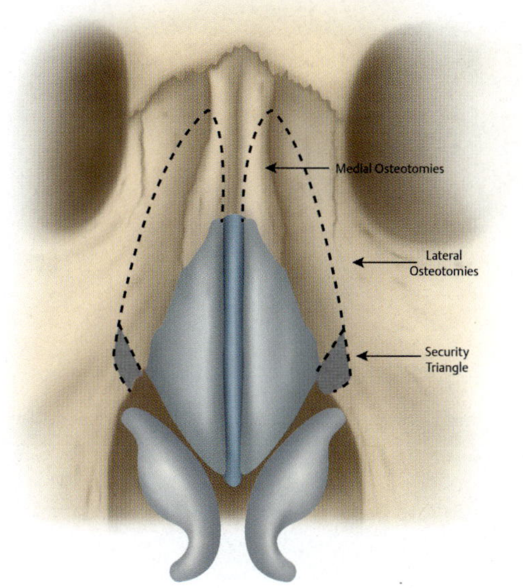

Fig. 6.6 Medial osteotomies are curved osteotomies that start at the midline just lateral to the dorsal septum and are angled laterally off the midline, heading in the direction of the medial canthus. Lateral osteotomies are performed using a high-low-high technique. This means a small triangle of bone is left intact at the base of the nose in the piriform aperture. This small triangle of bone will help prevent an external nasal valve collapse.

6.11.2 Anatomical Findings: Low Radix with Small Hump or Pseudohump

Surgical Technique: Radix Graft with or without Hump Reduction

Radix grafts using crushed cartilage are used to fill in the small concavity that is frequently seen in the dorsum of Mestizo patients. If, once the radix is filled in, there is still a prominence at the rhinion or a small bony hump, it can be lowered using osteotomes, rasps, or both. The cartilaginous portion of a hump is usually resected with a no. 15 blade until the dorsum is smooth. When the radix is going to be filled in with cartilage, a small, precise pocket is elevated and the space is filled in with the crushed cartilage. Care must be taken not to extend dissection too far laterally over the dorsum because cartilage fragments could end up positioned laterally, creating irregularities in the lateral nasal walls **(Fig. 6.7)**.[6]

6.11.3 Anatomical Findings: Low Nasal Dorsum

Surgical Technique: Dorsal Augmentation with Cartilage or Implants

Cartilage is the material of choice when dorsal augmentation is needed, and septal cartilage is preferred over auricular cartilage. In special cases where important augmentation is necessary or when there is no septal or auricular cartilage available, rib cartilage can be used. If patients refuse harvesting of rib (this happens more commonly in women), implants can be an option. Even though there are several implant options available in the market today, the author's preference is expanded polytetrafluoroethylene (Gore-Tex) sheeting. The complication rate is very low and the results are excellent if patients are chosen properly. Ideally, when implants are used, they are placed using an open rhinoplasty approach because the risk of infection is lower. The implant should be cut according to the patient's needs, soaked in antibiotic solution, placed in a precise pocket over the dorsum, and, when possible, fixed with sutures to the cartilaginous middle third of the nose. This keeps the implant in place and avoids shifting over time **(Fig. 6.8)**.[7,8]

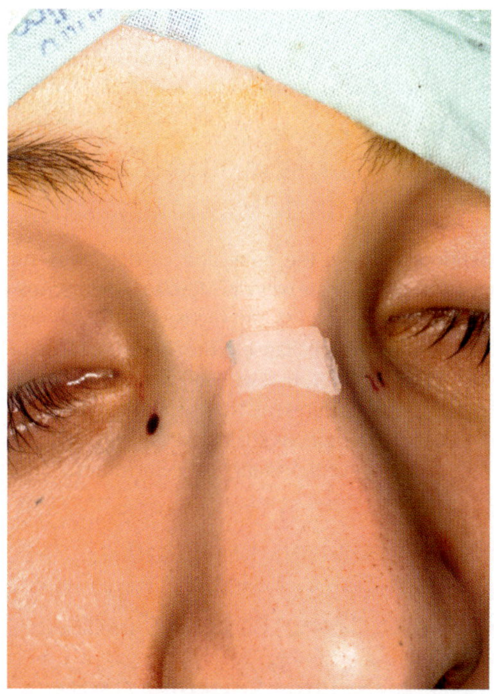

Fig. 6.7 Radix grafts are usually fashioned from crushed cartilage. This cartilage is placed in a small pocket in the area of the nasion. Crushing the cartilage slightly will help prevent irregularities and will make it easier to mold.

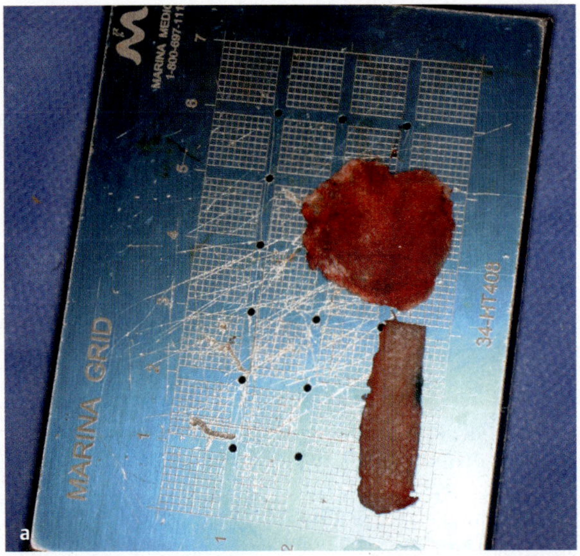

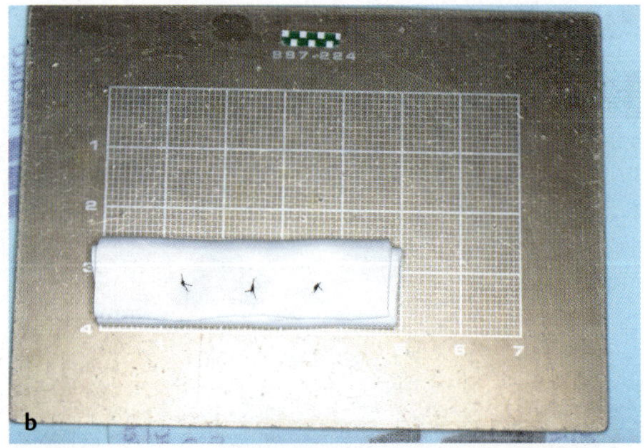

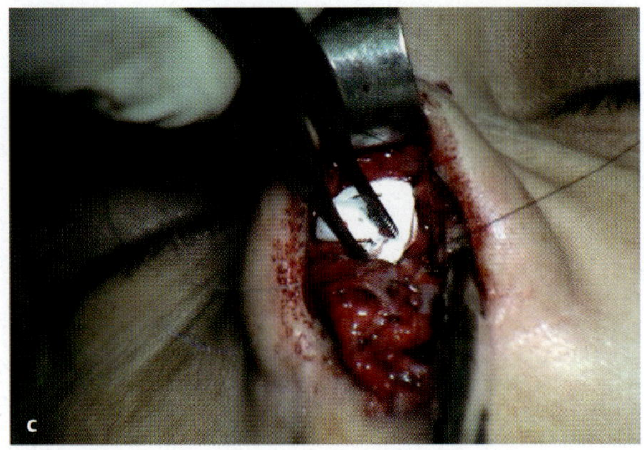

Fig. 6.8 Dorsal augmentation. **(a)** Augmentation ideally should be done with cartilage. Septum is the cartilage of choice. Edges should be beveled so no irregularities will be visible over time. **(b,c)** Gore-Tex is the implant of choice. The implant is carved according to the patient's needs and is placed in a precise pocket over the dorsum. If possible, it should be sutured in place.

6.12 The Middle Third of the Nose (Cartilaginous Dorsum)

As mentioned above, the bony and cartilaginous support structures of the nose are weak in Mestizo patients. Any work that is done to the dorsum can increase this weakness and result in deformities or collapse of the upper lateral cartilages, resulting in important functional and structural deformities. When deformities are present, they should be corrected, and, if middle third cartilaginous structures are weak, they should be reinforced to prevent postsurgical deformities.

6.12.1 Anatomical Findings: Flattened/Wide Middle Third of Nose and Weak Upper Lateral Cartilages

Surgical Technique: Spreader Grafts

Spreader grafts are rectangular, carved pieces of cartilage that are placed between the upper lateral cartilage (ULC) and the septal cartilage. Spreader grafts can be placed in only one side of the septum, can be placed bilaterally, and can be placed as a single graft or as a double. They should be tailored to the patient's needs, but the usual dimensions are: length, 18 to 25 mm; width, 3 to 5 mm; thickness, 1 to 3 mm. Grafts are sutured in place using absorbable Vicryl or PDS sutures. These grafts give additional support to the cartilaginous nasal vault. Their uses are many, and they can be used in primary or secondary rhinoplasty patients. They correct weak or buckling ULC, widen a narrow middle third of the nose, correct inverted V deformities, correct internal nasal valve collapse, and help align a crooked dorsal edge of the nasal septum (**Fig. 6.9**).

Surgical Technique: Mattress Sutures/Flaring Mattress Sutures

Mattress sutures using a 4–0 PDS or a nonabsorbable suture can be used to open up naturally weak ULC, to widen a slightly narrow middle third of the nose, or to help align slight dorsal deviations.

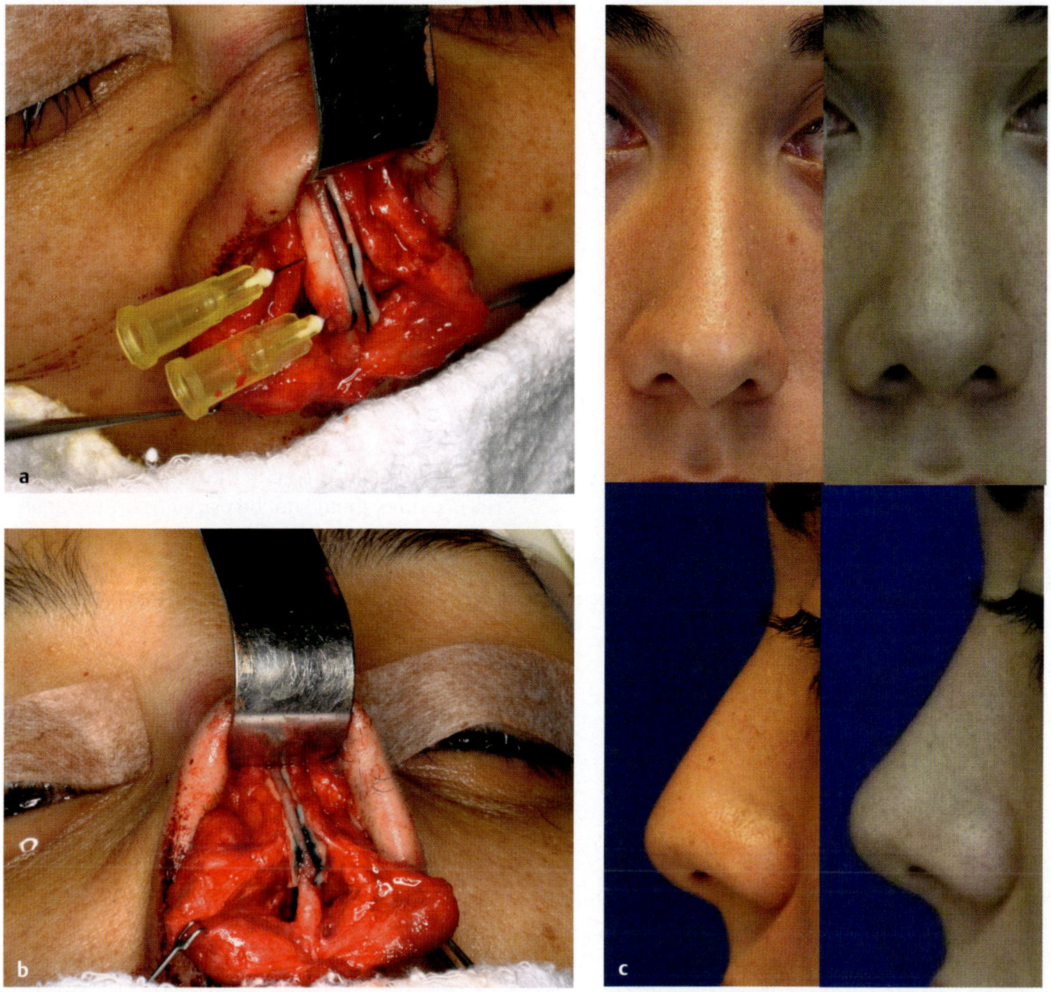

Fig. 6.9 Spreader grafts. **(a)** Rectangular pieces of cartilage are placed in a pocket between the upper lateral cartilage and the dorsal septum. They are sutured in place with 5–0 Vicryl or PDS using a 27 to 30 gauge needle. **(b)** The middle cartilaginous vault is closed, leaving upper lateral cartilages at the same level of the spreader grafts and the dorsal edge of the septum. **(c)** Presurgical and postsurgical frontal and lateral views of a patient with a narrow middle third of nose and a hump. The hump was lowered, the middle third of the nose was strengthened, and a normal configuration was restored using bilateral spreader grafts.

Surgical Technique: Onlay Grafts/Crushed Cartilage

Onlay grafts and crushed cartilage can be used to fill in and smooth out irregularities over the middle nasal vault. Grafts should be placed in precise pockets and fixed in place if possible.

6.13 Lower Third of the Nose (Nasal Tip)

The nasal tip is formed by the pedestal and the nasal tripod. The pedestal is an important support structure that is formed by the caudal edge of the septum and the nasal spine. The tripod is a flexible structure that is formed by the two conjoined medial crura and the diverging lateral crura. These two structures and the tip's covering, the S-STE, give the final shape to the nasal tip.

Following the structuring principle, it is important to strengthen the pedestal before any tip work is done. This way, changes made to the tripod will not be lost because of loss of support of the underlying pedestal.[9]

6.13.1 The Pedestal

Mestizo patients have noses with mesorrhine characteristics. The septum can be modest and relatively thin. Its thickness usually ranges between 2 and 3 mm. It is not uncommon to find a short, retrusive, caudal septum sitting on small nasal spines, resulting in a nasal tip with poor tip recoil, an acute nasolabial angle, and a short columella.

Anatomical Findings: Small Nasal Spine, Normal Caudal Septum, Flimsy Medial Crura

Surgical Technique: Columellar Strut

The columellar strut is the workhorse of rhinoplasty. It gives additional strength to the pedestal, helps maintain any changes in projection and rotation that are performed on the alar cartilages, and provides a stable base so that sutures and grafts can be used in the nasal tip. Struts ideally should be carved from septal cartilage, but conchal cartilage or rib cartilage can also be used with good results.

A pocket is made between the medial crura and the graft is sutured in place with absorbable 5–0 Vicryl sutures (**Fig. 6.10**). Recommendations for placing the graft include:

- The graft should not go all the way down to the nasal spine and should not overlap with the caudal edge of the septum. An uncomfortable clicking sensation can be produced when patients move their nasal tips.
- The medial crura should be aligned so that the domes are symmetrical before the graft is sutured in place.
- Sutures should be placed in the middle third of the crura. Sutures should not be placed near the domes, as this can efface the natural double break of the columella.
- Long struts can be used if extra support is needed. Care should be taken to fix the strut well over the nasal spine so it won't click or dislodge, creating a secondary nasal obstruction.

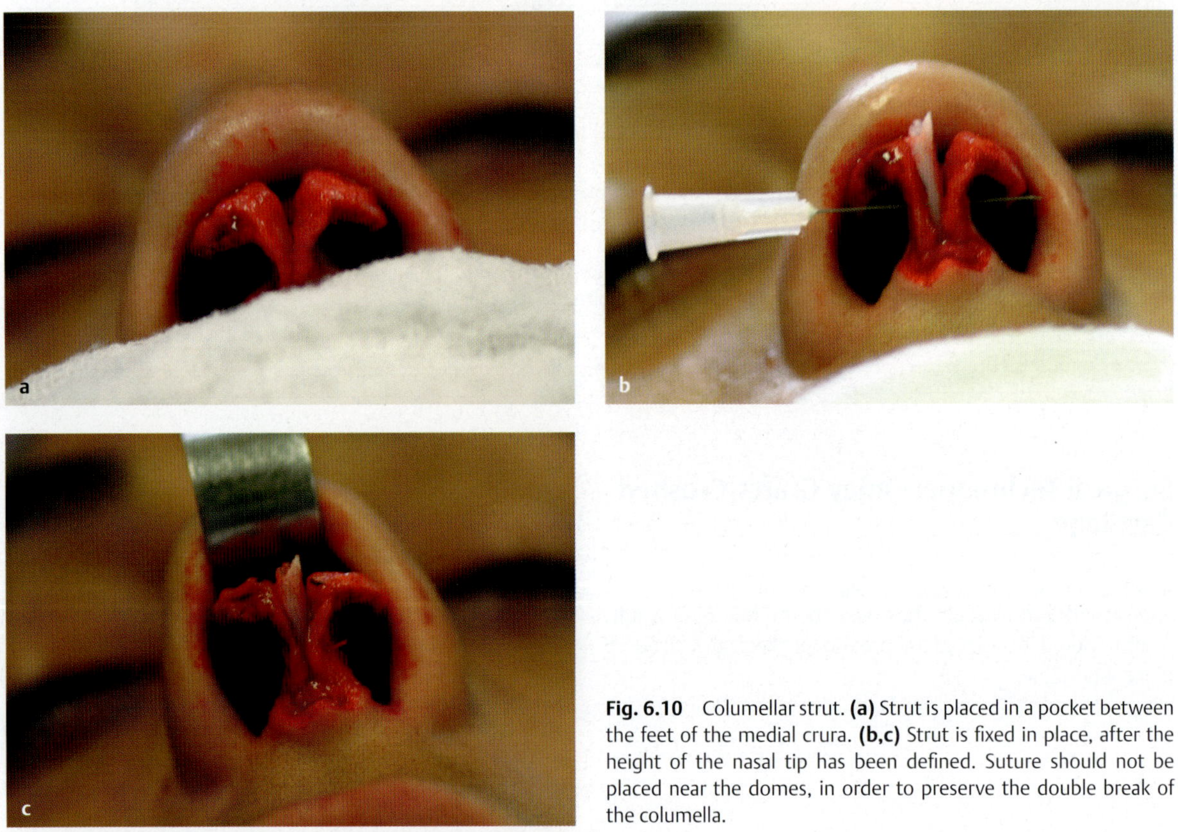

Fig. 6.10 Columellar strut. **(a)** Strut is placed in a pocket between the feet of the medial crura. **(b,c)** Strut is fixed in place, after the height of the nasal tip has been defined. Suture should not be placed near the domes, in order to preserve the double break of the columella.

Anatomical Findings: Small Nasal Spine, Short and Weak Caudal Septum, Acute Nasolabial Angle

Surgical Technique: Caudal Septal Extension Graft

The caudal septal extension graft is valuable in a Mestizo patient who has a severely acute nasolabial angle and a retrusive caudal septum for which we know a columellar strut will not give the necessary support and will not be strong enough to push out the nasolabial angle. Indications for using this type of graft are[10,11]:

- severely acute nasolabial angle with poor tip recoil
- retrusive caudal septum
- inadequate alar–columellar relationships (heavy alae with retrusive columella)

The ideal grafting material again is septal cartilage. In its absence, straightened conchal cartilage can be used, or rib cartilage. The graft is placed to overlap the caudal edge of the nasal septum. It is fixed in place inferiorly at the level of the nasal spine and superiorly at the level of the nasal septum. The overlapping portion of cartilage should be thinned out so that it won't produce nasal obstruction. Once the graft is sutured in place, the position of the nasal tip is defined by suturing the feet of the medial crura to this graft. How high or low the feet of the medial crura are placed will depend on how much rotation and projection of the nasal tip the surgeon wants to obtain. Grafts are usually carved in a rectangular shape, but, depending on the patient's needs, the graft can be wider at the top (to produce counter-rotation) or wider at the bottom (to produce rotation and to open the nasolabial angle) **(Fig. 6.11)**.

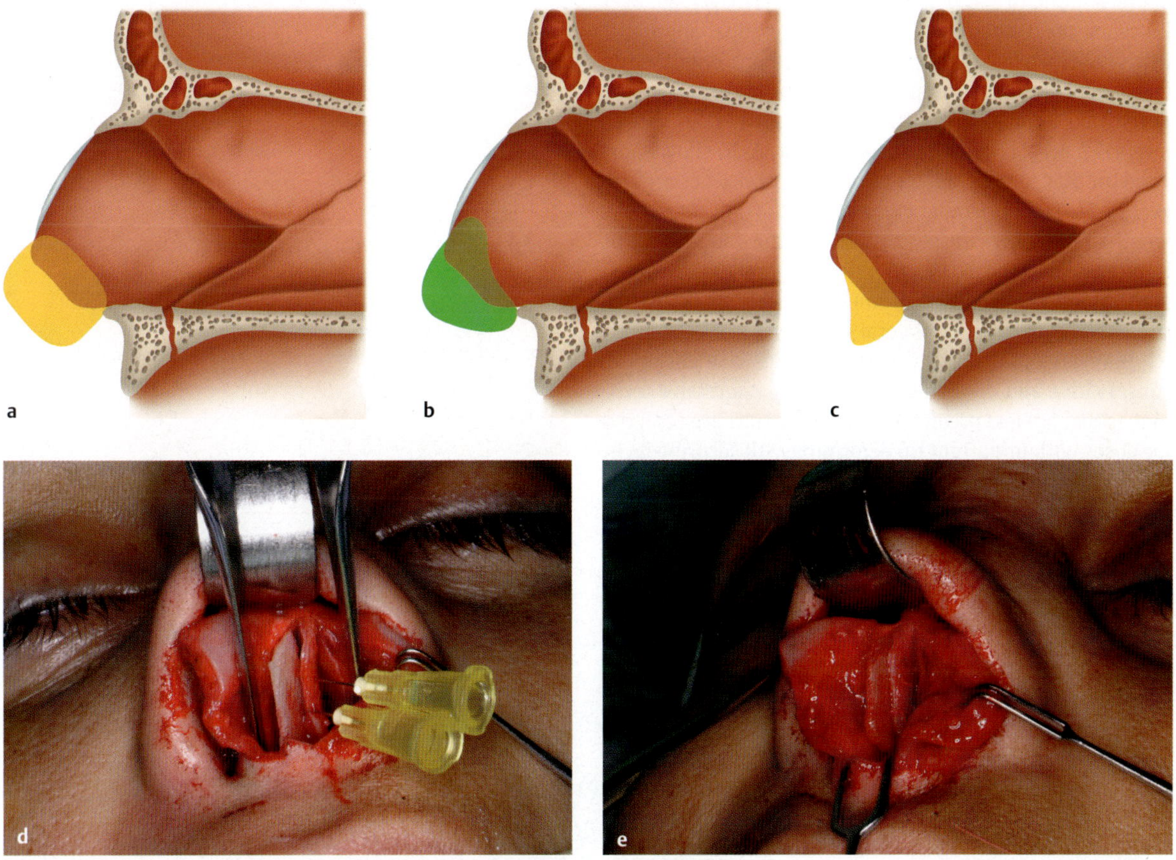

Fig. 6.11 Septal extension graft. **(a)** The graft ideally is carved from septal cartilage and has a rectangular configuration. It is sutured in place overlapping the existing caudal edge of the septal cartilage. The portion of the graft that overlaps the caudal edge of the septum is thinned out before suturing in place with absorbable 5–0 Vicryl sutures. **(b)** If counter-rotation is needed, the graft is carved wider in its superior portion. **(c)** To increase rotation and to open a narrow nasolabial angle, the graft is carved wider at the bottom. **(d,e)** Intraoperative images of rectangular extension graft being fixed in place.

6.13.2 The Nasal Tip

Once all the support structures of the nose have been strengthened, work can safely be performed on the nasal tip. The issue with most Mestizo nasal tips is that they are undefined and bulbous and have poor support. Alar cartilages, although wide, are usually thin and flimsy, with a tendency to collapse. To correct this problem, usually sutures and grafts are needed. Our patients want noses that have more definition but without necessarily looking bigger. This is a challenge for the surgeon because it means using grafts and sutures in such a way that the tip will have support but will not look big.

Anatomical Findings: Thick S-STE, Wide and Flimsy Alar Cartilages, Short Columella, Poor Projection and Rotation

In the nasal tip, the philosophy of using a structural approach means very little (if any) tissue resection (of alar cartilages) and the use of sutures and grafts to give contour, to create definition, and to add support to the alar cartilages. For over 20 years, the author has been using a "gradual approach" to the Mestizo nasal tip. Alar cartilages are evaluated in their vertical and horizontal dimensions and changes are performed depending on the anatomical findings at this level **(Fig. 6.12)**. The vertical component (A–B) shows how wide the alar cartilage is. Concavities or convexities are also evaluated. The horizontal component (C–D) evaluates the length of the alar cartilage, the width of the domal angle (is it too wide or too narrow and pinched?), and the definition of the dome (is it flattened, prominent, or asymmetric when compared with the contralateral side?).

Surgical options are chosen starting with the more conservative and predictable procedures. Aggressive techniques that are less predictable in their results are reserved for noses with important tip deformities. All suturing techniques are done using 5-0 PDS or a 5-0 nonabsorbable suture like Prolene or Ethilon.[11]

The author has divided the surgical techniques performed in the nasal tip into techniques to treat the vertical component and techniques to treat the horizontal component. Procedures can also be divided into complete strip procedures, incomplete strip procedures, and use of grafts **(Table 6.2)**.

Table 6.2 Gradual approach to the nasal tip

Anatomical problem	Surgical solution
Intact Strip Procedures	
Wide alar cartilage (vertical component)	Cephalic trim of lateral crura Lateral crural turn-in flap
Under-projection/under-rotation of nasal tip (horizontal component)	Lateral crural steal Dome-defining sutures Septocolumellar suture
Increased interdomal distance (horizontal component)	Lateral crural spanning sutures
Incomplete Strip Procedures	
Over-projected tip/long, plunging nose (horizontal component)	Lateral crural overlay technique Medial crural overlay technique
Grafts on the Nasal Tip	
Bulbous, undefined nasal tip	Shield graft Morcelized cartilage over nasal tip
Concave or convex lateral crura of alar cartilages (vertical component)	Lateral crural strut graft Alar batten grafts
Buckling or flaring of lateral alar sidewalls	Alar rim grafts

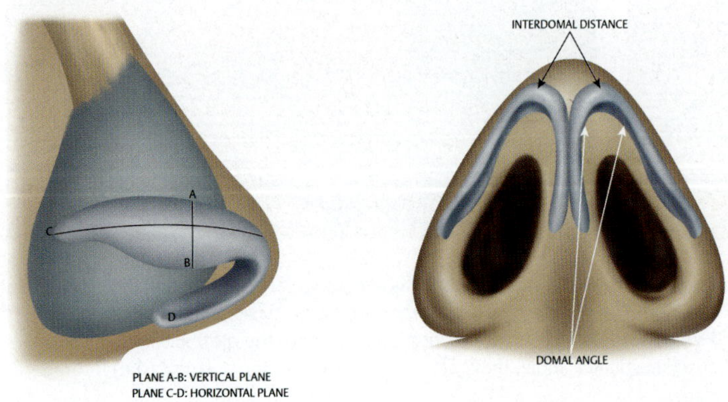

Fig. 6.12 Alar cartilage should be evaluated in vertical and horizontal dimensions. The vertical component (A–B) describes how wide the cartilage is and if it is concave or convex. The horizontal component measures how long the cartilage is (C–D) and also measures the interdomal distance and the domal angle.

Intact Tip Procedures

Intact tip procedures leave the whole strip of alar cartilage intact. The length of the cartilage is not changed. What can be modified is the width of the alar cartilage or the shape.

Reduction of the Width of the Alar Cartilage

Cephalic Resection of Alar Cartilages

The author usually preserves the entire width of the alar cartilages unless they are excessively wide. When this is the case and the cartilages are strong, conservative trimming of the cephalic edge is done, leaving at least 9 to 10 mm at the lateral crus and 5 to 7 mm in the domal area. The resection should not go all the way into the lateral portion of the lateral crus, as this can result in supra-alar pinching when the healing process is complete. This is especially true in patients with very thin and flimsy alar cartilages.

Lateral Crural Turn-in Flap of Cephalic Portion of Alar Cartilage

Currently, the cephalic trim is frequently replaced by the lateral crural turn-in flap. This technique is especially useful in patients with wide cartilages that are flimsy and lack support. In this technique, the cephalic portion is folded under the cephalic edge and sutured in place. This turn-in flap gives additional structural support to the area and prevents the postsurgical supra-alar pinching that is so commonly seen in our patients **(Fig. 6.13)**.

Suturing Techniques

The list of possible suturing techniques can be extremely long. Most techniques used by the author are used to refine, project, and rotate the bulbous, undefined nasal tip. They are reliable and predictable. The biggest advantage is that if the result is not satisfactory, things can be undone until the desired result is achieved. All sutures are done with 5–0 PDS; when this is not available, a 5–0 nonabsorbable suture is used.

Lateral Crural Steal

Lateral crural steal is one of the most frequently used suture techniques, especially in patients with bulbous, undefined nasal tips. Lateral crural steal increases rotation and projection and defines the nasal tip, creating a more triangular nasal base. For this technique, the existing dome is marked and the place of the new dome is also marked, usually 3 to 5 mm lateral to the original dome. With this maneuver, the medial crura is lengthened and the lateral crura is shortened, resulting in rotation of the dome **(Fig. 6.14)**.[12,13]

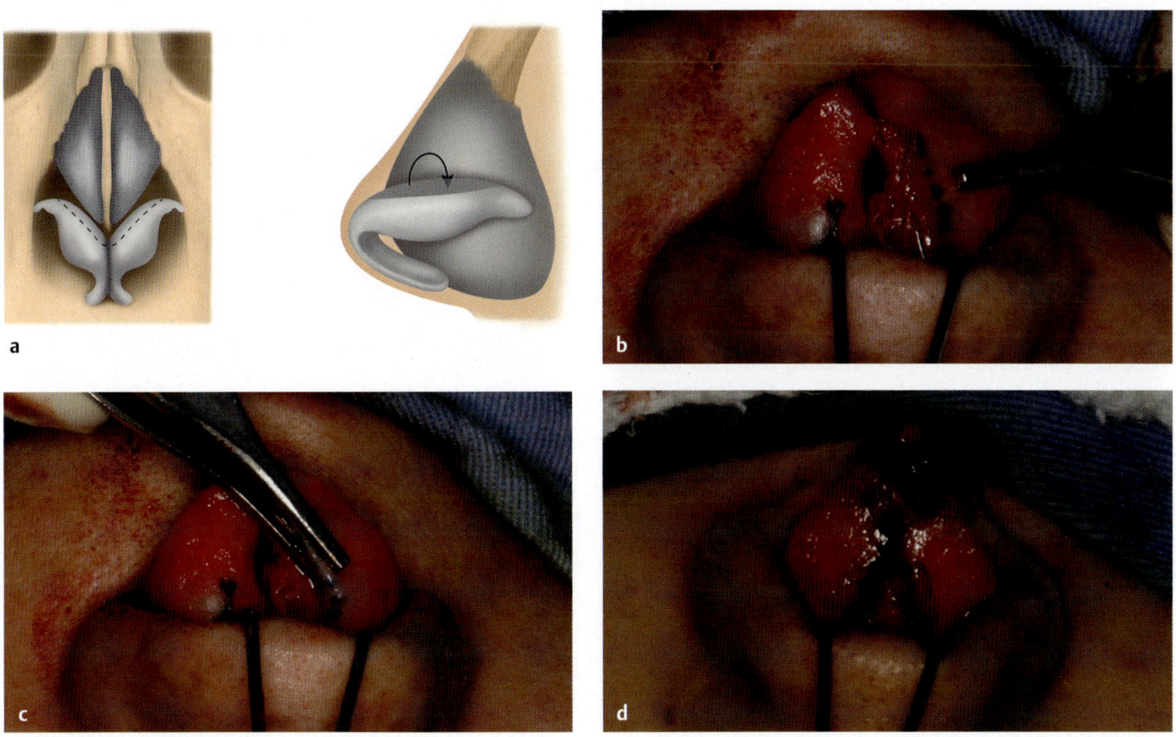

Fig. 6.13 **(a)** Schematic drawing of the lateral crural turn-in flap, showing how the cartilage is folded in on itself and is sutured in place. **(b)** This will give extra strength to the cephalic margin. **(c)** How much needs to be "turned in" is marked. **(d)** Cephalic margin is turned in. Turn-in flap is sutured in place.

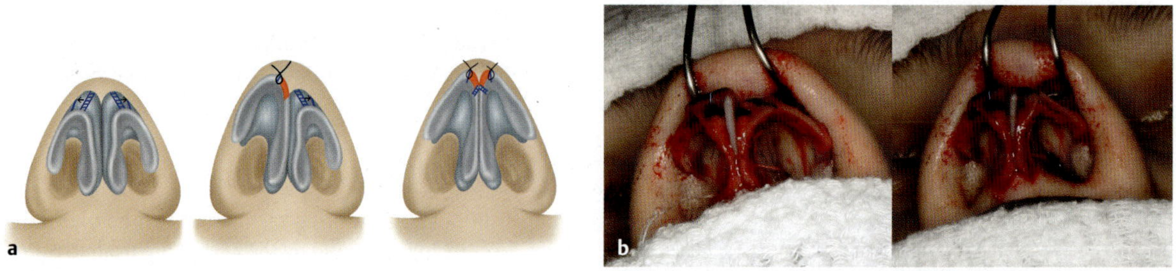

Fig. 6.14 **(a)** Schematic drawing of the lateral crural steal. The medial crura are lengthened at the expense of the lateral crura. This results in rotation and projection of the nasal tip. **(b)** Intraoperative images. In the left image, a lateral crural steal was done on the right alar cartilage, with the dome at a higher point than on the left side. In the right image, the procedure is complete. There has been an important gain in nasal tip rotation and projection.

Dome-Defining Sutures

Dome-defining sutures are used to define the nasal tip and to increase projection slightly. A mattress suture is placed at the level of the existing dome, narrowing the area. Sutures should not be knotted too tightly because this can produce pinching in the dome area. If a concavity is created lateral to the dome after the suture has been tied, a small piece of morcelized cartilage can be used to fill in the defect and again avoid postoperative pinching of the dome.

Alar-Spanning Suture

An alar-spanning suture corrects bulbosity in the lateral crus area. It can also increase rotation of the nasal tip. A mattress suture is placed in the cephalic margin of the alar cartilages directly behind the dome area and is tied in the midline. The suture will narrow a wide nasal tip, decrease the interdomal distance, and give slight additional projection to the nasal tip **(Fig. 6.15)**.[14]

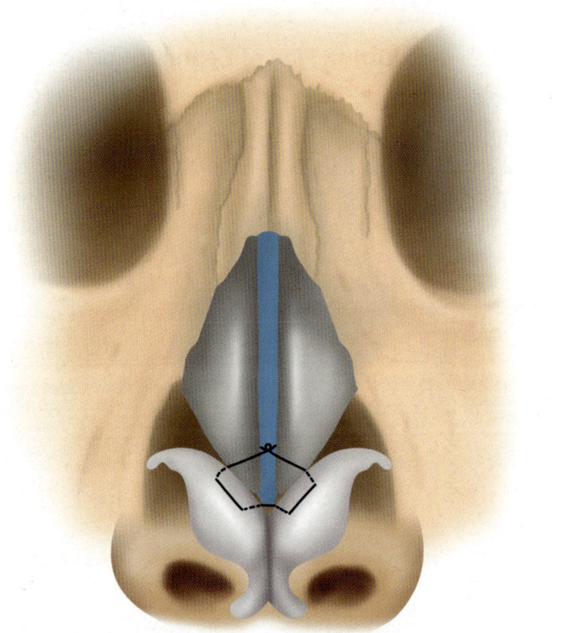

Fig. 6.15 The lateral spanning suture helps correct the lateral bulbosity of the nasal tip and increases rotation and projection if needed. A schematic drawing shows that a mattress suture is passed just posterior to the domes in the lateral crura and the knot is tied in the midline.

Septocolumellar Suture

The septocolumellar suture maintains and can increase projection and rotation of the nasal tip. The suture is usually performed after the tip work has been done. It requires a stable pedestal that should be clearly set in the midline. The septocolumellar suture is a loop suture that is introduced at a low point near the medial crural footplate on one side and is oriented upward and crossed to the other side at a point near the dorsal edge of the caudal septum; finally, it is taken out near the medial crural footplate of the contralateral side. The knot is tied in the midline between the medial crura. This pulls the medial crura–columellar complex up against the caudal septum, resulting in an increase in rotation and projection of the nasal tip **(Fig. 6.16)**.[11]

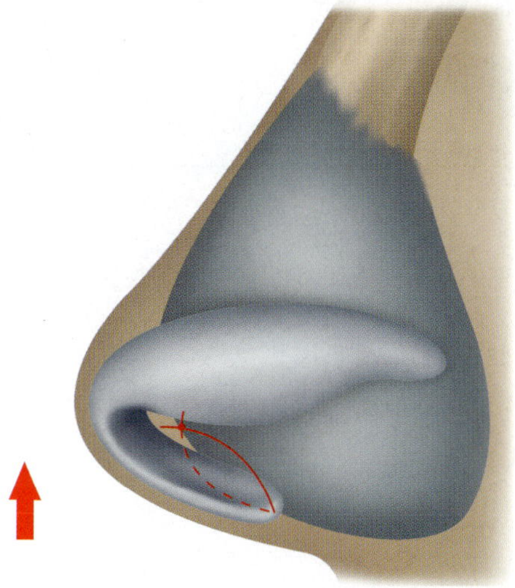

Fig. 6.16 Schematic drawing of the placement of a septocolumellar suture. A 5–0 suture of nonabsorbabe material is passed from a point low in the feet of the medial crura and high in the dorsal edge of the septum, crossing over to the other side. The suture is tied in the midline, bringing the crural–strut complex up against the caudal edge of the septum. This results in an increase of rotation and projection of the nasal tip.

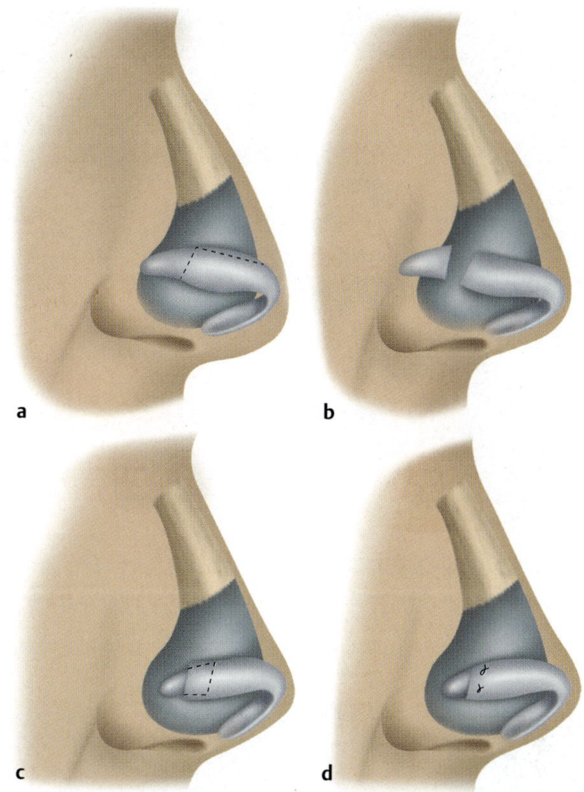

Fig. 6.17 (a–d) The lateral crural overlay technique is indicated for a long, plunging nasal tip. The lateral crus of the alar cartilage is sectioned 10 mm lateral to the dome and the two edges are overlapped, depending on how much rotation and/or shortening of the nasal tip is needed.

Incomplete Strip Procedures

It is not uncommon to find patients who have over-projected noses and long plunging tips that are the result of alar cartilages that are excessively long. In these cases, the techniques most commonly used by the author are the lateral crural overlay and the medial crural overlay. The lateral or medial crura are sectioned and the cut edges are overlapped and sutured in place. In this fashion, the strip of alar cartilage is shortened but at the same time it is reinforced by the overlapping edges.[11,13,14]

Lateral Crural Overlay

Lateral crural overlay is used for a plunging nasal tip where the lateral crura are much longer than the medial crura. The overlay results in shortening of the lateral crura, which produces upward rotation of the nasal tip and shortening of the nose. An incision line is marked on the lateral crus of the alar cartilage 10 mm lateral to the dome. The lateral crus is dissected from the underlying mucosa and the incision is done at the marked site. The proximal (medial) segment is superimposed over the distal (lateral) segment and is sutured in place. How much is superimposed will depend on how much rotation and shortening of the nasal tip is needed. Usually segments are overlapped between 3 and 5 mm (**Fig. 6.17**).

Medial Crural Overlay

The medial crural overlay is used in a patient with a long nose that has long medial and lateral crura, in patients with overly projected and overly rotated nasal tips, and in patients with asymmetric medial crura. An incision point is marked a few mm below the existing dome. Incised fragments are elevated, superimposed, and sutured in place. The technique results in counter-rotation of the nasal tip, lowering the height of the dome (**Fig. 6.18** and **Fig. 6.19**).

Grafts

When a structural philosophy is used in performing rhinoplasty, grafts are essential. Ideally, cartilage is harvested from the nasal septum, but when this is insufficient, the auricular concha or rib cartilage can be valid alternatives. Mestizo patients tend to have nasal tips that are bulbous and undefined. Grafts in this area are used for support, to create definition, to fill in, and to camouflage.

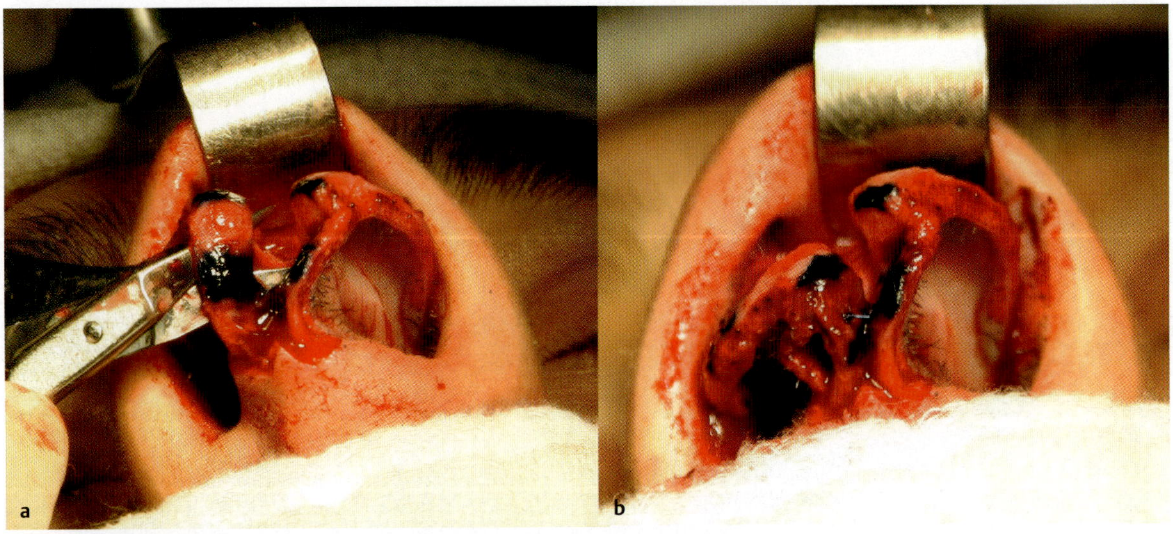

Fig. 6.18 (a,b) Medial crural overlay is indicated for an over-projected nose where the medial crura are overly long. The medial crura are sectioned below the domes and the edges are overlapped. This brings the nasal tip down.

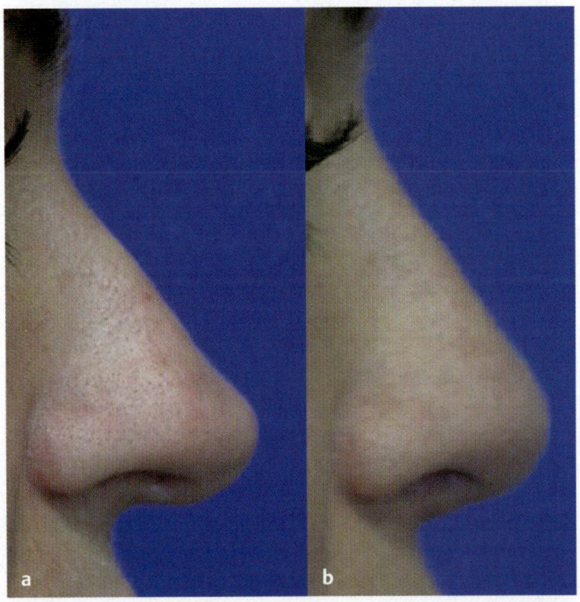

Fig. 6.19 (a) Preoperative and **(b)** postoperative lateral views of a patient in whom a lateral crural overlay and medial crural overlay were performed. The result is that the nose is smaller and rotation has been achieved.

Shield Graft

A shield graft helps to define the bulbous nasal tip, increases projection, and can help lengthen a short nasal tip slightly. The graft should ideally be carved from a straight piece of cartilage. If septum is not available, conchal cartilage or rib cartilage can also be used. The graft should be carved according to the patient's needs and dimensions will vary. Measurements usually range between 8 and 12 mm at the leading edge, 8 and 15 mm in length, and 1 and 3 mm in thickness. All edges should be carefully beveled. The final graft is sutured to the caudal edge of the medial–intermediate crura complex with 6–0 nonabsorbable sutures. The superior leading edge is set at the level of the domes or slightly higher in thick-skinned patients. The leading edge is then covered with morcelized cartilage, fascia, or perichondrium. Softening the leading edge will make edges less noticeable over time (**Fig. 6.20**).

Alar Strut Grafts

Alar strut grafts are rectangular, straight pieces of cartilage that are used as structural grafts in the lateral crura. They help support weak, flimsy lateral crura, help prevent lateral buckling when domal sutures are used to define the nasal tip, and help flatten concave or convex alar cartilages. The lateral crus of the alar cartilage is dissected from the underlying mucosa. A thin rectangular piece of cartilage is placed in the undersurface and sutured in place with absorbable sutures (**Fig. 6.21**).

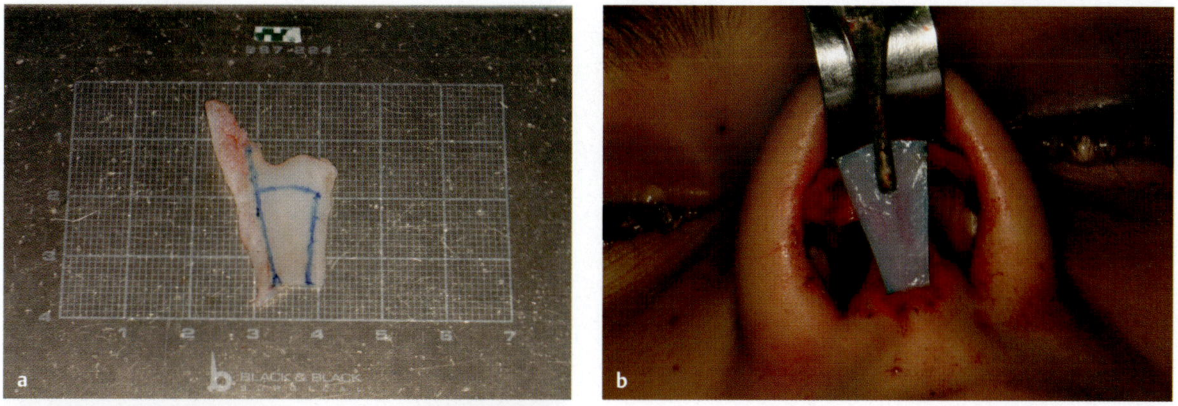

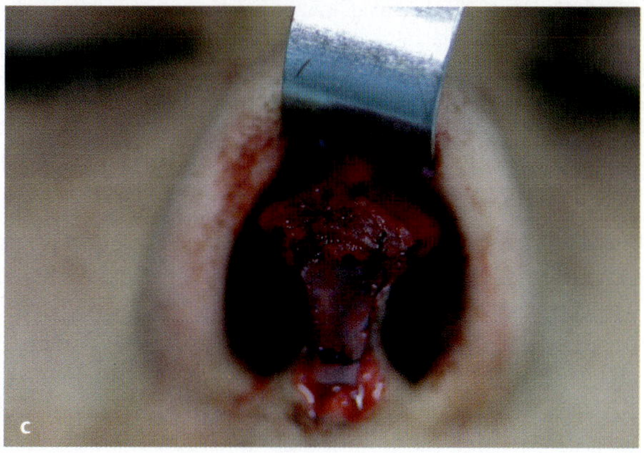

Fig. 6.20 **(a)** Ideally, the shield graft is carved from a straight piece of septal cartilage. **(b)** When carving is complete, the graft is fixed in place with 6–0 nonabsorbable sutures, placing the graft in front of the medial and intermediate crura and leaving the leading edge 1 to 2 mm above the dome area. **(c)** The leading edge is covered with morcelized cartilage or perichondrium, which will make the graft less visible over time and will soften any sharp edges that could have been left behind.

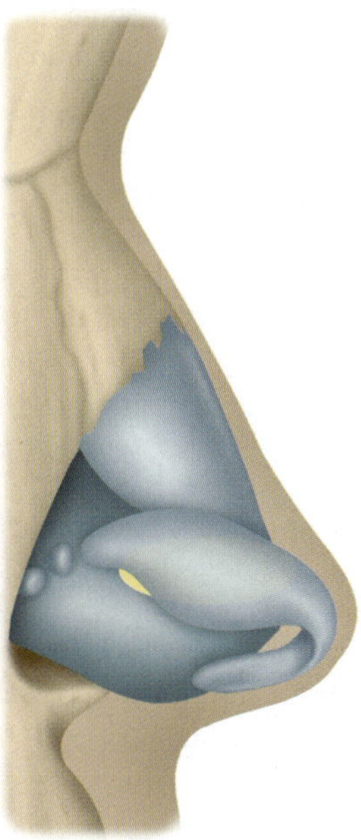

Fig. 6.21 Schematic drawing of the alar strut graft, which is a rectangular piece of cartilage that is placed underneath the lateral crus of the alar cartilage. The graft corrects buckling of the lateral crus, as well as any convex or concave deformities.

Alar Rim Grafts

Alar rim grafts are thin, long pieces of cartilage placed along the alar rim. They correct flaring and buckling and give support to the ala. With sharp scissors, a pocket is created along the alar rim, extending from just below the facets all the way down toward the base of the nose. A long, thin piece of cartilage is placed in a nonanatomical position in front of the caudal edge of the lateral crus of the alar cartilage. The graft is fixed in its pocket with a single absorbable suture. The superior leading edge can be gently crushed so it will not create any asymmetries in the area or become visible over time (**Fig. 6.22**).

Morcelized Cartilage/Crushed Cartilage

Crushed cartilage or cartilage chopped into tiny pieces is frequently used to fill in small defects. Morcelized cartilage is a piece of cartilage that is carefully crushed without causing it to disintegrate into small fragments. Morcelized cartilage is soft and pliable and can be manipulated as a single unit. It can be used anywhere in the nose to soften edges, to hide irregularities, and to fill in defects. It is more frequently used by the author over the nasal tip structures to help soften any sharp edges, to camouflage any changes

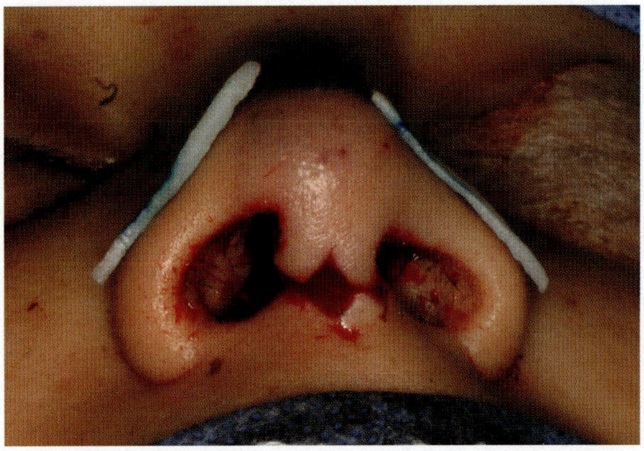

Fig. 6.22 Alar rim grafts are thin, long pieces of cartilage that are placed in a nonanatomical position along the alar rim. They correct flaring and buckling and give additional support to the alar rim.

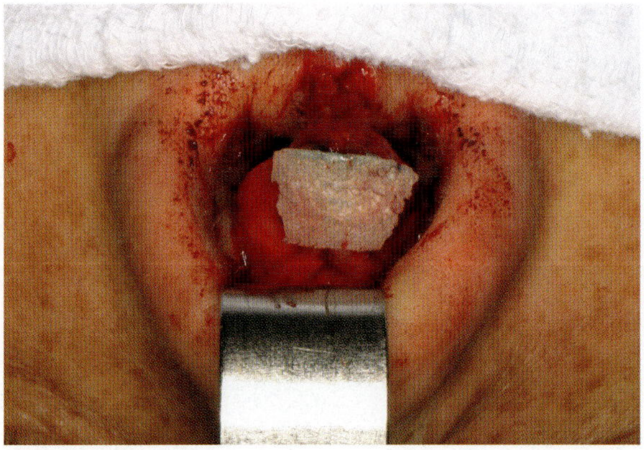

Fig. 6.23 Morcelized cartilage can be used in any part of the nose to fill in, to hide irregularities, and, if used in the tip, to give the tip a rounder look. It is important not to crush the cartilage excessively, because, if crushed too much, it can reabsorb.

done on the cartilage, and to fill in any defects that were not corrected with the other techniques used. The ideal material to morcelize is septal cartilage. Conchal cartilage has a tendency to break up into pieces when morcelized, and rib cartilage is very difficult to manipulate and to convert into something soft and pliable. Using a cartilage crusher, the cartilage is crushed, obtaining a piece of cartilage that is soft and pliable, that looks like a small Persian carpet, that will not break up easily if manipulated, and that can be used as a covering over the different areas of the nose. Whenever possible, it should be sutured in place **(Fig. 6.23)**.[12]

6.14 The Nasal Base

Once the rhinoplasty procedure is completed and incisions are closed, the alar nasal base is evaluated. It is not uncommon to find that, after completing all the surgery, the configuration of the nasal base has changed and the nostrils have acquired a more oval shape. Alar base reduction should be performed only if there is a need to decrease the alar flare, to reduce the alar base width, or both. The skin should be marked and incisions should be placed carefully so they won't leave any unsightly scars, which often become the telltale sign that the patient has had a rhinoplasty.

6.15 Postsurgical Follow-up

Postsurgical follow-up can be as important as the actual surgery. Stiches and cast are removed on day 8 and the nose is taped for an additional week. The skin is a priority in Mestizo patients due to its oily, acne-prone character. Acne breakouts, blackheads, and postinflammatory edema are common in our patients. Skin should be managed properly and sun should be avoided for at least 3 months after surgery. Because of the skin pigmentation in Mestizo patients, they should be warned that dark circles under the eyes can become more noticeable for a few months after surgery. Long-term follow up is essential for monitoring the patient's progress. Postsurgical photographs are taken at 6 months and 1 year after surgery and, if possible, every year after surgery. Postsurgical photographs allow the surgeon to evaluate the nose after inflammation has subsided **(Fig. 6.24)**.

6.16 Conclusion

Mestizo noses commonly have a poor osteocartilaginous framework and a thick S-STE. Nasal tips commonly are bulbous and undefined, with poor rotation and projection. The structural approach to rhinoplasty involves minimal tissue excision and adequate use of sutures and grafts to strengthen and, when necessary, to build up the underlying osteocartilaginous framework. The structural approach improves rotation and projection and defines nasal structures without compromising support. As surgeons, we should aim for a final result that brings patients closer to what they consider beautiful without compromising nasal form or function.

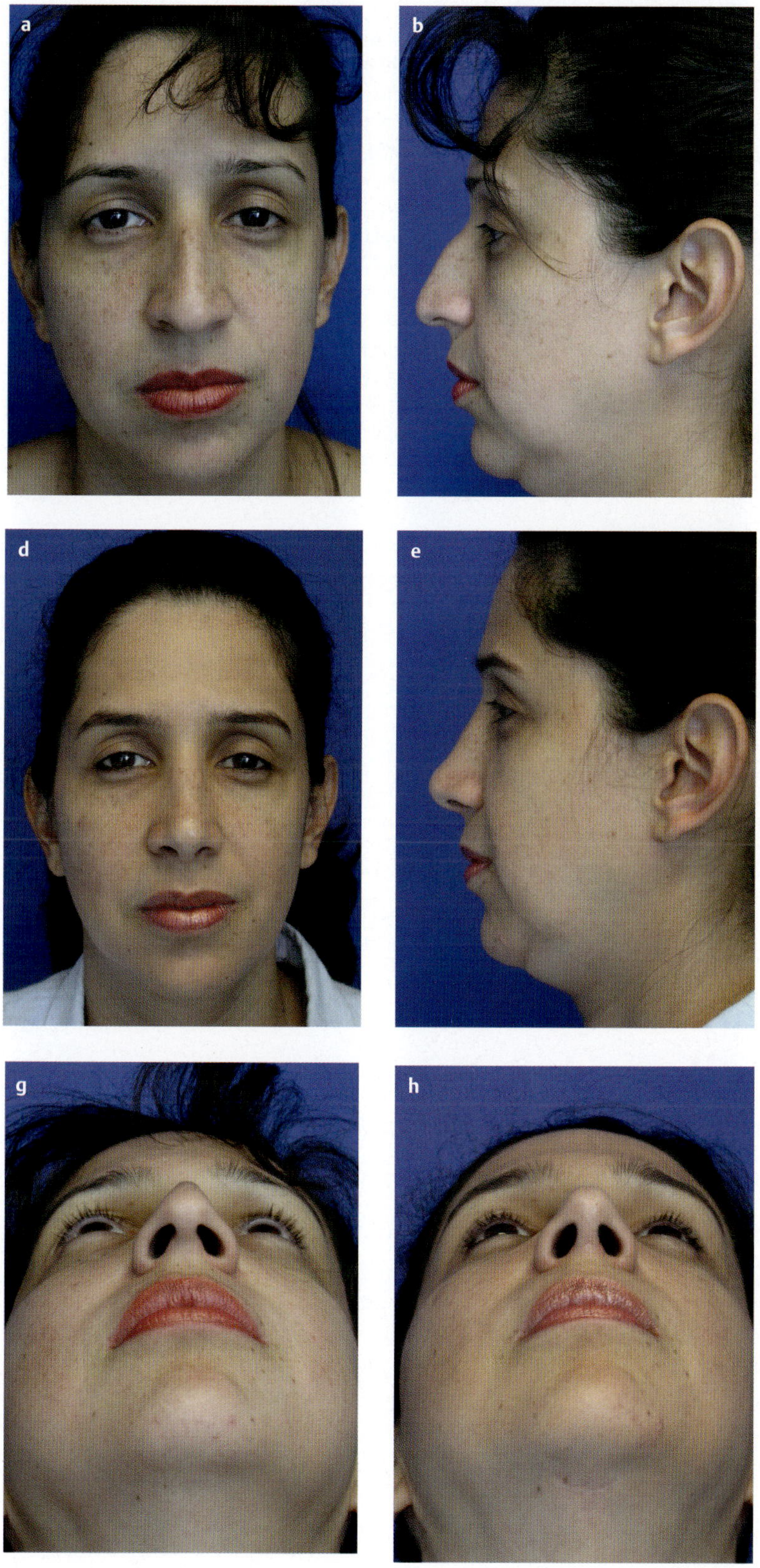

Fig. 6.24 (a,b,c,g) Presurgical and **(d,e,f,h)** postsurgical images of a Mestizo patient in whom the hump was removed and the middle third of the nose was strengthened with bilateral spreader grafts. Radix was filled in with morcelized cartilage. Definition, rotation, and projection of the nasal tip were obtained by performing a lateral crural steal and by using alar-spanning sutures. Alar rim grafts were used to give support to lateral sidewalls and morcelized cartilage was used to hide irregularities over the nasal tip.

References

1. Cobo R. Trends in facial plastic surgery in Latin America. Facial Plast Surg 2013;29(3):149–153
2. Fernández FL. Composición Étnica de las Tres Áreas Culturales del Continente Americano al Comienzo del Siglo XXI. Convergencia Revista de Ciencias Sociales 2005; 12(38):185–232
3. Ospina W. América Mestiza—El País del Futuro. Bogotá, Colombia: Villegas Editores; 2000:23–38
4. Hispanic Heritage Month 2014. Release Number: CB14-FF.22 Sept 2014. At: www.census.gov.
5. Cobo R. Structural rhinoplasty in Latin American patients. Facial Plast Surg 2013;29(3):171–183
6. Becker DG, Pastorek NJ. The radix graft in cosmetic rhinoplasty. Arch Facial Plast Surg 2001;3(2):115–119
7. Romo T III, Abraham MT. The ethnic nose. Facial Plast Surg 2003;19(3):269–278
8. Godin MS, Waldman SR, Johnson CM Jr. Nasal augmentation using Gore-Tex. A 10-year experience. Arch Facial Plast Surg 1999;1(2):118–121, discussion 122
9. Johnson CM, To WC. The tripod-pedestal concept. In: A Case Approach to Open Structure Rhinoplasty. 1st ed. Philadelphia, PA: Elsevier Saunders; 2005:9–20
10. Toriumi DM. New concepts in nasal tip contouring. Arch Facial Plast Surg 2006;8(3):156–185
11. Cobo R. Rhinoplasty in the Mestizo nose. Facial Plast Surg Clin North Am 2014;22(3):395–415
12. Cobo R. Nuances with the Mestizo tip. Facial Plast Surg 2012;28(2):202–212
13. Konior RJ, Kridel R. Controlled nasal tip positioning via the open rhinoplasty approach. Facial Plast Surg Clin North Am 1993;1:53–62
14. Perkins S, Patel A. Endonasal suture techniques in tip rhinoplasty. Facial Plast Surg Clin North Am 2009;17(1): 41–54, vi

7 Revision Rhinoplasty Techniques in Thick-Skinned Patients

Fernando Pedroza Campo and Luis Fernando Pedroza

7.1 Introduction

Mestizos are the product of racial mixing in Latin American countries and they are the predominant racial type in our country (Colombia). The Mestizo nose has demonstrable differences from, and is in marked contrast to, the Caucasian nose in dimensions, shape, and skin cover. Generally, Mestizo bone and cartilaginous structures are smaller and thinner than in Caucasian noses; the dorsum is wide and slightly convex, with a moderate hump, in contrast to a low and wide nasal base with a subprojected tip; and the nasal skin forms a thick layer, rich in glands and subcutaneous fat. Mestizo patients tend to have weak and thin alar cartilages, short and weak medial crura, a columella with subprojected tip, a retracted caudal septum, and wide and rounded nostrils. They have no discernible points of domes, and therefore no identifiable aesthetic Sheen triangle. The tip is usually ptotic and subprojected, lumpy and poorly protected, without definition.

Nasal tip revision remains one of the most challenging surgeries for facial plastic surgeons to perform. Changes in the support mechanisms, which are commonly disrupted by previous surgeries, as well as alterations in normal anatomy, make the procedure very difficult for many surgeons. Manipulation of the nasal tip to restore tip contour and nose function is one of the most difficult tasks to achieve.

For a successful rhinoplasty, it is necessary to understand the fundamental aspects of the complex nasal architecture that allow a global approach to the problem and its possible solutions. The dynamics of the nasal tip and its structures are the most important problems to solve in revision rhinoplasty patients.

In 1969, Anderson[1,2] described in a very didactic way how the structure of the tip cartilages resembles a tripod, with three important pillars of support. According to this analogy, the medial crura of the lower lateral cartilages together form the anterior arm of the tripod. Each lateral crus independently forms the rear pillars. Modification of the nasal tip by altering the components of the tripod is made possible by contemporary techniques in primary and secondary rhinoplasty.

The deformities that most frequently occur in revision rhinoplasty patients are external valve dysfunction, alar pinching, alar retraction, and lack of tip definition and projection, due to over-resected lower lateral cartilages. To correct these deformities, the surgeon must not only restore, but also replace, the tip framework.

In the management of the Mestizo nose, the deformity of the tip is higher, so structural cartilage grafts are required, and they are invaluable for influencing tip projection and definition.

In 1968, Sheen designed a graft technique for the nasal tip that, except for the shape and positioning of the graft, remains unchanged today.[3] Toriumi[4] reported the importance of reestablishing tip support by stabilizing the nasal base with a columellar strut, suturing the medial crura to the caudal septum, or using a caudal extension graft to maintain projection postoperatively.

Alar and tip asymmetries and contour deformities have been addressed with multiple graft types; for example, batten grafts,[5] lateral crural strut grafts,[6] composite grafts,[7] alar rim graft,[4] shield graft,[8] and suture techniques.[9,10]

Although numerous techniques to restore nasal tip structure have been proposed, no single structured graft that is capable of solving all of these major problems simultaneously has been described. The "seagull wing" technique[8] described previously by the senior author is designed to replace the lower lateral cartilages and to restore nasal tip contour. This graft technique has been found to improve tip projection, tip rotation, alar pinching, alar collapse, and alar retraction, but less improvement has been observed for columellar retraction. According to our results, columellar retraction was still present in 64% of patients after surgery.

In search of a graft structure that corrects major aesthetic aspects of the nasal tip contour, including columellar retraction, we created a structured graft that we have named the "tripod."[11]

The tripod graft is made by adding a complementary shield graft[8] to the seagull wing graft,[12] giving it the appearance of a tripod like the ones used in photography,[13] and as Anderson explained, it has a structure most similar to the normal cartilaginous nasal tip.[14] The tripod graft replaces the total cartilaginous structure of the nasal tip in cases where there is lack of the support mechanisms due to over-resection of nasal cartilages in previous rhinoplasties, and it improves nasal tip projection, tip rotation, alar pinching, alar retraction, and columellar retraction.

7.2 Surgical Technique

The tripod technique[11] consists of four steps: (1) marking the nasal tip; (2) harvesting the ear cartilage grafts; (3) sculpturing and molding the grafts; and (4) placing the tripod graft as a single block or as independent grafts.

7.2.1 Marking the Nasal Tip

The first step consists of marking the nasal tip. Determining a patient's domes, and the location of the remaining alar cartilages, is essential for surgical planning. The inferior nasal tip is pressed upward to rotate it cephalically to the desired position to define the level of the new dome,[10] and the new dome position is marked. The position of cartilage grafts and additional rhinoplasty techniques needed for the patient are also marked **(Fig. 7.1)**.

7.2.2 Harvesting the Ear Cartilage Grafts

The anterior surfaces of the cymba conchae and the cavum conchae are infiltrated with 1% lidocaine and 1:100,000 epinephrine. An incision is made with a no. 15 blade 2 to 3 mm below and anterior to the anthelix, from the anterior crus of the anthelix to the antitragus. A skin–perichondrium flap is elevated on the anterior surface of the concha.

The cartilage incision is made 1 mm below the skin incision to improve wound closure. The posterior perichondrium is harvested together with the cartilage. Removing the cymba conchae usually provides a cartilage strip of ~ 15 × 30 mm that will be used to shape the seagull wing graft.[12] The cavum conchae is always removed when using the tripod technique to shape the frontal shield graft. A 3 mm wide cartilage bridge is left between the cymba conchae and the cavum conchae to maintain good support to the ear **(Fig. 7.2)**. Two small drains are left in the field. The concha is packed with moistened cotton and is draped with Micropore strips.

7.2.3 Sculpturing and Molding the Grafts

After harvest of the ear cartilage, the cymba conchae is divided into two equal parts along its longer axis. The domes are marked and sutured with 910 polyglactin mesh (Vicryl 5–0, Ethicon, Inc., Somerville, NJ). The final size of this graft, which represents the alar cartilage, has ~ 10 mm of medial crus and 20 mm of lateral crus. The lateral crus is 7 mm wide in the central part, and 5 mm at the dome area. Each part of the graft constitutes one lower lateral cartilage. The two grafts are then sutured together through their medial crura with the polyglactin mesh. The intercrural stitches are first placed posteriorly, 2 to 3 mm below the domes, and then anteriorly, 6 to 8 mm below the domes. This configuration allows the creation of the aesthetic triangle of Sheen **(Fig. 7.3)**.[8] This forms the seagull wing graft.[8]

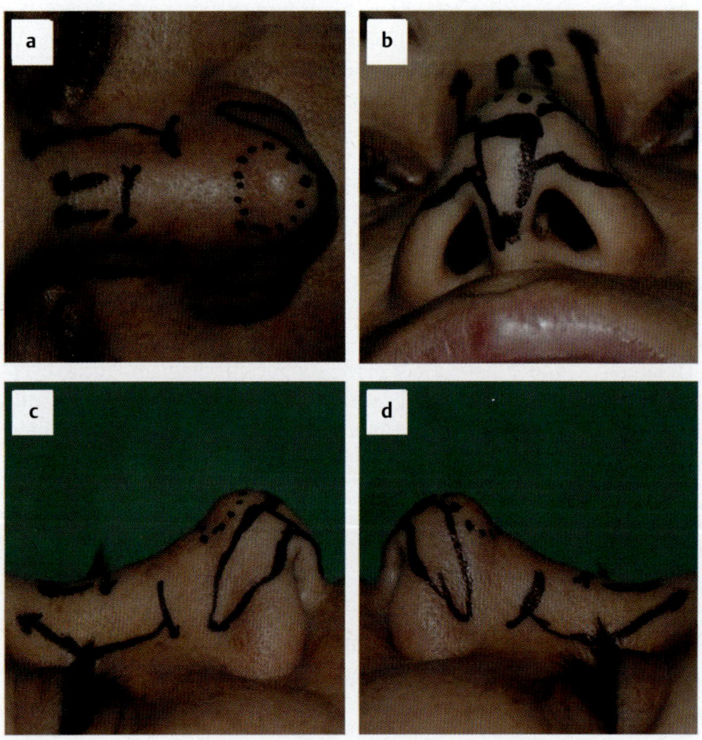

Fig. 7.1 (a–d) Marking the position of cartilage grafts and additional rhinoplasty techniques.

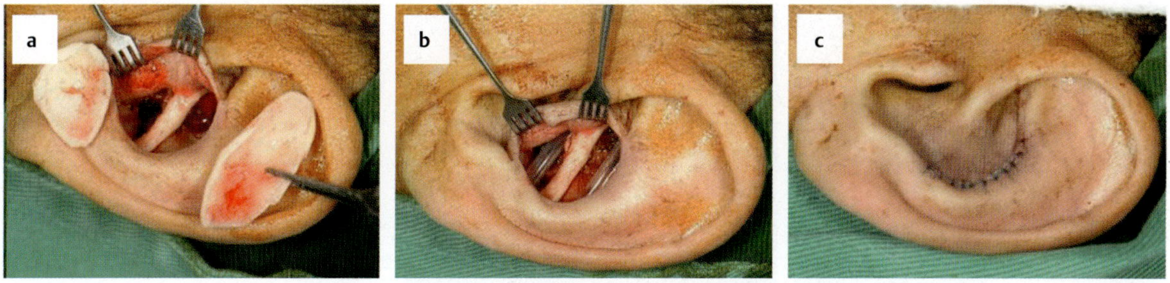

Fig. 7.2 Conchal cartilage harvest. **(a)** Cymba conchae and cavum conchae. **(b)** Drains. **(c)** Suturing the skin incision.

Then, the shield graft is sculpted from the cavum conchae. The approximate measurements depend on the individual patient, but usually range from 15 to 20 mm long and 7 to 8 mm wide at the superior border. Once the shield has been shaped, it is sutured to the caudal border of the domes and medial crura of the seagull wings to form a single block cartilage graft, called the tripod graft **(Fig. 7.4)**.

7.2.4 Placing the Tripod Graft

The whole graft can be inserted via an endonasal or external approach. The usual approach used is the endonasal via a precartilaginous or marginal incision 2 mm from the alar border **(Fig. 7.5)**.

Bilateral precartilaginous incisions are made, and pockets are formed above the remaining alar cartilages. The precartilaginous (marginal) incisions[10] are made at the caudal border of the lower lateral cartilage and are performed as follows: The double hook is placed at the edge of the naris while putting pressure with the finger on the alar cartilage, thereby everting and visualizing the vestibular skin. The caudal border of the lower lateral cartilage is identified and the incision made on the skin. The incision is made posteriorly to anteriorly following along the lateral crus, and then anteriorly along the caudal medial crus.

Then, pockets are formed above the remaining alar cartilages, and the graft is inserted through the incision and fitted into the pockets. The graft is placed anterior and superior to the patient's own alar cartilages to increase the length of the nose and to improve columellar retraction.

The graft is sutured to the remaining lower lateral cartilages and to the anterior skin of the precartilaginous incision with 5–0 polyglactin sutures. The skin incisions are closed meticulously.

If needed, the tripod can be assembled separately; the seagull wing graft can be independently added over the remaining alar cartilages and then the shield is placed and sutured to the seagull wings **(Fig. 7.6)**.

7.3 Discussion

The tripod technique[11] was designed to correct all nasal tip alterations derived from previous surgical procedures and is indicated in cases with poor nasal tip definition, tip under-projection, tip over-rotation, alar retraction, pinched ala, alar collapse, columellar retraction, and lack of support of the nasal tip. The technique can also be used to lengthen an over-rotated and short nose.

The tripod graft[11] replaces the total cartilaginous structure of the nasal tip; therefore, it provides excellent support

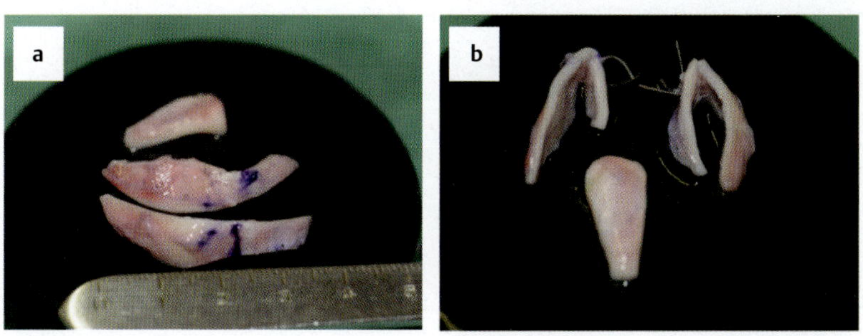

Fig. 7.3 (a,b) Graft sculpturing and molding: independent grafts.

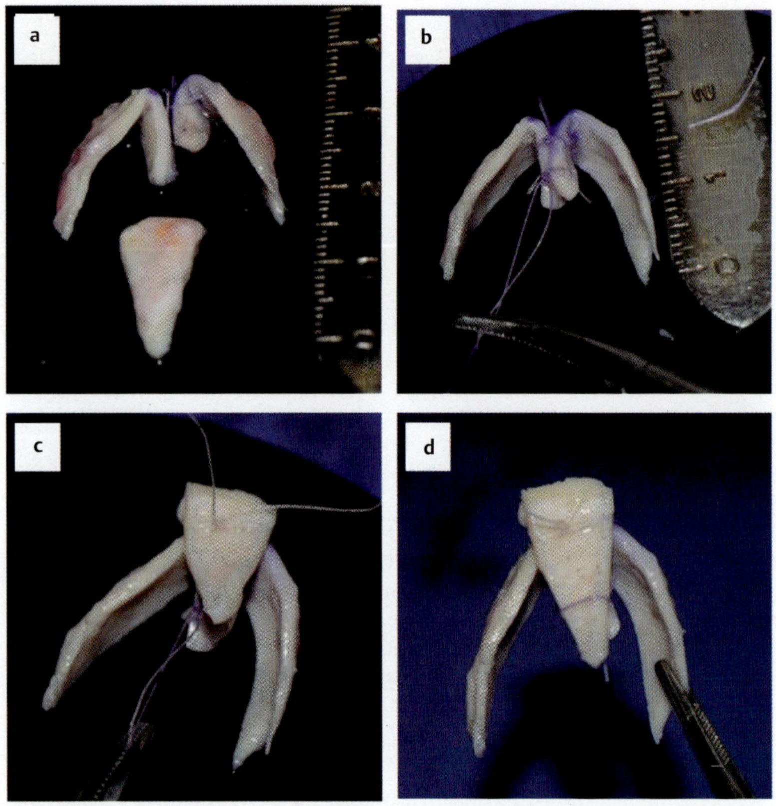

Fig. 7.4 (a–d) Graft sculpturing and molding: tripod graft in block.

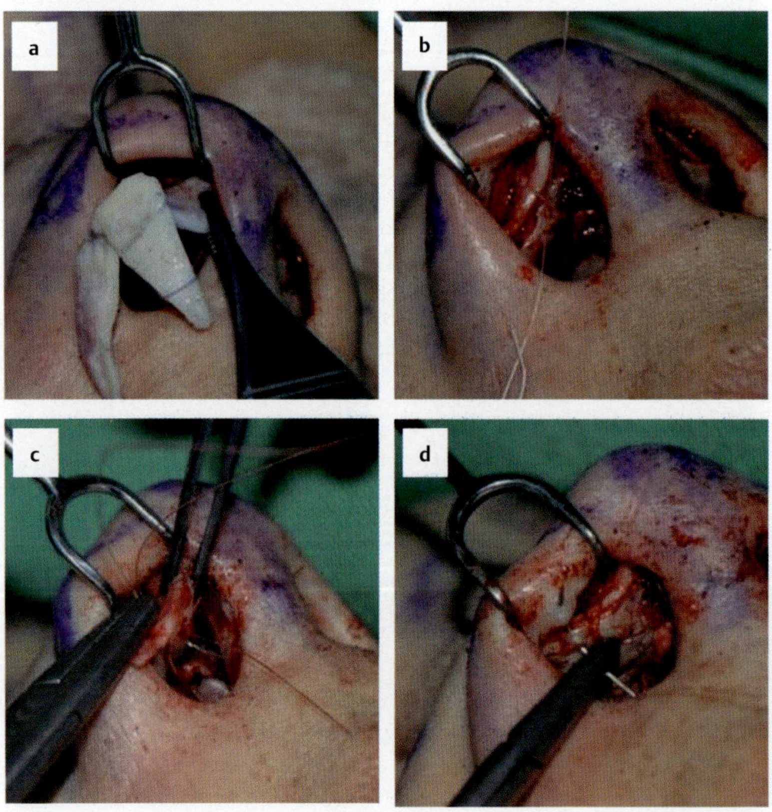

Fig. 7.5 (a–d) Tripod placement as one block.

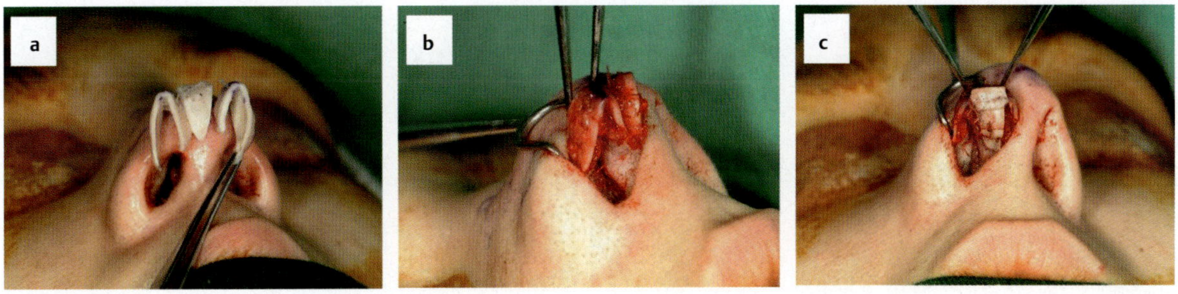

Fig. 7.6 (a–c) Tripod placement as independent grafts.

to the nasal tip, as well as a pleasing aesthetic appearance, and it recovers the functional aspects of the nose. The addition of the shield graft gives more support to the tip by adding strength to the medial crura and columella. It also improves nasal tip definition.

Most revision rhinoplasty techniques promote an open approach to correct the deformities, arguing for better visualization of the structures that must be corrected.[15] However, the tripod technique addresses all nasal tip structural, functional, and aesthetic problems using an endonasal approach, in which the graft can be correctly positioned and sutured to the alar remnants.

The tripod technique[11] can be used as a single framework to reproduce nasal tip structure and contour, correcting all the aesthetic deformities and functional problems derived from previous surgeries, producing a natural-looking nasal tip.

Columellar retraction, which is a common problem in revision rhinoplasty cases, is difficult to correct, but the addition of a shield graft[8] to the seagull wing graft[12] (the tripod graft) will correct the columellar retraction, in addition to correcting the other previously mentioned nasal deformities.

We believe that conchal cartilage is the best cartilage graft for recreation of the normal cartilage framework of the nasal tip because of its flexibility and similar thickness to the alar cartilages. Its natural shape facilitates the task of sculpting and molding the graft so that it will be similar to the original alar anatomy. Preserving one layer of perichondrium over the graft offers better nutrition to the cartilage and decreases graft absorption. It is also easy to sculpt, facilitating reproduction of the shape of the alar cartilages.

The only limitation of the tripod graft technique is when patients lack ear cartilage to harvest, due to resection in previous rhinoplasties.

The tripod technique[11] has been demonstrated to be clinically and statistically effective for correction of nasal tip rotation and projection, improvement of nasal tip definition, and correction of columellar retraction and alar deformities, such as pinching or retraction (**Fig. 7.7, Fig. 7.8, Fig. 7.9, Fig. 7.10, Fig. 7.11,** and **Fig. 7.12**). It also corrects functional problems, such as valvular collapse. The tripod technique is a reliable method of repairing nasal tip alterations in revision rhinoplasty cases in which cartilage overresection is an issue or in which there is a combination of aesthetic and functional problems that must be addressed.

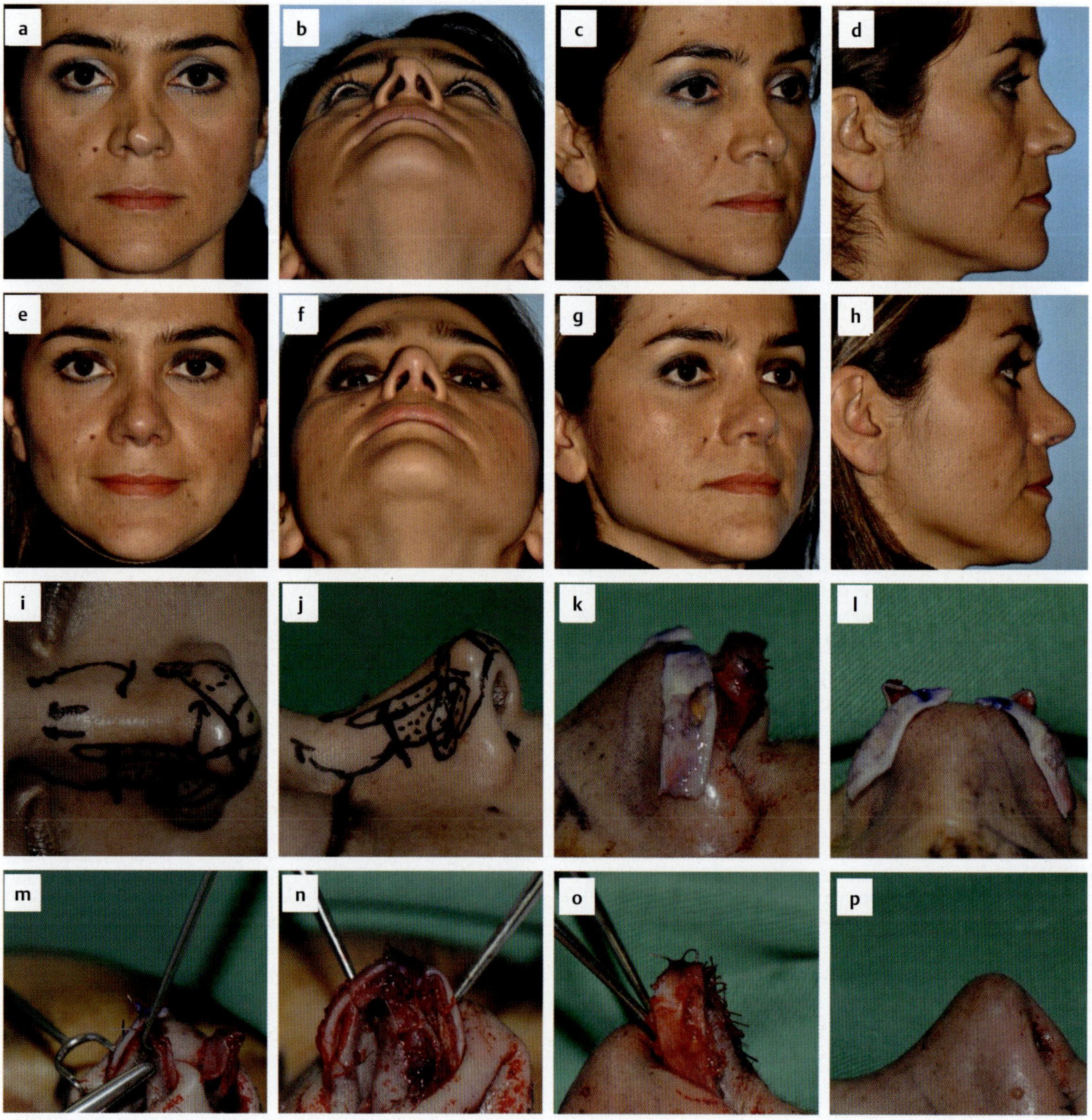

Fig. 7.7 Seagull wing technique as independent grafts. **(a–d)** Preoperative photographs. **(e–h)** Photographs taken 1 year after surgery. **(i,j)** Nasal surgical markings. **(k.l)** Independent seagull wing graft. **(m–p)** Placing the independent grafts as a seagull wing graft.

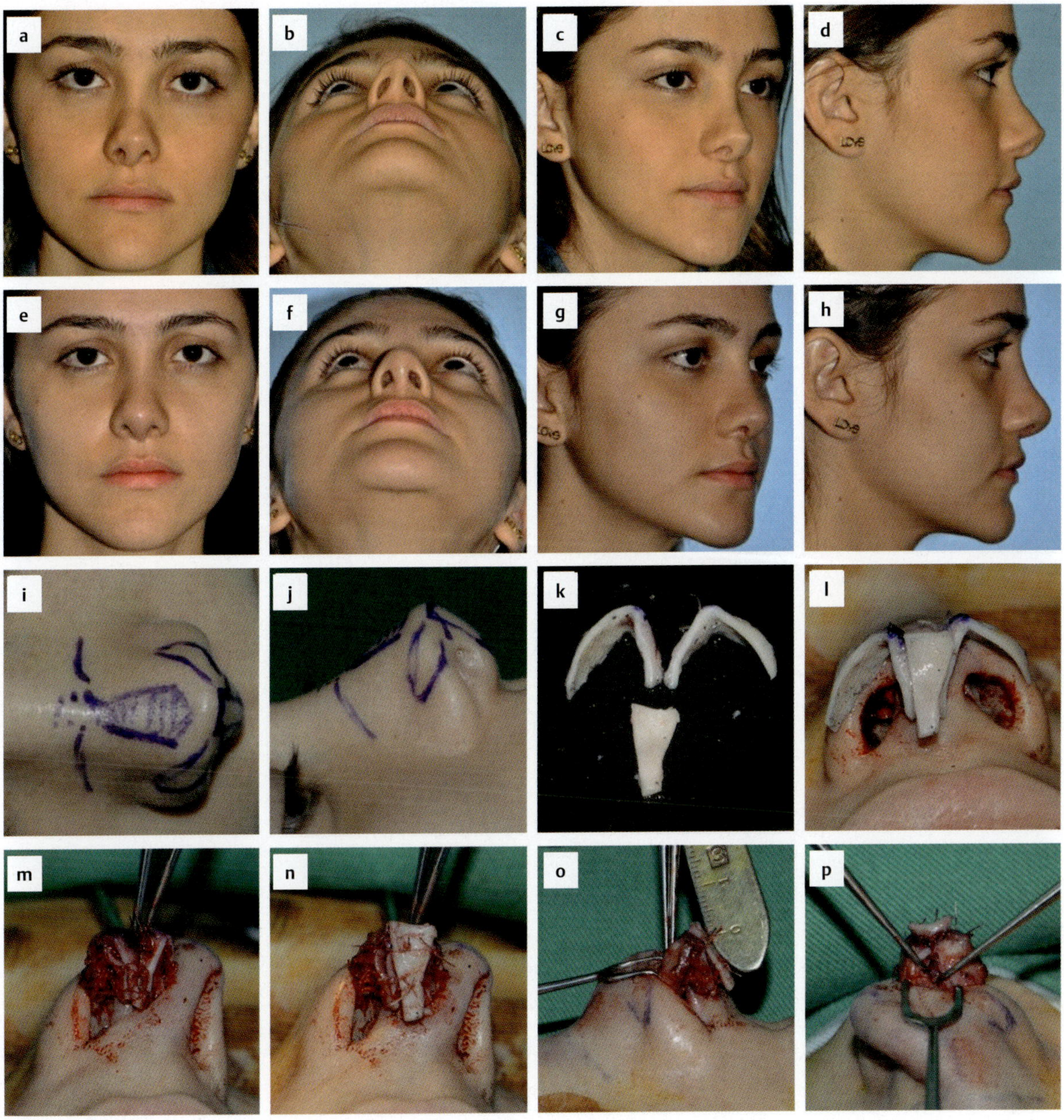

Fig. 7.8 Tripod technique as independent grafts. **(a–d)** Preoperative photographs. **(e–h)** Photographs taken 1 year after surgery. **(i,j)** Nasal surgical markings. **(k,l)** Independent tripod graft. **(m–p)** Placing the independent grafts as a tripod graft.

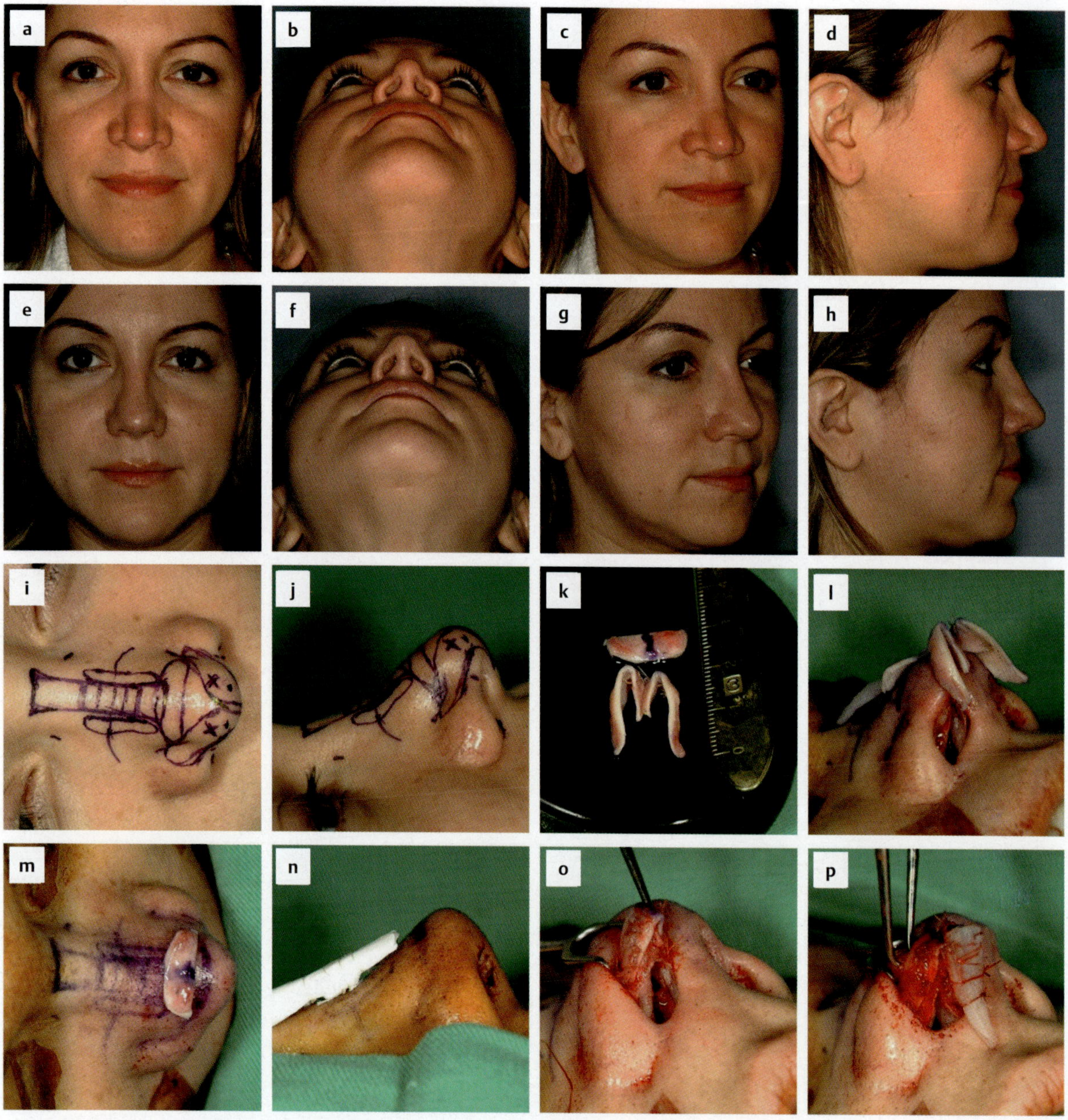

Fig. 7.9 Tripod technique as independent grafts. **(a–d)** Preoperative photographs. **(e–h)** Photographs taken 1 year after surgery. **(i,j)** Nasal surgical markings. **(k,l)** Butterfly graft and seagull wing graft. **(m)** Butterfly graft. **(n)** Gore-Tex (W. L. Gore and Associates, Newark, Delaware) dorsal implant. **(o,p)** Placing the independent grafts as a tripod graft.

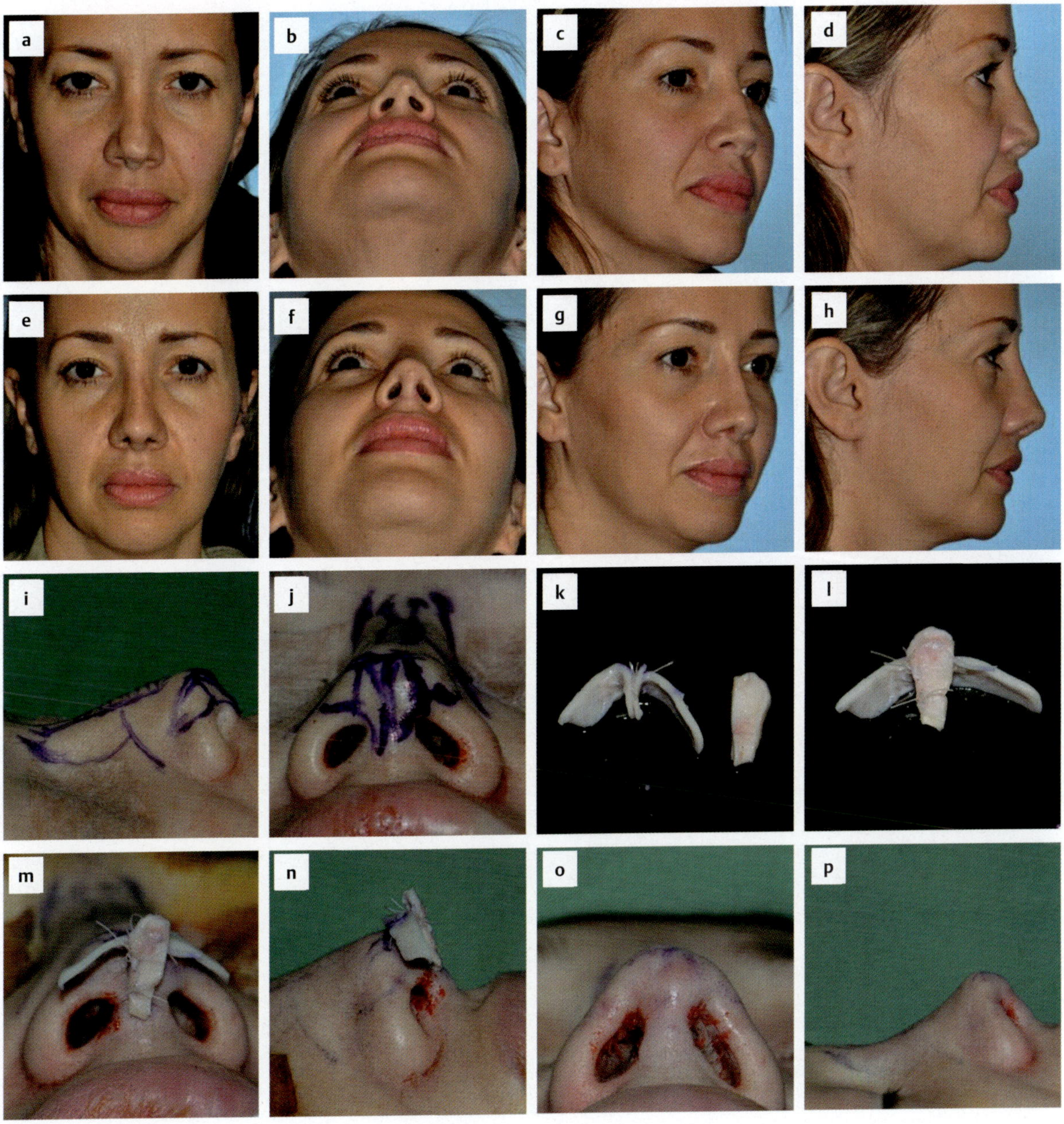

Fig. 7.10 Tripod technique in one block. **(a–d)** Preoperative photographs. **(e–h)** Photographs taken 1 year after surgery. **(i,j)** Nasal surgical markings. **(k,l)** Tripod graft in one block. **(m–p)** Placing the tripod graft in one block.

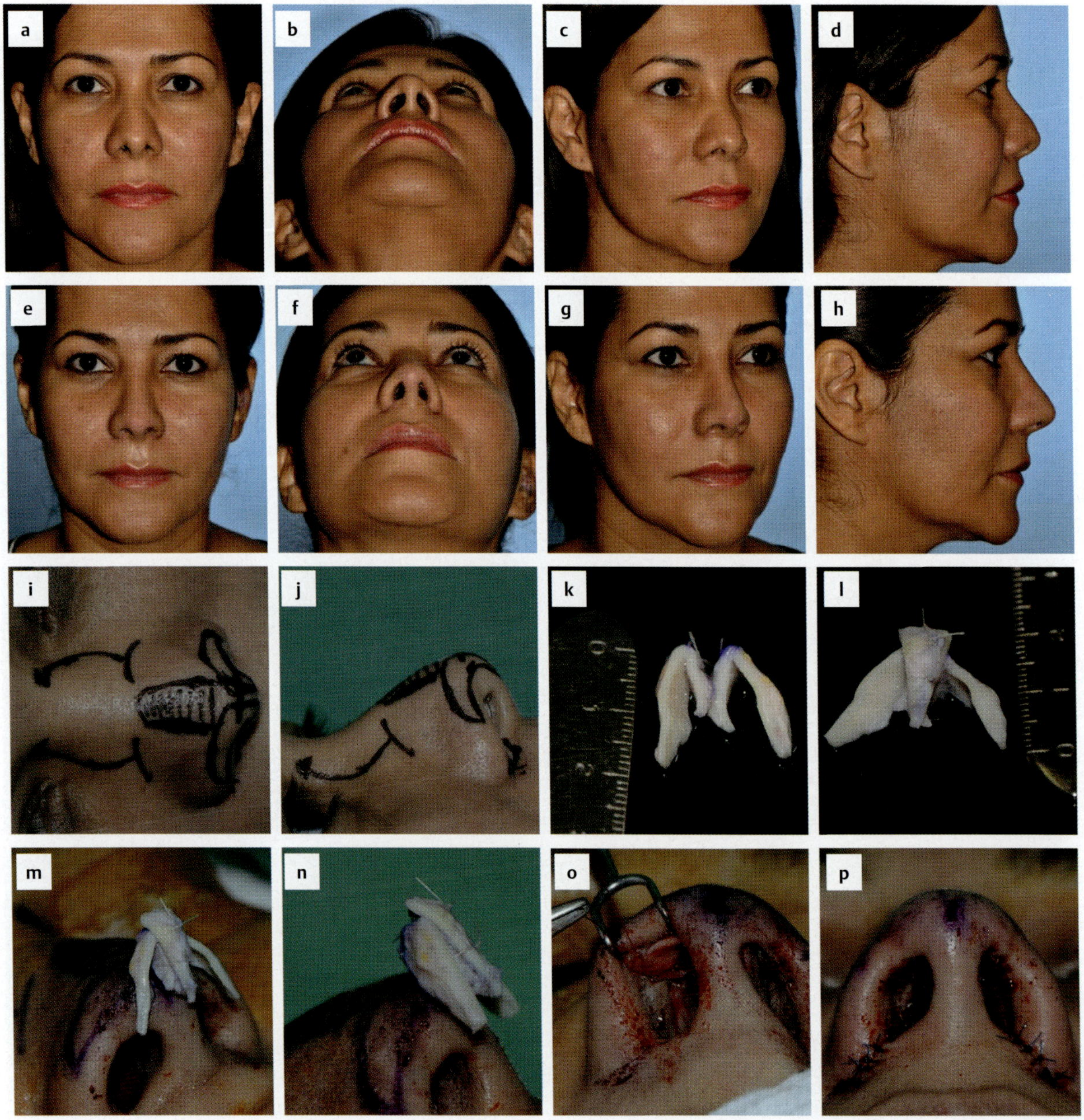

Fig. 7.11 Tripod technique in one block. **(a–d)** Preoperative photographs. **(e–h)** Photographs taken 1 year after surgery. **(i,j)** Nasal surgical markings. **(k,l)** Tripod graft in one block. **(m–p)** Placing the tripod graft in one block.

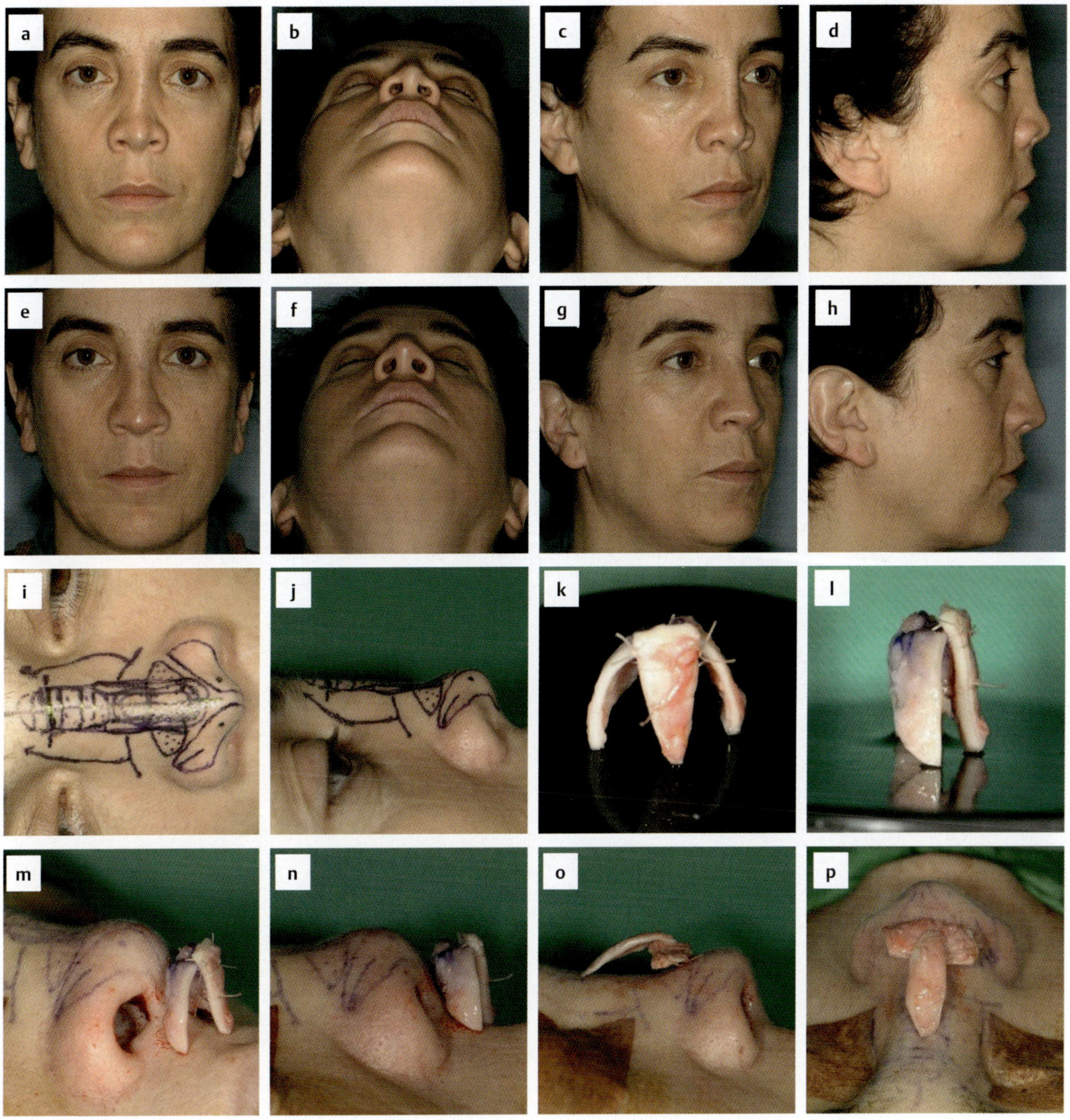

Fig. 7.12 Tripod technique in one block. **(a–d)** Preoperative photographs. **(e–h)** Photographs taken 1 year after surgery. **(i,j)** Nasal surgical markings. **(k,l)** Tripod graft in one block. **(m,n)** Placing the tripod graft in one block. **(o,p)** Butterfly graft and dorsal augmentation with conchal cartilage (airplane graft).

References

1. Anderson JR. The dynamics of rhinoplasty. In: Proceedings of the Ninth International Congress. Series, No.206
2. Anderson JR. A reasoned approach to nasal base surgery. Arch Otolaryngol 1984;110(6):349–358
3. Sheen JH. Achieving more nasal tip projection by the use of a small autogenous vomer or septal cartilage graft. A preliminary report. Plast Reconstr Surg 1975;56(1):35–40
4. Toriumi DM. New concepts in nasal tip contouring. Arch Facial Plast Surg 2006;8(3):156–185
5. Toriumi DM, Josen J, Weinberger M, Tardy ME Jr. Use of alar batten grafts for correction of nasal valve collapse. Arch Otolaryngol Head Neck Surg 1997;123(8):802–808
6. Gunter JP, Friedman RM. Lateral crural strut graft: technique and clinical applications in rhinoplasty. Plast Reconstr Surg 1997;99(4):943–952, discussion 953–955
7. Tardy ME Jr, Toriumi D. Alar retraction: composite graft correction. Facial Plast Surg 1989;6(2):101–107
8. Sheen JH. Tip graft: a 20-year retrospective. Plast Reconstr Surg 1993;91(1):48–63
9. McCollough EG, English JL. A new twist in nasal tip surgery. An alternative to the Goldman tip for the wide or bulbous lobule. Arch Otolaryngol 1985;111(8):524–529
10. Pedroza F. A 20-year review of the "new domes" technique for refining the drooping nasal tip. Arch Facial Plast Surg 2002;4(3):157–163
11. Pedroza F, Pedroza LF, Achiques MT, Felipe E, Becerra F. The tripod graft: nasal tip cartilage reconstruction during revision rhinoplasty. JAMA Facial Plast Surg 2014;16(2):93–101
12. Pedroza F, Anjos GC, Patrocinio LG, Barreto JM, Cortes J, Quessep SH. Seagull wing graft: a technique for the replacement of lower lateral cartilages. Arch Facial Plast Surg 2006;8(6):396–403
13. Larrabee WF Jr. The tripod concept. Arch Otolaryngol Head Neck Surg 1989;115(10):1168–1169
14. Anderson JR. The dynamics of rhinoplasty. Excerpta Med Int Cong Ser 1969;206:708–710
15. Quatela VC, Jacono AA. Structural grafting in rhinoplasty. Facial Plast Surg 2002;18(4):223–232

8 Approaches to the Midface in Heavy-Skinned Patients

Tomas G. Patrocinio, Lucas G. Patrocinio, and Jose Antonio Patrocinio

8.1 Introduction

Fullness of the cheek represents youthfulness. It is important to understand the anatomic changes associated with aging and to have a clear vision of what needs to be accomplished for correction. The aging process initiates during the third decade, affecting the lower lid and midface together, and in response to gravitational forces, the fat and soft tissues of the cheek drift downward in relation to the underlying bony skeleton. In this process of aging, a constant hollowness of the midface develops. As a result, a patient may appear tired, old, or sad.[1]

Weakening of the malar and orbital ligaments is a major component of the aging process. The result is a downward and medial displacement of the malar fat pad and other soft tissues over the fixed ligaments of the nasolabial fold. The fat over the malar eminence is left standing, accentuating the malar bag. Another anatomical change that occurs is weakening of the orbital ligaments, which contributes to hollowness under the orbit. The malar fat pad, which in youth was at the level of the orbital rim, falls downward and medially, producing hollowness. This concavity, which is below the convexity of the ocular globe and orbital fat, accentuates and no longer covers the bulge of herniated orbital fat. This produces the "double contour" deformity characteristic of the aging orbital/midface complex. The vertical aperture of the eye elongates, creating a more round shape with increasing scleral show. As tarsoligamentous laxity increases, the lateral commissure often descends, creating a more inferior slant from medial to lateral commissure. Eyelid tone decreases, as exhibited by skin and muscle laxity. An important volume loss of the midface also contributes to the aging process. Finally, the collapse of the zygomaticus major and minor muscles, which suspend the ligamentous and muscular connections of the midface, causes a droop of the corner of the mouth and deepens the labiomental fold **(Fig. 8.1)**.[2]

The purpose of the facelift procedure is to reverse the aging process that has occurred. This can be achieved through various techniques that have been developed to date. The evolution of face rejuvenation consists in deciding which facial plane is going to be accessed.[3]

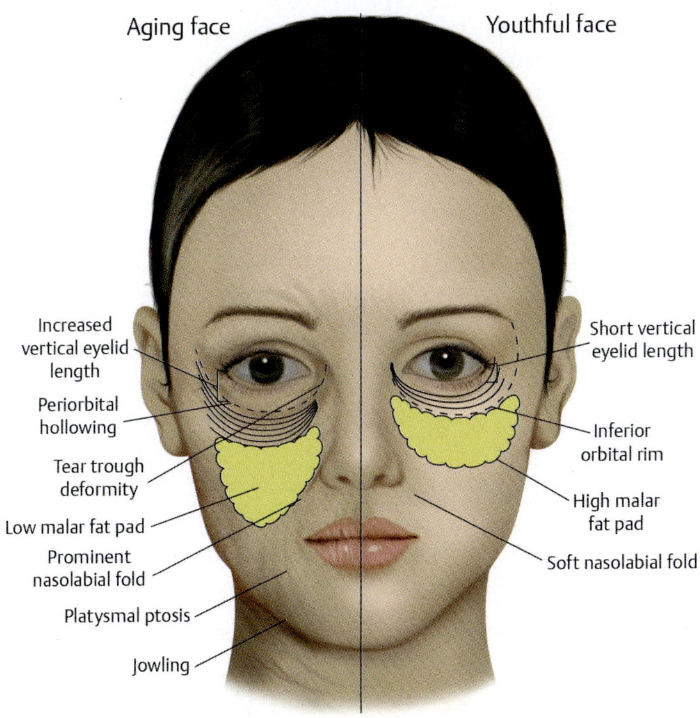

Fig. 8.1 Schematic representation of aged anatomical findings shown on the left and youthful contours shown on the right.

Previously, facial rejuvenation technique consisted of interrupted incisions placed both in front of and behind the ears in natural wrinkles, combined with limited strips of excised skin.[4,5] This technique was followed by the first descriptions of extensive skin undermining and lipectomy. More recently, the discovery of the SMAS (subcutaneous muscle-aponeurotic system) improved the technique (plication, suture, partial sectioning, etc.), with the goal of long-lasting results. In an effort to address the nasolabial fold, which had not been modified by other techniques, the deep plane and composite facelift were described. They consisted of a deep SMAS dissection to access the nasolabial fold; however, use of this technique has been increasingly questioned because of the risk of facial nerve injury.[6] Moreover, Barton, in 1992, showed with histologic sections as well as cadaver and clinical dissections that the SMAS is the investing fascia of the zygomaticus major and minor muscles in the medial cheek, providing support for the clinical finding that the nasolabial crease was minimally improved by traction on the SMAS.[7]

Recent studies emphasize the central third of the face, often referred as midface, the most difficult region of the face to effectively address. In 1979, Tessier[8,9] revolutionized the treatment of the aging face; he introduced a subperiosteal approach for reducing signs of aging in young and middle-aged patients. He applied his extensive experience in craniofacial surgery to aesthetic plastic surgery by utilizing the innovative subperiosteal approach in the upper and middle thirds of the face with an extensive coronal incision. Following the studies of Tessier, Psillakis,[10,11,12] Santana,[13] and others have improved the application of subperiosteal dissection in face rejuvenation. Isse[14] and Ramirez[15,16,17] led to the popularization of this technique in the United States with the introduction of the endoscope. Others described correction of midfacial aging using the transblepharoplasty approach.[18,19,20] To address the atrophy of soft tissues, particularly the subcutaneous fatty layer, other techniques were described.[21,22,23,24,25]

8.2 Preoperative Evaluation

Before any aesthetic surgery of the face, a complete medical history has to be obtained, including allergies, medications, medical problems, previous surgery, and drinking and smoking habits. Smoking cessation is advocated before and after surgery; however, patient noncompliance may not affect final results due to the thickness of the flap created during the subperiosteal facelift. Furthermore, emotional/psychological evaluation is important for elective aesthetic surgery. Preoperative photographs are essential for preoperative planning, intraoperative decisions, patient communication, and medicolegal documentation. At the preoperative consultation, the patient is informed about the planned procedure, with both written and oral information provided. Written informed consent is also obtained.[3]

8.3 Patient Classification and Approach Selection

A preoperative classification of patients is essential for both diagnosis and approach planning. Each of the categories in **Table 8.1** represents patients with specific lower lid and/or midfacial changes. In this chapter, we describe the transtemporal endoscopic subperiosteal facelift (Group 4), which is the technique we use more often to address the characteristics of our heavy-skinned patients.

The subperiosteal facelift is especially advantageous for patients who have undergone other facelift procedures, need skin resurfacing, need soft tissue augmentation, have skeletal disproportion, or need alloplastic implants. Combination with a forehead lift is common and produces excellent results.[26,27] Ramirez[15,16,17] and Psillakis[10,11,12] demonstrated that the subperiosteal facelift could be applied across the full spectrum of facial aging.

Table 8.1 Surgical group approach according to the lower lid/midface characteristics

Group	Characteristics	Surgical technique
1	Postseptal fat herniation with taut skin; no lower lid skin laxity or excess and no midfacial changes (young patients)	Transconjunctival blepharoplasty
2	Laxity and/or excess of lower lid skin, with or without postseptal fat herniation; minimal midfacial changes or vertical descent of the malar soft tissue	Transblepharoplasty fat reposition
3	Lower lid aging with descent of lid/cheek junction; skeletalization of the orbital rim and deepening of the nasolabial fold; no lower lid malposition or deformities of the lateral canthus	Subperiosteal transblepharoplasty Midfacelift + fat graft
4	Lower lid aging with descent of lid/cheek junction; skeletalization of the orbital rim and deepening of the nasolabial fold; lower lid malposition (scleral show)	Transtemporal midfacelift + fat graft

8.4 Surgical Technique

The surgery is usually performed with the patient under sedation, and local anesthesia (2% lidocaine with 1:100,000 epinephrine) is infiltrated in all areas of planned surgery for anesthesia and vasoconstriction. The surgeon is positioned above the patient's head with the video monitor on the left.

Important anatomical structures to consider are the frontal branch of the seventh cranial nerve and the infraorbital neurovascular bundle. The important dissection planes include dissection deep to the temporoparietal fascia along the deep layer of the deep temporalis fascia and the subperiosteal midface dissection. The surgical technique is divided into three major steps: (1) the endoscopic creation of a temporal pocket; (2) mobilization of the midface by subperiosteal dissection; and (3) elevation and suspension of the mobilized midface to the deep temporalis fascia.

In the temporal region, a 3- to 5-cm incision, perpendicular to the temporal line, is placed 3 cm behind the hairline. The dissection is performed to identify the deep layer of the deep temporalis fascia **(Fig. 8.2)**. As the pocket is enlarged, the endoscope is introduced for visualization. The frontal branch of the seventh cranial nerve is contained in the overlying temporoparietal fascia, which is analogous to the SMAS found in the lower face, facilitating the mobilization of the entire zygomatic arch periosteum and protecting the frontal branch of the facial nerve from injury. Identification of the superficial temporal fat pad is an important landmark that assures the surgeon that the frontal branch of the facial nerve is lateral to the endoscope.

The dissection continues medially and inferiorly, exposing the medial third of the zygomatic arch and orbital rim. An incision is made on the zygomatic periosteum and a lower subperiosteal elevation is performed to the malar eminence, gingival buccal sulcus, and nasolabial fold. It is important to respect the arcus marginalis, the confluence of the periosteum of the orbital rim and the periorbita, to minimize the risk of edema and lid eversion in the final result. Care is taken to avoid damage to the infraorbital nerve.

The dissection is extended to the piriform aperture medially, the oral vestibular mucosa inferiorly, and the superior/anterior border of the masseter muscle laterally. The dissection detaches the eyelids, external canthi and Lockwood ligaments, parotid fascia inferiorly and temporalis fascia superiorly, zygomatic muscles and levator labii superioris, and other muscles from their superior origins **(Fig. 8.3)**. The periosteum is very thin medially and a careful dissection avoids muscle injury. Complete periosteum release and division must be accomplished to avoid incomplete suspension.

The final step involves suspension of the mobilized midface to the deep temporal fascia using three 3–0 polyester sutures (Ethibond, Ethicon Inc., Somerville, NJ) to secure the cheek. The sutures are crossed and secured to the deep temporalis fascia, creating appropriate superior and lateral vectors of force. Systematization of the midface lifting is made at three main points: Bichat fat pad, malar fat pad, and sub-orbicularis oculi fat (SOOF) **(Fig. 8.4)**.

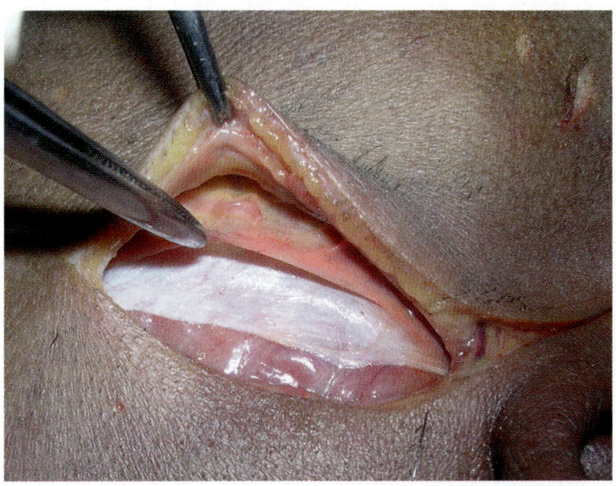

Fig. 8.2 Photograph of cadaver dissection showing the temporoparietal fascia (forceps) and the underlying deep temporalis fascia.

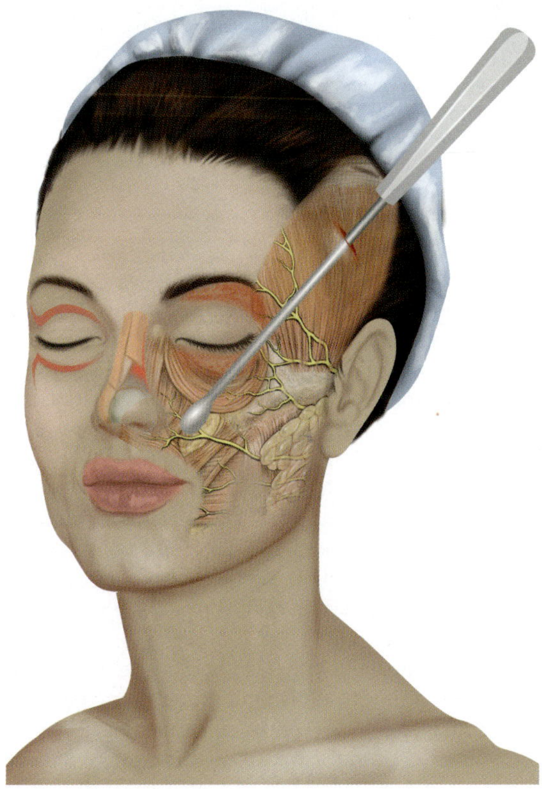

Fig. 8.3 Schematics showing the extent of undermining for the transtemporal subperiosteal facelift.

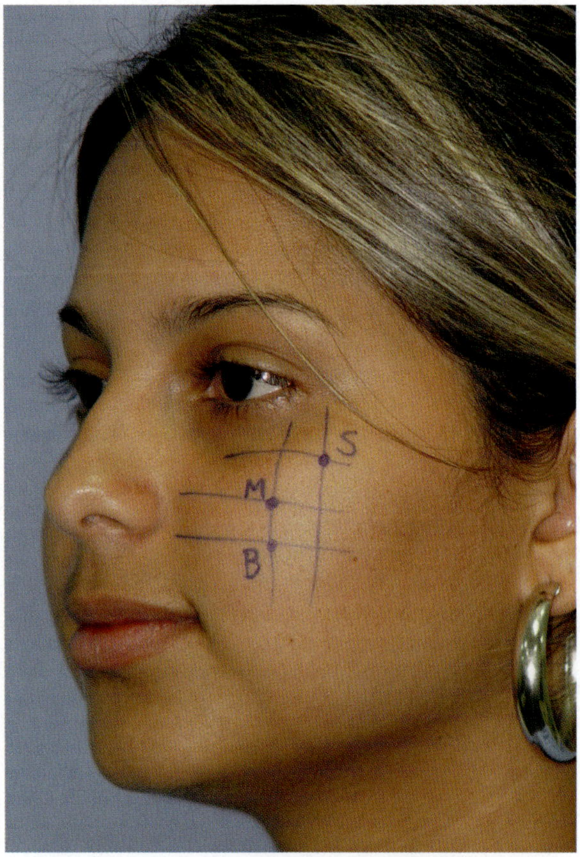

Fig. 8.4 Photograph showing the systematization of the three main points for midface lifting: Bichat's fat pad ("B point"), malar fat pad ("M point"), and sub–orbicularis oculi fat ("S point").

The first point, the "B point" (Bichat fat pad), is located at the intersection of a vertical line from the lateral canthus and a horizontal line from the nasal base. Suspension of this point promotes volumetric augmentation of the midface, elevation of the corner of the mouth, and restoration of a triangular face. The second point is the "M point" (malar fat pad), which is located at the intersection of the same previous vertical line and a horizontal line from the superior margin of the nasal ala. The third point, the "S point" (SOOF), is located at the intersection of a vertical line from the most lateral portion of the brow and a horizontal line from the inferior orbital rim.

These three previously marked points are lifted using a Casagrande needle[28] (similar to a Reverdin needle, but smaller) for passing the 3–0 polyester suture **(Fig. 8.4)**. The needle is introduced transcutaneously through the B point and, with an endoscopic view, is driven through the temporal incision. Then, the suture is passed through the needle's guide-hole and is returned to the Bichat fat pad area. Keeping the needle inside the soft tissues, a change of direction is performed to grasp more tissue, and the needle is driven to the temporal incision again. There, the suture is removed from the needle and is sutured to the deep temporalis fascia. The same procedure is performed at the M point and the S point, bilaterally **(Fig. 8.5)**.

At the deep temporalis fascia, the Bichat fat pad is suspended and sutured medially, the malar fat pad centrally, and the SOOF laterally. Such fixation lengthens the zygomatic muscles and the soft tissue of the cheeks, correcting tear-trough deformity and softening the nasolabial fold. The zygomatic area is also well modeled because the zygomatic muscle insertions are reinserted in a higher position. Both sides must be suspended and fixated concomitantly (interchanging one suture on each side) to avoid asymmetries **(Fig. 8.6)**.

The temporal scalp incision is closed by securing the temporoparietal fascia from the anterior edge of the incision to the deep temporalis fascia posteriorly. The skin is sutured with uninterrupted 4–0 nylon (Ethilon, Ethicon Inc., Somerville, NJ). In all cases, we use fat grafting to address the fat deflation.

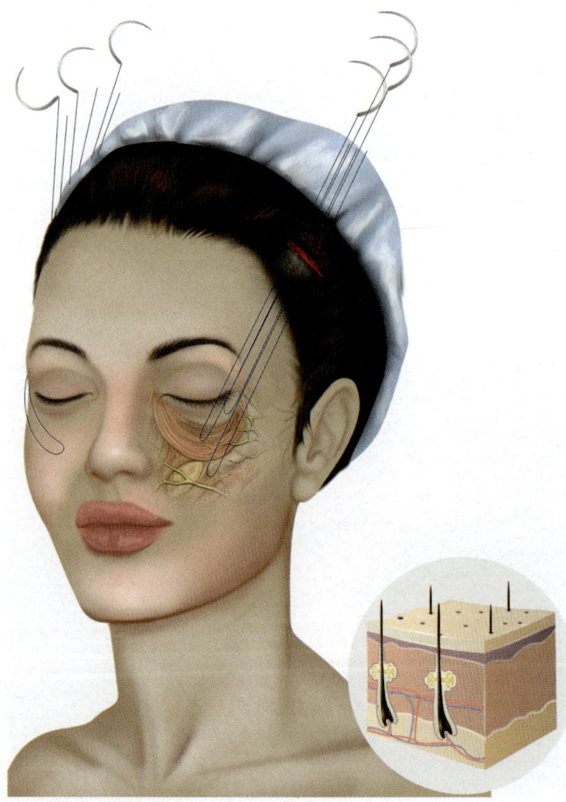

Fig. 8.5 Schematics showing midface suspension by sutures anchored to the deep temporalis fascia.

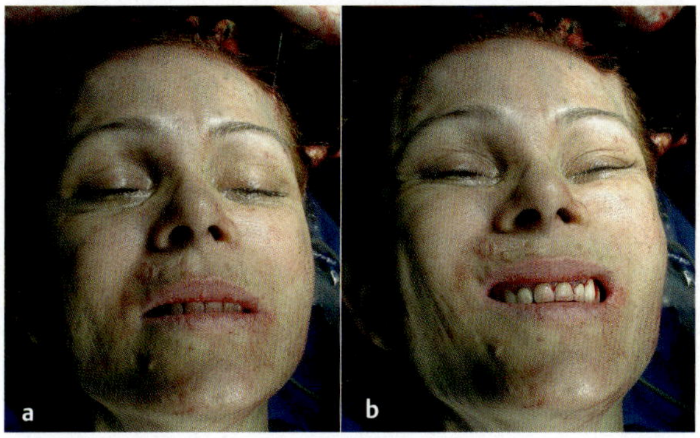

Fig. 8.6 Photographs showing **(a)** preoperative and **(b)** immediate postaoperative outcome of the midface lift when the surgeon pulls the sutures.

8.5 Postoperative Care

Proper postoperative care is as follows.

- Antibiotics are started prior to surgery and are continued for 7 days after surgery.
- A compressive bandage is used during the first 6 to 10 hours postoperatively.
- Supportive taping is placed for 7 days. (Another bandage is used for 7 days more after taping is removed.)
- Lid skin incision stitches are removed on the 7th postoperative day.
- Temporal skin incision stitches are removed on the 10th postoperative day.

8.6 Pitfalls and Complications

Prevention of complications is the best approach to managing them, but in spite of precautions during surgery, complications can occur. Well-recognized complications of facelift surgery include hematoma, hair loss, skin slough, hypertrophic scarring, infection, and motor nerve or sensory nerve injury. Major complications, including cardiopulmonary emergency, anesthetic disaster, and death, are fortunately extremely rare.[29,30]

Hematoma and seroma are the most common complications after facelift. Major hematomas occur in the first 10 to 12 hours postoperatively, due to hypertension, medication use, abnormal bleeding, intraoperative technique, cough, retching, and agitation. Expanding hematoma is a feared complication requiring prompt return to the operative room for inspection, hemostasis, supportive taping, and compressive dressing. Due to the bloodless plane of dissection, hematomas are extremely rare. Small hematomas and seromas can be either observed, needle aspirated, or rolled through openings in the incision.

Long-lasting edema, sometimes lasting more than 3 months, may occur and is due to the extensive undermining, especially at the zygomatic arch. It is advisable to avoid dissection over the whole zygomatic arch. Massage is recommended after the 7th postoperative day.

Nerve injury is one of the complications most feared by patients. Nerve damage is frequently transient, as a result of anesthetic infiltration, direct injection into the nerve, blunt dissection injury, edema of the nerve sheath, traction, or cautery trauma. Injury of branches of the facial nerve can be prevented with a careful dissection under the superficial layer of the deep temporal fascia, as the temporal branch of the facial nerve is located superficially within the temporoparietal fascia. Temporary numbness is caused by interruption of small sensory branches. Sensation always recovers, although it may take months to do so.

Hypertrophic scarring is frequently attributable to excessive tension on the incision closure. Nevertheless, some patients develop hypertrophic scars despite the best efforts of the surgeon. Diluted triamcinolone can be injected into the scars and usually improves the appearance of the scar considerably.

Asymmetries are rare. They are usually due to the learning curve of the procedure. Careful bilateral suture of the three points of suspension, using the lateral canthus as a parameter, is an important rule to follow. An augmentation of facial width may be noted, due to fat pads' repositioning superiorly and laterally.

When using the transblepharoplasty lowerlid approach, there are other concerns. Surgeons should be careful to avoid complications like lateral orbital skin excess, canthal deformity, and lower lid malposition.

Lateral orbital skin excess can be avoided by maximizing the lateral skin excision via temporal-brow incisions and by a wider preperiosteal lateral and superior undermining via lateral extensions of the lower lid incisions, allowing the lateral orbital tissues to more effectively redrape with elevation of the brow.

Lateral canthal anchoring procedures are used to provide excellent lid support and to avoid canthal deformity. A simple canthopexy is used in most of the cases. Canthotomy with horizontal lower lid shortening is used only in older patients who exhibit more severe degrees of laxity.

Lower lid malposition can be avoided by suture fixation of the musculoligamentous cheek flap to the periosteum of the lateral orbital rim and deep temporal fascia, providing secure elevation of the midface and minimizing postoperative midfacial descent. By performing the skin excision as usual for an isolated lower lid blepharoplasty, and before the subperiosteal cheek lift is performed, the amount of skin excision is reduced compared to the amount with performing the skin excision after the cheek lift and then stabilized to the lateral orbital rim, avoiding lower lid skin over-resection.

Patient satisfaction is imperative for facelift surgery. Although physicians try to help patients understand why complications occur, patients do not fully expect that complications will happen to them. Indeed, any complication detracts from the quality of the outcome; therefore, it is difficult for both surgeons and patients to accept complications.

8.7 Discussion

The earliest recorded contributions to the field of facial plastic surgery came from ancient Egypt and India over 25 centuries ago. In 1901, surgeons in Germany performed the first modern facelifts.[4] In these procedures, they excised ellipses of facial skin without any tissue undermining. In 1920 and 1921, Bettman[31] and Bourguet[32] were independently credited with the first subcutaneous rhytidectomy. Unlike previous procedures, this one consisted of extensive undermining and lipectomy. This subcutaneous facelift was the facelift most commonly performed prior to the 1970s. Subcutaneous dissection of a variably sized skin flap in the face and neck was performed, followed by redraping of the skin flap, excising the excess skin, and closing the incisions, and this surgery was mostly indicated on young, thin individuals with minimal ptosis of deep structures and no submental fullness. Advantages of this technique include ease of operation, limited postoperative edema due to limited dissection, no risk of facial nerve injury, and a smooth contour of the face immediately after the procedure. The major disadvantage of the subcutaneous lift was the fact that the deeper tissues of the neck were not lifted.

More recently, technique modifications have addressed the lack of long-term correction that occurred with the "classic" skin undermining procedures described in the early 1900s. In 1974, Skoog[33] describe a technique in which the fascia and platysma muscle were undermined to the level of the nasolabial fold and jowl in an attempt to address the lower third of the face. In 1976, the discovery of the superficial musculoaponeurotic system (SMAS) by Mitz and Peyronie[34] confirmed the existence of a fascial layer investing the facial mimetic musculature. It is also important to note that this was the first approach that advocated the effectiveness of imbrication as a rhytidectomy technique. The SMAS may be incorporated into the facelift operation in several ways. In an effort to obtain longer-lasting results, SMAS dissection and plication, or partial sectioning, can be done; however, the procedure has a longer learning period.

During the past 30 years, various modifications and changes to the traditional facelift techniques have been developed. They have varied in scope, incisions, and level of tissue dissection.

In 1979, Tessier applied his innovative and extensive experience in craniofacial surgery to aesthetic plastic surgery by utilizing the subperiosteal approach in the upper and middle thirds of the face.[9] His extensive use of the coronal incision allowed him to effect increased lifting of the temporal region and the lateral canthus by a subperiosteal dissection of the zygoma down to the maxilla, thereby reversing the changes in midfacial aging.

In the 1980s, the emphasis turned to improving the midface, traditionally the most difficult region of the face to effectively address. This was accomplished through the introduction of the deep plane and composite rhytidectomy, which was pioneered by Hamra.[35] He realized that by undermining the orbicularis oculi muscle through a lower blepharoplasty approach and joining this with the facelift dissection, he could create a composite flap that was composed of the orbicularis oculi, cheek fat, and platysma muscle. Repositioning the composite flap corrected these three ptotic areas while maintaining their relationship with each other and the skin. The SMAS and skin are dissected together as a single flap, rather than independently. The advantage of this procedure is that theoretically the flap is better vascularized and less likely to slough. The disadvantage of the technique is the magnitude of the procedure, the prolonged recovery period, and a higher risk of nerve damage.

Barton, in 1992, showed with histologic sections as well as cadaver and clinical dissections that the SMAS is the investing fascia of the zygomaticus major and minor muscles in the medial cheek, providing support for the clinical finding that the nasolabial crease was minimally improved by traction on the SMAS.[7]

Psillakis et al[10,11,12] described the subperiosteal midfacelift as an open, nonendoscopic procedure. Their technique involved subperiosteal dissection of the midface through a coronal incision in combination with an eyebrow lift. They thought that, since the SMAS was firmly attached to the periosteum through the facial muscles, the subperiosteal undermining was necessary for adequate mobilization of the cheek.

Isse[14] and Ramirez[15,16,17] were pioneers in developing the endoscopic approach to the midface. Ramirez noted that the midface dissection had several components, which required careful elevation of the suborbicularis oculi fat pad with the underlying periosteum along the inferior orbital rim and malar areas. By starting his dissection in the temporal area and creating a tunnel between the malar-zygomatic arch and the temporal pocket, he was able to suspend the midface suborbicularis oculi fat pad to the temporal fascia. He approached the zygoma from the superior direction along the deep temporalis fascia as Psillakis did. However, at 2 to 3 cm above the arch, he incised both the superficial and deep layers of the deep temporalis fascia to gain access to the zygomatic arch and to separate the periosteum and overlying soft tissue, as the frontal branch of the cranial nerve VII remained superficial to their dissection. He suspended the midface by placing sutures through the periosteum and the SOOF and the periosteum just superior to the zygomaticus major origin. Each suture was then secured to the deep temporalis fascia.

Several authors have advocated the nonendoscopic elevation of the midface through lower eyelid blepharoplasty incisions. In 1996, Hester, Codner, and McCord[18] published "The 'Centrofacial' Approach for Correction of Facial Aging Using the Transblepharoplasty Subperiosteal Cheek Lift." This technique was designed to correct midfacial aging by a central, direct approach, avoiding "extensive peripheral to central dissection in the subcutaneous, subSMAS, 'deep plane,' or subperiosteal plane." In 1996, Cardim described a subperiosteal blepharoplasty to correct midface aging.[19] Similar to this technique, in 1997 Paul published the periosteal hinge flap as a method of correcting midface aging.[20] This technique produced vertical elevation of the midface by suspending the subperiosteal cheek flap to a dissected orbital rim periosteal flap. Canthopexy was not routinely performed.

Moelleken[36] described a superficial subciliary cheek lift with the use of a single subciliary incision with suborbicularis dissection of the malar fat pad (superficial to the zygomaticus major and minor muscles) and fixation to the "intermediate" temporalis fascia located just lateral to the lateral orbital rim. Gunter and Hackney[37] presented a technique in which the cheek is undermined in the subperiosteal plane with fixation of the ptotic malar fat pad to the thick periosteum over the lateral orbital rim. They determine the amount of skin excision before the subperiosteal dissection is performed, avoiding lower lid malposition or having to perform a lateral canthoplasty.

The subperiosteal facelift fascinated many authors, since it raises the eyebrows, eyelid lateral corner, forehead, glabella, cheeks, and nasolabial fold, reaching the middle third of the face. This technique allows less incision, use of the endoscope, better fixation (especially of the cheeks), more ancillary procedures, repositioning of the Bichat fat pad, and jowl treatment.

The subperiosteal facelift is indicated for patients with significant aging and ptosis of the oval center of the face, tear-trough deformity, scleral show in severe malar pockets, past facial fractures, a need for simultaneous resurfacing, facial implants that need to be changed, or a need for soft tissue augmentation with fat transfer. It is even indicated in smokers.

As a result of the procedure, the cheek advances upward and backward and a tremendous amount of vertical lift is produced. The fat pad is repositioned, reducing the orbital hollow and the "double contour deformity." Volume augmentation is enhanced by meloplication that fills in both the "orbital hollow" and the "cheek hollow." The nasolabial fold is diminished. The "oral frown" is diminished, to a degree. Malar bags are diminished, to a degree.

The advantages of the subperiosteal facelift include: easier correction of prominent midface wrinkles, lateral orbital bulging caused by brow ptosis, and ptosis of deep soft tissue and orbital festoons; no compromise of the blood supply to overlying tissue, especially for cigarette smokers and those who have thinner tissue; and reduced possibility of facial nerve injury when compared with any other intermediate plane.

The subperiosteal facelift technique, as originally described by Tessier, has benefited from significant technological advances in medicine. The endoscope allows extensive subperiosteal undermining of facial soft tissue through minimal access incisions. Improved understanding of facial anatomy and the facial aging process allows surgeons to reposition and remodel the soft tissue envelope with excellent aesthetic results. Restoration of facial volume can be achieved with the subperiosteal techniques described and can be applied to the full spectrum of patients, with long-lasting results.

Correct diagnosis of age-related changes in the midface, therefore, dictates the most appropriate choice of surgical approach. If the findings are confined predominantly to the periorbital area, with only mild descent of the cheek structures evident, blepharoplasty utilizing a variety of techniques may be all that is required to restore a youthful appearance to the midface. Classical transconjunctival or skin–muscle blepharoplasty is effective when the problem is confined to fat pseudoherniation and skin excess, without deepening of the nasolabial fold. When mild cheek descent is present, with resultant thinning of the soft tissues over the infraorbital rim, and/or deep nasolabial folds are present, blepharoplasty with fat repositioning is more appropriate **(Fig. 8.7)**. Fat repositioning is especially indicated when a negative vector is present, and the bony orbital rim lies posterior to the plane of the cornea. These patients often have scleral show preoperatively, and scleral show can be exacerbated with fat removal, as in the traditional blepharoplasty.

As the distance from the infraorbital rim to the malar fat pad increases, the nasolabial folds deepen, and age-related perioral changes are evident, midface lifting should be considered along with blepharoplasty. The subperiosteal facelift is ideal because all areas of midface aging, from the lower eyelid to the perioral area, can be addressed with a single exposure, and the effects of gravity can be directly opposed by a 180-degree vertical vector. The transtemporal approach offers a good possible reversal of the effects of aging on the midface, especially when combined with a forehead lift **(Fig. 8.8, Fig. 8.9,** and **Fig. 8.10)**. On the other hand, the subperiosteal midface lift through a lower lid incision, combined with lateral canthal anchoring procedures, should be used when the patient presents with lower lid malposition (scleral show) and/or deformities of the lateral canthus.

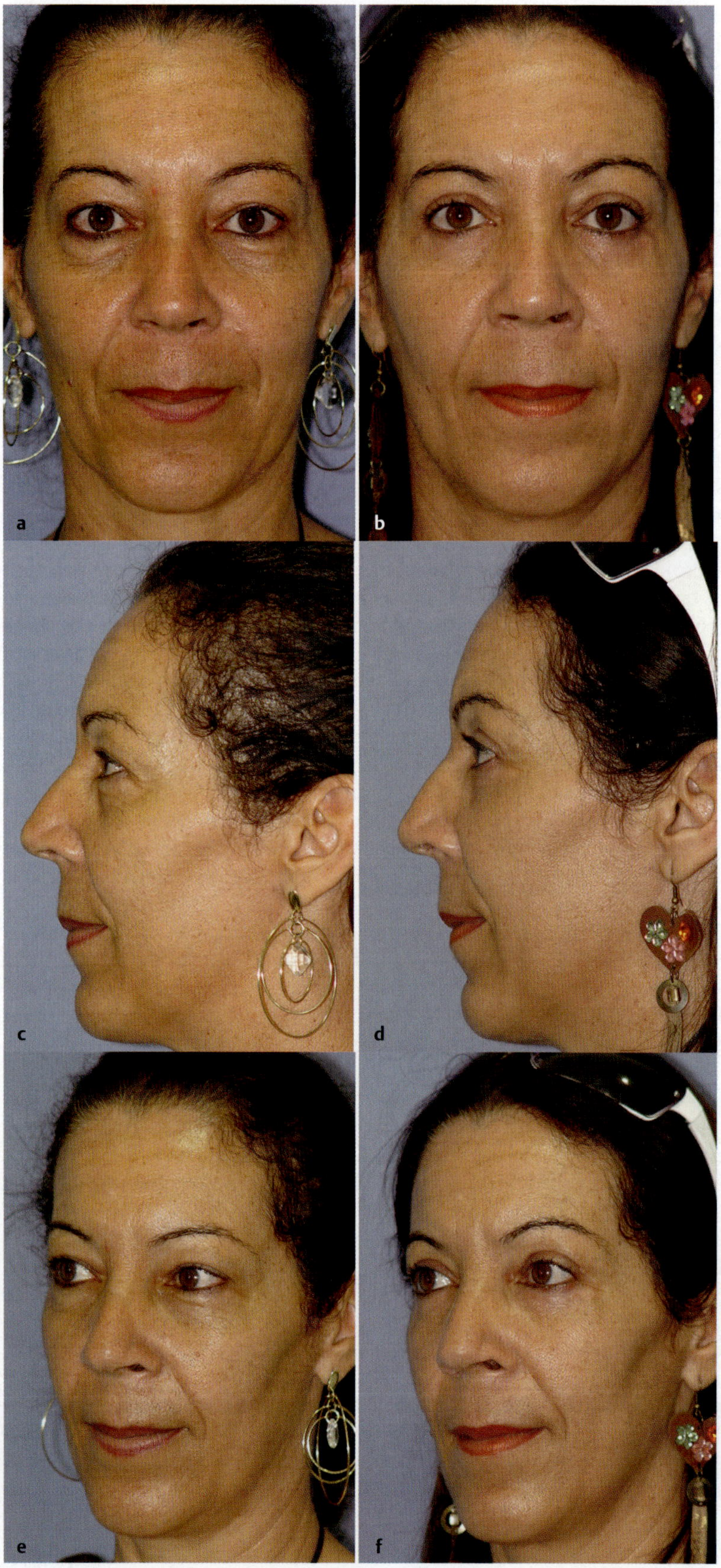

Fig. 8.7 (a,c,e) Preoperative and **(b,d,f)** 10-month postoperative photographs of a female patient who underwent blepharoplasty with fat repositioning.

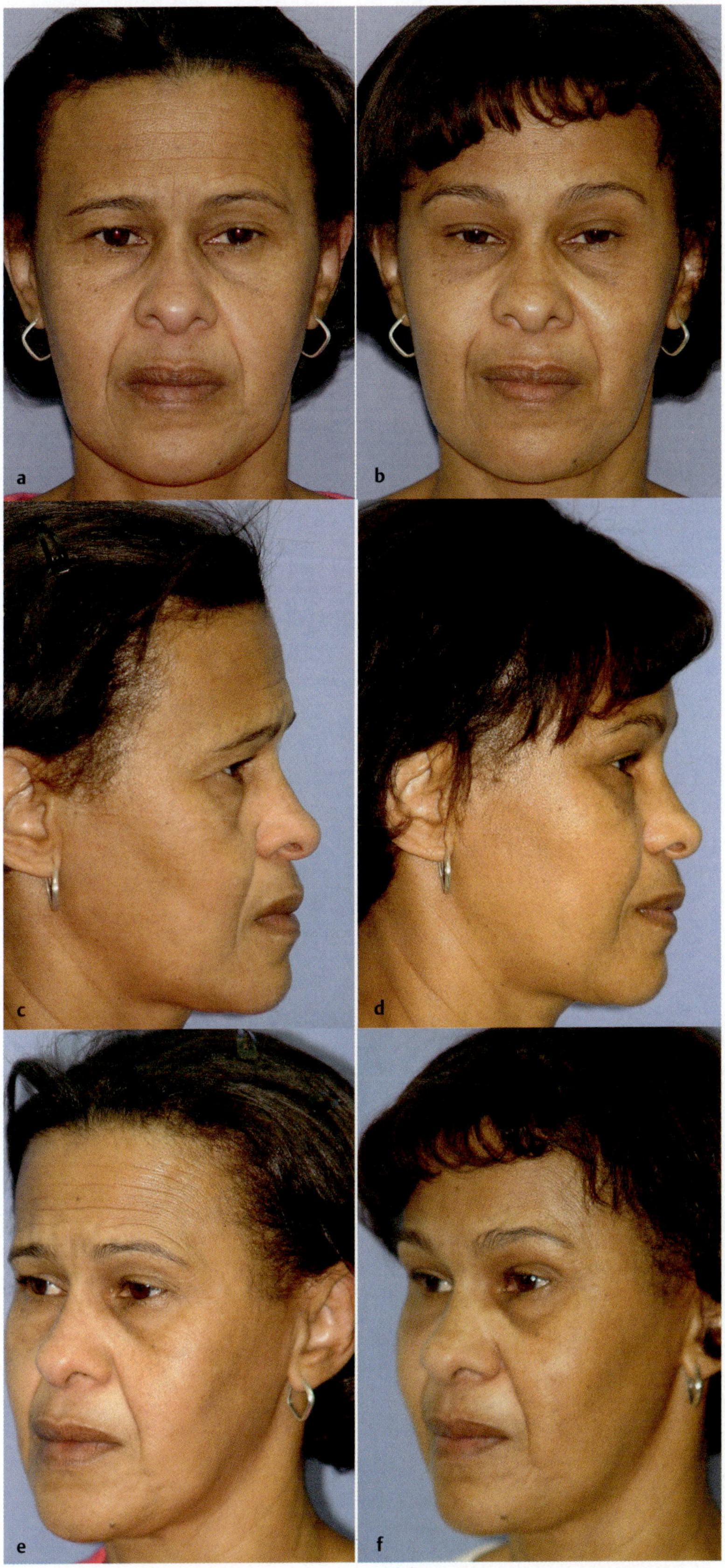

Fig. 8.8 (a,c,e) Preoperative and **(b,d,f)** 2-year postoperative photographs of a female patient who underwent subperiosteal midfacelift.

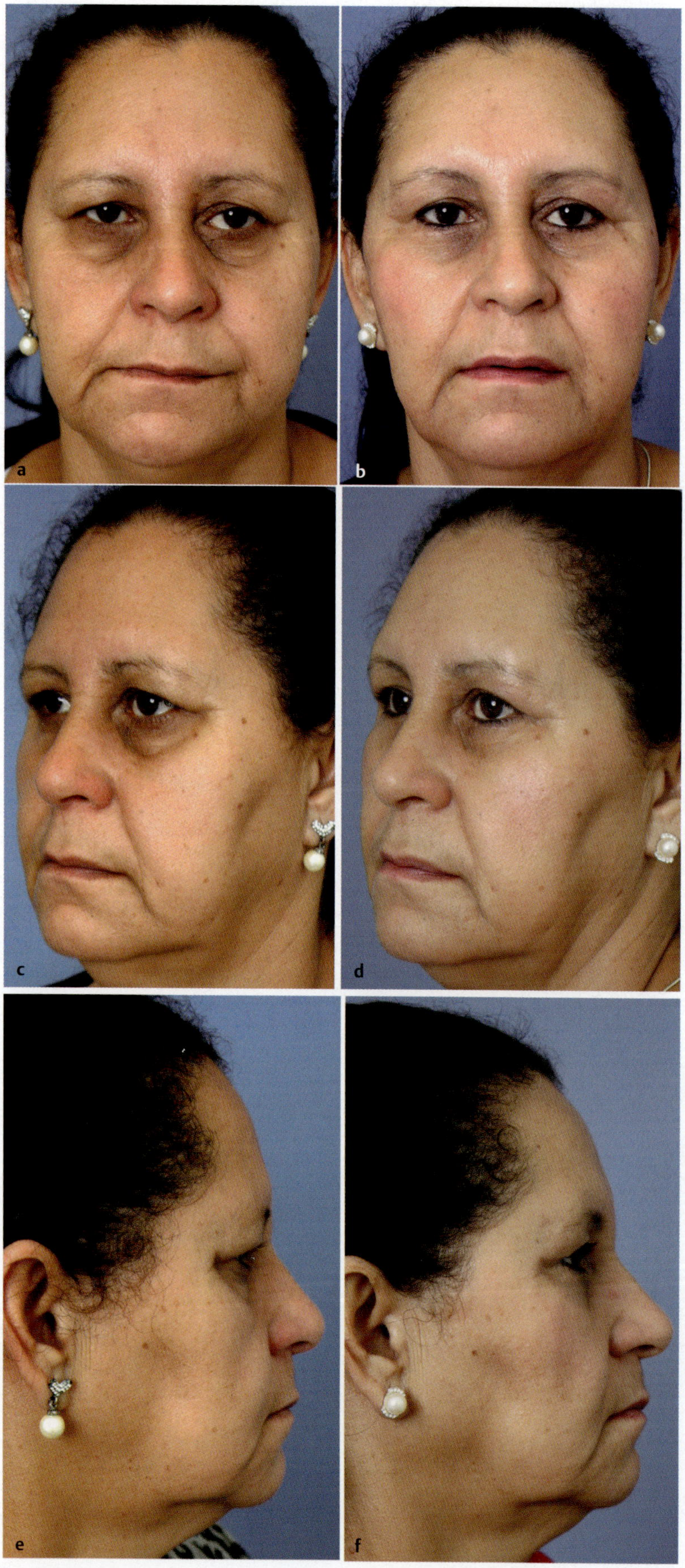

Fig. 8.9 (a,c,e) Preoperative and **(b,d,f)** 1-year postoperative photographs of a female patient who underwent subperiosteal midfacelift and endoscopic forehead lift.

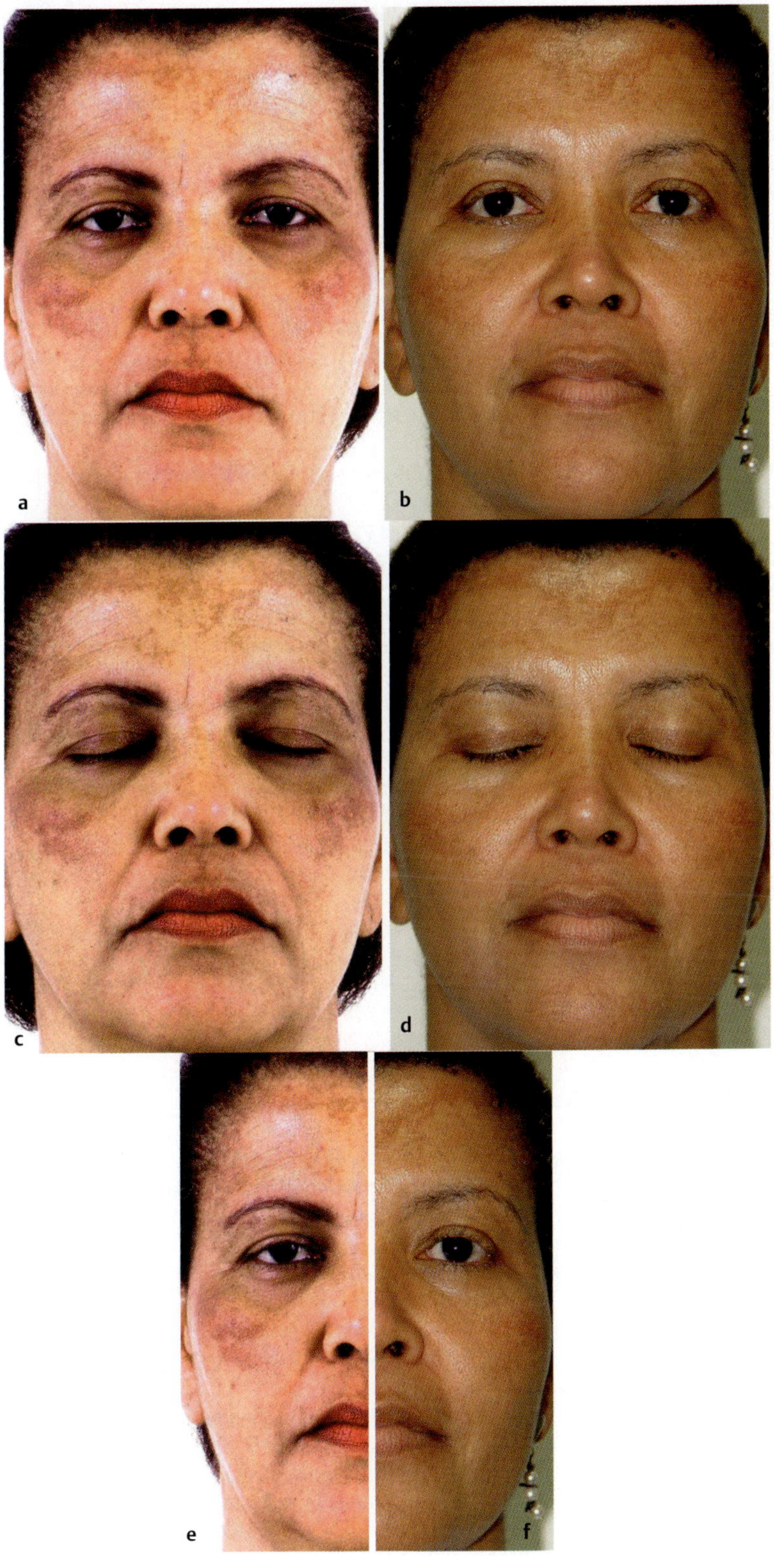

Fig. 8.10 (a,c,e) Preoperative and **(b,d,f)** 18-month postoperative photographs of a female patient who underwent subperiosteal midfacelift and injection of fat graft to the nasolabial folds.

Subperiosteal midface lift can be enhanced with injection of a fat graft (lipotransfer).[37] Coleman, in 1994, published his philosophy and technique of soft-tissue augmentation and lifting with fat grafting. He advocated that the technique of lipoinfiltration allows the surgeon to support and fill the periorbital region.[21] The graft helps to restore a youthful appearance in cases with more severe loss of midface volume. Ramirez also described his technique to address the atrophy of soft tissues, particularly the subcutaneous fatty layer. Three-dimensional endoscopic midface enhancement was achieved by adding volume to the midface while avoiding potential lower lid complications with temporal and intraoral access incisions.[24,25]

The demand for facelift surgery has increased dramatically in recent years as people from all socioeconomic levels become interested in facial rejuvenation. The evolution of surgical correction of the aging midface began with peripheral approaches and, as we began to understand the dynamics of midface aging, moved to a vector-based attempt to reposition ptotic soft tissues. Only later did the volumetric component of midface aging become a recognized essential clinical finding. The pathways developed to correct this component were repositioning of soft tissues when the displaced volume was adequate and were additive when more volume was required to recapture the soft tissue fullness of youth.

Anatomical knowledge, combined with a thorough understanding of the variety of techniques available, allows surgeons to provide patients with the best care possible. An important point to understand is that all techniques are simple to those familiar with them, and regardless of the procedure, the results will be better for those who adhere to the fine details and the art of the objective.

8.8 Conclusion

Subperiosteal facelift by the temporal approach is a procedure designed to rejuvenate the upper and middle thirds of the face. After subperiosteal detachment, the soft tissues of the cheek, forehead, jowls, lateral canthus, and eyebrows can be lifted to reestablish their youthful relationship with the underlying skeleton. The technique produces satisfactory cosmetic results in most cases, causing malar augmentation, nasolabial fold improvement, and mild jowl improvement.

References

1. Rees TD, Aston SJ, Thorne CHM. Blepharoplasty and facialplasty. In: MacCarthy J, ed. Plastic Surgery. Vol. 3. Philadelphia: W.B. Saunders; 1990:2320–2414
2. Patrocínio LG, Patrocínio JA, Couto HG, Muniz de Souza H, Carvalho PM. Subperiosteal facelift: a 5-year experience. Braz J Otorhinolaryngol 2006;72(5):592–597
3. DeFatta RJ, Williams EF III. Evolution of midface rejuvenation. Arch Facial Plast Surg 2009;11(1):6–12
4. Joseph J. Nasenplastik und sonstige Gesichtplastik nebst einen Anhang uber Mammaplastik. Leipzig: Kabitzch; 1931
5. Gonzaléz-Ulloa M. Facial wrinkles. Integral elimination. Plast Reconstr Surg Transplant Bull 1962;29(6):658–673
6. Adamson PA, Litner JA. Evolution of rhytidectomy techniques. Facial Plast Surg Clin North Am 2005;13(3): 383–391
7. Barton FE Jr. The SMAS and the nasolabial fold. Plast Reconstr Surg 1992;89(6):1054–1057, discussion 1058–1059
8. Tessier P. Face Lifting and Frontal Rhytidectomy. In: Ely JF, ed. Transactions of the Seventh International Congress of Plastic and Reconstructive Surgery. Rio de Janeiro, September; 1979
9. Tessier P. [Subperiosteal face-lift]. Ann Chir Plast Esthet 1989;34(3):193–197
10. French. PubMed PMID: 2473674. Psillakis JM. Ritidoplastia: nova técnica cirúrgica. Jornada de Carioca de Cirurgia Estética. Rio de Janeiro; 1982
11. Psillakis JM. Empleo de técnicas de cirugía craneofacial en las ritidoplastias del tercio superior de la cara. Cir Plast Iber Lat Am 1984;10:297
12. Psillakis JM, Rumley TO, Camargos A. Subperiosteal approach as an improved concept for correction of the aging face. Plast Reconstr Surg 1988;82(3):383–394
13. Santana PM. Craniofacial methods in rhytidoplasty. Cir Plast Ibero-Latinamer 1984;10:32
14. Isse NG. Endoscopic facial rejuvenation: endoforehead, the functional lift. Case reports. Aesthetic Plast Surg 1994;18(1):21–29
15. Ramirez OM, Maillard GF, Musolas A. The extended subperiosteal face lift: a definitive soft-tissue remodeling for facial rejuvenation. Plast Reconstr Surg 1991;88(2): 227–236, discussion 237–238
16. Ramirez OM. Endoscopic full facelift. Aesthetic Plast Surg 1994;18(4):363–371
17. Ramirez OM. Endoscopic facial rejuvenation. Perspect Plast Surg 1995;9:22
18. Hester TR, Codner MA, McCord CD. The "centrofacial" approach for correction of facial aging using the transblepharoplasty subperiosteal cheek lift. Aesthetic Surg Q 1996;16:51
19. Cardim VLM. Blefaroplastia subperiosteal. Rev Soc Bras Cir Plast 1996;11:7–14
20. Paul MD. An approach for correcting mid facial aging with a periosteal hinge flap. Aesthet Surg J 1997;17(1): 61–63
21. Coleman SR. Facial recontouring with lipostructure. Clin Plast Surg 1997;24(2):347–367
22. Little JW. Three-dimensional rejuvenation of the midface: volumetric resculpture by malar imbrication. Plast Reconstr Surg 2000;105(1):267–285, discussion 286–289
23. Ramirez OM. Full face rejuvenation in three dimensions: a "face-lifting" for the new millennium. Aesthetic Plast Surg 2001;25(3):152–164

24. Ramirez OM. Three-dimensional endoscopic midface enhancement: a personal quest for the ideal cheek rejuvenation. Plast Reconstr Surg 2002;109(1):329–340, discussion 341–349
25. Patrocínio LG, Reinhart RJ, Patrocínio TG, Patrocínio JA. Endoscopic frontoplasty: 3-year experience. Braz J Otorhinolaryngol 2006;72(5):624–630
26. Patrocinio LG, Patrocinio JA. Forehead-lift: a 10-year review. Arch Facial Plast Surg 2008;10(6):391–394
27. Casagrande C, Saltz R, Chem R, Pinto R, Collares M. Direct needle fixation in endoscopic facial rejuvenation. Aesthet Surg J 2000;20(5):361–367
28. Patrocinio JA, Patrocinio LG, Aguiar ASF. Complicações de ritidoplastia em um serviço de residência médica em otorrinolaringologia. Rev Bras Otorrinolaringol (Engl Ed) 2002;68(3):338–342
29. Sullivan CA, Masin J, Maniglia AJ, Stepnick DW. Complications of rhytidectomy in an otolaryngology training program. Laryngoscope 1999;109(2 Pt 1):198–203
30. Bettman A. Plastic and cosmetic surgery of the face. Northwest Med J 1920;19:205
31. Bourguet J. La chirurgie estetique de la face. Concours Med 1921;1657–1670
32. Skoog T. Plastic Surgery: New Methods and Refinements. Philadelphia, PA: W.B. Saunders; 1974
33. Mitz V, Peyronie M. The superficial musculo-aponeurotic system (SMAS) in the parotid and cheek area. Plast Reconstr Surg 1976;58(1):80–88
34. Hamra ST. Composite rhytidectomy. Plast Reconstr Surg 1992;90(1):1–13
35. Moelleken B. The superficial subciliary cheek lift, a technique for rejuvenating the infraorbital region and nasojugal groove: a clinical series of 71 patients. Plast Reconstr Surg 1999;104(6):1863–1874, discussion 1875–1876
36. Gunter JP, Hackney FL. A simplified transblepharoplasty subperiosteal cheek lift. Plast Reconstr Surg 1999;103(7):2029–2035, discussion 2036–2041
37. Coleman SR. Structural fat grafts: the ideal filler? Clin Plast Surg 2001;28(1):111–119

9 Minimal Incision Facelift Technique

Jaime Fandiño Izundegui

"We have to be able to grow up. Our wrinkles are our medals of the passage of life. They are what we have been through and who we want to be."
—Lauren Hutton

9.1 Introduction

The aging process is natural and unavoidable. Some of us accept the signs of aging as a natural part of growing older. Others believe that there is no good reason to look old and wrinkled, and they see cosmetic surgery as a way of regaining the smooth, tight facial appearance they enjoyed in their youth. It has been said that "youth is a gift, but age is an art."

Modern techniques in facial plastic surgery make it possible not only to tighten aging skin, but also to improve the underlying skeletal structures, to reduce superficial skin rhytids, and to treat skin lesions. With proper attention to each of the characteristics of the aging face (including the brow, eyes, ears, and neck), we can dramatically improve facial appearance while creating minimal telltale signs of rejuvenation surgery. Careful placement of incisions and judicious selection of procedures can result in the youthful appearance our patients often seek.

9.2 General Considerations

Major advances in facelift surgery over the past decade have allowed more natural-looking results. No one wants the "obvious" or "pulled" plastic surgery look caused by an overly aggressive or outdated surgical facelift technique. When performed by a skilled facial plastic surgeon, facelift surgery can take years off the face and help restore an overall more youthful appearance.

While it is not possible for us to completely reverse the signs of aging, we can achieve significant improvements. Our goal is to closely approximate the ideal while minimizing visible scars and ensuring the most long-lasting result possible. It is imperative that the surgeon aim for a balanced and harmonious result. Surgeons must inform the patient that addressing only the lower face will leave more stigmata of a lifted appearance. Potential benefits of browlift surgery, blepharoplasty, use of tissue fillers, etc., should also be discussed.[1]

The purpose of facial rejuvenation surgery is to elevate facial tissues that have descended with the aging process. A skin excision is performed, but this is not the sole goal. Most of the techniques rely on resuspension of the superficial muscular aponeurotic system (SMAS), through either the SMAS or the deep plane approach.[2]

The limited incision facelift, or short-scar facelift incision, begins at the bottom of the sideburn and follows into the ear, behind or anterior to the tragus, and ends just behind the ear lobe. Incisions are hidden, and signs of surgery disappear quickly **(Fig. 9.1)**. Patients can confidently appear in public 10 days after surgery. There is no scar in the hair, behind the ears, or in the neck, and women can wear their hair up without worrying about displaying telltale signs of traditional facelifts. Because the top of the incision is in the sideburn, there is no unsightly distortion of the hairline. The procedure reverses the loss of elasticity that has caused facial sagging and results in a firm, defined jawline.

Ancillary procedures include liposuction of the double-chin area and corners of the mouth, and fat transfer to the perioral area, lips, cheekbones, and chin. Use of fillers and eyelid surgery are done at the same time, when indicated **(Fig. 9.2)**.

9.3 Surgical Anatomy

Circulation to the facial skin is supplied by the external carotid artery, as well as by the superficial temporal artery, facial artery, transverse facial artery, and infraorbital artery. The internal carotid artery also contributes, with branches of the ophthalmic artery. The area that is routinely addressed during facelifting is the subcutaneous flap, which is based solely on the subdermal plexus, supplied by muscular cutaneous arteries, branches of the facial artery, and the infraorbital artery.

The SMAS is a fibromuscular layer that invests and interlinks the muscles of facial expression. The regional variations that are found in relationship to the SMAS are above the zygoma versus below the zygoma. Above the zygoma, the superficial temporal artery and frontal branch course through the SMAS. Below the zygoma, the SMAS fans out over the parotid gland and then above the masseter muscle before it surrounds the facial mimetic muscles.[3]

The SMAS has been noted to have several ligamentous supports, through which it adheres at specific points to the overlying dermis and underlying muscular or osseous attachments. These supports are the parotid masseteric ligament, the platysma auricular ligament, the zygomatic ligament, and the mandibular ligament.[3,4]

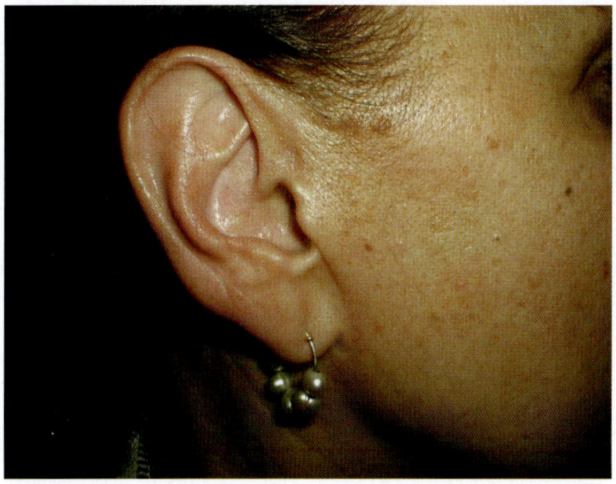

Fig. 9.1 Incisions are hidden, and signs of surgery disappear quickly. Lateral view of patient 6 months after surgery.

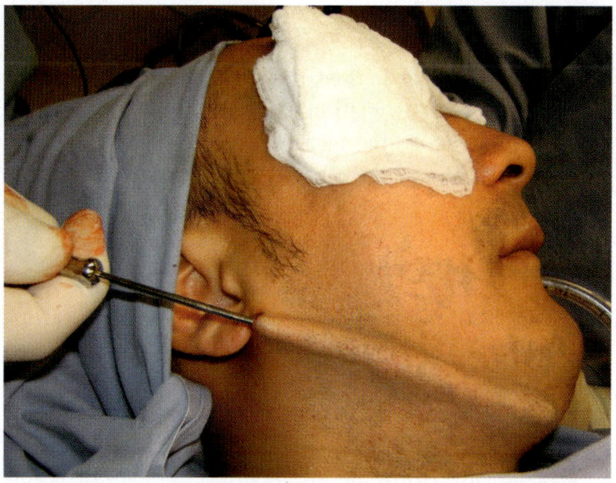

Fig. 9.2 Ancillary procedures like liposculpting of submental and submandibular fat can yield improved contouring in lower facial rejuvenation.

9.4 Preoperative Evaluation and Planning

The patient must understand that rhytidectomy helps correct excess skin, improves jowling, and provides redraping of the skin, but it does not change the quality of the skin itself. Patients who have good bony structure of the cheekbones, chin, and jaw during their youth will have the best results. The relationship between the hyoid bone and the mandible defines the course of the suprahyoid muscles in the floor of the mouth and can limit improvement in the cervicomental angle. A hyoid bone that has a high and posterior position will permit maximum elevation of the submental contour and definition of the submentum and will result in a neck with greater definition.[2]

The amount of actual skin excised, the tightness and completeness of the lift in the cheeks, the ability to contour and resuspend the neck, the smoothness of the submental region, and the degree to which the incisions can be camouflaged are all important considerations in achieving a natural, nonoperated appearance.[1,2]

9.4.1 Patient Categories

Based on Baker's classification, we have categorized candidates for minimal incision facelifts into four types[1,5,6]:

- **Type I:** The ideal candidate. Patients in their early 40s, with signs of aging primarily in the face, some slight cervical laxity, good skin quality, early presence of jowling, and submental and submandibular fat. The best approach for these patients is closed lipoplasty of the neck and jowls, wide subcutaneous skin undermining, and lateral SMASectomy. No retroauricular incision is necessary.
- **Type II:** The good candidate. Patients in their 40s to late 50s, with moderate jowls and moderate skin laxity, presence of submandibular and submental fat, and microgenia. Medial platysma bands are not present. The best option is lateral SMASectomy or plication and, if indicated, a chin implant. No retroauricular incision is required. If after closing all incisions a dog-ear is formed, this can be corrected with a small retroauricular incision.
- **Type III:** The fair candidate. Patients in their late 50s to early 70s. Presence of significant jowls, moderate cervical laxity, accumulation of submental and submandibular fat, and visible platysma bands on natural animation. The best approach is an open submental incision connecting subcutaneous undermining with the face and lateral neck. Open lipoplasty is performed to remove the submental and submandibular fat. A 4 to 5 cm wedge of platysma is removed and sutured in the midline. Retroauricular incision is performed when redundant skin is present.
- **Type IV:** The poor candidate. Patients in their 60s and 70s. They have significant jowls and active, lax platysma bands. Cervical elasticity is poor and skin folds with deep creases below the cricoid are often present. These patients are not good candidates for a short-scar rhytidectomy. It is common to have to extend the incision into the retroauricular area. Skin excess must be tailored into the retroauricular sulcus.

9.5 Marking

The patient has to be in the sitting position, gazing straight ahead, for a better evaluation of the descended tissues and effects of gravity on the face. Marking helps outline incisions, skin areas, and the severity of the descended tissue.

9.6 Surgical Technique

General anesthesia is preferred in an ambulatory setting or outpatient clinic center. Infiltration is done by predissecting facial areas with xilocaine with epinephrine, which improves hemostasis. The term "short-scar facelift" or "minimal incision facelift" refers to the type of incision used behind and below the ear. Patients who want to be able to wear a ponytail after surgery may choose this approach. There is a bit of trade off with the short incision, in that less neck lifting can be achieved. This trade off is acceptable for people who rate the importance of wearing a ponytail highly. Long-incision facelifts are sometimes recommended for people who require significant neck lifting. In most cases, incisions are located in well-concealed areas and are small enough to make scarring a minor issue **(Fig. 9.3)**.[7]

9.6.1 Incisions

The preferred incision is well within the temporal hair, making it necessary to excise a triangle of skin below the temporal sideburn at the level of the root of the helix. When the incisions are done properly, they heal well and camouflage scars. The incision does not have to extend higher than the frontotemporal hairline, allowing for the vertical elevation of the facial flap required even in a type III or IV patient.

The incision is curved anteriorly into the root of the helix, continuing inferiorly anterior to the tragus in a natural skin fold. When necessary, the incision can extend around the earlobe and behind the ear **(Fig. 9.4)**. Skin closure must be performed without tension. If a retrotragal incision has been performed, the flap of skin that overlies the tragus should be defatted, leaving only the dermis to preserve the anatomy in this area **(Fig. 9.5)**.

9.6.2 Skin Flap Elevation

Undermining is performed under direct vision to minimize trauma to the subdermal plexus and to preserve a significant layer of subcutaneous fat. Dissection extends across

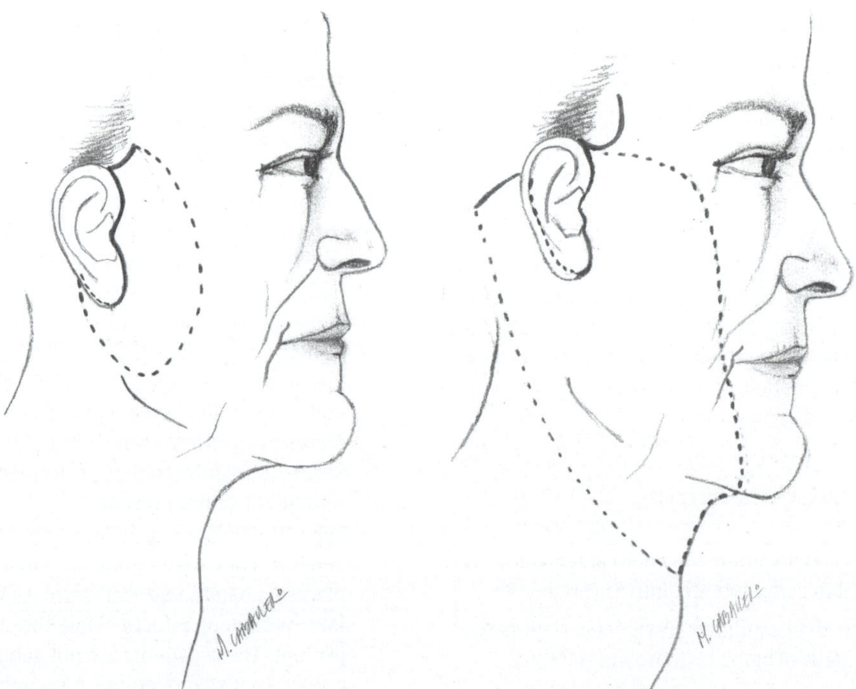

Fig. 9.3 The drawing on the left shows the typical short-scar facelift incision and the typical extent of the skin undermining with such a lift. The drawing on the right shows the typical incision pattern and the typical extent of skin undermining for a larger facelift.

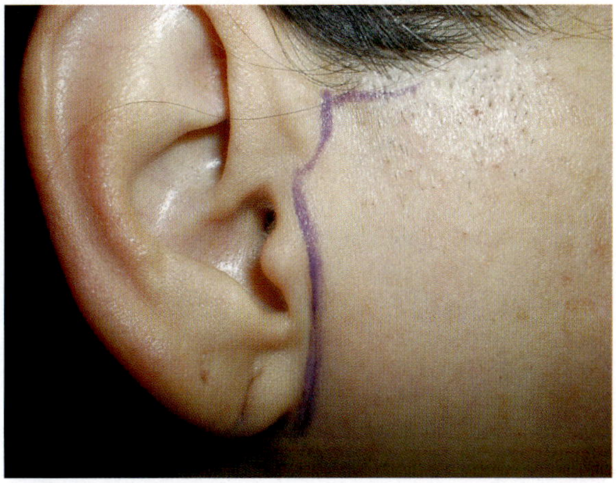

Fig. 9.4 Proposed incision outlined.

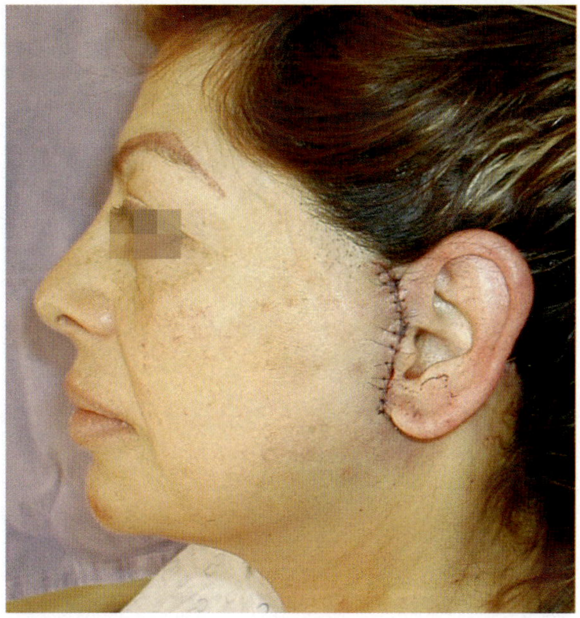

Fig. 9.5 Picture of patient 3 hours after surgery. No tension is on the wound. Notice the minimal bruising.

the zygoma to release the zygomatic ligaments but stops several centimeters short of the nasolabial fold. Subcutaneous dissection continues over the angle of the mandible and sternocleidomastoid muscle for 6 cm into the neck.[1,7,8]

9.6.3 Lateral SMASectomy, Including Platysma Resection

The incision line for the lateral SMASectomy is marked on a tangent that crosses from the lateral malar eminence to the angle of the mandible anteriorly, and to the edge of the parotid gland. Then, 2 to 4 cm of superficial fascia is excised. It is important to stay superficial to avoid parotid and facial nerve injury. To continue the lateral SMASectomy, a 1 cm strip of posterior platysma muscle is resected over the tail of the parotid and the anterior edge of the sternocleidomastoid muscle.

9.6.4 Vectors

SMAS suspension sutures are performed with 2–0 Prolene (Ethicon Inc.). The first SMAS suspension suture grasps the platysma at the angle of the mandible and advances it in a posterior direction to the fixed lateral SMAS overlying the parotid. This suspension suture lifts the cervical platysma and cervical skin. To close the rest of the lateral SMASectomy, interrupted 2–0 Prolene sutures are used **(Fig. 9.6)**.

Vectors are perpendicular to the nasolabial fold. The last suture lifts the malar fat pad, securing it to the malar fascia **(Fig. 9.7)**.

9.6.5 Skin Closure

After SMAS and platysma suspension, some tethering on the skin may appear because of the pull of the underlying SMAS. This tethering can also occur in the lower eyelid with elevation of the malar fat pad. Sometimes, subcutaneous undermining is necessary to free the tethers and to properly redrape the skin. When the SMAS layer is in its new position, it is impossible to close the skin flap without lifting and removing excess skin. Skin closure has to be done with minimal to moderate tension. When closing, the surgeon must pay special attention to eliminating the presence of any dog-ear formations of excess skin **(Fig. 9.8** and **Fig. 9.9)**.

Dog-ears may be present behind the earlobe, and they have to be trimmed and tailored into a short incision in the retroauricular sulcus. The most inconspicuous incision is a tragal incision along the free border of the tragus. One of the conspicuous signs of facelift occurs when skin tension pulls the tragus forward so that the ear canal is open. To avoid this, the last skin to be resected is in the region of the tragus. Final skin tailoring prevents tragal tension and distortion.[9,10,11,12]

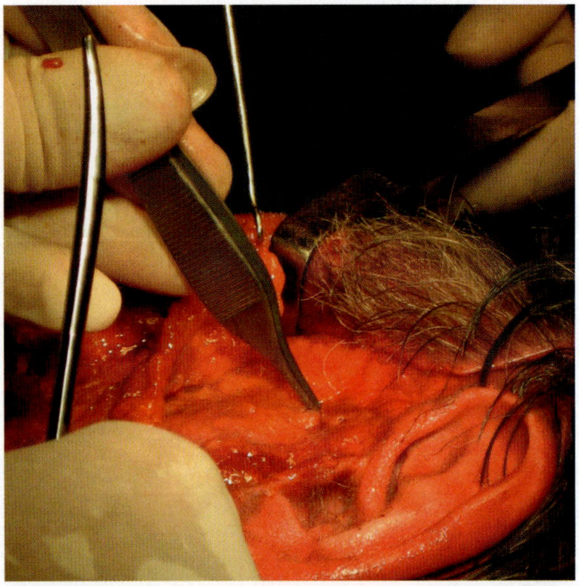

Fig. 9.6 SMASectomy is closed using interrupted 2–0 Prolene or nylon sutures.

9.7 Complications

Injury to any of the branches of the facial nerve and hematomas are the most common complications in facelift surgery. Injury of the facial nerve is a rare complication. The most vulnerable to direct damage is the frontal branch of the zygomatic-temporal division of the facial nerve, because of its superficial location. The most commonly injured nerve is the greater auricular nerve (sensory division of the facial nerve) because of its intimate association with the firm fascia surrounding the sternocleidomastoid muscle.

Hematoma is the most common and feared complication and requires immediate intervention to control bleeding and to evacuate and drain the newly dissected skin flaps. Smaller hematomas can be managed with serial needle aspirations and pressure dressings. The usual complaints are pain, unexpected swelling, chemosis, and firmness of the buccal region or neck area. To reduce the incidence of hematoma, careful attention to intraoperative hemostasis is very important.[2,7,8,11,12]

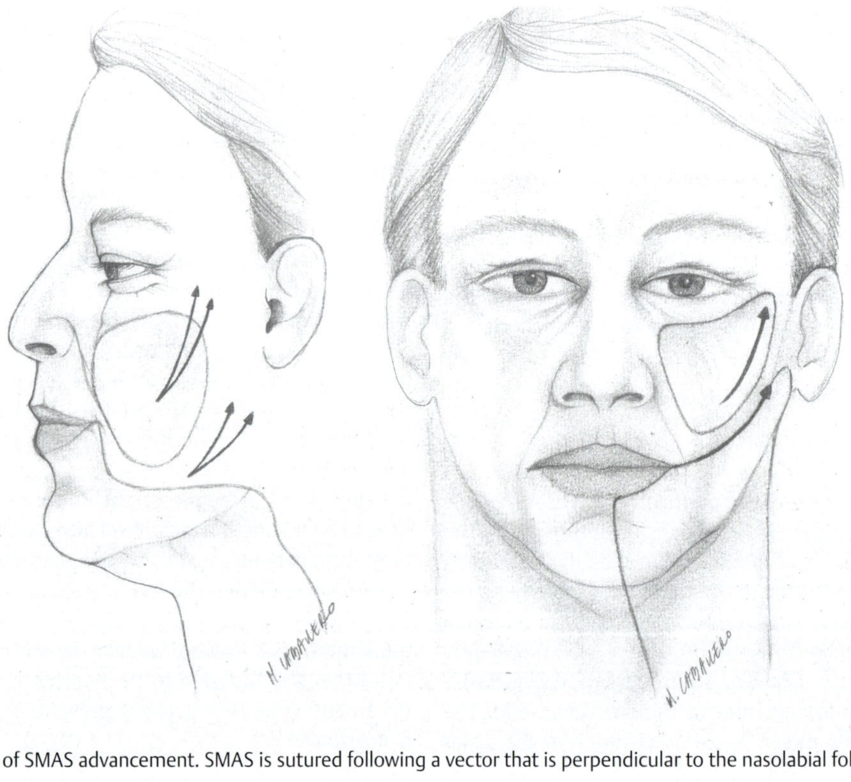

Fig. 9.7 Vectors of SMAS advancement. SMAS is sutured following a vector that is perpendicular to the nasolabial fold.

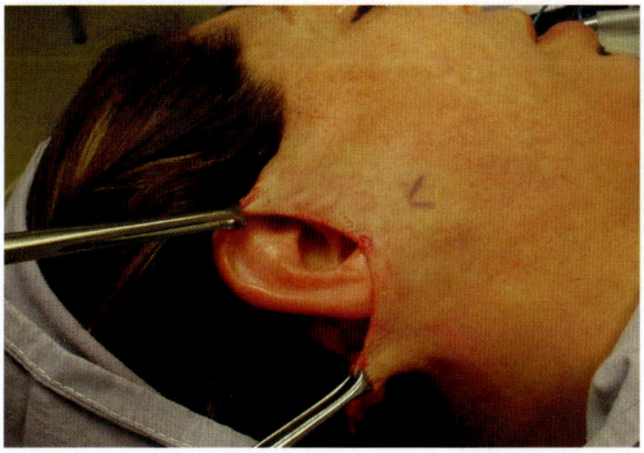

Fig. 9.8 Skin vectors. Redundant skin should be pulled in a superior and posterior fashion.

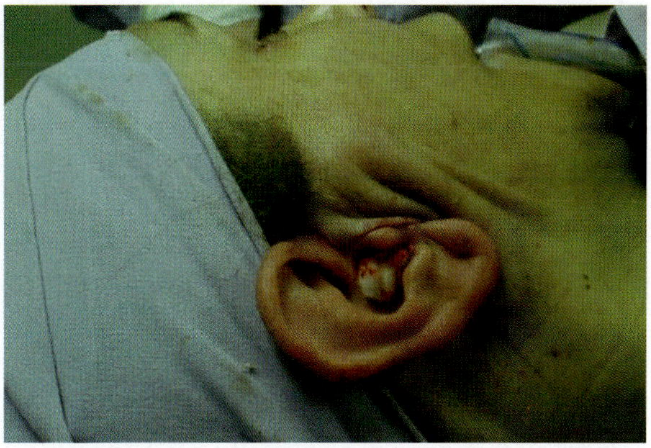

Fig. 9.9 When the SMAS is in the new place, it is impossible to close the skin flap without excision of redundant skin.

9.8 Postoperative Considerations

Postoperative care is relatively straightforward, barring unforeseen complications. A sizeable dressing, applied at the time of the operation, remains in place the first 6 hours, after which the dressing is removed and the wounds inspected. A minimal hematoma or seroma can be drained; if a hematoma is identified, then gauze may be used to roll out the blood. When necessary, sutures must be removed.

A lighter dressing that spans from the submental region to the top of the head, covering the exposed incisions, and one or two 3-inch bandage dressings are applied. The patient can then go home and may remove the dressing the following day.[13,14] Patients should be given instructions to call if they notice pain or any other discomfort. Sutures are removed between postoperative days 6 and 8. The patient is asked to return after 15 days, 1 month, 3 and 6 months, and then yearly. During these visits, anything needed to achieve better long-term results, like fillers, botulinum toxin, light peels, etc., can be done.

9.9 Conclusion

Our objective with all facial rejuvenation procedures is to obtain reasonable improvements with inconspicuous sequelae. It is not necessary to achieve phenomenal results in all cases. The most common untoward sequelae are altered hair patterns, deformed earlobes, and visible scars. We must plan our operations to incorporate strategically placed incisions to avoid these unaesthetic conditions (**Fig. 9.10** and **Fig. 9.11**).

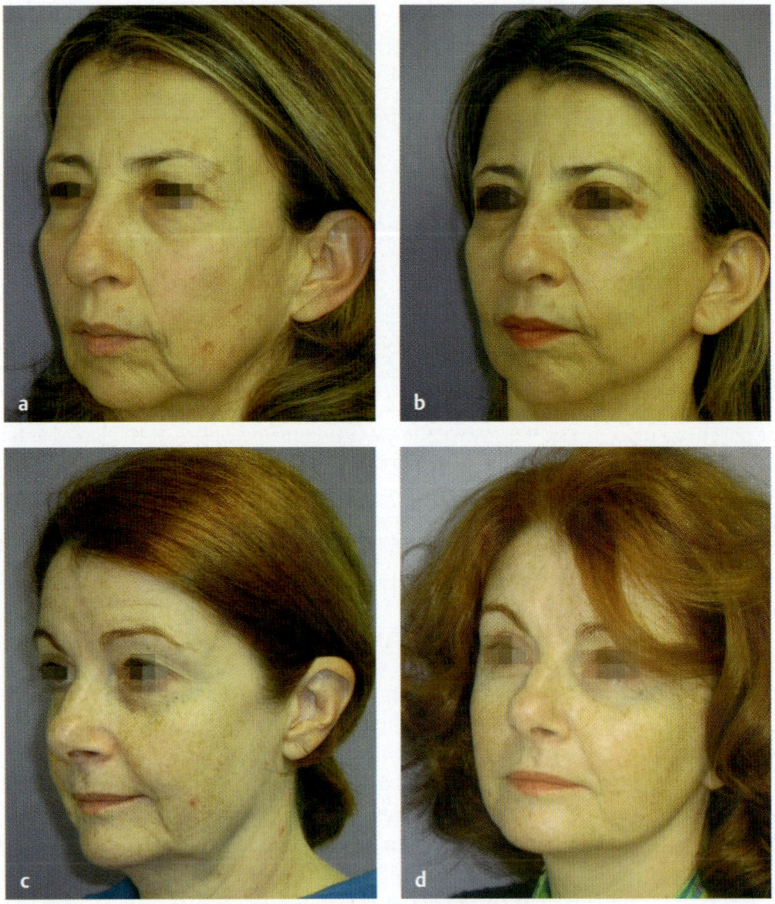

Fig. 9.10 **(a,c)** Preoperative images of patients before undergoing minimal incision facelift. **(b,d)** Results 3 months after surgery.

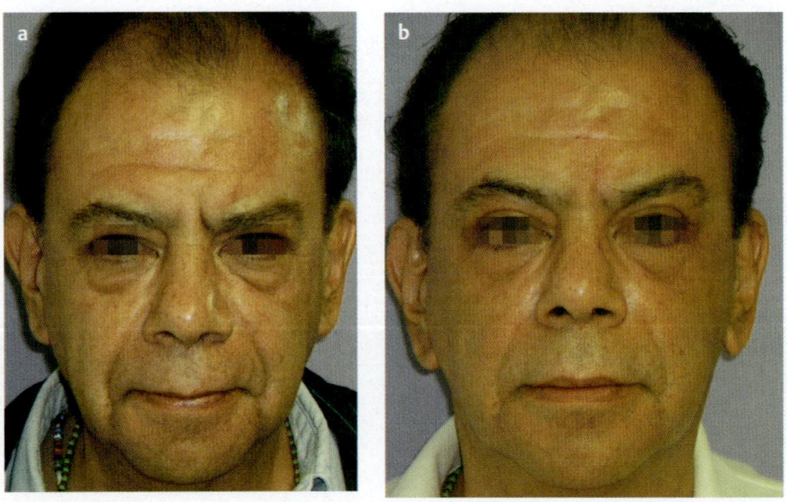

Fig. 9.11 **(a)** Preoperative frontal image of male patient. **(b)** Result 4 months after minimal incision facelift was performed.

References

1. Baker D. Lateral SMASectomy, plication and short scar facelifts: indications and techniques. Clin Plastic Surg NY USA 2008:533–550
2. Kridel R, Chacra Z. Rhytidectomy (Face-Lift). Bailey's Head and Neck Surgery, Otolaryngology. 5th ed. Baltimore, MD: Lippincott Williams and Wilkins; 2014:3103–3129
3. Larrabee WF Jr, Henderson JL. Face lift: the anatomic basis for a safe, long-lasting procedure. Facial Plast Surg 2000;16(3):239–253
4. Sherris DA, Larrabee WF Jr. Anatomic considerations in rhytidectomy. Facial Plast Surg 1996;12(3):215–222
5. Lambros V. Models of facial aging and implications for treatment. Clin Plast Surg 2008;35(3):319–327, discussion 317
6. Jacono AA, Rousso JJ. The modern minimally invasive face lift: has it replaced the traditional access approach? Facial Plast Surg Clin North Am 2013;21(2):171–189
7. Karam AM, Nayak LM, Lam SM. Short-scar purse-string facelift. Facial Plast Surg Clin North Am 2009;17(4):549–556, vii
8. Vincent D. Short scar rhytidectomy techniques. Atlas Oral Maxillofac Surg Clin North Am 2014;22(1):37–52
9. Zimbler MS, Mashkevich G. Pearls in facelift management. Facial Plast Surg Clin North Am 2009;17(4):625–632, vii
10. Fogli A, Desouches C. Less invasive face-lifting: platysma anchoring techniques. Clin Plast Surg 2008;35(4):519–529, vi
11. Nease CJ, Aldridge E, English JL. Adjunctive techniques in contemporary rhytidectomy. Atlas Oral Maxillofac Surg Clin North Am 2014;22(1):75–89
12. Adamson PA, Dahiya R, Litner J. Midface effects of the deep-plane vs superficial musculoaponeurotic system placation facelift: a comparative study. Arch Facial Plast Surg 2004;6:8
13. Farrior E. Aging-face surgery. In: Park SS, ed. Facial Plastic Surgery: The Essential Guide. New York, NY: Thieme; 2005:254–299
14. Lam SM, Williams EF III. Lower facial rejuvenation. In: Williams EF III, Lam SM, eds. Comprehensive Facial Rejuvenation. Baltimore, MD: Lippincott Williams and Wilkins; 2004:105–151

10 Eyebrow Lift Technique

José Roberto Parisi Jurado and Leila Freire Rêgo Lima

10.1 Introduction

Throughout history, in all civilizations, mankind has always looked for new ways to improve physical appearance. Youth has always occupied a prominent place in our minds.[1] In ancient Egypt, the dead were buried with pots of beauty creams, to immortalize their beauty even after death. In ancient Greece, men and women took pride in their physical appearance and would use oils, scents, and makeup to improve their looks. Regarding the Romans, beauty was reflected in the power to win battles and to expand their frontiers.[1]

With aging, there is a gradual loss of skin elasticity and weakening and increased laxity of the skin. In the face, this aging process results in the appearance of wrinkles, skin laxity, and presence of age spots, and irregular pigmentation in the skin. The upper third of the face is an area where the signs of aging can really become apparent. Exposure to sun, wind, and other external agents can result in brow ptosis and the presence of rhytids, giving patients a tired, sad, angry, and "old-looking" appearance.

Ptosis of the brows can have a functional or a cosmetic component. The eyebrow lift is a surgical procedure that aims to raise eyebrows that have descended because of a normal aging process or as a result of a functional problem. The eyebrows are structures composed of skin covered with hair and subcutaneous tissue, giving a particular aspect to the eye region. The eyebrow has three components: a head, a body, and a tail, with different characteristics depending on the gender. Having a clear understanding of the anatomy of the frontotemporal region is a must to give better results and avoid unwanted complications or unacceptable results.

10.2 Etiology

The aging process affects the skin and the deeper tissues through intrinsic and extrinsic factors.[2] Intrinsic aging factors are the result of the hormonal and biochemical modifications associated with the aging process on the skin.[3] There is a progressive loss of the organization pattern of collagen and elastic fibers (elastosis) and the weakening of underlying muscles.[4]

The most important extrinsic factor is the continuing force of gravity, which promotes displacement of the subcutaneous tissue, with drooping of facial features having an important impact on the forehead, the eyebrows, and the eyelids. Smoking and sun exposure are also key factors that are associated with the facial aging process, causing coarse wrinkles and a rough skin surface.[5]

Intrinsic and extrinsic factors include:

- Imbalance between the eyebrow elevator muscles and eyebrow depressors
- Decrease of collagen and elastin
- Menopause and andropause
- Sun exposure
- Smoking

10.3 Anatomy

The layers of the frontal region are as follows[5]:

- Skin
- Subcutaneous tissue
- Superficial fascia of the superficial musculoponeurotic system (SMAS)
- Musculature of the frontal region: frontal muscle, orbicularis oculi muscle, corrugators, supercilii muscle, and procerus muscle
- Deep fascia of the SMAS
- Pericranium
- Frontal bone

The facial muscles can be divided into two groups: muscles of mastication and muscles of expression. The muscles of expression, both deep and shallow, move the loose tissues of the face. It is through them that we express our emotions and feelings. They are also responsible for the presence of wrinkles and the formation of the "lines of expression" in the face.[6]

The movements of the frontal region are the result of the action of four muscles: frontal, procerus, corrugator supercilii, and the orbital portion of the orbicularis muscle.

The scalp consists of skin, subcutaneous tissue, galea or aponeurosis tissue, and areolar and periosteum tissue. Galea is a tough tendon blade that connects the frontal muscle to the occipital muscle. The galea is attached laterally to the temporoparietal fascia, which is aligned with the aponeurotic muscular system (SMAS) on the face.

The frontalis muscle originates from the galea and is attached to the skin of the forehead. It is the muscle responsible for raising the eyebrow and its innervations is stimulated by the temporal branch of the facial nerve. The depressor muscles of the eyebrow are the corrugator supercilii, orbicularis oculi muscle, and procerus.[7]

Lateral to the temporal line, on the temporal fossa, lies the temporal muscle, covered by its fascias. The superficial temporal fascia, or temporoparietal fascia, is located just under the skin and subcutaneous fat of the temporal region. Medial to the temporoparietal fascia, galea is attached. The temporoparietal fascia is continuous with the SMAS in the lower third of the face. Under the temporoparietal fascia lies the deep temporal fascia, or true temporal fascia.[7]

Signs of aging of the upper third of the face include: eyebrow ptosis, crow's feet, wrinkles in the lower eyelid, and fine and deep wrinkles on the forehead and glabela, as well as loss of elasticity.[8]

Patient assessment must be performed statically and dynamically. The patient should be placed in front of a mirror and asked to move the facial muscles. The real position of the eyebrows can be observed after asking patients to close their eyes for 10 to 20 seconds to allow total relaxation of the forehead musculature and, when the eyes are open, the real position of the eyebrow should be noted.[8]

Palpation of the eyebrow is another way that can be used to identify its real positioning. It must be noticed that there are particular differences between men and women. In women, the eyebrow should form an arch, 1 cm above the supraorbital foramen. The medial end should be on the orbital margin and the lateral end just above.

The upper limit of the eyebrow should match the lateral border of the limbus.[9] In men, the eyebrow should match its outline along the orbitary edge more horizontally straightened than in women. The distance between the mediopupilar line and the bottom edge of the eyebrow is 2.5 cm, and the distance from the top edge of the eyebrow to the anterior hairline is 5 cm.[10,11]

The medial portion or head of the eyebrow has its origin in a lower vertical line that extends to the alar-facial junction. The lateral extension of the eyebrow should reach a point where a line drawn from the lateral canthus reaches the ala of the nose.[12] The distance between the two medial ends of the eyebrows must be equal to the distance between the outside edges of the nostrils (**Fig. 10.1**).

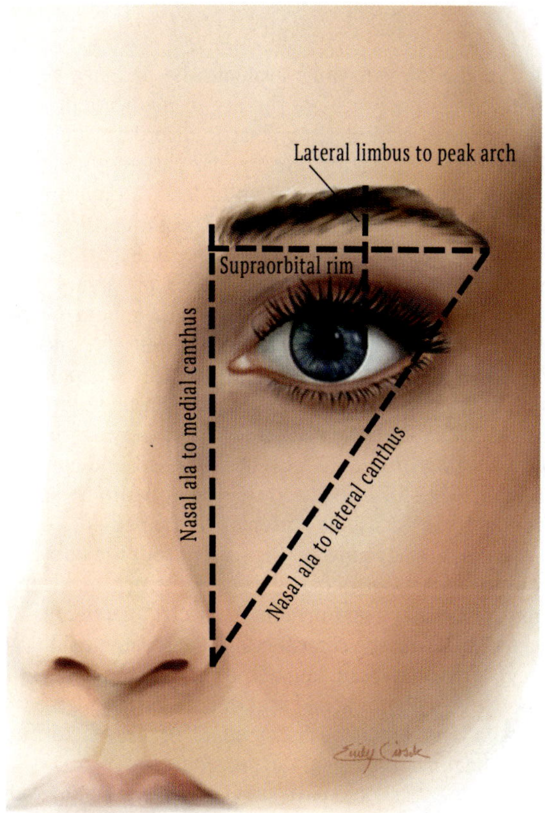

Fig. 10.1 Ideal brow position. In women the brow should lie slightly above the supraorbital rim. The brow ideally should be curved with its peak lined at the lateral limbus. The medial edge of the brow should be aligned vertically with the medial canthus and the lateral nasal ala. The lateral edge of the brow should be near an oblique line drawn from the lateral nasal ala passing the lateral canthus. In men brows are flatter and don't have the lateral peak.

10.4 Patient Evaluation

Accurate knowledge of anatomy, combined with static and dynamic clinical examination of the patient, make it possible to determine the timing and success of surgical treatment.[13,14] Regarding the facial aging process, especially in the forehead, skin ptosis can be significant, resulting in lax skin that moves into the upper orbit. This can produce the illusion of skin redundancy along the upper eyelid.[13] One of the most common errors is to perform an upper blepharoplasty when the desirable procedure would have been an eyebrow lift.

Eyebrow ptosis, clinically, has two main components: (1) low position of the eyebrow and (2) low position of the supratarsal fold.

10.4.1 Flower Sign

The flower sign describes how patients lift their eyebrows with their fingers to express their need for eyelid surgery.[14] This should alert surgeons to evaluate the frontal region and brow area, because many times what needs to be treated is this area instead of the eyelids.

10.4.2 Connell's Sign

A skin fold of the upper eyelid that protrudes laterally over the periorbital region is a hallmark of ptosis of the forehead. Therefore, it is important to distinguish problems between the upper eyelid and the forehead.[15]

10.5 Patient Selection

Initially, the surgeon must evaluate the patient's general health conditions, such as: the use of medications, allergies, previous surgeries, psychiatric disorders, and social habits, such as smoking. Ideally, the patient should stop using tobacco and nicotine from at least 1 month before umtil 1 month after the procedure. The patient's refusal to cooperate affects the result of the procedure and should be reason enough to turn down a candidate for surgery.[8]

An assessment of the patient's face should be performed. This consists of inspection in front of a mirror to check for and identify any asymmetries, as well as palpation of all facial structures. All findings should be pointed out and discussed with the patient before surgery. Limitations of the surgical procedure must be discussed, and nonsurgical alternatives like peels and the use of neuromodulators and fillers should also be presented to the patient.

Degrees of asymmetry originating from the bony skeleton and habits of personal behavior (such as sleeping habits or repeated and involuntary facial expressions) are discussed during the clinical evaluation.[8] Patient skin type is registered, and discussion of the possibility of a resulting hypertrophic and/or keloid scar in both African descent or Asian patients should be discussed. All of these factors may affect the final outcome of the procedure.

All patients should have standard clinical photographs taken. This will help the surgeon to identify any asymmetrries and will help in deciding what procedure will be performed.

10.6 Surgical Approaches

10.6.1 Eyebrow Lift with Limited Incision

The technique proposed by David M. Knize excludes the use of the endoscope.[10,11] Two fusiform incisions of 2.5 cm by 1 cm are performed lateral to the temporal lines, and, with the aid of a retractor, a dissection plane right on top of the deep temporal fascia is created and extended to the level of the orbital rim, where the periosteum is separated. This permits traction of the tail of the eyebrow with 3-0 Prolene (polypropylene; Ethicon Inc.).[13,14]

For this technique, the head of the eyebrow is treated by an upper blepharoplasty incision, then the eyebrow corrugator muscles are dissected and sectioned. Another option is that the surgeon can section the procerus muscle, although it is imperceptible at sight.

10.6.2 Coronal or Open Eyebrow Lift

A bitemporal incision is performed in the scalp region all the way down to the galea or the periosteum. A flap is elevated to the superior orbital rim. Eyebrow suspension to the desired level is done by fixation with absorbable or nonabsorbable suture threads to the adjacent temporalis muscle flap and resection of excess tissue.

The extensive scar is hidden behind the hairline, making the procedure technically simple and eyebrow suspension uniform. The disadvantages are: excessive bleeding during surgery, an extensive raw area, and increased recovery time when compared with other techniques. In bald patients, the scar is clearly visible.[16,17]

Criticisms of the use of open techniques include the possibility of a visible scar, alopecia along the incision site, and paresthesia on the forehead. Although any of these problems may occur, paresthesia can be avoided by protecting facial nerve branches.[15]

10.6.3 Surgical Description of Eyebrow Lift—Personal Technique

The surgical markings are performed with the patient sitting upright with the eyes open and looking forward. The temporalis lines, as well as the four incision sites, are marked: two fusiform incisions measuring 2.5 × 1 cm in the temporalis regions and two transverse incisions measuring 1 cm in posttrichialis parietal regions (**Fig. 10.2**).

Local infiltration is performed near the supraorbital and supratrochlear nerves, the incision sites, and the surroundings of the orbital rim with a solution of 1% lidocaine and epinephrine 1:40,000 (**Fig. 10.3**).

Incisions are made with a no. 15 blade. The temporal incision is dissected to the deep temporalis fascia, and the parietal incision is dissected to the periosteum (**Fig. 10.4** and **Fig. 10.5**). Tissue is elevated following the deep temporalis fascia and the subperiosteal plane, respectively.

Elevation of tissue planes (deep temporalis facia and subperiosteal plane) can be done under direct vision or using an endoscope (**Fig. 10.6**). Two 3 to 4 mm incisions are placed at the lateral brow area. A Reverdin needle is passed in a subcutaneous plane and is directed cephalically, and it exits through the temporal incision, where it is threaded with a 2-0 nylon suture. The same procedure is done to exit in the parietal incision (**Fig. 10.7**).

Once the needle is threaded with the suture, it is returned in the same subcutaneous plane to the small apertures at the level of the eyebrow. The needle that exits through the medial eyebrow incision is directed into the subperiosteal plane and then upward, where it exits in the parietal region. The needle that exits in the lateral incision is directed upward, following the deep temporalis fascia, and exits over the temporal region (**Fig. 10.8**).

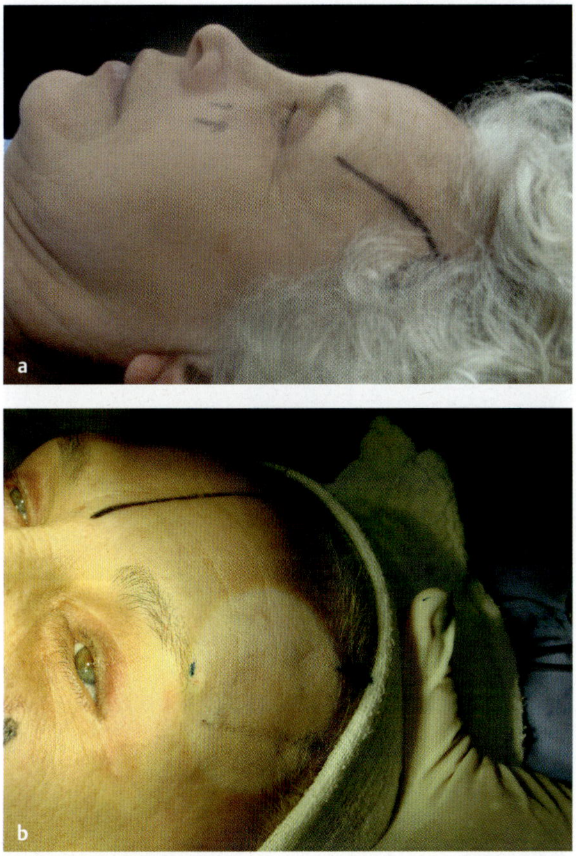

Fig. 10.2 **(a,b)** Incisions. An incision measuring 2.5 x 1 cm is marked in the temporal region and a transverse 1 x 1 cm incision is placed in the parietal region behind the hairline.

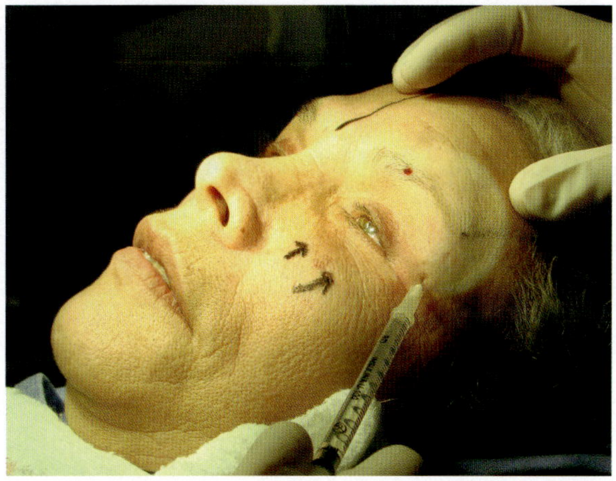

Fig. 10.3 Infiltration is performed near the supraorbital and supratrochlear bundles, around the orbital rims, and in the incision sites. A solution of 1% lidocaine and epinephrine 1:40,000 is used.

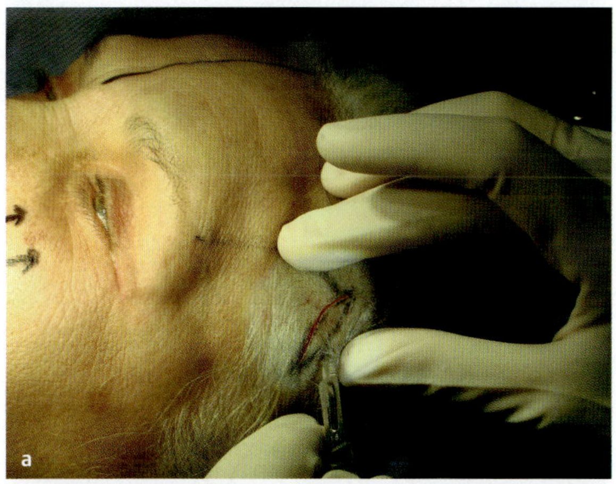

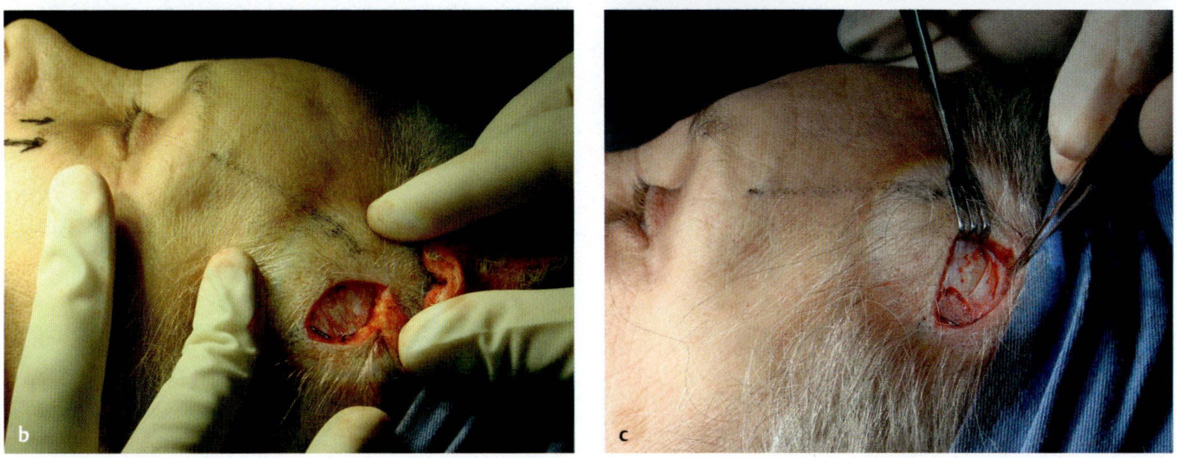

Fig. 10.4 **(a,b)** An elliptical incision is made using a no. 15 blade. **(c)** Dissection is done to the subperiosteal plane.

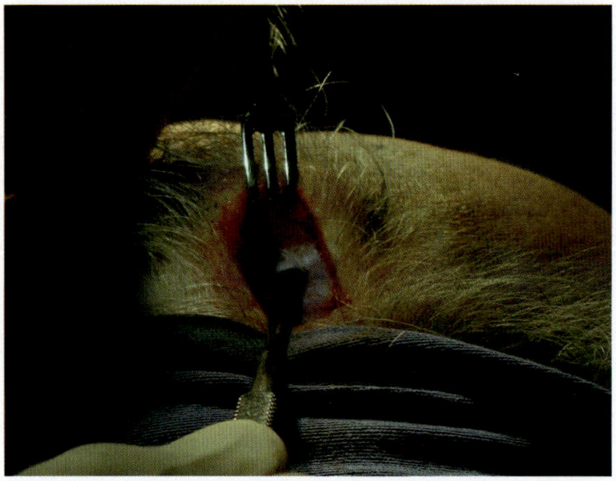

Fig. 10.5 An incision is made in the temporal area until the deep temporalis fascia is reached.

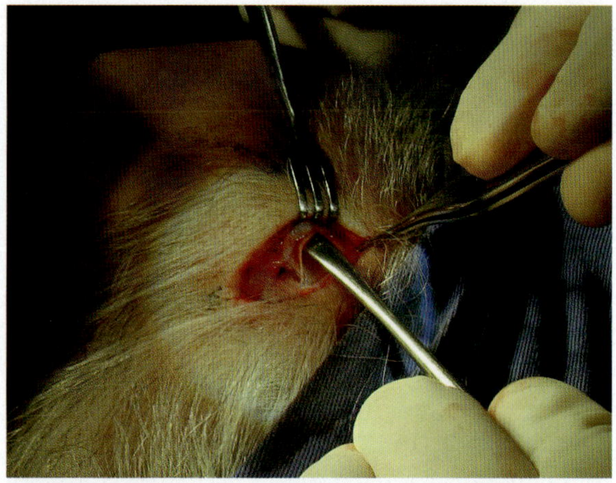

Fig. 10.6 Using direct vision or an endoscope, the deep temporalis fascial plane is reached. The dissection plane is connected.

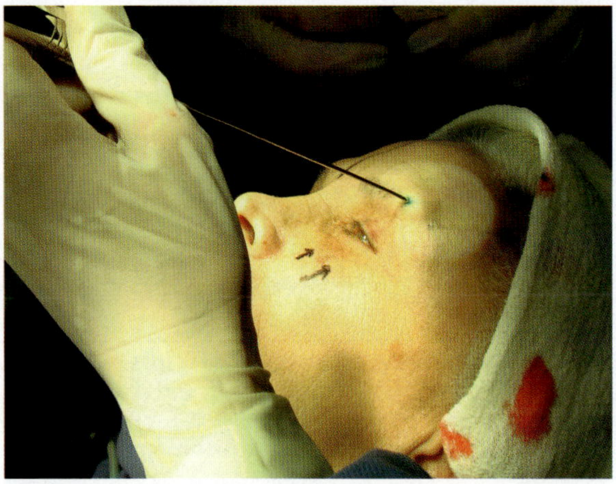

Fig. 10.7 Two 3 to 4 mm incisions are placed in the lateral brow area. A Reverdin needle is introduced and oriented cephalically to the temporal and parietal incision sites.

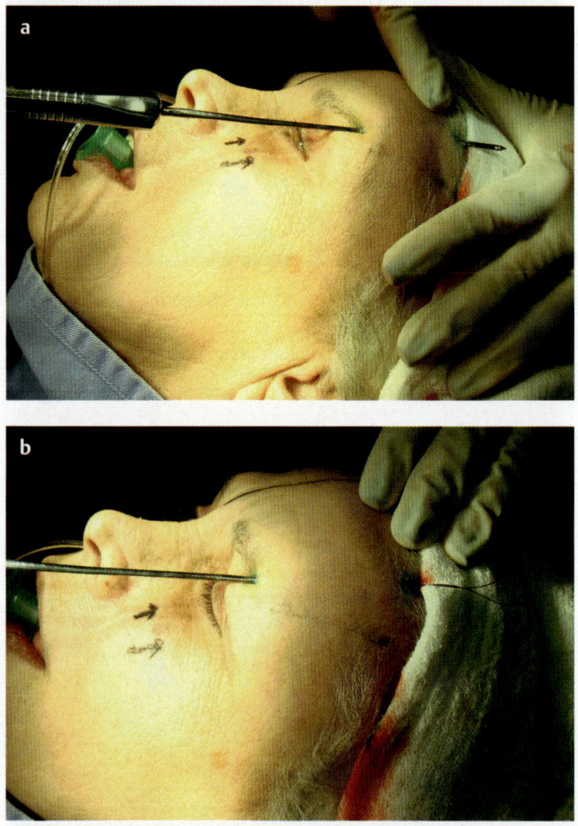

Fig. 10.8 **(a)** The Reverdin needle is introduced at the level of the brow and in a subcutaneous plane; it exits at the level of the parietal or temporal incision site. **(b)** The Reverdin needle is threaded with a 3–0 nonabsorbable suture. The needle is then lowered back to the eyebrow small incision site following the same subcutaneous plane. At this point, it is introduced into a subperiosteal plane or a deep temporalis fascial plane, exiting again in the temporal and parietal incision sites.

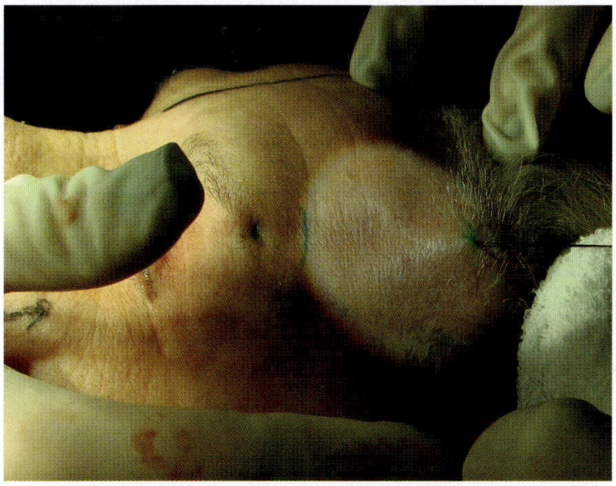

Fig. 10.9 The lateral brow area is suspended and the suture is tied in the deep temporalis fascia or the temporal muscle area. When necessary, it can also be suspended in the parietal bone using a bone tunnel.

The sutures are fixed to the deep temporalis fascia and temporalis muscle and when necessary to the parietal bone using bone tunnels. Using this technique, a durable lifting action is obtained. Temporal and frontal incisions are closed with 3–0 nonabsorbable sutures (**Fig. 10.9**). **Fig. 10.10** and **Fig. 10.11** show pre- and postoperative images of patients in whom this surgical procedure was performed.

10.7 Complications

The incidence of complications in eyebrow surgery is usually low. The most frequent complications or adversities include paresthesia of the scalp, incisional alopecia, unaesthetic scar, bruises, asymmetry, infection, and facial nerve injury. To prevent these complications, it is essential to have a clear understanding of the anatomy and to perform dissection in a precise and careful fashion.

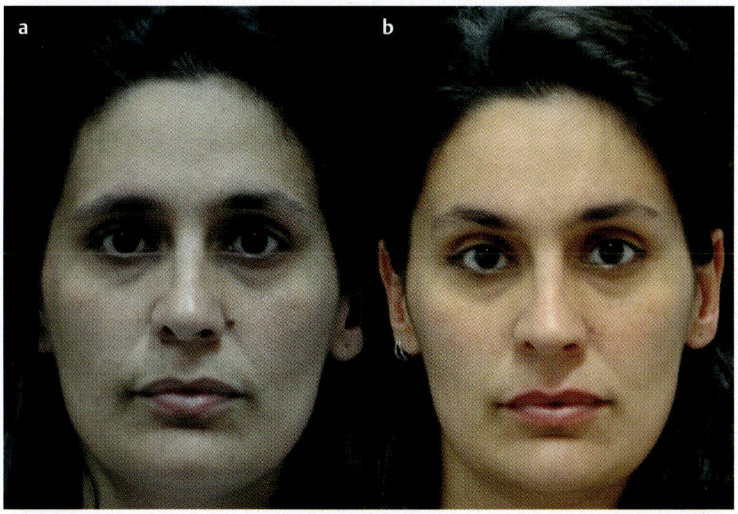

Fig. 10.10 (a,b) Preoperative and 2-year postoperative images showing brow elevation results. One can observe how much the area has improved and how symmetry has been achieved.

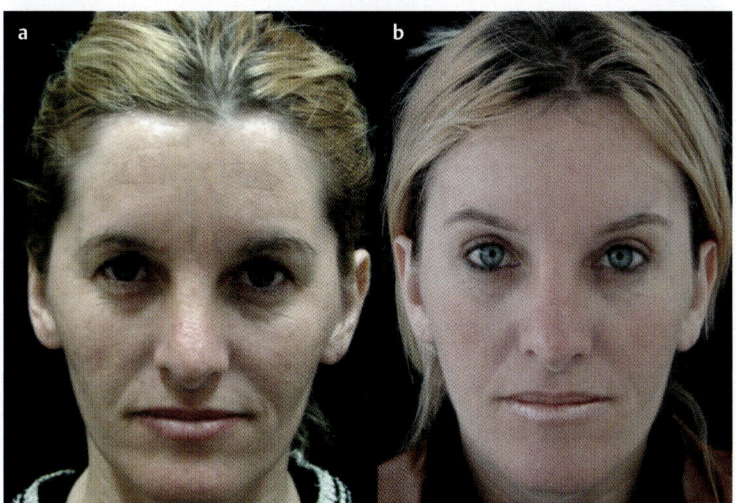

Fig. 10.11 (a,b) Preoperative and 2-year postoperative images showing brow elevation results. One can observe how much the area has improved and how symmetry has been achieved.

10.8 Conclusion

The eyebrow lift is a surgical procedure that can be performed on patients of different ages, genders, or ethnic groups. It may be recommended to patients who have suffered eyebrow ptosis over the years or even for young patients with inadequate brow positioning. It is a simple surgical technique that yields satisfactory results, thus bringing beauty and rejuvenation to the patient.

References

1. Badin AZD, Casagrande C, Saltz R. Rejuvenescimento Facial Cirurgia Videoendoscópica e Procedimentos Ancilares. Rio de Janeiro, Brazil: Revinter; 2003
2. Miller PJ, Wang TD, Cook TA. Rejuvenation of the aging forehead and brow. Facial Plast Surg 1996;12(2): 147–155
3. Montagna W, Carlisle K. Structural changes in aging skin. Br J Dermatol 1990;122(Suppl 35):61–70
4. Seify H, Jones G, Bostwick J, Hester TR. Endoscopic-assisted face lift: review of 200 cases. Ann Plast Surg 2004;52(3):234–239
5. Bolognia JL. Dermatologic and cosmetic concerns of the older woman. Clin Geriatr Med 1993;9(1):209–229
6. Connell BF, Lambros VS, Neurohr GH. The forehead lift: techniques to avoid complications and produce optimal results. Aesthetic Plast Surg 1989;13(4):217–237
7. Connell BF, Marten TJ. The male foreheadplasty. Recognizing and treating aging in the upper face. Clin Plast Surg 1991;18(4):653–687
8. Cook TA, Brownrigg PJ, Wang TD, Quatela VC. The versatile midforehead browlift. Arch Otolaryngol Head Neck Surg 1989;115(2):163–168
9. Dayan SH, Perkins SW, Vartanian AJ, Wiesman IM. The forehead lift: endoscopic versus coronal approaches. Aesthetic Plast Surg 2001;25(1):35–39
10. Ellis DAP, Masri H. The effect of facial animation on the aging upper half of the face. Arch Otolaryngol Head Neck Surg 1989;115(6):710–713
11. Howard BK. Aesthetic Surgery of the Upper Third of the Face: A Self-Instructional Package. Washington, DC: American Academy of Otolaryngology Head and Neck Surgery Foundation; 1998
12. Kede MPV, Sabatovick O. Dermatologia Estética. São Paulo, Brazil: Atheneu; 2004
13. Knize DM. Anatomic concepts for brow lift procedures. Plast Reconstr Surg 2009;124(6):2118–2126
14. Knize DM. Região Frontal e Fossa Temporal: Anatomia e Técnica Aberta e Endoscópica. Rio de Janeiro, Brazil: Revinter; 2007:91–99
15. Lapière CM. The ageing dermis: the main cause for the appearance of 'old' skin. Br J Dermatol 1990;122(Suppl 35):5–11
16. Troilius C. A comparison between subgaleal and subperiosteal brow lifts. Plast Reconstr Surg 1999;104(4): 1079–1090, discussion 1091–1092
17. Wang TD. Envelhecimento Facial. São Paulo, Brazil: Santos; 2007

11 Noninvasive Procedures in Mestizo Patients: What Works and What Patients Want

Frank Rosengaus Leizgold

11.1 Introduction

Beauty, the saying goes, is only skin deep. Not true. Skin is important, but so is what lies under it. In particular, the shape of a person's face, as determined by the subcutaneous tissue and the bone structure, contributes enormously to how beautiful one is. Mestizo patients have features that are unique and therefore they have different cosmetic concerns. For example, photoaging in the Mestizo population is not as pronounced as that seen in Caucasian patients, yet dyschromia is a more significant problem. Anybody dedicated to the beauty enhancement of the face must understand these differences and adapt his practice accordingly.

Although the terms *Mestizo, Hispanic*, and *Latino* are sometimes used interchangeably in English, they are not the same and comprise a variety of ethnicities. As a useful generalization, Hispanics have an increased bizygomatic distance, bimaxillary protrusion, a greater convexity angle, a broader nose, a broad and rounded face, and a receding chin. In persons of Mexican descent, the face is broad, with a prominent malar eminence, thick nasal skin, a broad nose, a short columella, and a widened alar base.[1]

Mestizo skin is considered to be phototype III–V according to the Fitzpatrick skin phototype system (**Table 11.1**).[2] Other differences in skin structure among different races are summarized in **Table 11.2**.[3]

In brief, whereas patients with lighter skin show more marked fine lines, wrinkles, laxity, and overall photodamage, Mestizo patients show much more hyperpigmentation and a greater tendency for a more uneven skin tone. In our experience, Mestizo patients do not have an increased risk of keloid formation after minimal injection procedures.[4]

The signs of facial aging in Mestizo patients tend to originate from volume loss from the deep fat pads, rather than the dermal layers, as in Caucasian patients. This is reflected in a tendency toward mid and lower facial aging, including upper lid laxity, sagging of the malar fat pads, and jowl formation, making Mestizo patients ideal candidates for volume replacement techniques.[5,6]

Table 11.1 Fitzpatrick skin phototype system

Phototype	Sunburn and tanning history (defines the phototype)	Immediate pigment darkening	Delayed tanning	Constitutive color (unexposed buttock skin)	UV-A MED (mJ/cm²)	UV-B MED (mJ/cm²)
I	Burns easily, never tans	None (–)	None (–)	Ivory white	20–35	15–30
II	Burns easily, tans minimally with difficulty	Weak ± (± to +)	Minimal to weak (± to +)	White	30–45	25–40
III	Burns moderately, tans moderately and uniformly	Definite +	Low +	White	40–55	30–50
IV	Burns minimally, tans moderately and easily	Moderate ++	Moderate ++	Beige-olive, lightly tanned	50–80	40–60
V	Rarely burns, tans profusely	Intense (brown) +++	Strong, intense brown +++	Moderate brown or tanned	70–100	60–90
VI	Never burns, tans profusely	Intense (dark brown) +++	Strong, intense brown +++	Dark brown or black	100	90–150

Data from Fitzpatrick TB. The validity and practicality of sun-reactive skin types I trough VI. Arch Dermatol 1988;124(6):869–871. (Labels –, ±, +, ++, +++ are a grading system explained in the text.)

Table 11.2 Racial differences in skin properties

Evidence supports	Insufficient evidence*	Inconclusive
– Increased melanin content and melanosomal dispersion in persons of color – Multinucleated and larger fibroblasts in black persons compared with white persons – pH black < white skin – Larger mast cell granules, increased PLS, and increased tryptase localized to PLS in black compared with white skin – Variable racial blood vessel reactivity	Racial differences in: – Skin elastic recovery/ extensibility – Skin microflora – Facial pore size†	Racial differences in: – TEWL – Water content – Corneocyte desquamation – Lipid content

Abbreviations: PLS, parallel-linear striations; TEWL, transepidermal water loss.

*Skin elastic recovery/extensibility, skin microflora, and pore size were classified as "insufficient evidence for" racial differences rather than "inconclusive" because only two studies or fewer examined these variables.

†Sugiyama-Nakagiri Y, Sugata K, Hachiya A, et al. Ethnic differences in the structural properties of facial skin. J Dermatol Sci 2009;53:135–139.

Adapted with permission from Wesley NO, Maibach HI. Racial (ethnic) differences in skin properties: the objective data. Am J Clin Derrmatol 2003;4:843–860.

To reduce the risk of adverse events during and after injection procedures like those for botulinum toxin and fillers, the author suggests the following:

- Try to minimize the number of points of entry by avoiding needle techniques like serial puncture or cross-hatching.
- An excellent option is the use of thin-walled microcannulas, which allow wide access through one or two strategically placed entry points.
- Try to stay subdermal in the superficial fat pads for most lines, wrinkles, and creases.
- To diminish postprocedure erythema, we recommend the use of topical cooling for a couple of hours after injection.
- We routinely recommend the use of sunscreen after the procedure to decrease the development of hyperpigmented macules.
- In patients with preexisting hyperpigmentation, hydroquinone may be used for 6 to 8 weeks after filler applications.

A fundamental requirement for performing high-quality injection procedures without complications is a thorough understanding of the anatomy of the region. The author uses topographic anatomy to identify the location, extension, and involvement of the different facial muscles and the distribution of the main vascular branches in the face and their companion nerves.[7] The main concepts are:

1. Lines, wrinkles, and creases are invariably perpendicular to the orientation of the muscle fibers.
2. Creases are defined by deeply situated vessels, while wrinkles are normally associated with superficial ones.
3. The muscle will consistently extend proximal and distal to the specific line, wrinkle, or crease.
4. Facial muscles are located between superficial and fat compartments, which are required to aid in their gliding.
5. Folds occur between adjacent fat compartments of varying thickness.
6. Anatomical units are determined by the anatomy of the underlying blood supply.

11.2 Botulinum Toxin

Long-term experience in the use of botulinum toxin for the treatment of facial wrinkles and expression lines has permitted the creation of consensus and general guidelines on its use.[8,9] In general, we abide by these principles, but we also consider that proper facial aesthetic botulinum toxin application requires individualization, including consideration of the patient's expectations.

There are currently three botulinum neurotoxin type A (BoNTA) formulations approved by the United States Food and Drug Administration (FDA): onabotulinumtoxin A (Botox, Botox Cosmetic), abobotulinumtoxin A (Dysport), and incobotulinum A (Xeomin). In this chapter, BoNTA is meant as abobotulinumtoxin A (Speywood Unit) and we consider the bioequivalent potency to onabotulinumtoxin A as 2.5:1.

Application sites and number of units per site are shown in the figures by anatomic area. The dark purple circles represent the most commonly recommended injection points and the light purple circles demonstrate application points that are more seldom used, and their indications are described in each figure legend.

Crow's feet are a major characteristic of an aging face. They are the result of the contraction of the orbital fibers of the orbicularis oculi muscle and therefore are an excellent indication for the use of botulinum toxin. The lateral extension of the wrinkles correlates with the width of the orbicularis oculi muscle **(Fig. 11.1)**.

Although there are few arteries or nerves in this area, the area-specific complication here is bruising.

The forehead muscle is the frontalis. It is large, broad, and vertically oriented, with insertions of fibers, and has interaction with the procerus, corrugator supercilii, and orbicularis oculi muscles. The horizontal forehead lines are mainly the result of the contraction of the frontalis muscle, but the tug of war between the elevator muscle (frontalis) and the depressor muscles (all the rest) is responsible for the positioning of the brow. Today, treatment of the forehead region with botulinum toxin needs to address both the lines and wrinkling, as well as brow position, brow shape, and brow symmetry. The latter requires a deep understanding of the regional muscles' interplay and fine-tuning of the injection points.[10]

In some patients, the frontalis muscle fibers don't intertwine in the midline. This can be easily observed if, when the patient is asked to elevate the eyebrows, no wrinkle is formed in the center of the forehead. In this case, the middle injection point is not necessary.

The basis of brow positioning and shaping is that any area of the frontalis that is left untreated will appear to be hyperactive; therefore, we can use this effect to elevate a specific portion of the brow, whether it be the cephalic part, the middle portion, or the tail. Be aware that, in some patients, their desire to have the tail of the brow elevated will be a trade-off, since additional lines might appear above it. On the other hand, elevated brows can always be corrected by applying extra units of botulinum toxin to the hyperactive area of the frontalis. Also, asymmetric brows will require additional compensation points for correction **(Fig. 11.2)**.

The area-specific complications here are brow ptosis and lid ptosis. To avoid them, injection points should be in the upper two-thirds of the forehead.

The glabellar area was the first, and until recently the only, area approved by the FDA for BoNTA treatments. (In 2013, the FDA approved the use of onabotulinumtoxin A for the treatment of crow's feet.) Treatment of the glabellar area is the treatment most sought after by Mestizo patients, because the creases and deep furrows in this region result in the patient's being incorrectly seen as angry, fatigued, upset, or aging. The glabellar muscle complex includes the vertically oriented procerus, which is responsible for the horizontal furrows on top of the bridge of the nose, the corrugator supercilii, producer of the vertical rhytids, and some depressor fibers of the orbicularis oculi muscle.[11]

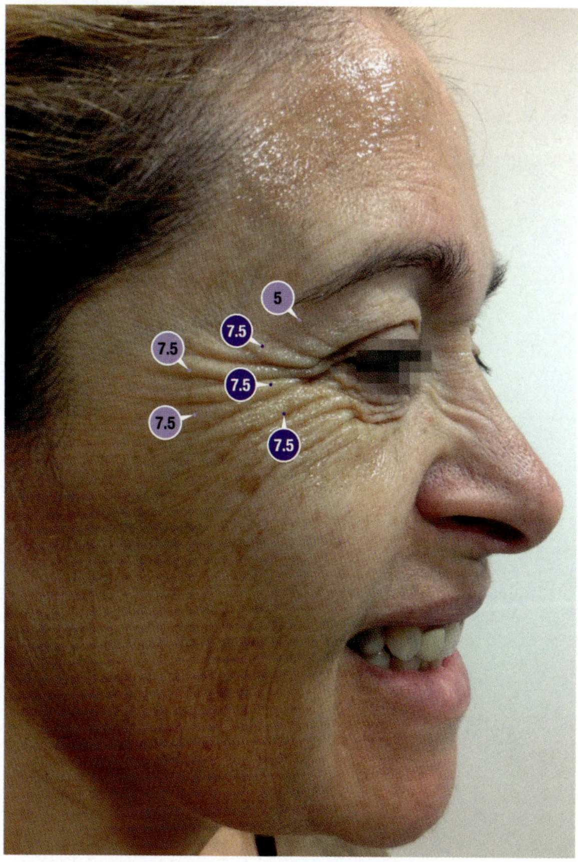

Fig. 11.1 Crow's feet. The more lateral point is used when wrinkles are seen even with no muscle activity and extend toward the temple area. The lateral subbrow injection point is used when extra elevation of the tail of the brow is sought. Botulinium toxin points (*dark purple*) indicate more standardized points. Additional injection points are indicated by *light purple*.

Facial topography is especially useful in the glabella, since by identifying the midline forehead crease, the corrugator crease, and the supraorbital crease, we can estimate the course of the central forehead artery and nerve, the supratrochlear artery and nerve, and the supraorbital artery and nerve, respectively. Furthermore, we can also define the lateral extension of the corrugator muscles and adapt our injection points accordingly **(Fig. 11.3)**.

The area-specific complication here is eyelid ptosis, involving the levator palpebrae superioris muscle. To avoid it, be sure that the injection points are 1 cm above the orbital rim (0.5 cm above the orbicularis retaining ligament) and medial to the mid-pupillary line.

The use of BoNTA in the treatment of wrinkles of the lower third of the face is not as generalized as in the upper third, but it could be very effective and safe for the proper indications. Because of the different muscle interactions in this area, we recommend it be practiced only by

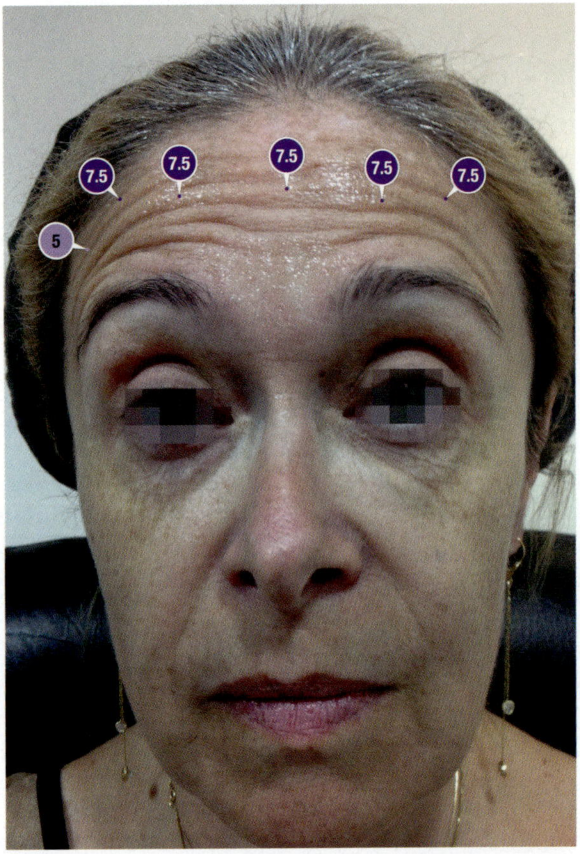

Fig. 11.2 Forehead treatment. The patient is seen before treatment, with forehead wrinkling at maximal upward gaze. Brow asymmetry is noted, with higher elevation of the right brow, as well as increased horizontal wrinkling. An additional injection point is applied to compensate for it (*light purple*). Botulinium toxin points (*dark purple*) indicate more standardized points.

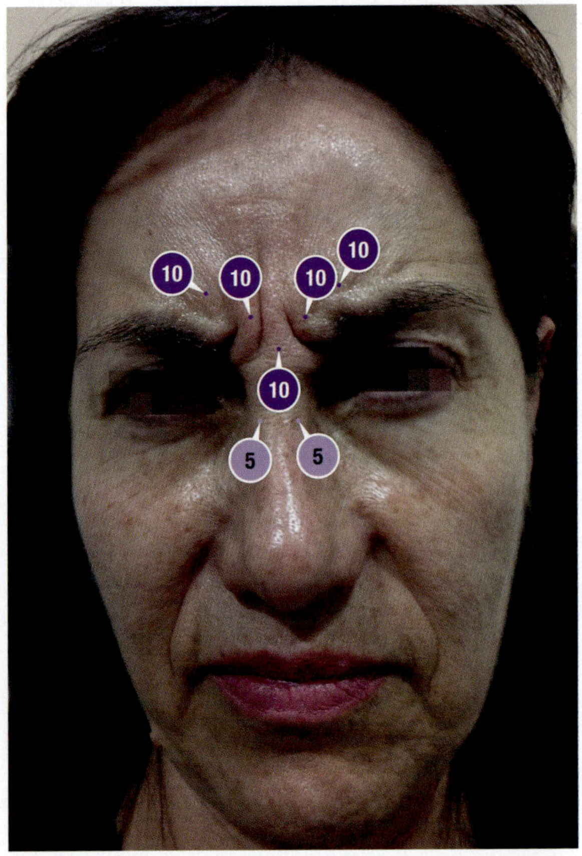

Fig. 11.3 Glabella and bunny lines. Some patients show marked nasalis muscle hyperactivity. In these cases, one injection point per side (*light purple*) is enough to reduce the appearance of bunny lines. *Dark purple* indicates standardized botulinum toxin points.

experienced injectors. A very small number of units is needed (even if dilution needs to be increased) to obtain results and to avoid complications **(Table 11.3)**.[12]

The perioral area encompasses several muscles, including the depressor anguli oris, which is responsible for the downward pull on the oral commissure, the orbicularis oris, which is accountable for the vertical rhytids of the upper lip, and the mentalis, hyperactivity of which is to blame for the dimpled chin. In our experience, these are the corrections most requested by Mestizo patients **(Fig. 11.4)**.

Overtreatment of the perioral area is an area-specific complication and can result in oral incompetence, drooling, and an asymmetric smile.

Recently, there has been more awareness in Latin America that BoNTA is a good treatment method for benign masseteric hypertrophy,[13] but, in contrast to Asia, the main objective for the Mestizo patient is aesthetic mandibular contouring to yield a more oval face. For this, even though the injection points are the same, we prefer to lower the dosage and to see the patient for additional treatments if necessary **(Fig. 11.5)**.

An area-specific complication, although rare, is oral dystonia or fatigue after vigorous chewing.

A paramount sign of senescent changes in the neck is the appearance of platysma bands. The platysma is a thin and broad muscle that originates in the upper chest, clavicle, and acromial regions and continues superolaterally to join the superficial muscular aponeurotic system. With aging, platysma bands result in the characteristic vertical neck cords or "turkey gobbler" deformity **(Fig. 11.6)**.[14]

Area-specific complications of platysma treatment include dysphagia and cervical dystonia. To avoid them, do not make the injection point near to, or lower than, the hyoid bone.

Table 11.3 Use of botulinum toxin type A on the middle and lower face, neck, and chest region

Indication	Dose per injection point (s.U)	Number of injection points	Total dose (s.U)	Injection site	Injection technique
Lower eyelid wrinkles	1–2.5	One to two per side (two to four total)	5	At the mid-pupillary line, ~ 2 mm below the lower eyelid border	Very superficial intradermal injections parallel to the skin, to create a white papula
Bunny lines	5–10	One per side (two total)	10–20	About 1 cm above the upper lateral part of the nostril	Superficial perpendicular injections (45° angle to the nasal bone) to the first third of the needle
Drooping nasal tip	10	One	10	Just below the nasal tip, at the base of columella	Perpendicular injection to at least the middle third of the needle
Perioral wrinkles	1–2	Total of four to six	4–12	Vermilion border of the lips and at least 1.5 cm from the mouth corners	Very superficial intramuscular injections perpendicular to the skin with just the tip of the needle
Masseter hypertrophy	10–20	Three per side (six total)	60 for Caucasians and 120 for Asians	Masseter muscle	Intramuscular perpendicular injection to at least the middle third of the needle
Drooping mouth corner	5–10	One per side (two total)	10–20	Slightly internal to a line extending from the nasolabial fold to the jaw line	Superficial intramuscular and perpendicular injections to the middle third of the needle
Dimpled chin	5–10	Two	10–20	Two points close to the center at the bony jaw line	Superficial intramuscular and perpendicular injections to the middle third of the needle
Platysma bands	5–10	Fewer than 10 per side	Maximum dose 50 per side	Start at the jaw line and go down every 2 cm until at least the middle part of the bands	Very superficial intramuscular injections on the bands with horizontal orientation, to the first third of the needle
Décolleté wrinkles	7.5–10	Five to six per side	75–120	V-shaped technique	Perpendicular injections at least 4 mm deep

Abbreviation: s.U, Speywood units.
Used with permission from Ascher B, Talarico S, Cassuto D, Escobar S, et al. International consensus recommendations on the aesthetic usage of botulinum toxin type A (Speywood units). Part II: wrinkles on the middle and lower face, neck and chest. J Eur Acad Dermatol Venereol 2010;24(11):1285–1295.

11.3 Pearls

- Apply topical anesthetic (lidocaine 7%, tetracaine 7%) at least 10 to 15 minutes before initiating the procedure.
- Precool the treatment area immediately before injection, both for further anesthesia and for vasoconstriction to reduce ecchymosis.
- Mark the injection points by asking the patient for all the facial expressions needed.
- Angle the needle depending upon the area to be injected. For example: glabella at 90°, forehead at 45°, crow's feet at 10°.
- Be systematic. Start the application on the same area with every patient and follow through in the same order.
- After treatment, apply a cooling mask to reduce erythema and inflammation.

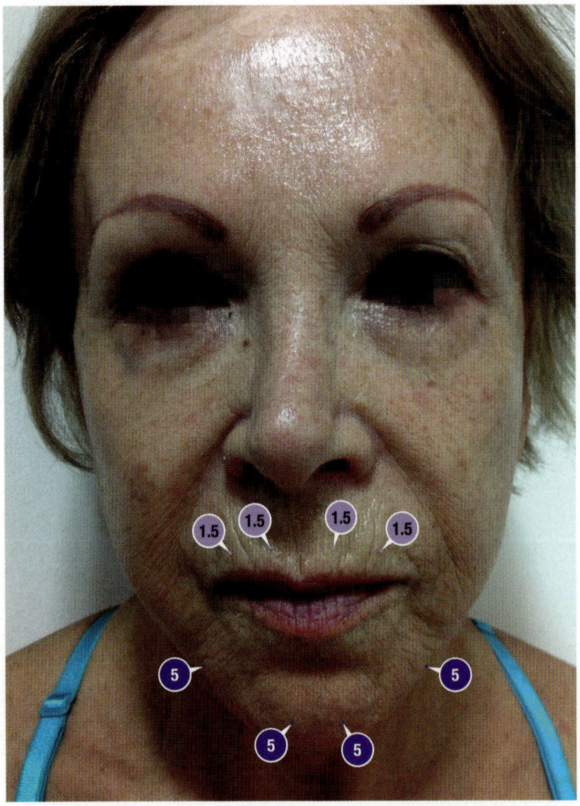

Fig. 11.4 Lower face treatment. To identify the depressor anguli oris muscle (DAO), push the jowl to the midline; the limit of displacement marks the labiomandibular ligament. The injection point should be slightly medial to, and 0.5 cm above, the mandible border. Botulinium toxin points (*dark purple*) indicate more standardized points. Additional injection points are indicated by *light purple*.

11.4 Fillers

Facial soft tissue augmentation has undergone a dramatic evolution in the last few years due to the confluence of several circumstances.

Our better understanding of how the face ages has created the opportunity to move from a "surgical model," where we assumed that facial skin and fat "fall" and that the treatment is excision and lifting, to a more integral model that takes into account the extremely important fact of the loss of facial volume that occurs as a person gets older.[15] A young face is not an old face with tight skin. As mentioned at the beginning of the chapter, the Mestizo patient is particularly prone to loss of midface volume with age.

Although not as significant as fat volume reduction in overall facial volume loss, facial bone, and therefore skeletal morphology, changes with time and contributes to the appearance of the aging face. This should be kept in mind when volumizing, especially in the periorbit.[16]

Innovative reevaluation of the facial subcutaneous fat layer showed distinctively that the fat is highly compartmentalized into subunits, with its own connective tissue boundaries. Comprehension of an individual fat pad's behavior during aging is leading to a better understanding and greater accuracy in evaluating the patient's volume needs.[17]

There are a variety of soft tissue augmentation biological products, but there is no perfect filler. The ideal filler should be biocompatible, nonimmunogenic, noncarcinogenic, nonmigratory, inexpensive, easily obtained and stored, easy to administer, able to produce cosmetically beneficial results with no side effects, easy to remove in the

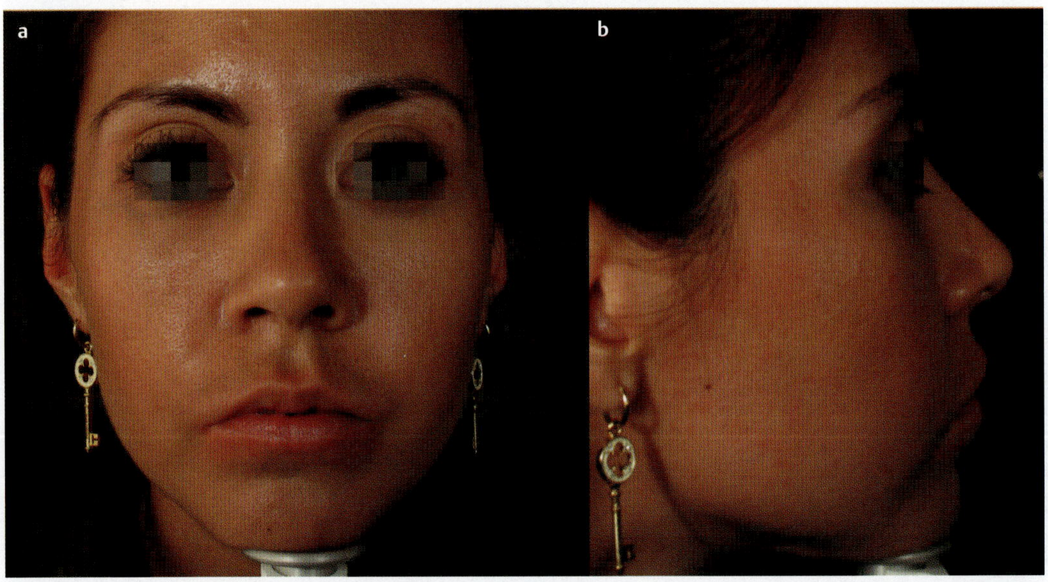

Fig. 11.5 **(a,b)** For the masseter muscle, a total dosage of 25 units per side is used, and is repeated if necessary. The medium point requires more units and should be injected deeper.

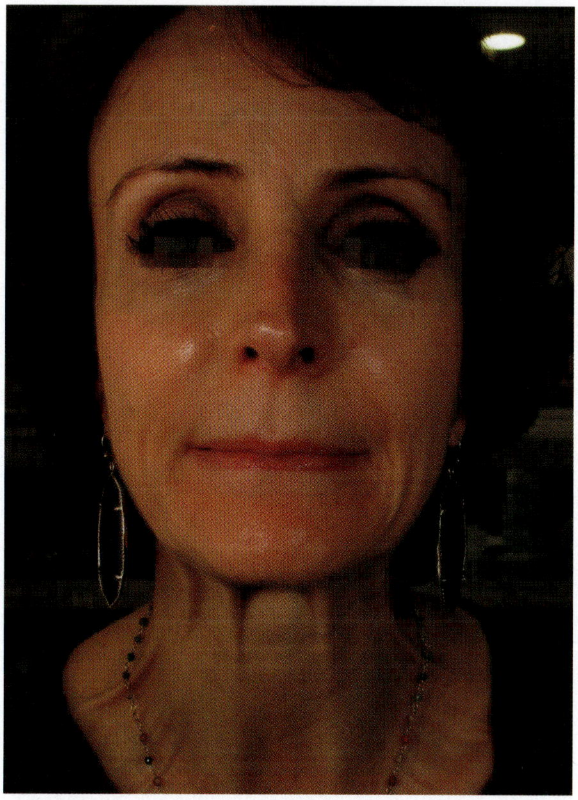

Fig. 11.6 Neck with platysma bands. No more than five injection points per side should be used. For better injection technique, bands should be held between two fingers and the needle should be applied vertically and superficially.

event of poor cosmetic outcome, and able to be used for multiple purposes. Fillers are normally classified as permanent (silicon, polyacrylamide, polymethylmethacrylate) or temporary (hyaluronic acid, calcium hydroxyapatite, collagen, polylactic acid, etc.). We strongly advise not to use permanent fillers, since they have a higher incidence of complications.

Autologous fat transfer is a technique with vast reconstructive and cosmetic potential, but the high variability of the procedure results in unpredictable clinical outcomes. Despite this, there has been a big resurgence in its use with the emergence of therapies using adipose-derived stem cells (ADSC). Autologous fat is biocompatible, can be applied in big volumes, and is the most accessible product. Unfortunately, stem cell–based regenerative medicine has been plagued with a lot of fraudulent and unsubstantiated claims. Today, fat transfer involves three distinctive steps: harvesting, some form of processing, and replacement into the new location. All of the steps have unresolved issues that need to be addressed to preserve fat viability and to increase procedure predictability.[18] Even so, this technique can yield impressive clinical results **(Fig. 11.7)**.

Compared with a few years ago, today we have a multiplicity of approved commercial hyaluronic acid (HA) dermal fillers (availability differs by country). They all contain HA obtained by bacterial production and most of them are stabilized by cross-linking. Despite their similarities, HA fillers have varying specific physical characteristics like viscoelasticity, firmness, lifting capacity, particle size, etc., that make them behave clinically in different ways, and therefore each one also has distinct indications.[19]

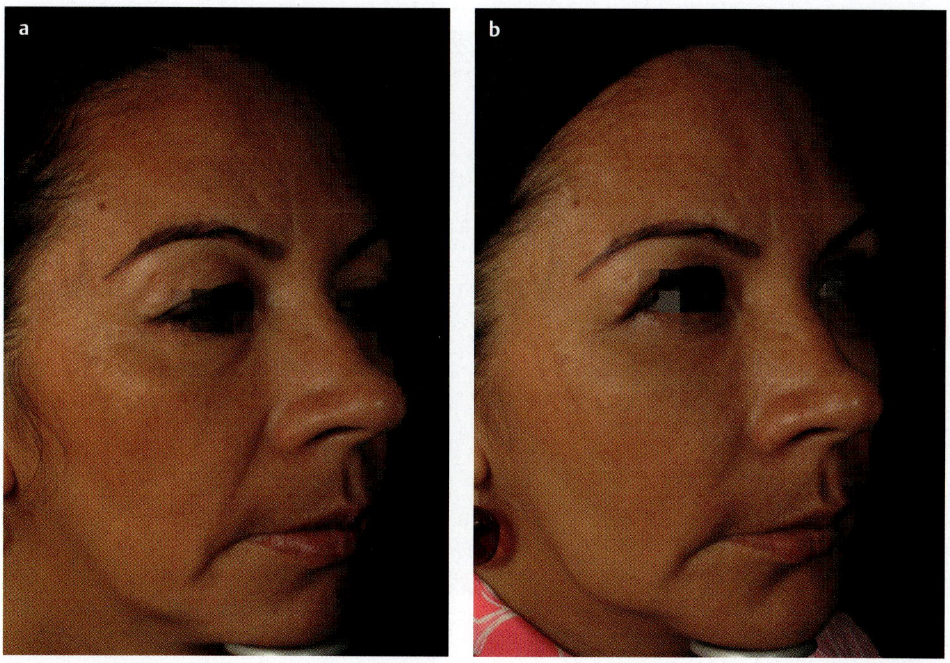

Fig. 11.7 (a,b) Fat autologous transfer. This 50-year-old patient received a total of 42 mL of fat harvested from the lower abdomen and flanks. Recipient sites include nasolabial folds, temporal area, brow, malar are, posterior jaw line, and tear trough.

The thin-walled, high-gauge microcannula has been a helpful addition to our armamentarium as a tool to apply soft augmentation fillers into deep layers while being less traumatic. Hexsel et al undertook a double-blind, randomized clinical trial comparing the use of needles and microcannulas and found that the use of the latter had fewer complications like hematomas, edema, redness, and pain.[20]

In the past 10 years, all of the above have helped fillers to become the second most popular noninvasive procedure in the United States, after botulinum toxin injection.[21] Because HA has most of the properties of an ideal filler, it is by far the most widely used filler worldwide (more than 80%). All the case examples in this chapter were treated with non-animal stabilized HA.

Before we review the use of dermal fillers in specific facial areas, we must add a word of caution. The subtle, natural, three-dimensional shaping of facial soft tissue with a tool like a needle or microcannula is more challenging than normally thought. Steer clear of overcorrection and expect a learning curve.

Since we strictly adhere to the concept that facial volume loss is primarily the result of fat compartments' deflation, we think that the best way to naturally augment the soft tissue is by weaving the filler back into the fat compartments. After reviewing the anatomy, the surgeon faces the question, Into which fat compartment should the injection go? The general principle is that to correct lines, creases, and wrinkles, fillers should be injected into the superficial fat compartments, but to correct a fold or to volumize an area, we need to use a deep fat pad. Actually, there are many cases where both are needed. We can give volume to the malar area by injection into the deep medial cheek fat pad (below the zygomaticus minor muscle) and deal with the nasomalar fold by filling the medial cheek fat pad (above the zygomaticus minor muscle). This is what some authors call 3D volumizing and I call facial harmonization.

Nasal remodeling with HA has become a widely solicited office procedure with an important "wow" effect on the patient. It is strictly reserved for selected patients who are either bad candidates for surgery or who are not interested in having surgery but are still bothered by the aesthetics of their nose. Good candidates are mainly noses with no previous rhinoplasties, a low dorsum, an inadequate nasofrontal angle, minor bossa or asymmetries, minor dorsal deviations, some tip ptosis, columella retraction, and an acute nasolabial angle.

In Mestizo patients, who have thick nasal skin, we use a high HA product. If the skin is thinner, a more malleable, medium HA can be used. Use a 27 gauge needle. Inject independently at each point at 90° and, especially in the bony dorsum, make sure the injection is supraperiosteal. Stop and evaluate. Never apply more than 0.1 mL per injection point and preferably no more than 0.5 to 0.7 mL in one session. HA can be used to mimic Sheen grafts, columella struts, spreader grafts, etc. Attention to detail is mandatory, as is the need for a secondary retouching consultation 2 to 3 weeks postprocedure. Results should last between 9 and 12 months (**Fig. 11.8** and **Fig. 11.9**).

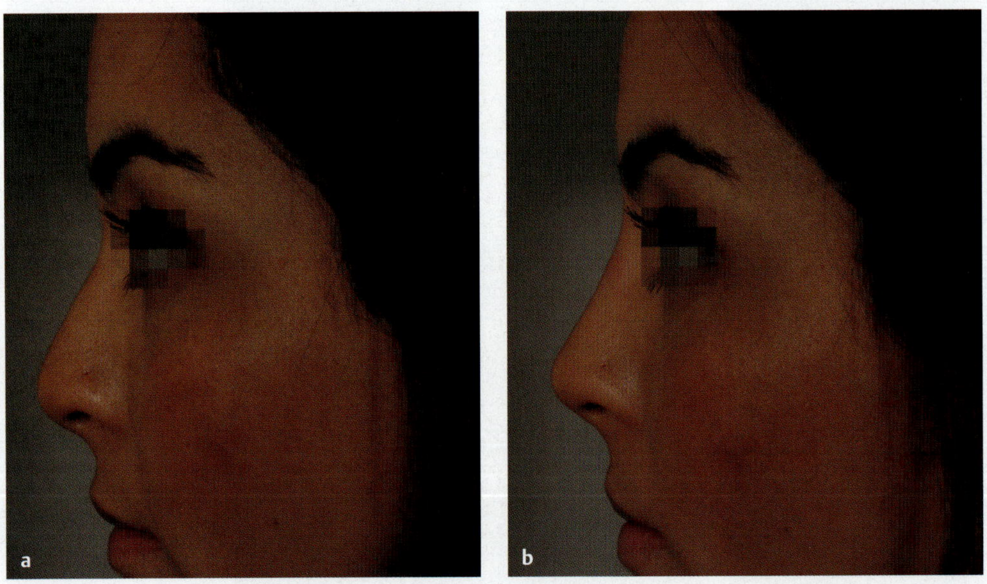

Fig. 11.8 Nasal remodeling. **(a)** A 28-year-old patient with lack of tip projection and a low nasion. **(b)** Correction was made with the application of 0.2 mL of low HA at the tip and 0.1 at the nasion.

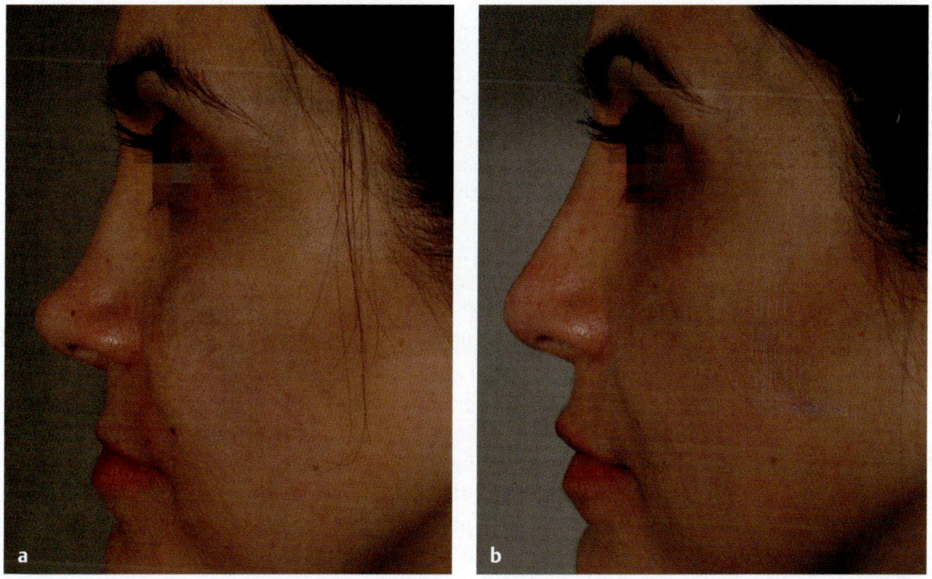

Fig. 11.9 (a) Nasal remodeling patient with a secondary rhinoplasty, an over-resected dorsum, and a pseudo tip excessive projection. **(b)** Using low HA, 0.6 mL was applied to the supratip and dorsum.

What to avoid: look out for immediate blanching, bluish skin color, or unusual pain, since they portend vascular compromise of the area, which requires preventive treatment.

Mental augmentation with HA can produce a natural and predictable correction of a receding chin. It can also show the patient what a permanent chin implant would look like. A high HA product is injected into the inferior chin fat compartment and is extended laterally. The amount of product used depends on the desired projection, but customarily between 1 and 2 mL are required **(Fig. 11.10)**.

What to avoid: under-correction of the prejowl sulcus, with the undesirable appearance of a "witch's" chin. For this reason, the point of entry for the microcannula is lateral, behind the labiomandibular ligament.

Patients with tear-trough deformity, or "nasojugal groove," often present complaining of dark circles under

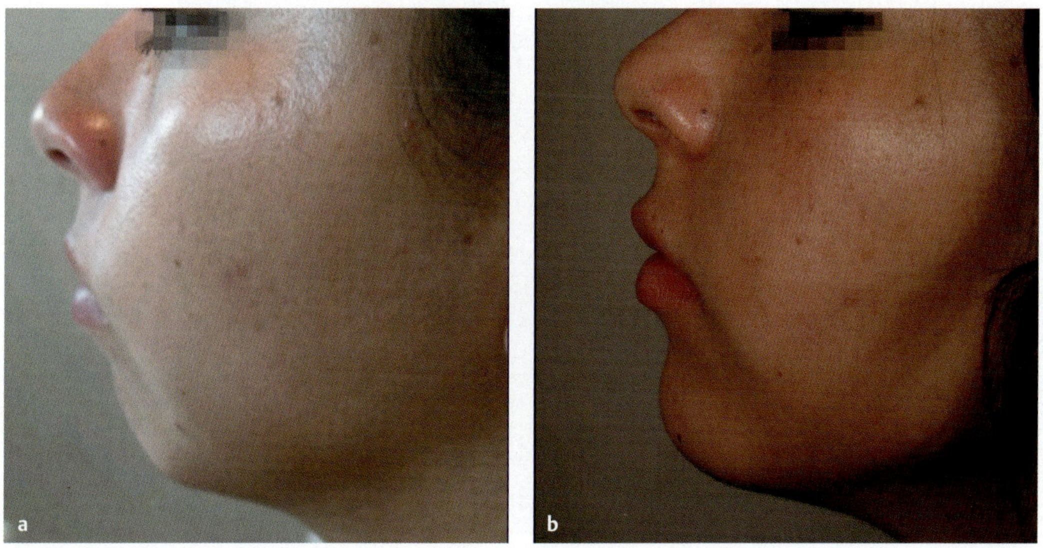

Fig. 11.10 (a,b) Chin augmentation. An 18-year-old patient with a receding chin received 2 mL of high HA. Results lasted around 18 months.

the eyes, a tired, aged look, and/or an aesthetically displeasing depression in the region. Anatomical descriptions have been put forward since the 1960s,[22] but what is important and specific to note is the scarcity of fat tissue in this area, which explains the necessity for depositing the filler below the orbicularis oculi muscle, in order to decrease visibility and the Tyndall effect. Injection technique should be in a retrograde, discontinuous fashion. An amount of 0.2 to 0.3 mL per side is sufficient in most patients. Tear-trough deformity can occur in conjunction with lower lid bags, which, if not too prominent, can be camouflaged with the treatment. Other options include fat grafting, skeletal implants, and fat transposition. In this area, use of a blunt-tip cannula has reduced side effects. We prefer a medium HA for this procedure, and the expected HA longevity in this area could be more than 2 years. Attention should also be paid to the lateral orbital rim **(Fig. 11.11)**.

What to avoid: over-correction. Always under-correct and massage the area gently toward the inner canthus. Ask the patient to sit up and then reevaluate. Remember to mention to the patient that some swelling will occur in the 48 hours postinjection, depending on the hydrophilicity of the HA being used.

If there is a universal facial feature that is aesthetically pleasing, it is the prominent, high cheekbone. From Cambodians to South Koreans, to Middle Eastern or Mestizo patients, it confers a youthful convexity to the middle face. Filler should be place at the deep medial cheek fat compartment close to the periosteum. The malar mount normally requires no or a very small increase in projection. We prefer to enter laterally and to use a 25 g microcannula. Approximately 0.5 mL of a very high HA product per side usually gives enough good results in an initial session, but more may be needed to meet the patient's expectations **(Fig. 11.12)**.

What to avoid: lateral volume placement and projection, especially when the patient smiles. Draw a vertical line from the outer wall of the lateral orbit and, to be safe, stay medial to it.

Full brows look younger. Ideal patients have visible, rounded orbits and hollow-looking eyes. Both anterior projection and a little lifting can be achieved with the right technique. Injection of a high HA with a 25 g microcannula is initiated around 1 cm lateral to the tail of the brow, into the retro orbicularis oculi fat compartment (ROOF) close to the periosteum and above the insertion of the orbital retaining ligament (ORL), which normally is 2 to 3 mm above the supraorbital ridge. An amount of 0.3 to 0.5 mL is applied per side and is thoroughly massaged. Reevaluate after 1 week.

What to avoid: low product placement with a resulting unnatural, heavy-looking eye.

Marionette lines are long, vertical lines that laterally circumscribe the chin. They originate at the corners of the mouth and might end all the way down at the mandibular border. They give the face an expression of being sad, grim, or scornful. Expansion of the premasseter space and the descent of the superficial jowl fat pad and deep buccal fat pads are thought to explain jowling.[23] The perioral area has a very thin layer of subcutaneous tissue and extra myodermal attachments; therefore, we prefer to do a subcision with a microcannula and create the necessary space for

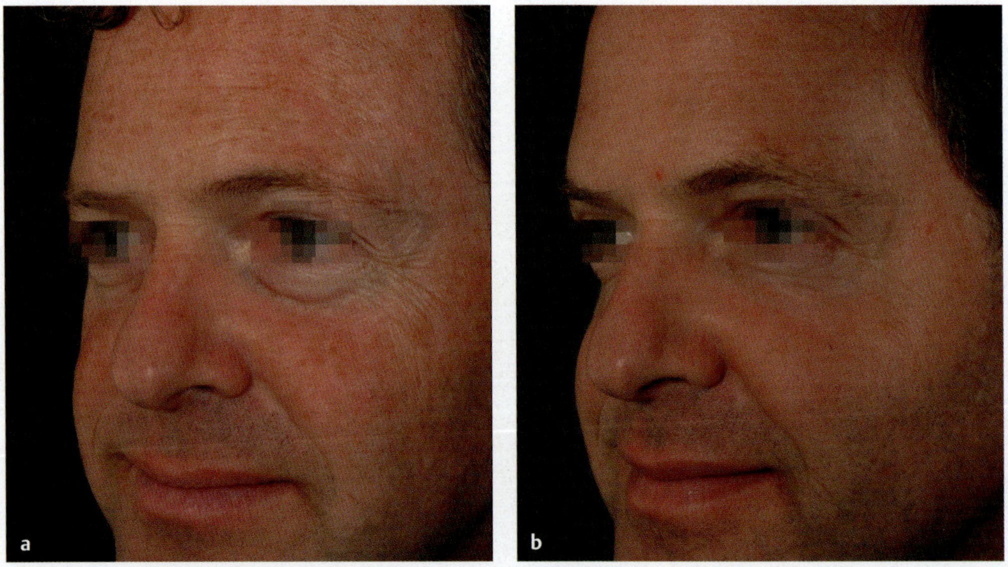

Fig. 11.11 (a,b) Tear-trough deformity. Injection of 0.2 mL of medium HA was done on two consecutive visits, for a total of 0.4 per side.

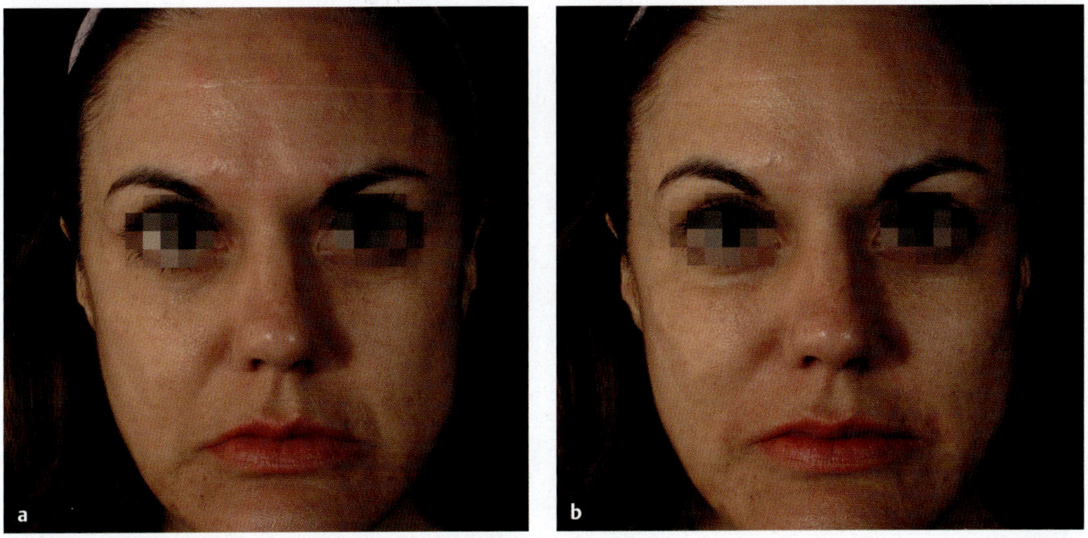

Fig. 11.12 (a,b) Malar area injection of 0.5 mL of very high HA per side. The goal is to have a uniform anterior convexity from the orbital rim to the nasolabial fold.

the filler. We call the correction of the drooping oral commissure and marionette lines the "happy face" treatment, which is performed as follows.

Mark the area with the patient sitting down. Select a high HA. Enter laterally in a line that extends from the lower lip to cross the nasolabial fold. A 25 gauge microcannula is directed toward the commissure. The labiomandibular ligament is traversed. With the same cannula, a subcision is undertaken, including the lip lateral compartment and 1 to 2 cm medial to the mandibular ligament, all the way to where a step-off is present between the mental and jowl areas. Do not include the prejowl sulcus, which needs augmentation on a deeper plane. Once space for the filler is created, apply the product in a retrograde fashion, from the lower marionette line toward the angle of the mouth (**Fig. 11.13**).[24]

The most common mistake is to administer the filler too laterally, into the jowl fat compartment, making it

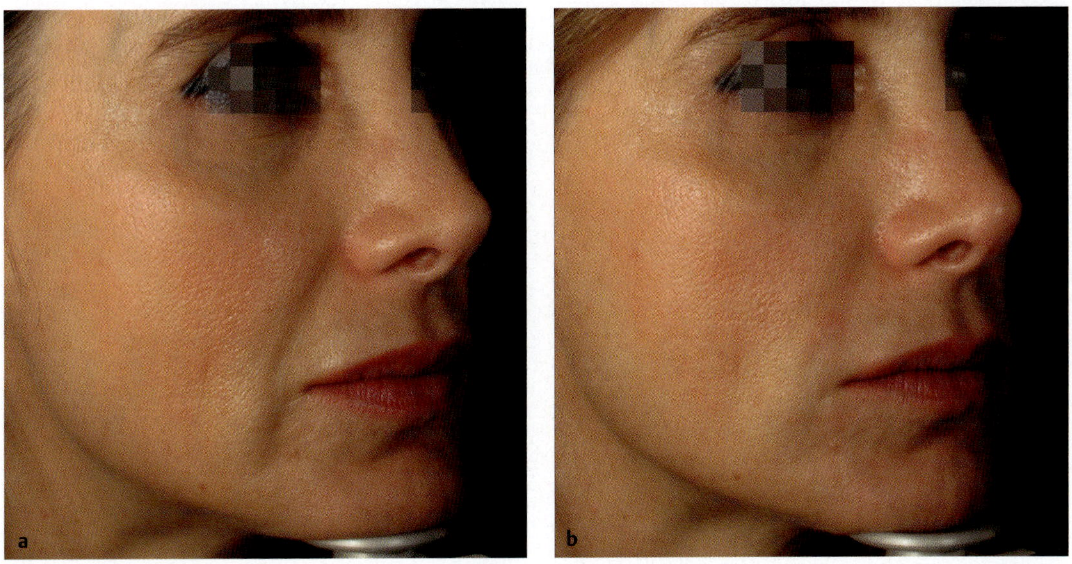

Fig. 11.13 (a,b) Immediate result of "happy face" treatment of the oral commissures and marionette lines in a 48-year-old patient.

even more apparent. It is wise to advise the patient that the product will be "felt" but not seen for some days and some bruising could appear, especially around the oral commissure.

The last specific area we address is soft tissue augmentation of the temporal fossa, which requires special considerations. Hollow temples give the impression of a narrowing of the upper third of the face, losing the oval form that is the ideal and contributing another sign of aging. Because the temporal area is such a wide area to fill, a homogeneous surface with no visible irregularities is the challenge. Therefore, we concur with other authors[25,26] that using diluted/reconstituted HA is an excellent option for obtaining a convex, smooth surface in the temple area. In our experience, it is best to dilute every 1 mL of HA with 1 mL of 1% lidocaine with epinephrine and 1 mL of normal saline. We use at least 1 mL of HA per/side (3 ml diluted total), but possibly more, and evidently some overfilling is needed due to reabsorption. We prefer the use of a microcannula to avoid bruising. Depth should should be at the deep subcutaneous tissue and should be under the superficial temporal vessels. Compression is recommended after treatment, but not massage, and the patient should be aware that some volume displacement and/or ecchymosis may be observed in the lower eyelid and cheek area.

Caution is necessary around the lateral orbit and above the arch, since this is where the hollow is deeper and an unaesthetic step-off can be noticed. A small, well-placed extra quantity of product usually resolves the problem.

11.5 Pearls

- Use only approved long-term dermal fillers, preferably HA for its low incidence of complications and the availability of hyaluronidase as an eraser.
- Be sure to select the right product with the correct rheological properties for the specific treatment area.
- Mark the lines, folds, and especially the area to be volumized. Take into consideration asymmetries and compensate for them.
- Except for the nose and posttreatment retouching, learn to use thin-walled microcannulas. In 80% of cases, you will need a 25 or 27 gauge microcannula.
- Always use one hand to inject and the other to palpate and protect.
- Being in the right plane means the microcannula slides easily with very little patient discomfort.
- To minimize the risk of intravascular injection, always apply the filler with low pressure, in a discontinuous manner, and with a retrograde technique.

11.6 Complications

Although in-depth consideration of complications is outside the scope of this chapter, they include:

- Overcorrection
- Lumps and bumps
- Tyndall effect
- Nodules and granulomas
- Allergic reactions
- Herpetic outbreaks
- Vascular occlusion, dermal necrosis
- Biofilm

11.7 Conclusion

There is no doubt that facial volume replacement is at the forefront of facial rejuvenation. A better understanding of the process of facial aging, of facial anatomy, and of physiology has provided the foundation for solid science-based treatments. A wider range of products and tools has provided the means to get the results. Facial soft tissue augmentation is a promising avenue that shows us the way we ought to be going.

References

1. Ortiz-Monasterio F, Olmedo A. Rhinoplasty on the Mestizo nose. Clin Plast Surg 1977;4(1):89–102
2. Fitzpatrick TB. The validity and practicality of sun-reactive skin types I through VI. Arch Dermatol 1988;124(6): 869–871
3. Wesley NO, Maibach HI. Racial (ethnic) differences in skin properties: the objective data. Am J Clin Dermatol 2003;4(12):843–860
4. Odunze M, Cohn A, Few JW. Restylane and people of color. Plast Reconstr Surg 2007;120(7):2011–2016
5. Jackson BA. Cosmetic considerations and nonlaser cosmetic procedures in ethnic skin. Dermatol Clin 2003; 21(4):703–712, ix
6. Harris MO. The aging face in patients of color: minimally invasive surgical facial rejuvenation—a targeted approach. Dermatol Ther 2004;17(2):206–211
7. Pessa J, Rohrich R. Facial Topography: Clinical Anatomy of the Face. St. Louis, MO: Quality Medical Publishing, Inc.; 2012
8. Carruthers J, Fournier N, Kerscher M, Ruiz-Avila J, Trindade de Almeida AR, Kaeuper G. The convergence of medicine and neurotoxins: a focus on botulinum toxin type A and its application in aesthetic medicine—a global, evidence-based botulinum toxin consensus education initiative. Part II: incorporating botulinum toxin into aesthetic clinical practice. Dermatol Surg 2013;39(3 Pt 2):510–525

9. Ascher B, Talarico S, Cassuto D, et al. International consensus recommendations on the aesthetic usage of botulinum toxin type A (Speywood unit)—Part I: Upper facial wrinkles. J Eur Acad Dermatol Venereol 2010;24(11): 1278–1284
10. Lorenc ZP, Smith S, Nestor M, Nelson D, Moradi A. Understanding the functional anatomy of the frontalis and glabellar complex for optimal aesthetic botulinum toxin type A therapy. Aesthet Plast Surg 2013;37(5):975–983
11. Macdonald MR, Spiegel JH, Raven RB, Kabaker SS, Maas CS. An anatomical approach to glabellar rhytids. Arch Otolaryngol Head Neck Surg 1998;124(12):1315–1320
12. Ascher B, Talarico S, Cassuto D, et al. International consensus recommendations on the aesthetic usage of botulinum toxin type A (Speywood unit)—Part II: Wrinkles on the middle and lower face, neck and chest. J Eur Acad Dermatol Venereol 2010;24(11):1285–1295
13. Kim NH, Park RH, Park JB. Botulinum toxin type A for the treatment of hypertrophy of the masseter muscle. Plast Reconstr Surg 2010;125(6):1693–1705
14. Matarasso A, Matarasso SL, et al. Botulinum A exotoxin for the management of platysma bands. Plast Reconstr Surg 2003;112(5, Suppl):138S–140S
15. Lambros V. Models of facial aging and implications for treatment. Clin Plast Surg 2008;35(3):319–327, discussion 317
16. Shaw RB Jr, Katzel EB, Koltz PF, et al. Aging of the facial skeleton: aesthetic implications and rejuvenation strategies. Plast Reconstr Surg 2011;127(1):374–383
17. Rohrich RJ, Pessa JE. The fat compartments of the face: anatomy and clinical implications for cosmetic surgery. Plast Reconstr Surg 2007;119(7):2219–2227, discussion 2228–2231
18. Longaker MT, Aston SJ, Baker DC, Rohrich RJ. Fat transfer in 2014: what we do not know. Plast Reconstr Surg 2014;133(5):1305–1307
19. Stocks D, Sundaram H, Michaels J, Durrani MJ, Wortzman MS, Nelson DB. Rheological evaluation of the physical properties of hyaluronic acid dermal fillers. J Drugs Dermatol 2011;10(9):974–980
20. Hexsel D, Soirefmann M, Porto MD, Siega C, Schilling-Souza J, Brum C. Double-blind, randomized, controlled clinical trial to compare safety and efficacy of a metallic cannula with that of a standard needle for soft tissue augmentation of the nasolabial folds. Dermatol Surg 2012;38(2):207–214
21. American Society for Aesthetic Plastic Surgery online data 2013. http://www.surgery.org/media/statistics
22. Flowers RS. Tear trough implants for correction of tear trough deformity. Clin Plast Surg 1993;20(2):403–415
23. Mendelson BC, Freeman ME, Wu W, Huggins RJ. Surgical anatomy of the lower face: the premasseter space, the jowl, and the labiomandibular fold. Aesthet Plast Surg 2008;32(2):185–195
24. Rosengaus F. The happy face treatment. Presented at IMCAS Paris 2014
25. Fagien S, Cassuto D. Reconstituted injectable hyaluronic acid: expanded applications in facial aesthetics and additional thoughts on the mechanism of action in cosmetic medicine. Plast Reconstr Surg 2012;130(1):208–217
26. Lambros V. A technique for filling the temples with highly diluted hyaluronic acid: the "dilution solution." Aesthet Surg J 2011;31(1):89–94

Section III

The African Perspective

12 Aesthetic, Ethnic, and Cultural Considerations and Current Cosmetic Trends in the African Descent Population

Monte Oyd Harris

"To be sure of one's self, to be counted for one's self, is to experience aliveness in its most exciting dimension."
Howard Thurman

12.1 Location Is Everything

This is most likely the first book chapter on the topic of facial plastic surgery written from a location of African centeredness. In researching perspectives on cosmetic trends in the African descent population, I found very little in the surgery literature that truly originated from a place of African centrality. Even in the seminal textbook *Ethnic Considerations in Facial Aesthetic Surgery*, edited by W. Earle Matory, the premise of African beauty was largely determined through comparison to neoclassical aesthetic proportions based upon European standards.[1] For most physicians, African beauty has been beholden to an objective ability to see, to measure, and to compare with a presumed Eurocentric ideal.[2,3,4,5] African centrality, however, prioritizes a view that there is much more to beauty than meets the eye. Aesthetics, from a location of African centeredness, is established by a dynamic interwoven relationship between the physical and the metaphysical. Thus, African-centered beauty matters not only for what it looks like, but also for what it does spiritually and how it is expressed through the individual as a way of life.

For all that is lacking in the cosmetic surgery literature, a wealth of resources exists on the subject of African aesthetics in arts and culture. My evolving appreciation for the spirituality of African and African diaspora aesthetics has been nourished through my relationship with the renowned artist, educator, and curator David C. Driskell. Within his extensive body of work, Driskell has expressed the cultural DNA of an authentic African diaspora aesthetic (**Fig. 12.1**). The radiant light of Driskell's life force and creative practice has illuminated my path for navigating the uncharted terrain of African centeredness in the context of facial plastic surgery. Ongoing conversations with Leslie King-Hammond, graduate dean emerita and founding director of the Center for Race and Culture at the Maryland Institute College of Art, have also helped to shape my understanding of the aesthetic and cultural connections between Africa and the African diaspora. In the groundbreaking exhibition "The Global Africa Project," co-curated by King-Hammond and Lowery Stokes Sims, the truly global—and extraordinarily variant—nature of being African, or African-descended, in the contemporary context is explored through the expression of individual creativity.[6] While the field of aesthetics has largely been dominated by European canons, an expanding global awareness has emerged that allows space for new perceptions of beauty and being "African" in the world today.

For the purposes of this chapter, *African* referemces people of African descent whose lives have been influenced by some or all of the following: the transatlantic slave trade, European colonialism, Western imperialism, racism, and global migration. The notion of African centeredness is rooted in Afrocentric philosophy, notably championed by African American studies scholar Molefi Kente Asante. Asante asserts, "Afrocentricity is about location precisely because African people living in Western society have largely been operating from the fringes of the Eurocentric experience. Whether it is a matter of economics, history,

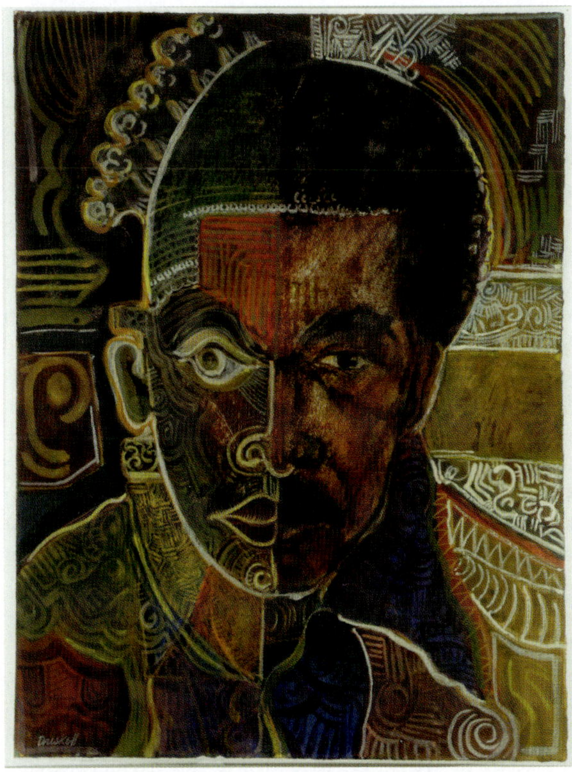

Fig. 12.1 David C. Driskell, *Self Portrait as Beni* ("I Dream Again of Benin") 1974; egg tempera, gouache, and collage; © David C. Driskell, 2015; photography by Greg Staley; from the David C. Driskell Center Collection; purchase from David C. Driskell; 2012.12.002

politics, geographical concepts, or art, Africans have been seen as peripheral to the real activity."[7] Afrocentricity emerges as a process for cultivating consciousness—a contemporary mind-tool for crafting new ways of discovering one's true self. Contemporary beauty culture has largely catered to the desires of a Euro-American audience, relegating African aesthetic perspectives to a distant periphery. To begin a healing shift in location, we must ask the question: What impact does this longstanding off-centeredness have on the minds of African patients pursuing facial cosmetic enhancement? Equally as important, What impact has a Eurocentric mindset had on the clinical practitioners offering aesthetic care to African individuals?

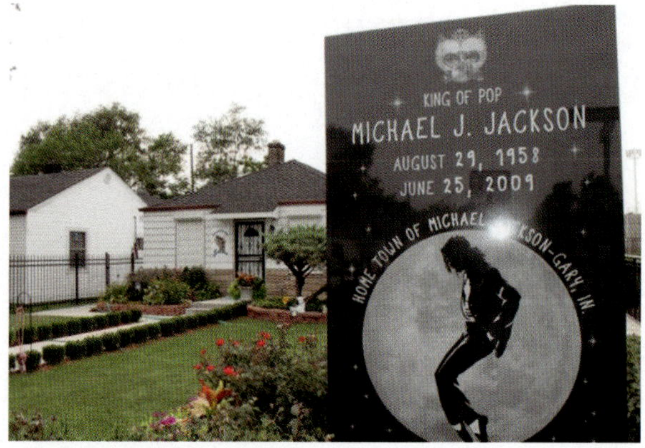

Fig. 12.2 Michael Jackson's childhood home in Gary, Indiana. (Courtesy of Monte Oyd Harris.)

12.2 Michael Jackson and Well-Being Disfigurement

For many, off-centeredness has resulted in a dislocated aesthetic consciousness, resulting in misalignment between a sense of beauty, health, and identity. This multidimensional misalignment is a primary cause of a modern "well-being disfigurement" that desperately warrants the restorative talents of the aesthetic community, as a whole.

I was raised in Gary, Indiana, the birthplace of Michael Jackson. So Michael Jackson's life story has always played very close to my own sense of identity and purpose as a facial plastic surgeon. I've often said that my professional purpose was to ensure that there were "no more Michael Jacksons"—that is, individuals of African descent who end up scarred or disfigured by elective facial cosmetic surgery. For the first decade of my professional career, I worked diligently and passionately toward that humanistic goal by cultivating my own technical expertise in rhinoplasty surgery for African patients, sharing knowledge through presentations at national and international meetings, and writing articles on the subject of rhinoplasty for patients of African descent.[8,9] In the midst of my growing a successful practice and becoming a well-respected rhinoplasty surgeon, Michael Jackson died on June 25, 2009, complicating my calling of "no more Michael Jacksons," since Michael, himself, was no more (**Fig. 12.2**). His untimely death forced me to think even deeper about identity scars and the notion of "well-being disfigurement," meaning the invisible emotional scars that are often present in our patients but that ultimately compromise their sustainable health and happiness. It became evident that Michael's life had been a dangerous dance, which he ultimately failed to master, of misaligned beauty, health, and identity: when this misalignment takes center stage in the great life performance, it is a definite show stopper. So my aesthetic focus has broadened to explore more openly the visible and invisible manifestations of a scarred identity (with the intent of developing new approaches for holistic identity scar revision). I hope that this chapter heightens awareness for the inherent complexity in achieving optimal aesthetic outcomes in patients of African descent. I encourage surgeons to explore the invisible motivators of their patients who seek visible change and, where indicated, to be a conscious participant in the process of cultivating health and wholeness.

Michael Jackson personified the hidden, misaligned aesthetic desires of many individuals of African descent, albeit in the most extreme manifestation. Jackson's assault on his African presence (performed by himself and cosmetic ground troops) offers lessons on many levels. The universal take-home message for my patients of African descent who present for rhinoplasty has been, "I don't want to look like Michael Jackson." I have often wondered why patients thought it was necessary to voice what in my mind was an obvious conclusion—as if anyone in their "right mind" wanted to look like Michael. I don't think that Michael actually wanted to look like Michael as the severity of his cosmetic narrative unfolded. My question now is: How can we shift patients from a focus on what they don't want to look like, or whose nose they desire (e.g., Beyoncé's), to looking at themselves and considering how they can beautifully express their best vision of self? Without a conscious African centeredness, this question is difficult to answer for both the patient of African descent and the aesthetic practitioner who is called upon to deliver care.

12.3 Plastic and Psychic Unity

Much of what has been written on the subject of African aesthetics, particularly in the facial plastic surgery literature, has been crafted in service of Eurocentric technique. In other words, the focus has been on the technical "how" and not the existential "why." I hope to provide cultural enlightenment by prompting the reader to visualize the cosmetic landscape from a fresh position—that is, with African aesthetic traditions in a position of centrality. This chapter cultivates aesthetic consciousness by highlighting Afrocentric concepts to realign the relationship between how one looks (physical beauty), how one feels (mental and physical health), and how one lives a good life, which ultimately determines identity.

I must be honest. It has been difficult to strike the right balance of tone and message in this chapter. How do you craft a chapter for a textbook on facial plastic surgery and place the foundational emphasis not on physical change but on the nonphysical determinants of a successful aesthetic outcome without sounding too much like a mystic? (While recognizing that may not be such a bad thing?) In many ways, facial plastic surgery relies on an undercurrent of psychic fragmentation to exist and thrive. We, as surgeons, along with our patients, are often misled into thinking that focusing on "the physical" in relative isolation can create sustainable well-being, without integrating therapy to enhance the mind or spirit. We all too readily accept the incomplete notion of physical change over metaphysical transformation. We can realize the strength of an African-centered approach to facial plastic surgery by actively embracing what is not seen (the invisible) and acknowledging the spiritual aesthetics of humanistic well-being.

Our highest aspiration as facial aesthetic practitioners should be stewardship of wholeness—body, mind, and spirit. The American artist Robert Motherwell once commented that the purpose of his art was to "unify the plastic and psychic" **(Fig. 12.3)**.[10] As aesthetic surgeons, we too easily accept the role of technician, utilizing our artistic talents to shape and mold only that which can be touched and visualized. The pioneering Sri Lankan art historian and collector Ananda Coomaraswamy's notion of "the way of life and the way of work being one and the same" should be a source of universal inspiration for the modern aesthetic practitioner.[11] We all have the capacity to undergo our own redemptive psychological process by opening our minds to a new aesthetic belief system—in this case, African-centered aesthetics. For Coomaraswamy, the true artist strives to "know and to live in the spirit."[11] Opening oneself to the power of the spirit is an essential principle of African-centered aesthetic thought. Africa provides an intersection that can give new form to an evolving quest for well-being through the integration of Eastern and Western healing philosophy. In particular, African-centered aesthetics offers an opportunity for physicians to assume an avant-garde role as Afrocentric metaphysicians, working artistically to create health and wholeness in their patients. In an essay on the African American aesthetic as optimal consciousness, Linda James Myers states, "From ancient times within African cultures the role of the artist has been one of elevating the consciousness of the people. Providing them signs and symbols of higher forms of life and human functioning, the aesthetician encouraged, educated, and reflected those aspects of being to which humanity must aspire to fulfill its purpose."[12] As facial plastic surgeons, we hold the esteemed title of being contemporary "artists of the head and neck." We have the ability to adopt an African-centered consciousness and to use our artistic talents in service of humanity.

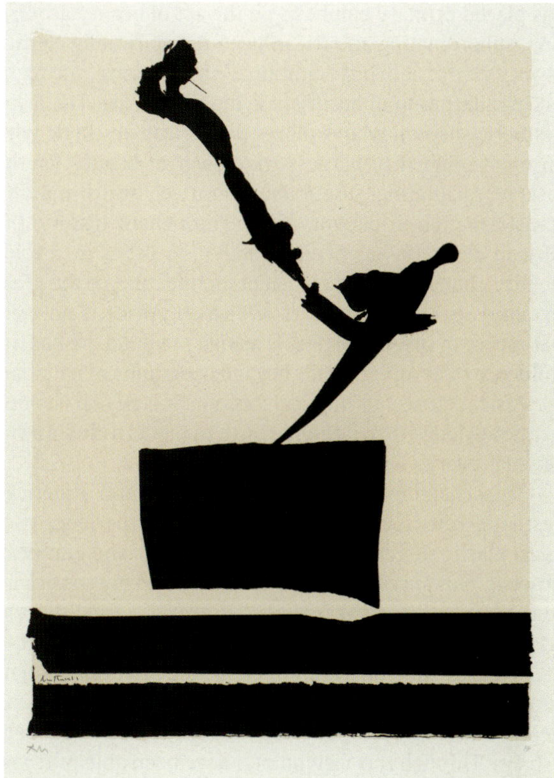

Fig. 12.3 Africa 5, 1970, Robert Motherwell (January 24, 1915–July 16, 1991). Screenprint on paper. 807 × 605 mm. Art © Dedalus Foundation/Licensed by VAGA, New York, NY. Photo ©Tate, London 2015.

Surgical textbooks are traditionally assembled to facilitate the acceleration of technical proficiency. I write, however, to enlighten, in the hope of accelerating self-actualization. Aesthetics, by definition, has both sensory and extrasensory triggers for the expression of beauty and goodness. The sensory component that most often takes precedence is sight—the focus on what can be seen (i.e., the visible). I argue that, when dealing with the patient of African descent, true artistry and aesthetic acumen are often manifested through one's ability to enhance what is not seen, the emotions (i.e., the invisible). In light of this counterculture idea, I ask: Is there a place for African-centered aesthetics in a Euro-dominant elective cosmetic landscape? Without any doubt, I say Yes.

Cosmetic pursuits are largely undertaken from the location of a fragmented mindset and not with the intent of restoring wholeness. Our materialistic modern culture has placed primary emphasis on the act of beauty acquisition, subordinating an African-centered spiritually elegant beauty expression. In a traditional African sense, the highest manifestation of beauty is living a good life. The facial aesthetic surgeon who explores the African aesthetic with an open mind may harness the power of beauty for the task of facilitating sustainable, positive, health-mindful transformation in patients' lives. Throughout history, the African aesthetic has been a catalyst to usher in revolutionary change. From the ancient architecture of the great pyramids to the modern art of Picasso, Africa is an eternal source of inspiration for a creative mankind. Just as the influence of Europe extends beyond geographical boundaries, Africa transcends physical location. It is not far-fetched to acknowledge that, by giving birth to modern civilization, Africa is everywhere.

This chapter arises from my African and American aesthetic consciousness born out of life experience as a facial plastic surgeon of sub-Saharan African and European descent. This ancestral hybridity has created my sensitivity to the space that exists between Afrocentric and Eurocentric aesthetics. My cultural identity as an African American facial plastic surgeon has afforded me the privileged opportunity to interact with a vast array of individuals of African descent seeking cosmetic enhancement to bolster self-esteem. Through this viewpoint, I have been able to recognize the subtleties of ethnic intersection and integration, as well as the differences in perspective between the center and periphery in the discourse around African and European aesthetics. The ability to harness the untapped beauty energy that exists between the center and periphery is a powerful resource that is accessible to all individuals, particularly those of African descent. Few recognize it, and even fewer have figured out how to access the restorative energy as fuel for personal growth. The simple colloquialism of being able to "put oneself in the shoes of another" has far-reaching implications in the facial plastic surgery community as we work to design inclusive aesthetic solutions aligned with health and well-being. As facial plastic surgeons, we must challenge ourselves not to accept limiting ethnocentric perspectives as a universal truth. It is not a healthy and nurturing location for all people.

12.4 The Need for Change

Individuals of African descent now actively and aggressively pursue elective facial cosmetic enhancement. Whether these cosmetic pursuits have a sustainable, positive effect on self-esteem and well-being over the long haul remains an open question. What we do know, however, is that the desire for physical change remains fueled by Eurocentric aesthetic prejudice and Western socioeconomic motivators. The undertaking and offering of elective facial cosmetic procedures is largely driven by a Euro-dominant beauty industry. Consider: If an African aesthetic was at center, how desirable would skin lightening, rhinoplasty, Botox, and injectable fillers be in the eyes of mainstream society? This question highlights the inherent contradiction we face when dealing with the patient of African descent who presents for cosmetic treatment as a means to enhance self-awareness, self-confidence, and self-acceptance. Does it really make any sense?

To a large degree, the mind of the contemporary cosmetic patient of African descent has been colonized by a Eurocentric consciousness that subjugates African-centered aesthetic thought. The contemporary African dance choreographer and scholar Kariamu Welsh insists that "Africans modifying their physical features to appear more European suggest a distorted view of aesthetic function."[13] Difficulties arise in the cosmetic care of patients of African descent on at least two significant levels: first, as a consequence of the presence of the Eurocentric aesthetic mindset, and second from the reality that, more often than not, neither the patient nor the physician can relocate themselves to make aesthetic judgments from a place of African centrality. Steven Dayan offered a commentary on this in his best selling book *Subliminally Exposed*.[14] I include the entire narrative here because it clearly encapsulates the metaphysical challenges that I have alluded to above.

> Late last year I met a young man from Nigeria who came in for a consultation. He had moved to the United States and was making a life for himself in Chicago. Recently married and starting to plan a family, he wanted to undergo a nasal reshaping procedure to make his nose smaller. I was curious why he insisted on having it done so soon and prior to attempting to get his wife pregnant. Upon further discussion, I came to understand his motive for undergoing rhinoplasty. He was concerned that his children would have a wide nose like his, which he thought would make it difficult for them to blend in with friends and others in the community. To assure they didn't get his nose, he wanted to reduce its size before they were conceived. He had not been taught the concept of genetic inheritance, and I had to advise him that even if he did undergo a nasal surgery, his children would still inherit the genetic traits for the noses that have been in his family lineage for over hundreds of thousands of years. But the good news was that because he was marrying a Caucasian woman with a narrower nose, his children would likely have noses that were a blend of the two of them.

When I first read the story, I was deeply disturbed by the implied messages. The story is indeed shocking, but it also subliminally exposes the Eurocentric location of the surgeon's aesthetic consciousness and the dislocation of the Nigerian patient from a place of African centeredness. The irony of this particular case is that both the patient and surgeon are operating from a constraining ethnocentric perspective, despite both having ancestral and cultural ties to the diverse rich traditions of Africa. (Dayan is of North African ancestry—Morocco—and the patient, as stated, is an immigrant from Nigeria.) The example perpetuates negative stereotypes associated with Africa—in this case, the idea that the African aesthetic is less desirable than a Caucasian or European alternative. This aesthetic dislocation nourishes the roots of self-hatred in individuals of African descent. Asante defines self-hatred as a particular orientation of African people, or any people, who have been so destabilized by being "off-center" and "out of location" within their own culture that they have lost all sense of direction.[7] Asante astutely recognizes that "it is probably in the area of aesthetics where Europe has most undermined the self-confidence of Africa."[15] Dayan suggests that there is good news in this story because the Nigerian man was "marrying a Caucasian woman with a narrower nose" and consequently, his implied *bad* genes would likely be balanced by her *good* genes to create a socially acceptable blend in the offspring. From an African-centered viewpoint, there is no good in this story. The implied acceptance of the superiority of Caucasian features over those associated with African ancestry shines light on an aesthetic prejudice that lies at the heart of misaligned African diaspora identity. We have an opportunity to confront this dislocated consciousness "head on" and to redirect patients to a healing place of African centeredness, and thus provide a new framework for constructing healthy self-esteem. The mindset of African-centered aesthetics is dynamic, not constricted by one dogmatic vantage point or singular frame of reference. My delight with African-centered aesthetics rests in its physical and metaphysical fluidity to enlighten and to function as a cultural (re)locator. In the facial plastic surgery community, the notion of African beauty is often relegated to limiting physical features, such as a shape of nose, texture of hair, or shade of skin, but Afrocentric beauty exists more expansively as a spiritual unity connecting individuals of African descent through tradition and culture across the diaspora. For example, African centeredness acts as a unifying aesthetic link providing a common thread to weave together the Nigerian Afrobeat of Fela Kuti with the Brazilian Afro Samba of Bossa Nova, to the Caribbean rhythms of AfroCuban jazz to the American Cool of Hip Hop. By adopting a transnational, transcultural aesthetic consciousness, individuals of African descent can begin to view themselves in a central position within a global community.

12.5 Africa As Inspiration—A Humanistic Catalyst

The African is frequently called upon to place a humanizing element on the ills of modern society. Humanitarian efforts to eliminate world hunger and global poverty functionalize the aesthetics of men, women, and children of African descent to raise social consciousness and to stimulate a caring call to action. Global missions to restore facial deformities, such as Operation Smile in Kenya, harness the technical expertise of plastic surgeons to improve the quality of life for patients suffering from cleft lip and cleft palate. The basic techniques that repair a cleft palate (physically and metaphysically) construct a path for a better life in the patients and families who benefit from the benevolent care. In this scenario, facial aesthetic work is directly linked to the beauty and goodness of improved health and well-being. This humanitarian consciousness does not have to be confined to "mission" work on the continent of Africa. We have the opportunity to be uplifted as humanitarians in our daily interactions with all patients by adopting traditional African-centered concepts into the practice of facial plastic surgery.

The fundamental premise of this chapter is to encourage the "artist of the head and neck" to open a mind's eye to the creative possibilities fueled by an expanded African-centered consciousness. This is not a totally new idea. As much as a century ago, avant-garde artists and photographers like Picasso, Matisse, Modigliani, Klee, Stieglitz, and Man Ray looked to Africa for new sources of creative inspiration.[16] In some ways, this inner eye's turning to Africa was a humanizing response to the transformation of daily life propelled by the rapid industrialization of Europe and America. The dehumanizing mechanization of modern living brought with it a spiritual longing for a life untainted by industry. Not everyone agreed with the idea that machines were a means to attaining a better world.

Picasso's *Les Demoiselles d'Avignon* is often heralded as the impetus for a major conceptual shift in the world of European art—and the subsequent development of modern art in the West (**Fig. 12.4**).[17] In her 2009 examination of Man Ray and African art, Wendy Grossman notes, "The assimilation of styles and motifs from African cultural artifacts into the work of avant-garde artists was a means of challenging conventional Western aesthetic values." Grossman further asserts "By looking to pre-industrial cultures to reinvigorate their own creative visions, these artists discovered new ways of seeing. At a time when traditional Western art was thought by some to have exhausted its potential, alternatives offered by novel forms of African and other indigenous cultures liberated European artists from the constraints of their own academic traditions and infused vitality into a radically new aesthetic vision."[17] Metaphorically, African plastic arts functioned as a regenerative "fountain of youth" for an aging Eurocentric aesthetic practice.[18]

The search for renewal through African aesthetics adopted by the European artistic avant-garde during the first half of the twentieth century has important implications for how we may consider the present moment and need for healing. The beginning of the twenty-first century brings with it a similar contextual array of challenges characterized by a struggle to find peace and balance in daily

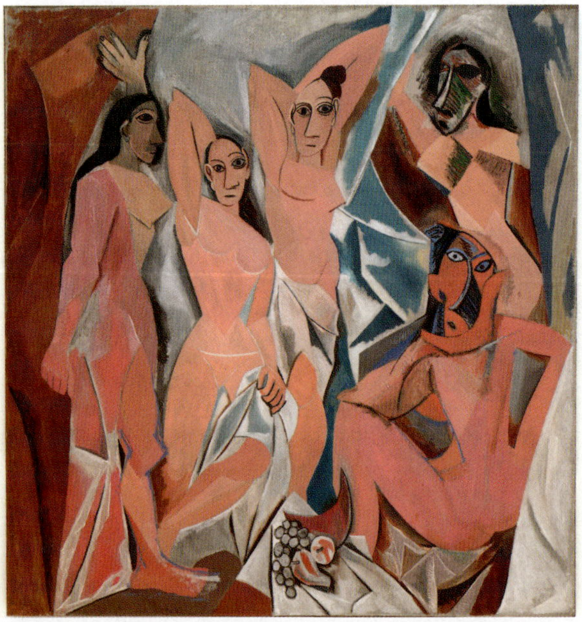

Fig. 12.4 Picasso, Pablo (1881–1973): Les Demoiselles d'Avignon (Paris, June–July 1907). New York, Museum of Modern Art (MoMA). Oil on canvas, 8′ × 7′8″ (243.9 × 233.7 cm). Acquired through the Lillie P. Bliss Bequest. 333.1939 © 2015. Digital image, The Museum of Modern Art, New York/Scala, Florence. © 2015 Estate of Pablo Picasso/Artists Rights Society (ARS), New York.

life. Instead of mechanical industrialization, we now face a psychosocial imbalance boosted by the expansive influence of the Internet and mobile digital technology. As we search for happiness in a digital world, it is time again to deconstruct aesthetic values and to create something fresh and new. African-centered principles may offer balancing aesthetic insight for the design of holistic approaches to achieve individual health and well-being. I offer three examples of African-centered aesthetic thought to consider for inspiration—the Gabonese Reliquary Ensemble, the Mende concept of *nyande*, and the Yoruba idea of the head as center of life.

12.6 The Guardian Reliquary Figure: Muse of Modernity

It should inspire present-day "artists of the head and neck" that the artifact revered by the early twentieth century artistic avant-garde was the reliquary figure of West and Central Africa. Several traditional African societies, including the Punu and Kota peoples in Gabon and the Fang peoples of Gabon, Equatorial Guinea, and Cameroon, honored their ancestors by keeping physical remnants of them as relics **(Fig. 12.5)**.[19] Portions of the skull and other bones were preserved in a barkwood box or woven basket to which a carved guardian reliquary figure or head was affixed.

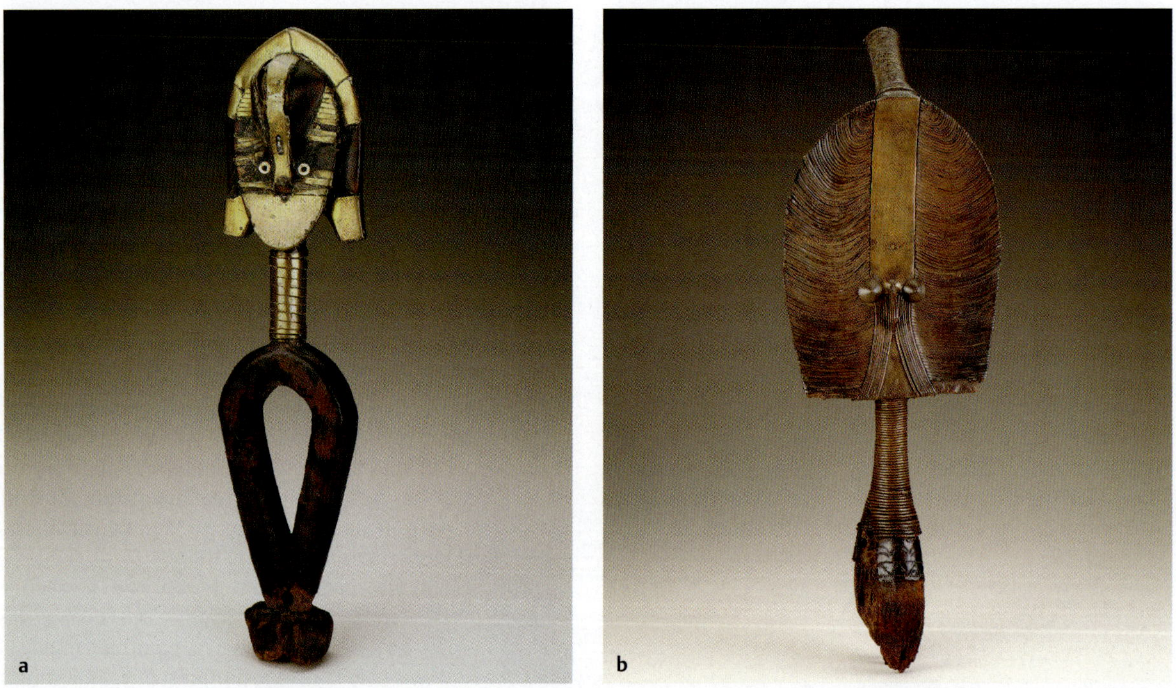

Fig. 12.5 **(a)** Reliquary guardian figure (*ngulu*). Kota peoples; Gabon; early 20th century; wood, brass, copper alloy, pigment, eggshell, encrustation; H × W × D: 41.9 × 11.7 × 5.1 cm (16½ × 4⅝ × 2 in); gift of Mr. and Mrs. George Lois; 83–17–1; photograph by Franko Khoury; National Museum of African Art, Smithsonian Institution. **(b)** Reliquary guardian figure (*bwiti*). Hongwe peoples; Gabon; 19th century; wood, copper, brass; H × W × D: 60 × 21.9 × 12.1 cm (23⅝ × 8⅝ × 4¾ in); acquisition grant from the James Smithson Society and museum purchase; 88–4-1; photograph by Franko Khoury; National Museum of Africa Art, Smithsonian Institution.

At the turn of the twentieth century, however, these African sculptural artifacts were progressively distanced from their traditional significance and were most often displayed as an ethnographic complement to abstract art **(Fig. 12.6)**.

The appropriation of the reliquary figure illustrates the conceptual differences between African-centered and Eurocentric aesthetic thought. The Reliquary Ensemble (guardian figure and ancestral basket) served as a familial altar tied inextricably to spiritual rituals and the well-being of the traditional African community. As noted by Alisa La Gamma, "Ancestral relics related to the most distinguished members of as many as nine generations of an extended lineage were contained within. The opening of the reliquary by elders was an opportunity to reflect on family history."[20] For the traditional African, the Reliquary Ensemble embodied the notion of balance in all things—the dynamic relationship between the living and the dead, the child and the elder, the individual and the community. The Eurocentric interest in the reliquary, however, was largely confined to its sculptural beauty or its role as a physical representation of imperial conquest.

The reliquary figure exhibited as a distinct entity separate from the ancestral container hints at the broader challenges that we face today in the context of visual objectification and functional misappropriation. In modern society, we often place emphasis on what is outwardly visible (the physical) without fully appreciating the unseen nature of wholeness—the invisible (metaphysical) things that make up our essential being. Our contemporary challenges with well-being are often directly related to an inability to appreciate "authentic life functionality," in other words, life purpose. Traditional African-centered aesthetics are by nature communal, functional, and holistic. From a location of African centeredness, we may interpret the reliquary guardian figure and ancestral container in its traditional context as a tool for the preservation of social order. There is an emphasis on the idea that physical beauty, such as in the case of the sculptural reliquary figure, has a spiritual role to keep people in harmony with nature and community. Through this (re)location of the reliquary back to traditional African-centered thought, we see how physical beauty and metaphysical goodness are inextricably interwoven in traditional African aesthetics.

12.7 Beauty and Goodness

For many African Americans who are descendants of the transatlantic slave trade, there is a deep longing to reconstitute the broken genealogical link to an African ancestral heritage. Genetic ancestry testing has become an increasingly popular tool for facilitating this African-centered goal. Through DNA testing, I recently discovered that I shared maternal mitochondrial DNA with individuals living in present-day Sierra Leone and who self-identified as Mende **(Fig. 12.7)**.

The Mende are an ethnic group of about one million persons, mainly agriculturists, who live in southern and eastern Sierra Leone, on the West Atlantic coast of Africa. Sylvia Ardyn Boone contributed immensely to scholarly knowledge of traditional Mende aesthetics through her influential book *Radiance from the Waters: Ideals of Feminine Beauty in Mende Art*.[21] She opens the book with a Mende proverb: "Hani gbė lewe ma ngele ya nja gbili kaango kpowa ėė to"

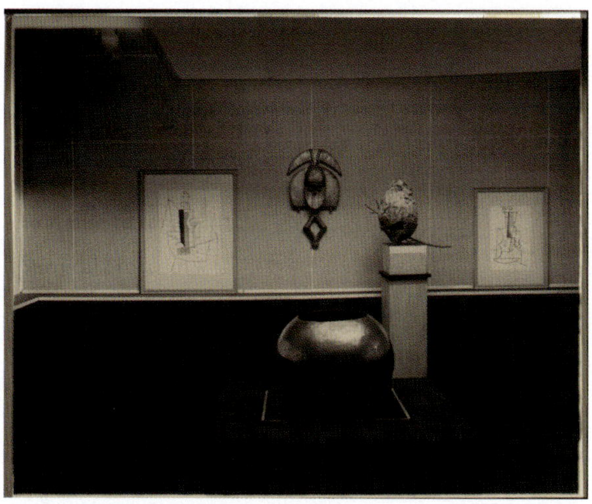

Fig.12.6 Stieglitz, Alfred (1864–1946): Picasso-Braque Exhibition at '291', 1915. New York, Museum of Modern Art (MoMA). Platinum print 7 11/16 × 9 11/16 (19.5 × 24.6 cm). Gift of Charles Sheeler. Acc.n.: 633.1941. © 2015. Digital image, The Museum of Modern Art, New York/Scala, Florence. © 2015 Georgia O'Keeffe Museum/Artists Rights Society (ARS), New York.

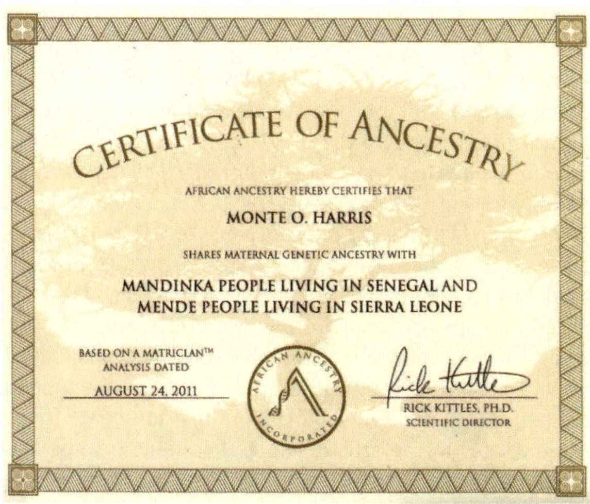
CERTIFICATE OF ANCESTRY
AFRICAN ANCESTRY HEREBY CERTIFIES THAT
MONTE O. HARRIS
SHARES MATERNAL GENETIC ANCESTRY WITH
MANDINKA PEOPLE LIVING IN SENEGAL AND
MENDE PEOPLE LIVING IN SIERRA LEONE
BASED ON A MATRICLAN™ ANALYSIS DATED
AUGUST 24, 2011
AFRICAN ANCESTRY INCORPORATED
RICK KITTLES, PH.D.
SCIENTIFIC DIRECTOR

Fig. 12.7 African Ancestry Certificate. (Courtesy of Monte Oyd Harris.)

("There is a thing passing in the sky; some thick clouds surround it; the uninitiated sees nothing"). The proverb introduces the reader to Mende aesthetic thought through the idea of initiation as a determinant for seeing. Boone comments that the "eyes" of the initiated are "metaphysical: an informed intellect, a widened vision, and a deepened discernment." The ability to see what is "surrounded by clouds," or not obvious, can be likened to the act in facial plastic surgery of cultivating the subjective "inner eye" or insight. Boone's reference to the metaphysical is important because it speaks to a recurrent theme in African-centered aesthetics: the role of initiation as a rite of passage for the cultivation of insight. I ask: What are the modes of initiation for the contemporary "artist of the head and neck"? If they were left up to the capitalist forces of a consumptive world, I'm pretty sure that the aesthetic rites of passage would be connected to digitally answering self-objectified questions on Web-based information-sharing networks or lending professional credibility for product promotional purposes in service of cosmetic industry needs.

In many traditional African societies, beauty and goodness are often represented as a unified entity with a singular term, such as *nyande* in the Mende from Sierra Leone and *nefer* in ancient Egyptian language. Our contemporary idea of beauty as separate from goodness implies that beauty may exist without functionality, suggesting a location for beauty for beauty's sake. *Beauty for beauty's sake* can be likened to the European modernist idea of art for art's sake. *Art for art's sake* expresses a philosophy that the intrinsic value of art, and the only "true" art, is divorced from any didactic, moral, or utilitarian function. Afrocentric theorists have asserted that art for art's sake originates from a Eurocentric location and had no place in traditional African culture. Art or handicraft was purposeful, imbued with functionality for the well-being of the community. African sculptural arts, as in the case of the reliquary guardian figure, served the purpose of ritual connectors to the spirit world. To some degree, contemporary society has transferred the individualistic premise of art for art's sake to the concept of beauty. Beauty pursuits have taken on a presumed stand-alone value without any moral value—their purpose being only to pleasure the eye. If art for art's sake had no place in traditional African society, is there a place for beauty for beauty's sake in the aesthetic care of patients, particularly those of African descent, in today's world?

The physical aspects of beauty in a traditional African-centered aesthetic are intimately related to the metaphysical aspects of goodness. The metaphysical qualities are manifested through a concern for function, ethics, and morality. Beauty, for instance, in traditional Mende society is judged for its goodness. "Beauty is closely inspected all the time to make sure it is good."[21] Goodness in the traditional African sense relates to the artistic expression, functionality, and moral character. "Mende assume that a beautiful exterior enshrines the most useful something. It is a big disappointment for something to be physically beautiful to look at but not good, not useful."[21] Linking beauty to goodness within an aesthetic framework is aligned with African-centered thought. Carrying this African-centered aesthetic mindset into cosmetic practice forces clinicians to critically reassess their relationship with patients by contemplating what goodness may come from the performance of any cosmetic procedure. In her description of Mende aesthetics, Boone succinctly states, "Beauty without a dimension of goodness is hollow, without substance, a deception."[21] By adopting an African-centered consciousness, we may (re)locate our perspectives around beauty to recognize cosmetic treatments as a humanistic means to adorn the physical and metaphysical qualities of goodness. At the highest level of conceptualization, the unity of beauty and goodness is represented by the human qualities of kind-heartedness and generosity, a sympathetic interest in the well-being of others, and a compassionate readiness to give.[21]

12.8 The Head as the Center of Life

Over the past 20 years, my professional life has been dedicated to understanding, exploring, preserving, and enhancing the essential organs that most directly determine our interactions with the outside world—the eyes, ears, nose, and mouth—which are, of course, all housed in the head. A focus on the head, and more recently on hair as an extension of the head, is aligned with my notion of African centeredness.

Like many traditional African societies, the Yoruba of western Nigeria regard the human head (*ori*) as the most vital part of a person.[22] The head is symbolically linked to notions about destiny, individuality, intellect, and personal power.[23] The head is of immense importance in Yoruba art and thought. In sculpture, its size is often enlarged in relation to the body to convey its position as the site of a person's essential nature. The prominence given to the head derives from both physical and metaphysical qualities. According to African scholar Babtunde Lawal: "While the Yoruba recognize the physiological importance of the head, they place a higher premium on its metaphysical significance as the source of life and the essence of human personality."[24] Inner qualities or metaphysical qualities should rule outer or physical ones, especially such qualities of the mind such as inner calm, self-control, and patience.[22]

The Western approach to life from ancient to modern times has placed overwhelming emphasis on the physical body. From the ancient Greeks and Romans to contemporary Euro-American beauty culture, the admiration and pleasure received from bodily pursuits is perceived as second to none. In search of new solutions to well-being, attention has gradually begun to shift from the Western body construct to an Eastern body, mind, and spirit consciousness. Eastern notions have been mythologized in the ancient healing traditions of Ayurveda and Chinese medicine. The irony of it all lies in the fact that as the West adopts a more Eastern consciousness for daily life rituals, many Eastern individuals are attaching themselves to the destructive patterns of a materialistic, visually objectified, Western lifestyle.

12.9 Cosmetic Trend—Going Natural

African-centered aesthetic expression is inspired and driven by a deep connection to nature. The relationship to the Earth is an ever-present source of creative inspiration, health maintenance, and spiritual renewal. There is a growing demand in the cosmetic and beauty industry for natural-looking results and organic products infused with ingredients derived from the Earth. Organic awareness is part of a larger mindfulness movement comprised of individuals seeking a balanced, health-conscious, and purposeful life. Daily beauty rituals are becoming more respectful of nature and sensitive to the sustainability of the planet.

An exciting cosmetic trend for women of African descent involves *going natural*, a cultural term used by black women who decide to stop chemically straightening their hair. Many women of African descent have not seen their hair in its natural textured state since childhood. The act of chemically processing the hair to conform to Eurocentric beauty standards has been a method of acculturation for women of African descent since the early twentieth century. Today, the modern woman of African descent is uniquely situated to personify an organic avant-garde by celebrating a renewed relationship with the beauty of natural textured hair.

Excessive chemical hair straightening, coupled with other traumatic grooming practices, can be considered a form of cosmetic abuse that insidiously leads to beauty, health, and identity misalignment over time. Traumatic grooming practices are practiced by women of all ethnicities—whether it's coloring the hair to eliminate gray, bleaching to achieve the blond ideal, adding extensions for length, or straightening to relax tightly wound curls. Unfortunately, for women of African descent, an alarming incidence of hair loss accompanies these beauty pursuits. Hair loss has become an epidemic, particularly for women whose hair has been traumatized by chemicals and damaging hairstyles. For many women of African descent, hair loss is a serious, life-altering condition. A recent study undertaken by the Cleveland Clinic showed the prevalence of hair loss among African American women to be nearly 30%.[25] So, the notion of "going natural" is a contemporary cosmetic trend that has both physical and metaphysical implications for the woman of African descent. The natural-hair movement goes beyond a simple desire for a new style; it is often fueled by a desire to live a healthy, balanced life.

Cosmetic pursuits should strengthen mental and physical well-being by reaffirming the best in oneself and nature. I have found that the aesthetic journey that women of African descent take to restore a relationship with their natural hair is a positive marker of a reaffirmation process (**Fig. 12.8, Fig. 12.9** and **Fig. 12.10**). The natural-hair trend is one that has far-reaching effects on well-being by establishing a healthy homeostasis between beauty and identity. By shunning the chemical demands of a Eurocentric hairstyle, women of African descent are in many ways adopting an African-centered location and a stable foundation for building up healthy self-esteem.

12.10 Call to Action

So, where's the growing edge in our effort to preserve our health, happiness, and well-being? For all that we do know in the West and in the East, there is still much that we have not learned about the traditions of Africa, our most diverse and vast continent. The ancients knew that out of Africa, always comes something new. A recurrent theme in African-centered thought is a reverential acknowledgment of the power that resides in what is not seen. The visible largely functions as a tool to assess the inner spiritual realm. For aestheticians who can (re)locate to African centeredness, I would argue that health, happiness, and wholeness reside in a head, mind, and spirit approach to life.

We have the ability to adopt an African-centered consciousness and to use our artistic talents in service of beauty and goodness. An African-centered aesthetic consciousness places emphasis on both the physical and metaphysical aspects of beauty. With this mindset, we may creatively explore new ways of unifying beauty and goodness. Cosmetic pursuits should harness the power of beauty to functionalize the goodness of life performance. This is a point of view that places African aesthetic thought at the center. This elevated Afrocentric consciousness is multidimensional and not limited to individuals of African descent. Just as individuals outside of the Eurocentric mainstream in America have adopted a Euro-American consciousness, I challenge aesthetic practitioners of today—of all ethnicities and cultural backgrounds—to open their mind and spirit to the beauty of traditional African-centered thought.

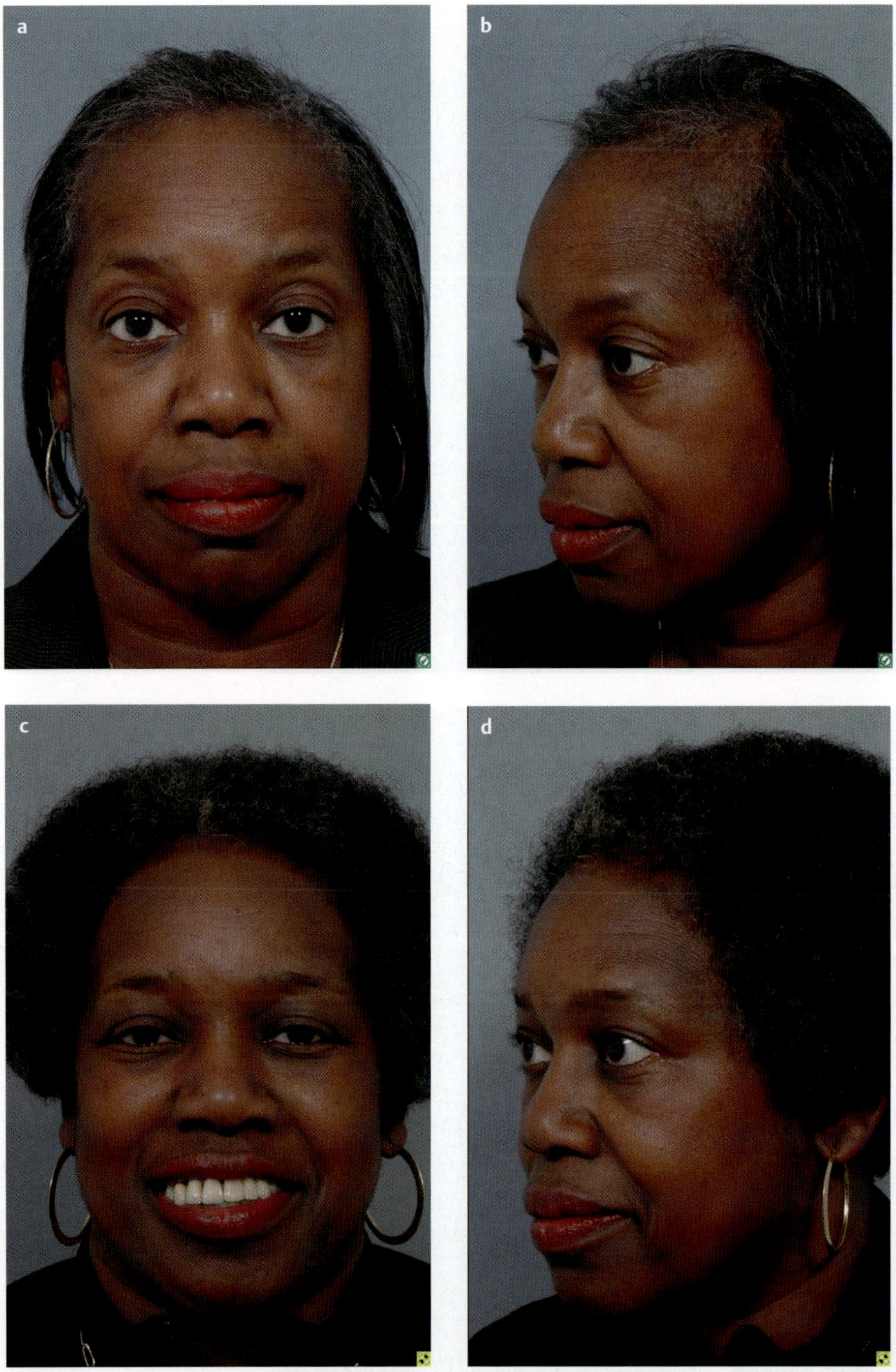

Fig. 12.10 (a–d) Visual narrative of "going natural" as illustrated by an African American woman who has undergone a transition to naturally textured hair. The physical changes align with an enhancement of overall self-image and a healthy state of mental consciousness. In this example, transition to naturally textured hair followed follicular unit hair transplantation. The patient underwent a single transplant procedure of ~ 1600 1–3-hair follicular unit grafts.

References

1. Matory WE. Definitions of beauty in the ethnic patient. In: Matory WE, ed. Ethnic Considerations in Facial Aesthetic Surgery. Philadelphia, PA: Lippincott-Raven; 1998:61–83
2. Grimes PE. Aesthetics and Cosmetic Surgery for Darker Skin Types. Philadelphia, PA: Lippincott Williams & Wilkins; 1998
3. Harris MO. Intrinsic skin aging in pigmented races. In: Halder RM, ed. Dermatology and Dermatological Therapy of Pigmented Skins. Boca Raton, FL: CRC Press; 2006: 197–208
4. Harris MO. The aging face in patients of color: minimally invasive surgical facial rejuvenation—a targeted approach. Dermatol Ther 2004;17(2):206–211
5. Porter JP, Olson KL. Anthropometric facial analysis of the African American woman. Arch Facial Plast Surg 2001;3(3):191–197
6. Sims LS, King-Hammond L. The Global Africa Project: Contemporary Design, Craft, and Art. Munich, Germany: Prestel Publishing; 2010:11–37
7. Asante ME. Afrocentricity: notes on a disciplinary position. In: Asante WE. An Afrocentric Manifesto. Cambridge, UK, and Boston, MA: Polity Press; 2007:31–32
8. Harris MO. Rhinoplasty in the patient of African descent. Facial Plast Surg Clin North Am 2010;18(1):189–199
9. Harris MO. Cultivating a global aesthetic consciousness. Arch Facial Plast Surg 2009;11(6):420–421
10. Taylor B. Motherwell's risk. In: Davidson S. Robert Motherwell: Early Collages. New York, NY: The Solomon R. Guggenheim Foundation; 2013:33
11. Jahanbegloo R. Ananda K. Coomaraswamy: A Metaphysical Critique of Modernity. 15 Oct 2012. Available at http://jahanbegloo.com/content/ananda-k-coomaraswamy-metaphysical-critique-modernity. Accessed 13 Mar 2015
12. Myers LJ. The African American aesthetic as optimal consciousness. In: Welsh-Asante K, ed. The African Aesthetic: Keeper of the Traditions. Westport, CT: Praeger Publishers; 1993:21
13. Welsh-Asante K. The aesthetic conceptualization of Nzuri. In: Welsh-Asante K, ed. The African Aesthetic: Keeper of the Traditions. Westport, CT: Praeger Publishers; 1993:5
14. Dayan SH. Subliminally Exposed: Shocking Truths about Your Hidden Desires in Mating, Dating and Communicating. Use Cautiously. New York, NY: Morgan James Publishing; 2013
15. Asante M. Location theory and African aesthetics. In: Welsh-Asante K, ed. The African Aesthetic: Keeper of the Traditions. Westport, CT: Praeger Publishers; 1993:57
16. Biro Y. African Art, New York, and the Avant-Garde: Exhibition Overview. Tribal Art Magazine 2013;(3):10–19
17. Grossman WA. African art between the modern and the "primitive." In: Grossman WA. Man Ray, African Art, and the Modernist Lens. Produced by International Arts & Artists, Washington DC. Minneapolis, MN: University of Minnesota Press; 2009:11
18. Blair C. Perspective on African art criticism: a brush with Western bias. Black World 1975;24(9):72
19. Freyer BM, Geary CM, Lifchitz E, et al. Selected Works from the Collection of the National Museum of African Art. Volume 1. Washington, DC: Published for the National Museum of African Art by the Smithsonian Institution Press; 1999:103–105
20. LaGamma A. Art from Gabon. Tribal Art Magazine. 2013; 3:26–35
21. Boone SA. Radiance from the Waters: Ideals of Feminine Beauty in Mende Art. New Haven, CT: Yale University Press; 1986:140–143
22. Drewel HJ. The splendor of ancient Ife: art in an early West African state. In: Drewal HJ, Schildkrout E. Dynasty and Divinity: Ife Art in Ancient Nigeria. New York: The Museum for African Art. Seattle: University of Washington Press; 2009
23. Arnoldi MJ, Kreamer CM. Focus on twelve African hats. In: Arnoldi MJ, Kreamer CM. Crowning Achievements: African Arts of Dressing the Head. Los Angeles, CA: Fowler Museum of Cultural History, University of California; 1995:27–51
24. Lawal B. Ori: The significance of the head in Yoruba sculpture. J Anthropol Res 1985;41(1):91–103
25. Kyei A, Bergfeld WF, Piliang M, Summers P. Medical and environmental risk factors for the development of central centrifugal cicatricial alopecia: a population study. Arch Dermatol 2011;147(8):909–914

13 Dorsal Augmentation Techniques in the African Descent Platyrrhine Nose

Thomas Romo III, Tara E. Brennan, and Ignacio Viza-Puiggros

13.1 Introduction

The platyrrhine nose has certain ethnic characteristics that are distinct from the Caucasian nose and important to take into consideration when performing rhinoplasty. The platyrrhine nose is typically characterized by thicker skin and a larger subcutaneous tissue pad,[1] characteristics that tend to obscure definition of the nasal tip.[2] The African platyrrhine nose was described by Schultz in 1913 as more broad and flat, with diminished nasal bones and cartilages, and less dorsal projection than the Caucasian nose.[3] The nasal alae are wider, and the nostrils are more horizontally oriented. The typical nasal tip is also more flat and round, and the alae and nostrils are more flared. The bony and cartilaginous support of the septum is often relatively lacking. The premaxilla and nasal spine also tend to be more hypoplastic, creating a more acute nasolabial angle **(Fig. 13.1)**. Characteristics of African nasal valve physiology have also been documented by several authors. Canbay and Bathia measured nasal valve resistance following decongestion using rhinomanometry, and they demonstrated a statistically significantly higher decrease in the mean total airway resistance among African American patients compared with Caucasians.[4]

The ethnic differences in nasal anatomy are important to take into account when analyzing a nose and planning a rhinoplasty, because the rhinoplasty surgeon has to pay more attention to structural support to address the typical aesthetic concerns of the rhinoplasty patient. Importantly, one must keep in mind that the skin–soft tissue envelope (S-STE) cannot be reduced sizably, and to create further refinement and definition of the nasal tip, structural augmentation is typically required to stretch and thin out the S-STE. This often involves a combination of grafts to augment the dorsum and lower third of the nose. Significantly, using grafts for augmentation not only improves the appearance of the nose by providing more shape and definition, but it also often improves its function as well.

Numerous implants and grafts are available for use in platyrrhine rhinoplasty to accomplish the goals of structural augmentation and refinement, although no ideal grafting material exists. The ideal graft is:

- Readily available
- Inexpensive
- Inert
- Sterile
- Structurally similar to native tissue
- Sculptable

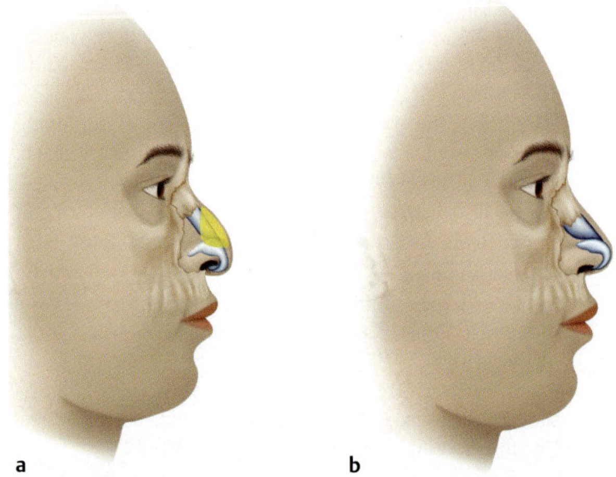

Fig. 13.1 **(a,b)** Lateral view comparing the anatomic features of a generalized ethnic nose and a Caucasian nose. In this representation, the diminished nasal bones and cartilages are shown, as is the prominent subcutaneous fibrofatty pad of the typical platyrrhine nose. The premaxilla and nasal spine are notably hypoplastic. Overall, the nose is less projected and has a less defined nasal tip.

- Resistant to trauma, infection, and extrusion
- Integrated with surrounding tissue
- Easy to remove

The surgeon must know the benefits and disadvantages of each grafting and implant material to obtain the best outcome.

13.2 Treatment Goals and Planned Outcomes

The most important goals in the typical platyrrhine rhinoplasty are structural augmentation and tip refinement.[5] Numerous autologous and alloplastic materials are available to facilitate structural grafting.

Autologous grafts include cartilage and bone. Cartilage is used more commonly, and it may be harvested from the patient's nose, ear, or rib. Cartilage is an ideal autologous grafting material for structural augmentation in the nose.

Septal cartilage is the most useful, as it matches the underlying framework one is attempting to augment, but it can be in short supply in the setting of prior surgery, trauma, or congenital deformity. Unfortunately, the platyrrhine nose often lacks enough native septal cartilage to fashion the grafts required to achieve structural augmentation, which leaves the surgeon searching for alternate material. Auricular cartilage is curved and relatively weaker than septal cartilage. Costal cartilage is also available to be harvested and abundant but requires a separate donor/surgical site, which can be associated with donor-site morbidity, including pain, chest-wall deformity, scarring, and pneumothorax. Additionally, costal cartilage has a tendency to warp, and experience is necessary to learn to predict the warp and to use the warping to one's advantage in effecting structural change in the nose. Fixation techniques are also important to master to minimize the warping.[6]

Autologous cartilage may be carved into boat-shaped dorsal grafts; long, straight segments to be used as extended spreader grafts; shorter, straight segments for columellar strut grafts; or triangle-shaped tip or shield grafts. It may also be morcelized and placed into discrete pockets to augment the dorsum or premaxilla.[7,8]

Autologous bone grafts harvested from the iliac crest or calvarium are options but less commonly used, as they have a tendency to fracture, can partially resorb, and tend to confer a more rigid feel to the nose.[9] In addition, associated potential complications of calvarial bone harvest include dural injury, intracerebral injury, subdural hematoma, cerebrospinal fluid leaks, and sagittal sinus lacerations.

Homografts like irradiated (cadaveric) rib cartilage may also be used, and good results have been obtained in rhinoplasty using this material.[10] Homograft rib cartilage has the advantages of not being limited in supply and not incurring additional donor-site morbidity. Its disadvantages include potential for disease transmission, although no such cases have been reported. Resorption, warping, and mobility within the nose if not stabilized are other disadvantages that irradiated rib cartilage grafts share in common with autologous rib cartilage grafts.[11]

Definitively, autologous cartilage has an advantage over synthetic materials in that it is associated with less chance of infection or extrusion, particularly when dealing with revision operations.[12,13] As septal cartilage is often in short supply in the platyrrhine nose, an additional cartilage donor site is often required if autologous cartilage is desired **(Table 13.1)**. Synthetic materials for augmentation rhinoplasty are often discussed when the patient and/or surgeon would like to avoid the morbidity of an additional surgical site.

Alloplastic implants include preformed synthetic grafts made of silicone or porous polyethylene, and they have been used for more than 50 years in nasal surgery. They are attractive alternatives to autologous grafts because of their abundant supply, ease of use, predictable biologic response,

Table 13.1 Nonsynthetic grafts for nasal reconstruction

Type	Pros	Cons	Recommended uses
Autogenous grafts			
Cartilage			
Septum	Consistent results, low extrusion rates, low infection rates, may be used for structural support and soft tissue augmentation	Limited availability in revision cases	Dorsal onlay, tip grafts, columellar strut, alar batten
Auricular	Easily harvested, concavity similar to lower lateral cartilage	Limited supply, separate donor site, warping	Alar battens, dorsal onlay, tip grafts
Costal	Ample supply	Separate donor site, potential for warping	Dorsal onlay, tip grafts, columellar strut, alar batten
Bone			
Split calvarium	Ample supply, biocompatible	Potential for resorption, separate donor site, potential for fracture, palpability	Dorsal onlay, columellar strut, alar batten
Homologous graft			
Irradiated rib	Ample supply, biocompatible	Resorption, warping, patient stigma	Dorsal onlay, tip grafts, columellar strut, alar batten

and lack of need for an additional surgical donor site, with its inherent morbidity. Drawbacks include the additional cost of the implant, and an often-cited greater chance of infection than with autologous grafting materials. The senior author, however, has had negligible negative experiences with synthetic grafting materials in rhinoplasty, and porous high-density polyethylene (PHDPE), or Medpor, in particular, over the last 20 years of experience.

Synthetic materials are used as implants in other parts of the body without controversy. Calcium hydroxylapatite is used with titanium mesh to repair skull base and calvarial defects relatively commonly, for example. Silicone implants have been used for breast augmentation for many years. The nose, however, is mobile. It is used for breathing and is relatively animated, since the SMAS layer is intimately adherent to the overlying skin, as are the muscles of facial expression. Fixation of implants, therefore, is a relatively unique consideration when choosing a synthetic implant to use in the nose.

Synthetic implants have the advantage of being readily available and easy to use, and they effect predictable aesthetic results. Synthetic implants do not carry the risk of warping inherent to costal cartilage grafts; however, they can be expensive and they have a small but higher tendency for infection and extrusion when compared with their autologous graft counterparts. As with their autologous graft counterparts, special attention needs to be paid to stabilizing the synthetic implant in the nose to prevent asymmetry.

Silicone in its solid form (Silastic; Dow Corning Corporation) can provide a smooth and natural-feeling structural augmentation to the nasal dorsum. It is easily sculpted as well. However, it is smooth and not porous, and therefore does not lend itself to surrounding soft tissue ingrowth. This results in a graft that has a greater tendency to move within the nose. Characteristically, a fibrous capsule forms around silicone implants, which, if traumatized, can lead to infection or fluid accumulation. Removal of the implant is sometimes required in these cases. Another disadvantage of using silicone implants in the nose is their risk of extrusion, particularly when placed under tension and under a thin skin envelope. In general, rates of extrusion are higher when implants are placed in the columella (up to 50%) as opposed to the nasal dorsum.[14]

Expanded-porous polytetrafluorethylene (e-PTFE; Gore-Tex) is another synthetic polymer that has been widely used in general surgery (e.g., mesh for abdominal hernia repair) and has also been used in nasal dorsal augmentation. Macroscopically, it is soft and pliable, and it is useful when soft volume filling is necessary, but it is not recommended when structural grafting material is needed.[15] e-PTFE differs from silicone in that it is porous and therefore permits soft tissue ingrowth.[16] However, its pores are small, ranging from 10 to 30 µm, which leads to less soft tissue integration and fixation to the surrounding tissues. It has a significant risk of extrusion, and infection rates are relatively high, especially in thin or scarred skin.[17,18] It is also very costly compared with other synthetic materials and, more recently, not readily available from the manufacturer for use as a nasal implant.

Porous high-density polyethylene (PHDPE) implants are robust, synthetic, porous, inert carbon polymer grafts that can be used for dorsal augmentation in rhinoplasty. These implants have large pores (ranging from 100 to 250 µm), which allow for soft tissue ingrowth, affording stability to the implant and reducing the chances it will move once placed into the nose. PHDPE implants come in a variety of shapes that can be used to create a variety of grafts in the nose. They come in canoe-shaped implants that can be carved and placed on the dorsum for augmentation, and they are also available as straight sheets (1.1 mm) that can be used for fashioning a columellar strut or nasal tip grafts. Concave oval sheet (0.85 mm) PHDPE grafts are also available to be used as alar batten grafts. PHDPE implants have a firm but cancellous consistency, which affords easy sculpting but confers a significant rigidity to the nose on palpation.

The most frequent complication of PHDPE implants is infection, with rates between 2.6 and 7.4% and usually requiring implant removal,[12] although Scalfani and colleagues demonstrated that implant infection and partial exposure can often be treated conservatively, with antibiotics and conservative debridement.[19] Notably, removing an infected implant can prove extremely difficult to do without compromising the thickness, vascularity, and integrity of the overlying S-STE of the nose, and this task can be quite a challenge to the rhinoplasty surgeon confronted with a revision case requiring removal of a synthetic implant (**Table 13.2**).

13.3 Preoperative Planning and Preparation

Complete presurgical evaluation is the first requirement in platyrrhine nose surgery. It is important to understand patients' concerns and expectations and to elicit their motivations for seeking a rhinoplasty. Their concerns may be cosmetic, functional, or a combination of the two. It is paramount to communicate that the goals of rhinoplasty are to effect the desired cosmetic changes without compromising nasal function. Often, structural augmentation rhinoplasty will result in not only an improved appearance of the nose but also improved function. Augmentation rhinoplasty (for example, dorsal augmentation with placement of a columella strut and a tip shield graft) may have a refining effect on the nose by stretching out the overlying S-STE, thereby providing more definition to the underlying structure of the nose. Usually, the platyrrhine patient has a thick S-STE, which lends itself well to structural augmentation

Table 13.2 Synthetic implants

Type	Pros	Cons	Recomended uses
Expanded-porous polytetrafluoroethylene (Gore-Tex)	Tissue ingrowth, soft/pliable, sculptable	Limited structural support, expensive	Dorsal onlay, tip grafts
Porous high-density polyethylene (Medpor)	Tissue ingrowth, sculptable	Difficult to remove, palpability	Dorsal onlay, tip grafts, columellar strut, alar batten
Silicone, solid form	Easy to insert, soft/pliable, sculptable	Extrusion potential (lifetime), capsule formation, no tissue ingrowth	Dorsal onlay

Data from Romo T III, Kwak E. Nasal grafts and implants in revision rhinoplasty. Facial Plast Surg Clin North Am 2006;373–387.

rhinoplasty.[2] The thicker skin, itself, also reduces the chance of implant extrusion or infection.

A focused history is important in preoperative planning. The surgeon should note if the patient has a history of nasal trauma, however remote, and any prior nasal surgeries. Prior operative reports are helpful but are not required. Current medications, particularly blood thinners, are important to note and to stop prior to surgery if medically cleared. History of cocaine use or rhinitis medicamentosa is also notable, because these conditions compromise healing and increase the patient's risk of infection, nasal septal perforation, and implant extrusion. One should approach revision surgery patients and those with a history of nasal cocaine use with extreme caution, especially if one is considering alloplastic implants, as these patients are at a heightened risk of complications. History of chronic rhinitis, particularly atrophic rhinitis, is also important to note, especially if septoplasty or turbinate surgery is part of the surgical plan.

A focused exam is also important, and it should include analysis of the nose in several views, an intranasal exam with endoscopy, and palpation of the nose. The nose should be analyzed in several views, and professional-grade photographs should be taken in frontal, side, oblique, and base views. Views with and without smiling are helpful to assess for the presence of a premaxillary crease, which may be affected by rhinoplasty maneuvers that anchor grafts to the nasal spine. Views of the nasal base with and without inspiration are also helpful to assess for external nasal valve collapse. This may also be assessed using a Cottle maneuver. The internal nasal valve angle (formed by the nasal septum, caudal border of the upper lateral cartilage, and the head of the inferior turbinate) should also be assessed, as this may be affected by septoplasty, submucosal inferior turbinate reduction, spreader graft placement, and external nasal valve strengthening maneuvers like alar batten or lateral crural strut graft placement, if required. The nose should also be palpated so that the strength of the lower lateral cartilages may be assessed. Deficiency of the caudal nasal septum, not uncommon in the platyrrhine nose, should also be noted, as should any premaxillary deficiency. The body should be examined for keloids, as history of keloid formation definitely increases the patient's risk of having this complication in rhinoplasty.[5]

Once the surgeon understands the patient's goals and a complete examination has been performed, he or she must present the surgical plan. The surgeon should explain to the patient how the plan will achieve the patient's goals, the limitations of the proposed procedure, expected postoperative care and follow-up, and potential complications. The importance of managing patients' expectations cannot be overstated. Computerized three-dimensional imaging is often very helpful in demonstrating to patients the results they may expect with a given operation.

13.4 Procedural Approach

The rhinoplasty example shown here illustrates characteristics of the typical platyrrhine nose, including thick, sebaceous skin, deficient caudal septum, relatively deficient nasal dorsum (cartilage and bone), weak nasal tip (deficient caudal septum and thin lower lateral cartilages), and deficient premaxilla/nasal spine area. Overall, the nasal dorsum and tip are not well defined underneath a thickened overlying S-STE. Structural augmentation of the nasal dorsum and tip are key for this patient; furthermore, because the nasal septal cartilage is deficient for grafting and the patient prefers not to undergo autologous cartilage harvest from a separate surgical site, alloplastic augmentation is planned (**Fig. 13.2**).

An open rhinoplasty technique is preferred in this example so that the grafts may be fixated under superior visualization. Preoperative marking is performed to

At this point, the dorsum is addressed, with or without osteotomies. Typically, a large dorsal PHDPE implant is chosen and is carved to the desired size and contour using a no. 10 blade. A sheet of AlloDerm may be used to camouflage any subtle irregularities or to soften the transition between the dorsum and nasal sidewalls of the implant. The implant is placed in a tight dorsal pocket. If it is not completely stabilized, temporary transcutaneous 4–0 Prolene stitches may be used to anchor the implant in place **(Fig. 13.7)**.

Finally, a tip shield graft may be placed. It is typically fashioned from septal cartilage, and smooths the transition between the tip and the columella. It is secured in place using a 6–0 Prolene suture.

Closure begins with the columellar incision. One interrupted 5–0 Vicryl (Ethicon Inc.) stitch is placed in the deep tissue, followed by interrupted 6–0 nylon sutures for the skin closure. Marginal incisions are closed with interrupted 5–0 chromic sutures. After closure, alar base reduction may be performed, if desired, and the incisions are closed with 5–0 Vicryl deep sutures and 6–0 nylon sutures through the skin. It is important to avoid placement of these incisions in the nasal/alar crease itself, as those incisions heal less favorably than ones placed more medially **(Fig. 13.8)**.

At the conclusion of the operation, Steri-Strips are placed over the nasal bridge, and an Aquaplast splint (Patterson Medical Products Inc.) is placed over them, stabilizing the nasal dorsum. Intranasally, Silastic sheet splints may be used to promote healing, especially if the mucoperichondrial flaps were traumatized substantially during elevation. Telfa-wrapped Merocels coated with bacitracin are then positioned anteriorly in bilateral nares; they are removed 1 to 2 days postoperatively **(Fig. 13.9)**.

13.5 Potential Complications and Treatment

The vast majority of ethnic patients undergoing dorsal augmentation using this technique are satisfied and enjoy a complication-free recovery. However, complications are possible and need to be discussed with patients beforehand.

As mentioned above, infection is more common among patients undergoing revision operations or those with a history of intranasal cocaine abuse. Thinner-skinned patients are more susceptible to implant infection and extrusion, and infection rates of up to 50% have been cited among alloplastic implants used in the columella.[20] However, Romo and Shapiro[5] reviewed 187 patients (35.4% non-Caucasian) who underwent rhinoplasty with PHDPE implants and found only one patient who required revision (the case involved revision of a dorsal implant). It is possible that their practice of soaking the implant in gentamycin solution prior to its implantation may have played a role in the low infection rate.

Scarring is always a possibility with any surgery, and non-Caucasian patients are more prone to this complication, including keloid formation. Prolonged nasal tip edema is also possible, especially in the setting of thickened skin. Nasal asymmetry or implant migration is also a possibility, which is why special attention should be paid to implant fixation during the procedure.

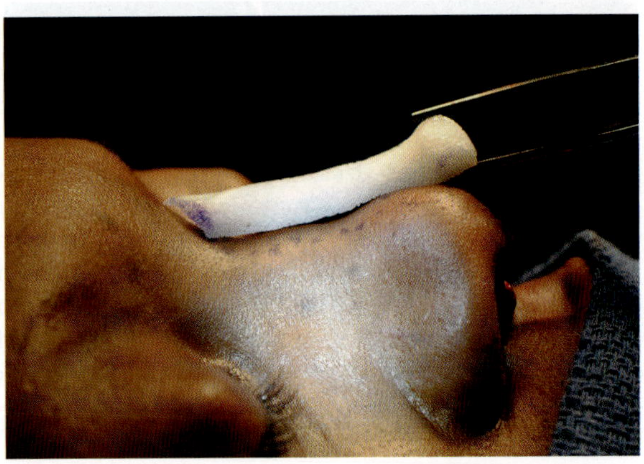

Fig. 13.7 Intraoperative placement of dorsal graft.

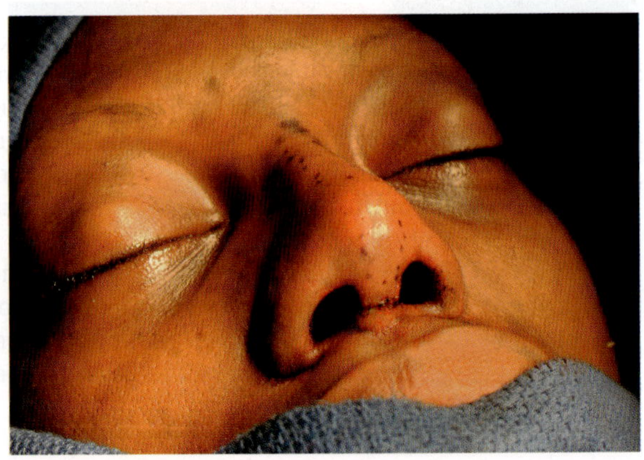

Fig. 13.8 Intraoperative three-quarter view after placement of grafts.

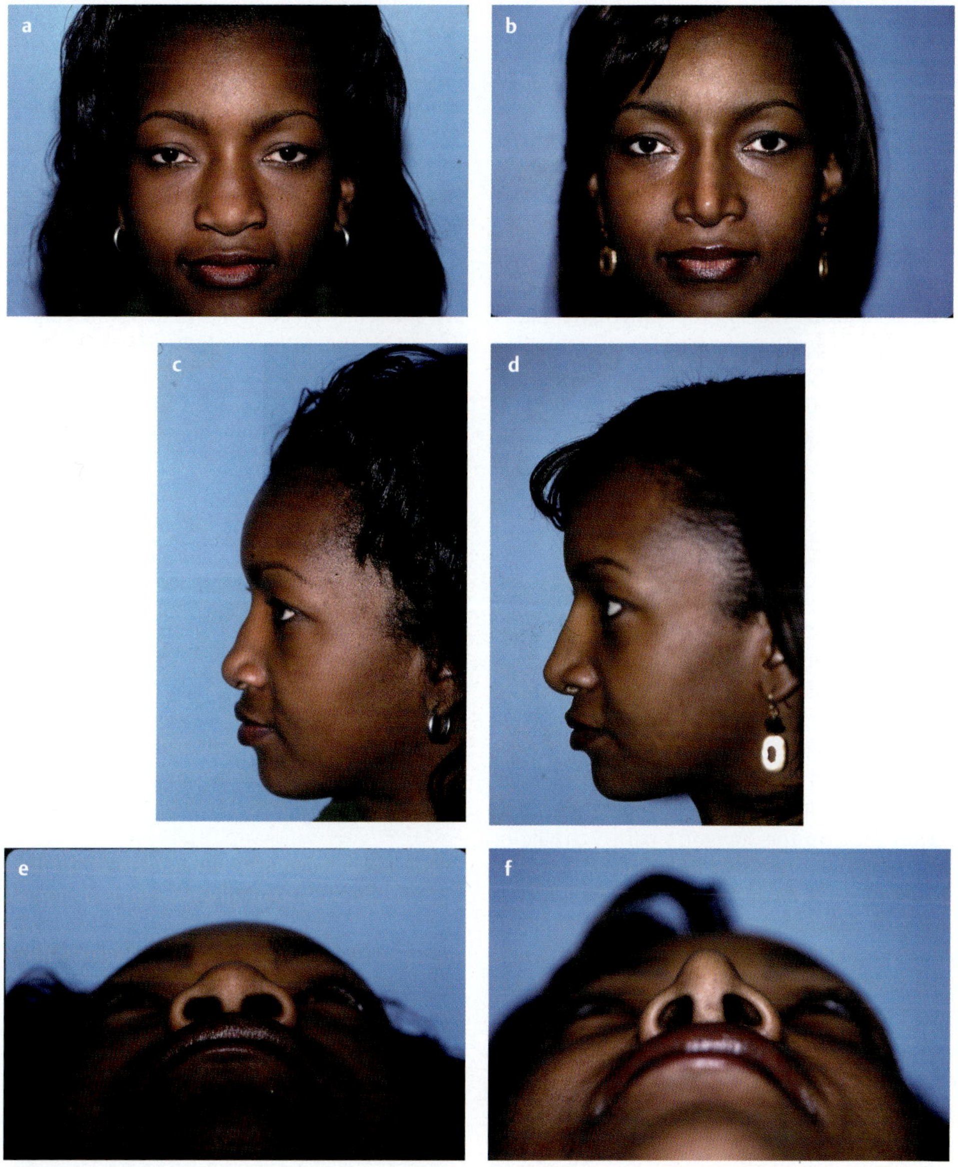

Fig. 13.9 **(a)** Preoperative frontal view. **(b)** One year postoperative, frontal view. **(c)** Preoperative lateral view. **(d)** One year postoperative, lateral view. **(e)** Preoperative base view. **(f)** One year postoperative, base view.

13.6 Postprocedural Care

Antibiotic-coated Telfa-wrapped Merocel packs should be removed 1 to 2 days postoperatively. Patients are sent home with oral antibiotics for 1 week. Patients should begin nasal saline sprays and irrigations 2 days after surgery and perform them conservatively. The Aquaplast dorsal splint, internal Silastic splints, and nonabsorbable stitches are removed 5 to 7 days after surgery. It is important that the patient avoid any heavy lifting or intense exercise in the week following surgery. Care should be taken to avoid nasal trauma as well.[21]

13.7 Recovery and Follow-Up

Recovery is swift among the majority of patients. A small amount of oozing from the nares is expected, but brisk bleeding is uncommon and should warrant prompt attention from a physician. Periorbital swelling and bruising is possible, especially if osteotomies were performed. Pain medication is prescribed and should be used as needed.

Patients will note that their nose feels firmer than it did prior to surgery due to the firm consistency of the grafts. Patients should be advised that postoperative swelling is normal and can be prolonged, lasting for a few months after a rhinoplasty, particularly among thick-skinned patients. Steroid injections are sometimes utilized to reduce swelling and scar formation in the nasal tip and to effect increased nasal contouring.

13.8 Outcomes

The senior author has enjoyed excellent cosmetic results and satisfaction among his ethnic rhinoplasty patients undergoing structural augmentation using alloplastic, and specifically PHDPE, implants. Alloplastic implants in rhinoplasty have been a subject of controversy, with some surgeons preferring to use autologous cartilage exclusively when augmentation is required; however, this option requires a second surgical site, with its inherent morbidities, and a certain comfort level on the surgeon's part. Warping of autologous rib cartilage is also an often-cited concern, and experience is necessary to learn to use the rib's inherent tendency to warp to one's advantage in effecting change to the nose during rhinoplasty. Irradiated cadaveric rib cartilage is also relatively popular, but it carries a risk of warping akin to autologous rib cartilage. Moreover, alloplastic implants have achieved good results with relatively little morbidity when used in the correct patient and site.

It should be noted that thin-skinned patients and patients undergoing revision operations have higher risk of complications related to alloplastic implants. Alloplastic implants placed in the columella have a higher chance of infection and complication than those used for dorsal augmentation, likely secondary to the increased movement associated with this area of the nose.[20] Patients with a history of nasal cocaine use should also be treated very conservatively. For the vast majority, however, PHDPE is a readily available, reliable material for structural augmentation rhinoplasty with minimal complication. Further studies are warranted to investigate longer-term follow-up of PHDPE augmentation rhinoplasty to further validate its safety.

13.9 Conclusion

Dorsal augmentation in the platyrrhine nose may be reliably performed with PHDPE implants. This material is often desirable in the setting of deficient nasal septal cartilage, and it may serve as an alternative to harvesting autologous cartilage from additional surgical sites (i.e., ear or rib). It becomes stable in the nose due to soft tissue ingrowth into its porous substance, and it lacks the risk of warping inherent to rib cartilage. It is strong and abundant in supply, and it has not been shown to resorb. Candidates for this procedure should be carefully selected, with the risks and benefits of the operation fully disclosed and alternative options discussed. Caution should be used in formulating a surgical plan for patients presenting for a revision operation, patients with a history of severe trauma, or those with nasal cocaine use. Autologous grafts should be used for columellar augmentation, if available. Implants should be soaked in antibiotic solution prior to placement, and patients should keep their incisions coated in antibiotic ointment in the initial postoperative period. Close follow-up should be observed, with any complications noted.

References

1. Matory WE Jr, Falces E. Non-Caucasian rhinoplasty: a 16-year experience. Plast Reconstr Surg 1986;77(2):239–252
2. Romo T III, Abraham MT. The ethnic nose. In: Fedok F, Nolst-Trenité GJ, Becker DG, et al, eds. Facial Plastic Surgery. New York, NY: Thieme; 2003:269–277
3. Schultz AH. Relation of the external nose to the bony nose and nasal cartilages in whites and Negroes. Am J Phys Anthropol 1913;1:329–339
4. Canbay EI, Bhatia SN. A comparison of nasal resistance in white Caucasians and blacks. Am J Rhinol 1997;11(1):73–75
5. Romo T III, Shapiro AL. Aesthetic reconstruction of the platyrrhine nose. Arch Otolaryngol Head Neck Surg 1992;118(8):837–841
6. Toriumi DM. Autogenous grafts are worth the extra time. Arch Otolaryngol Head Neck Surg 2000;126(4):562–564
7. Cárdenas-Camarena L, Guerrero MT. Use of cartilaginous autografts in nasal surgery: 8 years of experience. Plast Reconstr Surg 1999;103(3):1003–1014
8. Ortiz-Monasterio F, Olmedo A, Oscoy LO. The use of cartilage grafts in primary aesthetic rhinoplasty. Plast Reconstr Surg 1981;67(5):597–605
9. Romo T III, Jablonski RD. Nasal reconstruction using split calvarial grafts. Otolaryngol Head Neck Surg 1992;107(5):622–630

10. Kridel RWH, Krause WM. Grafts and implants in revision rhinoplasty. Facial Plast Surg Clin North Am 1995; 3(4):473–486
11. Murakami CS, Cook TA, Guida RA. Nasal reconstruction with articulated irradiated rib cartilage. Arch Otolaryngol Head Neck Surg 1991;117(3):327–330, discussion 331
12. Costantino PD, Friedman CD, Lane A. Synthetic biomaterials in facial plastic and reconstructive surgery. Facial Plast Surg 1993;9(1):1–15
13. Romo T III, Sclafani AP, Sabini P. Use of porous high-density polyethylene in revision rhinoplasty and in the platyrrhine nose. Aesthetic Plast Surg 1998;22(3):211–221
14. Deva AK, Merten S, Chang L. Silicone in nasal augmentation rhinoplasty: a decade of clinical experience. Plast Reconstr Surg 1998;102(4):1230–1237
15. Neel HB. Implants of Gore-Tex: comparisons with Teflon coated polytetrafluorethylene carbon and porous polyethylene implants. Arch Otolaryngol Head Neck Surg 1983;109:427–433
16. Conrad K, Gillman G. A 6-year experience with the use of expanded polytetrafluoroethylene in rhinoplasty. Plast Reconstr Surg 1998;101(6):1675–1683, discussion 1684
17. Mass CS, Monhian N, Shah SB. Implants in rhinoplasty. Facial Plast Surg 1998;13(4):279–290
18. Godin MS, Waldman SR, Johnson CM Jr. Nasal augmentation using Gore-Tex. A 10-year experience. Arch Facial Plast Surg 1999;1(2):118–121, discussion 122
19. Sclafani AP, Thomas JR, Cox AJ, Cooper MH. Clinical and histologic response of subcutaneous expanded polytetrafluoroethylene (Gore-Tex) and porous high-density polyethylene (Medpor) implants to acute and early infection. Arch Otolaryngol Head Neck Surg 1997;123(3):328–336
20. Winkler AA, Soler ZM, Leong PL, Murphy A, Wang TD, Cook TA. Complications associated with alloplastic implants in rhinoplasty. Arch Facial Plast Surg 2012;14(6):437–441 10.1001/archfacial.2012.583
21. Romo T, Abraham MT, Pafford W. Rhinoplasty in the multiracial nose. In: Shiffman MA, Di-Giuseppe A, eds. Advanced Aesthetic Rhinoplasty. New York, NY: Thieme; 2013:197–206

14 Approach to the Nasal Base in Patients of African Descent

Christian P. Conderman and Russell W. H. Kridel

14.1 Introduction

Patients of African descent pose a unique challenge in rhinoplasty. Significant differences in anatomical characteristics yield a nose that is distinctive from what has over the years been considered an attractive nose in people of Caucasian or European descent. Historically, African noses have been categorized into an "ethnic rhinoplasty" grouping with noses of Asian and Latin descent. This categorization has proven wholly inadequate to describe the unique morphologic features of each of these groups. Furthermore, characterizing a nose as ethnic is largely a question of perspective and can be relative. For instance, this description likely has a significantly different meaning to someone in Asia than it does to someone in Europe or Africa. Attempts to create a more Caucasian or Caucasoid nose without incorporating an individual's desires into the surgical plan have also largely resulted in undesirable outcomes. Sensitivity and awareness of the individual and ethnic differences are of paramount importance in achieving a desirable surgical outcome in alar base surgery in patients of African descent.

Individual and ethnic differences, as well as features unique to patients of African descent, have been described in several studies.[1,2,3,4,5,6] In general, the uniquely African features include a shorter nose with a wider dorsum, acute columellar and nasolabial angles, thicker skin, a bulbous nasal tip, weak lower lateral cartilages, and large nostrils in both the vertical and horizontal dimensions (with nostrils that in some cases have an inverted orientation). Additionally, the alar base tends to be wider in these patients and requires special attention.

These nasal features are the result of great heterogeneity within the population of African descent. The heterogeneity is attributable to the varied ethnic groups that contribute to nasal features in particular, and to the great variability in the population in general. African, Native American, and Northern European origins and influences contribute in varying degrees to the characteristic nasal morphology. In 1993, Ofodile studied 201 African American noses and further classified the noses into three subgroups based on morphologic features.[1] He termed the groups the African, Afro-Caucasian, and Afro-Indian noses. Of the three groups, the African nose is the most common and has the features traditionally associated with a platyrrhine nose. Afro-Caucasian and Afro-Indian noses are less common but are marked by variations in the height of the nasal dorsum, as well as the shape and orientation of the nostrils. These structural differences are thought to be the result of climate-driven adaptations. In colder climates, a long and narrow nasal passageway provides more surface area for humidification of inhaled air. In contrast, in a warmer, more humid climate, a wider, narrower nose is more suitable because the requirements for humidification of inspired air are not as great.[2,7,8]

Ofodile's classification provides a framework for understanding anatomical variations in patients. Nonetheless, with interracial marriage becoming more common, the morphologic distinction between groups is becoming more arbitrary. As a result, individualized preoperative evaluation and analysis are critical in determining the appropriate approach to the alar base. Preoperative assessment includes an awareness of the aforementioned ethnic characteristics and how they may diverge from classical aesthetic ideals. As cosmetic facial surgery is becoming more desirable across all ethnic groupings, preservation of natural beauty within a cultural, ethnic, and societal framework should be considered a primary surgical goal. The surgical plan should be formulated to preserve facial harmony while also responding to the individual patient's desires. In patients of African descent, this can be accomplished with the use of a graduated and algorithmic approach to the alar base, with resultant aesthetic outcomes that comply with cultural standards of beauty in a consistent and reproducible manner.

14.2 Nature of the Problem

In patients of African descent, noses can show a great variety of anatomical features, as noted above. This variety has been the subject of detailed analysis and has been compared to normative values associated with neoclassical canons of beauty.[1,9,10,11,12,13] As discussed above, Ofodile was one of the first to describe these features in terms of the overall appearance of the nose, while also specifically characterizing the nostrils and alar base. In the African nose, found in darker pigmented individuals, the interalar width was wider, with more flaring of the alae. The nostrils were also described to have a more horizontally oriented axis. In the Afro-Caucasian nose, the nostrils were oriented more vertically, with a narrower base and less alar flare. The Afro-Indian nose, the third and the least common type of nose that Ofodile described, has an "aquiline" shape, with more projection, a high and wide dorsum, and alar flaring. Despite outlining the differences and describing three different types of nose, Ofodile advised a tailored rhinoplasty approach based on individualized preoperative assessment.

Approximately 10 years before Ofodile's description of noses in patients of African descent, Farkas described a classification system for nostril types based on morphometric analysis of 156 Caucasian, 55 Asian, and 32 African American noses.[10] This classification was based on the inclination of the medial longitudinal axis of the nostrils and generally followed the Topinard system for facial analysis described in the late nineteenth century.[10,14] In Ofodile's African nose type, nostril types V and VI predominate (**Fig. 14.1**, nostril axis more horizontally oriented, with an angle of inclination of 25–39 degrees and 10–24 degrees for nostril types V and VI, respectively)[10] and alar base correction can require partial resection of the sill in addition to traditional alar wedge excision. This is the result of the orientation and inclination of nostril types V and VI. Afro-Caucasian noses, however, were noted to have narrower nostrils with a more vertically oriented axis, and alar base reduction was less reliant upon excision of the nasal sill. In Afro-Indian noses, where nostril shape falls somewhere between those of the African and Afro-Caucasian nose, a combination of the two methods is usually required. Despite the differences detailed above, the importance of preoperative evaluation and a surgical approach that addresses a patient's unique anatomical findings cannot be overemphasized. In a subsequent analysis of African American facial proportions, Porter noted that nostril types III, IV, and V (as defined by Farkas et al)[10] were most common in the African American population of the United States. Porter cited the prevalences of types III, IV, and V to be 28.7%, 25.0%, and 25.0%, respectively.[12]

Ofodile later described average anthropometric values in 69 of the original 201 patients whom he had used to classify the three subtypes outlined above.[11] His calculations showed mean values of 41.4 mm and 30.3 mm (1.36:1) for interalar and intercanthal widths, respectively. He was therefore able to show objectively that lateral alar attachments in patients of African descent are generally found lateral to the anatomical location of the medial canthus.[11] More recently, Porter has largely corroborated these findings and compared facial proportions of Americans of African descent with neoclassical guidelines and proportions found in American Caucasians.[9,12,13] She noted significant variations in her own results and stated there were some limitations in applying Ofodile's grouping to her results. She specifically noted that the differentiation between Afro-Caucasian and Afro-Indian noses could be arbitrary. She also lamented the broad age range in Ofodile's initial study (ages 18–87) and cited senescent changes as a confounding factor in the categorization of African noses.[12]

Additional morphometric analysis performed largely by Porter et al added to the existing literature characterizing the alar base and interalar width in African American males and females.[9,12,13] The investigators compared African American males and North American Caucasian males and found that, in African American males, in contradistinction to the neoclassical canon that dictates a 1:1 ratio between the interalar width and intercanthal width, the ratio is closer to 1.3:1, with the interalar width being greater than the intercanthal width.[9] Porter et al noted a wider nasal base in 99% of African American subjects. Nostril orientation was found to be vertical in most subjects, while a horizontal orientation was second most common.[9] Porter et al also found that, from the base view, the African American nose had a more oval configuration, with a

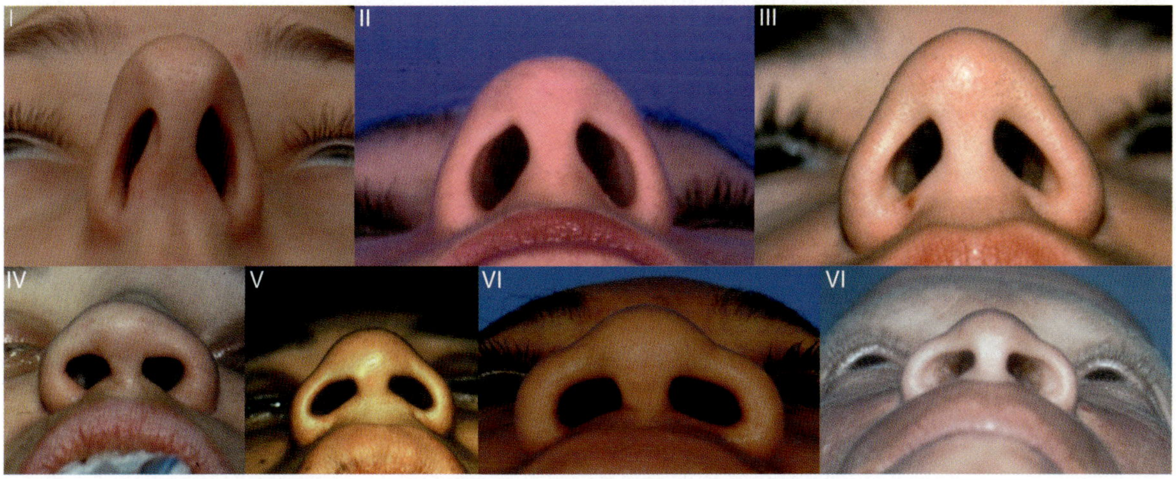

Fig. 14.1 Ethnic variations in the nostril axis. The Farkas classification of nostril types as adapted to our patients. Top row: types I, II, and III. Bottom row: types IV, V, and two examples of type VI nostril. (Nostril type VII, inverted nostril, not shown.) As nostril axis becomes more horizontally oriented, consideration must be given to sill reduction in addition to standard alar wedge excision.

distinct breakpoint between the nasal lobule and ala. In addition to this specific morphometric finding, the breakpoint can have surgical implications, as alterations in the alar base can produce or exacerbate notching at the alar-lobular junction. Anthropometric differences between the African American and Caucasian females were also recorded and revealed differences in the nasal dorsum and in terms of overall nasal width. The African American female's nose was wider, with less inclination of the dorsum. Again, it was noted that the interalar width was greater than the intercanthal width (5:4 or 1.25:1).[12] Both studies confirmed that African American facial analysis and metrics do not fall neatly into the confines of the neoclassical canons. Porter concluded that, in general, horizontal measures of facial analysis had more interracial variation, particularly when considering metrics applied to the nose.

14.3 Applied Anatomy

Excessive alar base width has multiple causes and requires the understanding and application of a variety of techniques to correct alar width and/or flare. Alar base reduction can be considered when the interalar width exceeds the intercanthal distance. The result is what has traditionally been considered ideal in the Caucasian nose; however, as outlined above, these norms are not necessarily applicable to patients of African descent. This is due to the larger interalar to intercanthal ratio in a large percentage of these patients as outlined in the above analyses. While guidelines serve as a useful reference, patient desires should be the critical influence in terms of surgical decision-making in alar base reduction.

In addition to excessive sill width and interalar distance, alar flare is another indication for reduction of the alar base. This is defined as the lateral aspect of the alae extending significantly (≥ 2 mm) beyond the alar-facial groove **(Fig. 14.2)**.[15,16] This is best seen on the preoperative base view. In addition to alar flare's occurrence as a preoperative or native anatomical finding, it can result from rhinoplasty maneuvers that de-project or retro-displace the nasal tip. This may cause the alae to assume a more lateral position without causing a change in the interalar width or nostril size **(Fig. 14.3)**.

In some instances, the nasal sill in isolation (i.e., without flaring) may contribute to an overly wide alar base. A relative indication for sill reduction is an enlarged nostril with a horizontal axis.[15] This can often be seen in the African or platyrrhine nose, especially in the setting of nostril types V and VI as described by Farkas.[10] In contrast to a horizontally oriented nostril, with a more vertically oriented nostril, i.e., types I to III, great care should be taken when alar base surgery is planned. If the alar base is narrowed excessively in this setting, aesthetic outcomes can be poor.

If the alar base is too wide due to a lateral alar-facial insertion, as is common in patients of African descent, a V-Y

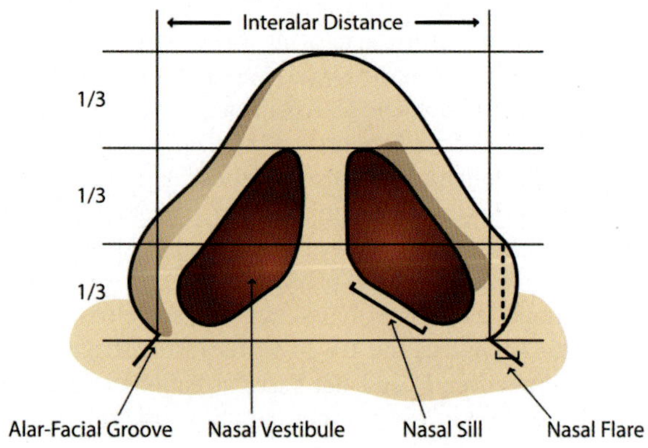

Fig. 14.2 Alar base anatomy. Excessive alar flare is noted when the lateral aspect of the alae extends significantly beyond the alar-facial junction. (Adapted with permission from Kridel RW, Castellano RD. A simplified approach to alar base reduction: a review of 124 patients over 20 years. Arch Facial Plast Surg 2005;7(2):81–93.)

advancement flap of the lateral alae can be used to correct this. Bernstein popularized this method of alar base reduction,[3] and when it is combined with correction of alar flare and excessive width of the nostril sill, it has shown good results in patients with this anatomical configuration.[15]

In summary, the varying causes of alar base excess require an algorithmic approach for appropriate reduction and correction of a specific anatomical deformity. Correction can include narrowing an excessively wide interalar distance, reducing alar flare, reducing excessive nasal sill width, with or without a horizontally oriented nostril axis, and/or a combination of the above **(Fig. 14.4)**.

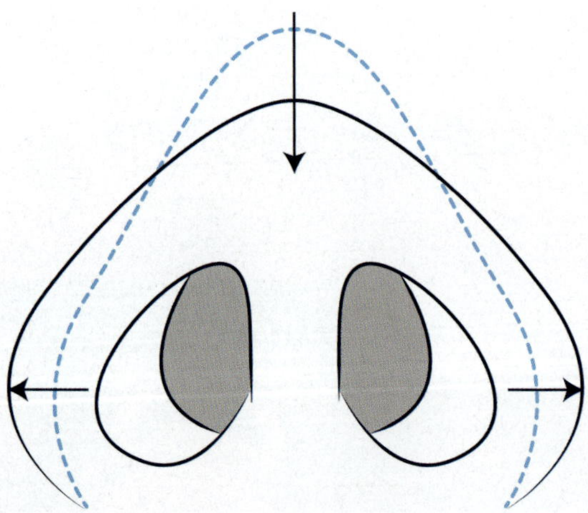

Fig. 14.3 De-projection or retro-displacement of the tip can lead to an increase in alar flaring. Conversely, an increase in projection can lead to a reduction in alar flaring.

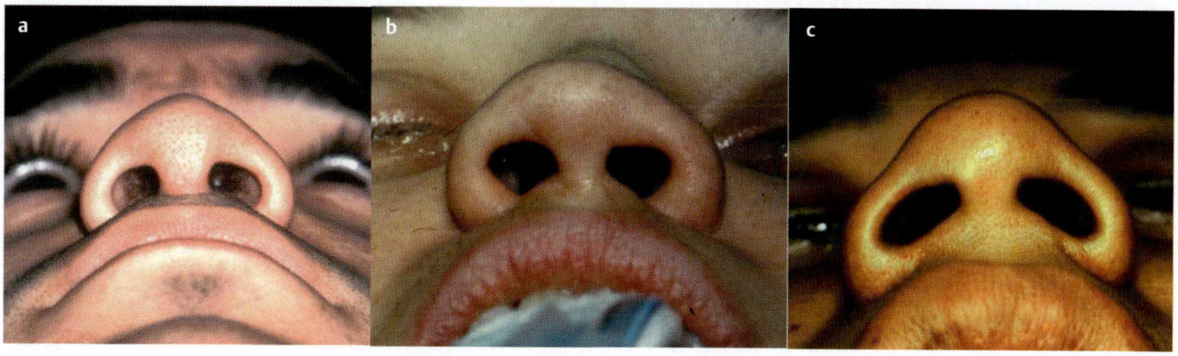

Fig. 14.4 **(a)** Excessive interalar width. **(b)** Excessive alar flare. **(c)** Excessive width of the nasal sill with horizontally oriented nostril axes.

14.4 Treatment Goals and Planned Outcomes

Correction of alar base disproportion in patients of African descent must be performed in a systematic manner that addresses a clearly defined anatomical defect in line with an understanding of ethnic features and individual patient desires. A clear preoperative plan is necessary for achieving natural results. The plan should include an assessment and diagnosis of what is causing the base to be widened, i.e., excessive flaring, excessive horizontal width of the nasal sill, true excess of the interalar width, or a combination thereof. By keeping these factors in mind, appropriate narrowing in line with ethnic, cultural, and racial features can be achieved while preserving nasal-facial harmony. Computer imaging can serve an integral role in communication of surgical goals between the patient and surgeon and should be used to clearly define a proposed treatment plan and possible surgical outcome.

14.5 Preoperative Planning and Preparation

A targeted history and physical should precede any nasal surgery. This includes a detailed history of specific nasal complaints, such as congestion and drainage, nasal airway obstruction, prior nasal trauma, and a history of nasal allergies and/or sinusitis. Patients should also be queried regarding any history of excessive bleeding or bruising and hypertrophic or keloid scarring following prior surgeries, and in particular nasal surgeries. Current medications should be discussed, including the use of over-the-counter and herbal medications. Aspirin and NSAIDs, as well as known anticoagulants like warfarin and heparin, can predispose the patient to postoperative bleeding and complications. Similarly, ginkgo, garlic, fish oil, and vitamin E may increase a patient's postoperative risk of hemorrhage.

Preoperative physical examination should include a thorough facial examination, with close inspection of the nose. Dysmorphic and/or disproportionate features should be noted. The nasal examination should include a close inspection of both the external and internal components. The nasal dorsum and cartilages should be palpated and assessed for strength and support. Intranasally, the septum and turbinates should be evaluated to assess for any deviations or other factors contributing to nasal obstruction. Evaluation of the nose should include documentation of the size, shape, and symmetry of the nostrils, the width and length of the columella, the relationship between the columellar length and height of the lobule, and the thickness and contour of the alae.[15] The base view should be examined to assess for the aforementioned anatomical findings, including alar flaring; excessive interalar width; the size, shape, and orientation of the nostrils; and nasal sill width. The columella should also be evaluated, as flaring of the medial crural footplates or deviations of the caudal septum can contribute to preoperative asymmetry. This asymmetry should be discussed with the patient prior to surgery. Additionally, the junction of the alae and lobule should be evaluated for alar notching. This finding may be worsened by a reduction in alar base width and may necessitate concomitant placement of an alar rim graft for correction of the deformity. As noted above, changes in the alar base can result in the creation of, or exacerbation of, this defect, and its presence or absence should be noted at the time of the initial evaluation. Rhinometry can serve as a useful adjunctive measure to assess preoperative airflow before and after application of a topical decongestant, and it provides an objective evaluation of airway patency.

Preoperative photographic documentation is necessary in all facial cosmetic procedures. Photos include standard documentation of frontal, oblique, profile, base, and sky/overhead views. Additional close-up photographs can be taken of any nasal lesions and/or the naso-facial junction/peri-alar area. Computer imaging should also be performed in all patients prior to rhinoplasty. This allows the physician to depict the changes that he/she is proposing, including modifications of the alar base and how they might affect the overall appearance of the nose from frontal and base views. Additionally, this gives the patient the opportunity to state his/her desires with regard to the rhinoplasty procedure. Some patients may desire a nose more in line with neoclassical canons, whereas others may prefer to maintain varying degrees of ethnic expression.[2]

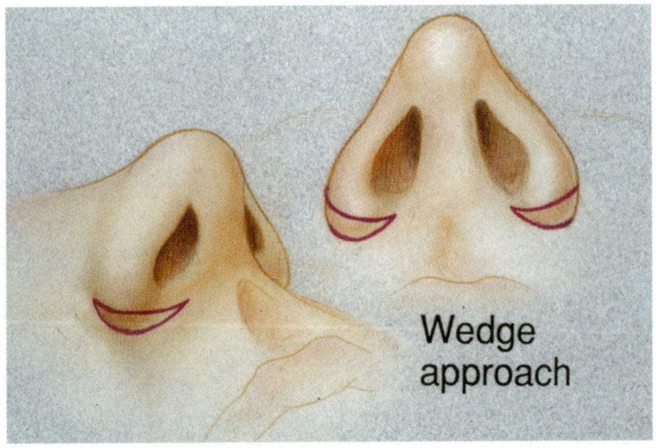

Fig. 14.5 Alar wedge excision. This is used to correct a wide alar base when alar flaring alone is the cause of excessive width. Wedges should be excised in a symmetrical fashion without violation of the vestibule or nasal sill. (Used with permission from Kridel RW, Castellano RD. A simplified approach to alar base reduction: a review of 124 patients over 20 years. Arch Facial Plast Surg 2005;7(2):81–93.)

14.6 Patient Selection

Appropriate patient selection is critical in achieving satisfying outcomes for both the surgeon and patient. Moreover, communication between the surgeon and patient is of paramount importance in that a perfectly executed alar base reduction can still lead to patient dissatisfaction if it is not what the patient had in mind prior to undergoing the procedure. Therefore, it warrants repeating that preoperative expectations must be properly assessed and explicitly defined prior to embarking on any surgical procedure. The surgeon must be aware of inherent differences in his or her own perceptions and expectations and should clearly define the goals of surgery.[15] Most patients of African descent desire nasal refinement in line with ethnic characteristics.[2,5,6,17] Nonetheless, some patients may wish to achieve a narrower alar base that more closely approximates a 1:1 intercanthal to interalar ratio. A patient's wishes should be clearly defined prior to alar base reduction, and computer imaging is effective in minimizing the risk of miscommunication between patient and surgeon. In addition, patients should be made aware of the possibility of visible scars at the locations of the alar base modification. Finally, and most importantly, patients should have reasonable expectations for the outcome of rhinoplasty and alar base correction.

14.7 Procedural Approach/ Surgical Approaches

Once the need for surgical correction of a wide alar base has been established, a combination of three basic techniques is used to achieve this goal. Excessive alar flaring is addressed using a modified Weir excision (**Fig. 14.5**, **Fig. 14.6**, and **Fig. 14.7**).[18] This technique spares entry into the nostril, thereby avoiding violation of the natural curvature of the internal nostril border.[15] The goal of a wedge excision designed in this manner is to avoid over-straightening the ala, with preservation of its natural curve, and to avoid telltale incisions into the nostril opening. While this technique is effective in isolation, it can be combined with nasal sill reduction if there is excessive sill width in the setting of a horizontally oriented nostril (**Fig. 14.4c**, **Fig. 14.7**, **Fig. 14.8**, and **Fig. 14.9**). Similarly, if the lateral insertion of the alae is responsible for excessive nasal base width, the wedge excision can be combined with a V-Y advancement, as described by Bernstein,[15,19] to narrow the interalar width while simultaneously reducing alar flare (**Fig. 14.10**, **Fig. 14.11**, **Fig. 14.12**, and **Fig. 14.13**).

Considering the above factors, alar base reduction should be approached in a conservative manner as overresection can be extremely difficult to correct. Therefore, if there is any doubt about the need for alar base reduction, it is best to defer the procedure, as it can suitably be

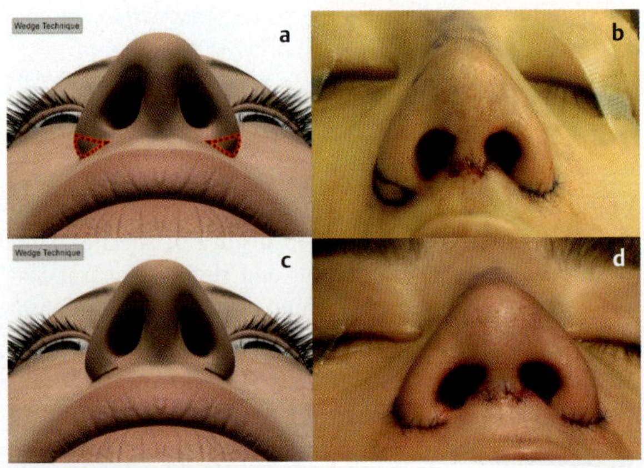

Fig. 14.6 Alar wedge excision. **(a,c)** Schematic showing alar wedge design and postexcisional narrowing of alar base. **(b)** Intraoperative view showing completed alar wedge excision on the left and design of wedge excision on the right. **(d)** Alar wedge excision completed on both sides, with narrowing of alar base.

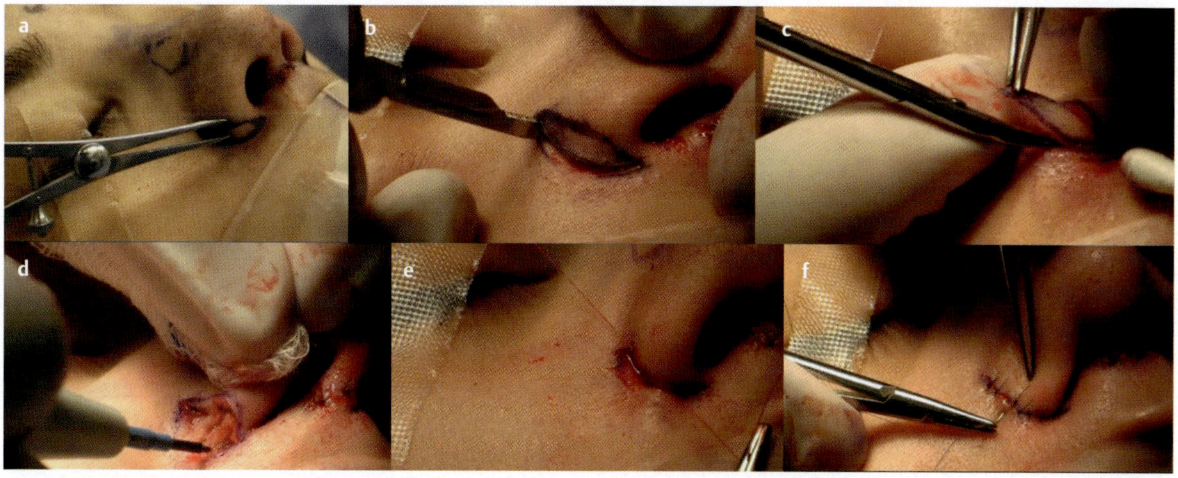

Fig. 14.7 Steps of alar wedge excision. **(a)** Measuring alar wedge with surgical calipers. **(b)** Excision of alar wedge with scalpel. **(c)** Tenotomy scissors used to complete excision. **(d)** Hemostasis using monopolar cautery. **(e)** Deep 5–0 Vicryl suture used to reapproximate edges of incision. **(f)** Superficial closure with interrupted 6–0 Prolene sutures.

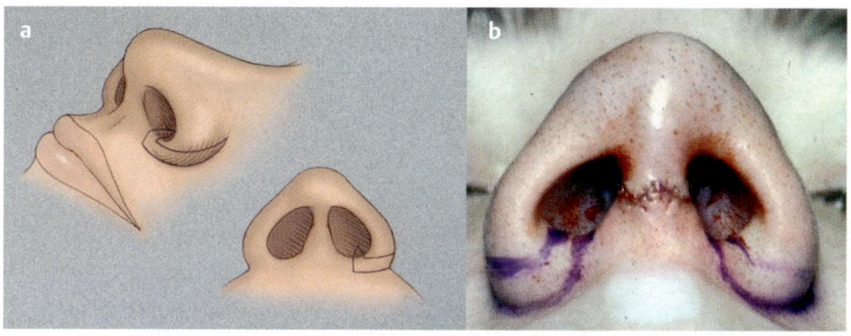

Fig. 14.8 Combined wedge and nasal sill excision. This method of alar base reduction is used to correct excessive width as a result of alar flaring combined with an excessively wide nasal sill. Undermining of the vestibular tissues is required and eversion of the incision at the sill is critical to avoid postoperative notching at this location. **(a)** Schematic showing design of wedge and sill excision. **(b)** Intraoperative view showing design of excision that is medial to the long axis of the nostril without violating the natural curve of the ala. (Used with permission from Kridel RW, Castellano RD. A simplified approach to alar base reduction: a review of 124 patients over 20 years. Arch Facial Plast Surg 2005;7(2):81–93.)

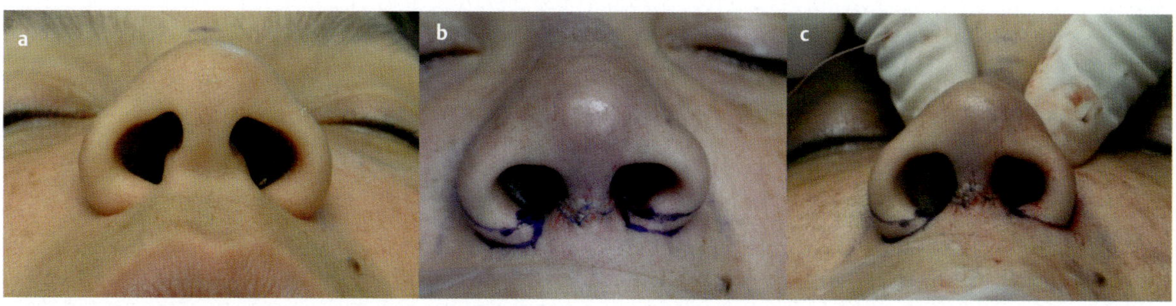

Fig. 14.9 Wedge and sill excision for wide nasal sill. **(a)** Preoperative base view. **(b)** Design of wedge and sill excision (see also **Fig. 14.8**). **(c)** Intraoperative view of completed left wedge and sill excision, with reduction of alar base and sill width, and preservation of natural alar curve.

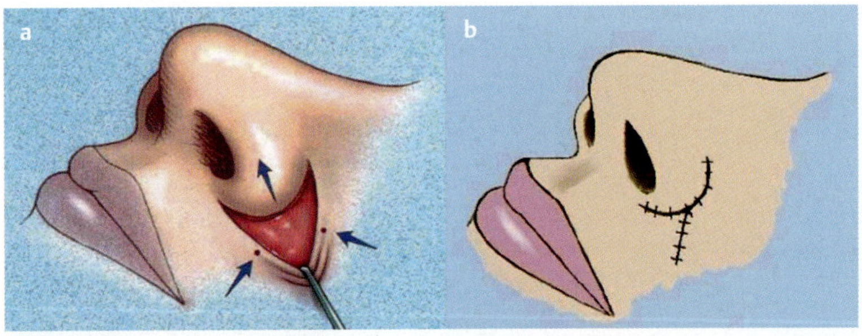

Fig. 14.10 V-Y advancement combined with alar wedge excision. **(a)** The crease incision is lateralized with a skin hook. The V shape of the wedge incision is converted to a Y by retracting laterally. The midportions of the skin edges, with the dots shown in the drawing, are then sutured to one another, creating the Y-leg. This technique is used to correct a wide alar base that is the result of alar flaring coupled with excessive interalar width. This is done to medialize the alae. **(b)** After closure. Additional sutures placed along the stem of the Y will lead to additional medialization. (Used with permission from Kridel RW, Castellano RD. A simplified approach to alar base reduction: a review of 124 patients over 20 years. Arch Facial Plast Surg 2005;7(2):81–93.)

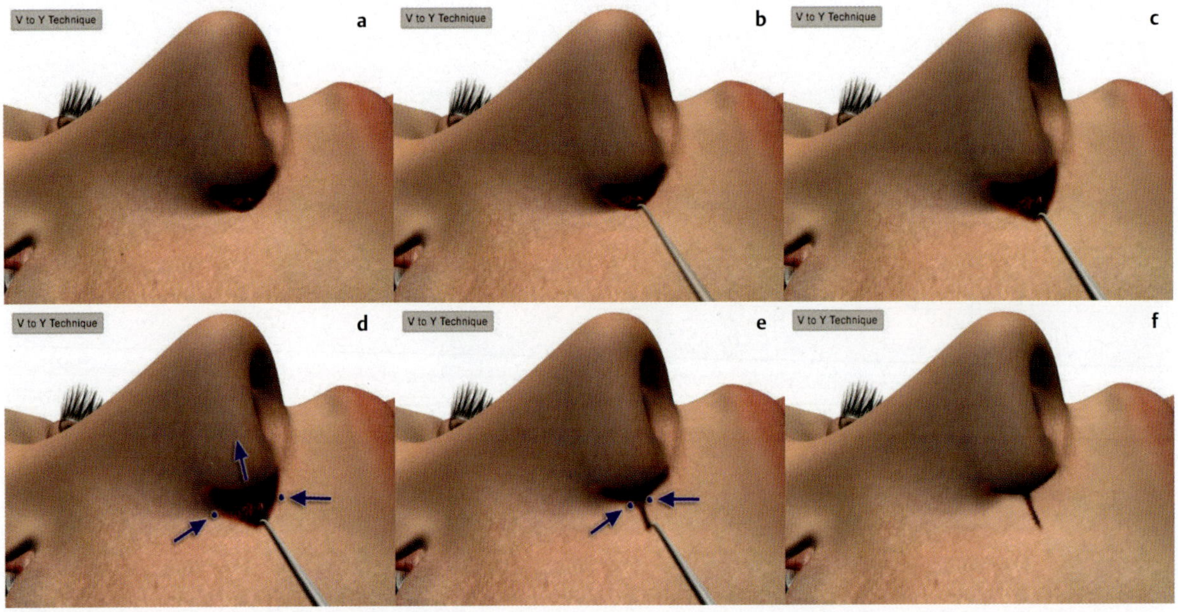

Fig. 14.11 Schematic showing steps of V-Y advancement of alar base for narrowing of interalar width. **(a)** Alar wedge excision completed. **(b)** Hook in place at nasolabial fold. **(c)** Lateral retraction of hook. **(d)** Location of suture placement and medial displacement of alar-facial junction. **(e)** Suture placed for medialization. **(f)** Completed V-Y advancement for narrowing of alar base. More narrowing of the alar base will result when more sutures are placed in the stem of the Y during advancement.

done in the office under local anesthesia with or without mild sedation. If it is done at the time of the rhinoplasty, it should be the last maneuver performed during the operation. Projection and de-projection of the nose can have a significant effect on alar flare, as outlined above (**Fig. 14.3**).

Given the general tendency toward under-projection in noses of African descent, we prefer to perform alar base reduction after the completion of all other rhinoplasty maneuvers. The transcolumellar and marginal incisions are closed prior to addressing the alar base. As stated above, one of the principal goals in surgery of the nose in these patients is to achieve more projection and tip refinement. This is usually achieved using dorsal onlay grafts, columellar strut grafts, the creation of a double dome after lateral

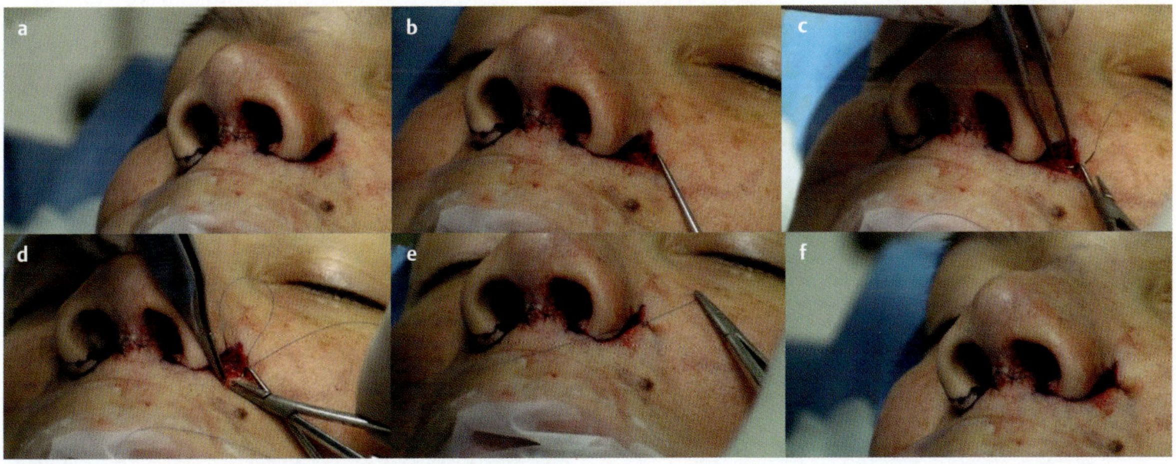

Fig. 14.12 Intraoperative views of V-Y advancement. **(a)** Wedge and sill reduction completed. **(b)** Lateral retraction of hook in nasolabial fold. **(c)** Suture placement in superior aspect of wedge excision. **(d)** Suture placement in inferior aspect of wedge excision. **(e)** Suture tied resulting in medialization. **(f)** Completed V-Y advancement of left alar base.

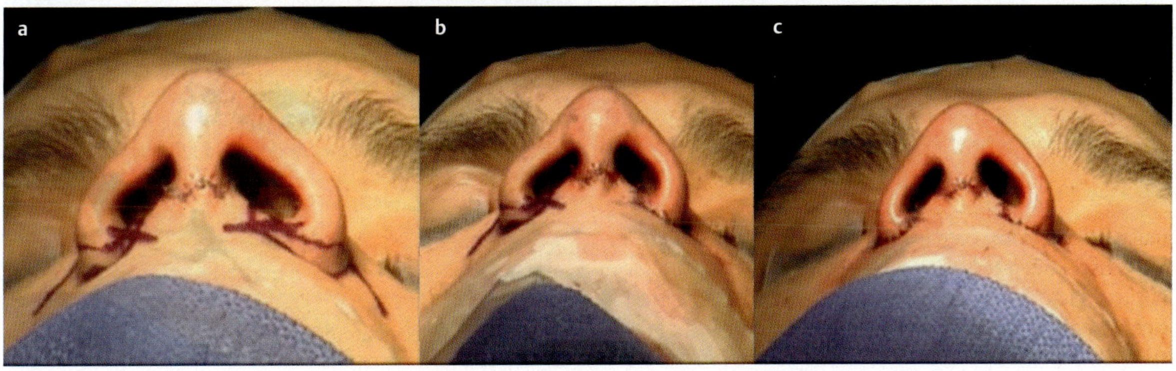

Fig. 14.13 Wedge and sill with V-Y advancement for narrowing of alar base. **(a)** Intraoperative view before alar base reduction. **(b)** Left wedge and sill with V-Y advancement completed on patient's left. Correction of excessive sill width and wide interalar distance on left can be seen with preservation of natural alar curve. **(c)** Completion of wedge and sill with V-Y advancement on both sides. Narrowing can be seen, with improvement of nostril asymmetry.

crural steal, and other maneuvers that may increase projection. With increased projection, there may be a "tent-pole" effect that leads to changes in the anatomical positioning of the alar base and mandates reevaluation prior to undertaking alar base reduction. If an increase in nasal projection has led to a correction of the alar base by reducing alar flaring, treatment of the alar base may be obviated. By focusing on alar flare, sill excess, and overall base width, an algorithmic approach, as outlined in **Fig. 14.14**, can be followed for an appropriately tailored approach to each patient.

The first step in alar wedge excisions is appropriately marking skin incisions in the alar-facial groove. This is done to preserve the (natural) curve of the ala, and to prevent a postoperative teardrop or Q-deformity of the nostril (see below, **Fig. 14.15**). The importance of symmetrical preoperative marking cannot be overstated, and the use of surgical calipers can facilitate the task. One should avoid excising too much tissue in this location or an excessively straight appearance of the ala at the alar–facial jnction may result. Finally, as noted above, the excision should not go above the supra-alar groove, or the dominant blood supply to the nasal tip, in the form of the lateral nasal artery, may be compromised.

After injection of local anesthetic (usually 1% lidocaine with 1:100,000 epinephrine), a no. 15 scalpel is used to

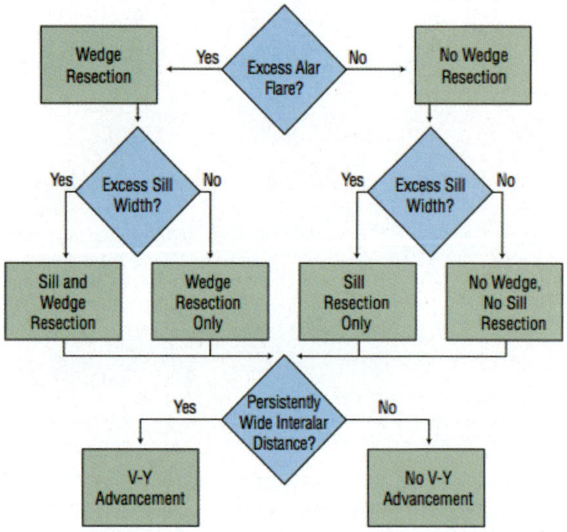

Fig. 14.14 Algorithm used in determining the appropriate surgical technique for correction of a wide alar base. (Used with permission from Kridel RW, Castellano RD. A simplified approach to alar base reduction: a review of 124 patients over 20 years. Arch Facial Plast Surg 2005;7(2):81–93.)

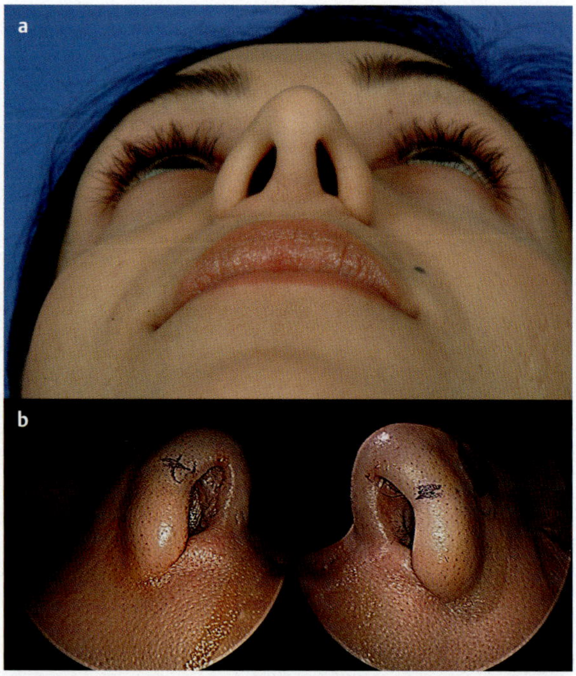

Fig. 14.15 Q (or teardrop) deformity of the nasal sill caused by reducing the alar flare and entering into the nostril when unnecessary. **(a)** Base view of a patient who underwent rhinoplasty at another institution with bilateral Q deformity of the alar base/nostrils. **(b)** Intraoperative views of right and left alar-facial junction showing Q deformity.

make the incisions. Care is taken not to violate the underlying muscle deep to the skin. Similarly, care must be taken not to violate the vestibular mucosa or notching can result. Needle-point cautery can then be used to achieve hemostasis. Meticulous reapproximation of the incision edges is necessary to avoid step-offs, and this is best achieved by placing one or two buried, interrupted deep 5–0 Vicryl sutures. Then 6–0 Prolene is used in a simple interrupted fashion to close the cutaneous layer. If flattening or over-straightening of the ala has occurred as a result of the closure, one should consider a modest V-Y advancement, as outlined below, to recreate the alar-facial groove (**Fig. 14.7** and **Fig. 14.11**).

Sill excisions are not often performed in isolation, and are typically combined with wedge excisions with or without V-Y advancement (see algorithm for specific indications for each, **Fig. 14.14**). When planning the incision for the enlarged nasal sill, the most natural results occur when the resection of the sill does not extend laterally past the long axis of the nostril or does not include too much of the vestibular lining.[15] When performing sill excision, additional undermining of the sill and vestibular tissues is recommended to avoid any notching or bunching of tissue. A 6–0 Prolene suture is used to precisely reapproximate the nostril border, and a deep 5–0 Vicryl suture is used to evert the skin edges at the nasal sill (**Fig. 14.8** and **Fig. 14.9**).[15] Everting the skin edges is critical in this location because improper suture technique can result in a notched appearance of the nasal vestibule.

If indicated, V-Y advancement is performed after either of the two previously described maneuvers has been completed but prior to closure of the incisions. Prior to V-Y advancement, the nostril sill must first be reapproximated with a single 6–0 Prolene suture if nasal sill excision was performed.[15] The lateral aspect of the open alar wedge incision is then drawn into the nasolabial fold with a single-pronged skin hook. Simple, interrupted 6–0 Prolene sutures approximate the V to create the stem of the Y within the nasolabial crease. The more sutures that are placed along the stem of the Y, the further the ala will be medialized (**Fig. 14.10, Fig. 14.11, Fig. 14.12,** and **Fig. 14.13**). In 3 days, every other suture is removed, and at 5 days, all sutures are removed.[15]

14.8 Potential Complications and Treatment

Alar base reduction can usually be achieved safely with minimal residual untoward effects. Nonetheless, certain risks exist, including infection, bleeding, scarring, and other cosmetic deformities that can result from poor technique. Visible scarring can result from improper placement of incisions, and incision placement is critical in achieving nearly imperceptible scars. We prefer to place the incisions into the alar-facial junction, as this results in the best camouflage and preservation of the curve. Nonetheless, noticeable scars and hypertrophic scarring can occur in this area due to the increased density of the sebaceous glands at the alar-facial junction. For correction of scarring in this location, dermabrasion can be performed under local anesthesia in the office and it has resulted in a high degree of patient satisfaction. We found that patients who underwent wedge and sill excision were more likely to require postoperative dermabrasion.[15] Additional indications for dermabrasion are noticeable or irregular scars present 6 weeks after surgery.[15] Similarly, one patient in our series had noticeable suture tracking that necessitated postoperative excision with scar revision. Proper timing of suture removal and avoidance of excessive tension on wound edges can minimize the chance of this complication.

In addition to the external scar of the wedge excision, incisions that violate the nostril can result in step-offs or notching of the nasal sill or internal alar margin. Failure to achieve exact epithelial alignment in these locations can lead to a Q or teardrop deformity of the nostril as viewed from the base (**Fig. 14.15**). As noted above, incisions should be extended into the nostril only when excessive nasal sill width is present and then only through the horizontal portion of the nasal sill and not via a lateral approach.[15] Another factor believed to contribute to notching of incisions is violation of the deep muscular layer in the alar base, and this is best avoided during dissection and excision of the alar wedge.[20] Keloid formation is also a concern in patients with Fitzpatrick skin types IV, V, and VI; however, in our experience, as in other studies, this has not been a problem.[2,4,5,6,15]

In addition to scarring, alar base asymmetry and/or excessive reduction can result from improper preoperative planning. Marking and measurement of the alar base excision should be done systematically, with calipers as a guide for symmetrical removal of tissue. Excessive alar wedge excision can result in an overly straight alar-facial junction, without the natural and desirable curve in the alae.[15,21] In our series, we removed an average of 4.6 mm of tissue from the alar wedges and 3.4 mm from each side during sill reduction. There were no significant complications with this amount of tissue excision.[15] Excessive reduction of the alar base can also lead to a noticeable notch at the junction of the alar and lobular nasal aesthetic subunits. Therefore, we recommend assessing the base view after excision has been completed but prior to complete closure of the incisions. An alar rim graft can be placed via the marginal incision or via the alar base excision if needed. Excessive narrowing of the alar base may also lead to ethnic incongruities. Finally, functional airway problems can result from excessive narrowing of the external valve, with resultant stenosis or collapse.

While we did not encounter any problems with the viability of the tip skin, damage to the vascular plexus of the tip is a theoretical risk when combining open rhinoplasty with alar base reduction. Recent studies have shown that this combination can be performed safely in both primary and revision rhinoplasty if the superior extent of the alar wedge excision is not taken beyond the supra-alar groove.[22,23] Additionally, dissection in the avascular plane immediately superficial to the lateral cartilages does not violate the major blood supply to the nasal tip from the lateral nasal artery (2–3 mm above the supra-alar groove).[24,25] Excessive debulking of the nasal tip is also discouraged as violation of the subdermal plexus can occur with overly aggressive thinning in the layer superficial to the nasal superficial muscular aponeurotic system.

14.9 Postoperative Care, Recovery, and Follow-up

As noted above, we prefer to perform alar base reduction as the last part of any rhinoplasty. After the procedure is completed, we apply a standard dressing and splint to the nasal dorsum as well as antibiotic ointment to any exposed incisions. The skin of the dorsum is cleaned and a liquid adhesive, such as Mastisol (Ferndale Laboratories, Ferndale, MI), is applied, followed by a layer of Micropore tape (3M, St. Paul, MN) to the dorsum and tip. A metallic tin splint is then applied, followed by a second layer of tape.

We advise all patients to keep their incisions clean and covered with a thin layer of antibiotic ointment at all times in the immediate postoperative period. Patients are usually seen on postoperative day 3, and every other alar Prolene suture is removed. The patient is again seen on postoperative day 5, and the remaining alar sutures and transcolumellar sutures are removed. The splint is taken down and, after inspection, the dorsum is usually retaped for a total of 10 days. Postoperative taping may need to be left in place for longer than usual in patients of African descent. Given the thick, fibro-fatty nature of the skin and soft tissue envelope in these patients, edema may be more prolonged than in Caucasians and thinner-skinned individuals.[5] We will often have the patient switch from an antibacterial ointment to a petroleum-based or mineral oil–based compound like Aquaphor (Beiersdorf US, Wilton, Connecticut) to reduce the risk of contact dermatitis and other local skin reaction.

The patient is followed closely for the first month postoperatively and then every 2 to 3 months for the first year. Supratip fullness can be treated with Kenalog (triamcinolone) injections and can be done as early as 1 week postoperatively.[2] Generally, no more than two to three injections of Kenalog 10 mg/mL are necessary for this purpose.[4] Similarly, if there are noticeable or irregular scars at 6 weeks post-op, dermabrasion can be performed. When necessary, it is done on both the alar and sill scars. We prefer using a hand-held dermabrader with a pear-tipped diamond fraise. The scar is treated until pinpoint bleeding is noted, indicating that the papillary dermis has been reached.

14.10 Outcomes

In 2005, the senior author published data from the 20-year review of 124 medical charts in his practice of patients who underwent alar base surgery. Inclusion criteria were history of wedge resection, nasal sill excision, and/or V-Y advancement during rhinoplasty. Exclusion criteria were those patients who did not follow up at the practice.[15] Of these patients, 16 were of African descent. Six patients underwent wedge excision alone, three underwent wedge and sill excision, one underwent wedge excision with V-Y advancement, and six underwent combined wedge and sill excision with V-Y advancement.[15] Patients ranged in age from 23 to 54 years and dermabrasion was required in 5 of 16 (31%).

The hallmark of surgery in patients of African descent is augmentation of the osseo-cartilaginous framework using grafts to increase dorsal projection and reduce nasal width. The alar base was appropriately narrowed using the techniques outlined above, with minimal complications and a high degree of patient satisfaction. **Fig. 14.16**, **Fig. 14.17**, and **Fig. 14.18** are representative examples of surgical cases and outcomes when alar base reduction is combined with rhinoplasty in patients of African descent. Other studies have shown similarly good outcomes in achieving harmonious results in patients of African descent when alar base reduction has been performed.[5,6,21,26]

14.11 Conclusion

Patients of African descent can have a great deal of variability in the anatomical characteristics of their noses. This goes significantly beyond the platyrrhine classification that has been used to define all noses in this group. When addressing alar base disproportion, an individualized approach to each patient will yield the best surgical outcomes. An algorithmic approach tailored to the specific anatomical deformity is outlined above and has shown satisfactory long-term outcomes in this patient population. Finally, patients of African descent often seek nasal refinement in the framework of ethnic identity, and preoperative evaluation should include a clear discussion with the patient about his or her surgical goals. As Porter has summarized, the goal should be to obtain an aesthetically pleasing result that is congruent with the patient's ethnicity and heritage,[9] while also accounting for a patient's individual desires.

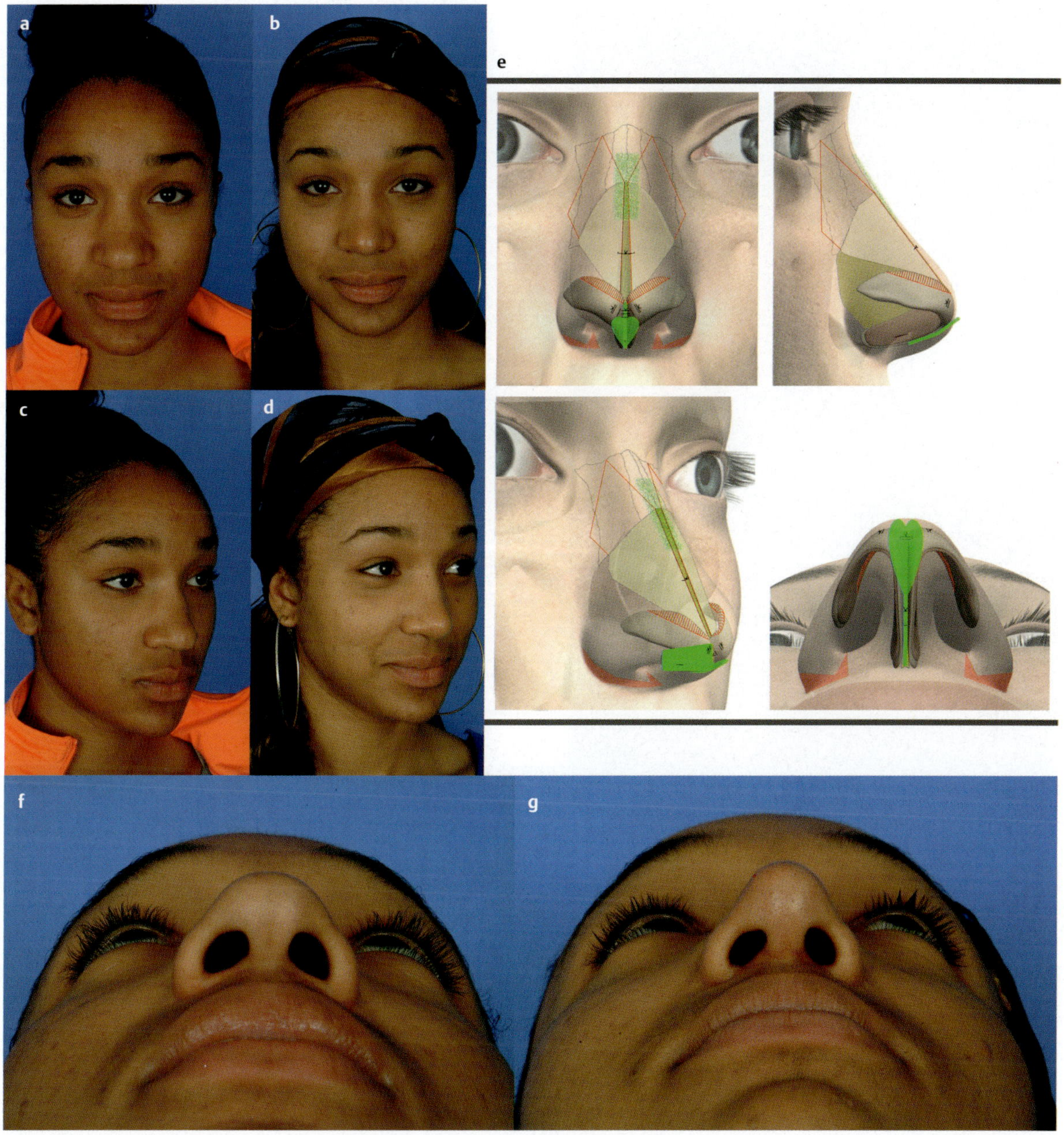

Fig. 14.16 (a,c,f) Preoperative views. **(b,d,g)** Postoperative views. **(e)** Nasal schematic depicting rhinoplasty in an African American patient. Alar base corrected with alar wedge and sill reduction. **(f,g)** Preoperative and postoperative base views demonstrate reduction in alar flare and horizontal width of nasal sill.

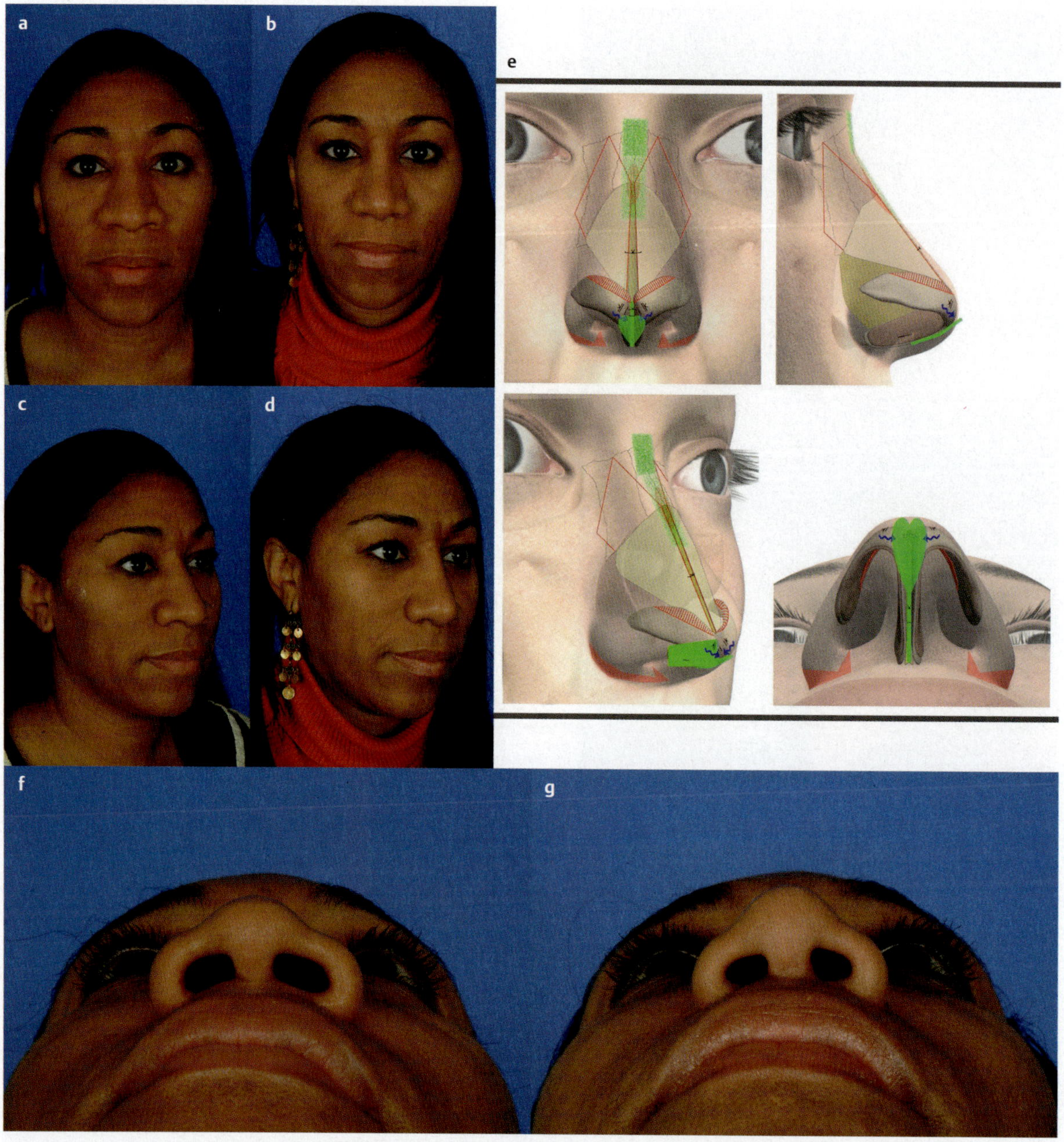

Fig. 14.17 **(a,c,f)** Preoperative photos. **(b,d,g)** Photos at postoperative month 2. **(e)** Nasal schematic of primary rhinoplasty for an African American woman. Wedge and sill reduction performed to correct excessive alar base width. **(f,g)** Base views demonstrate reduction in alar flare and horizontal width of nasal sill.

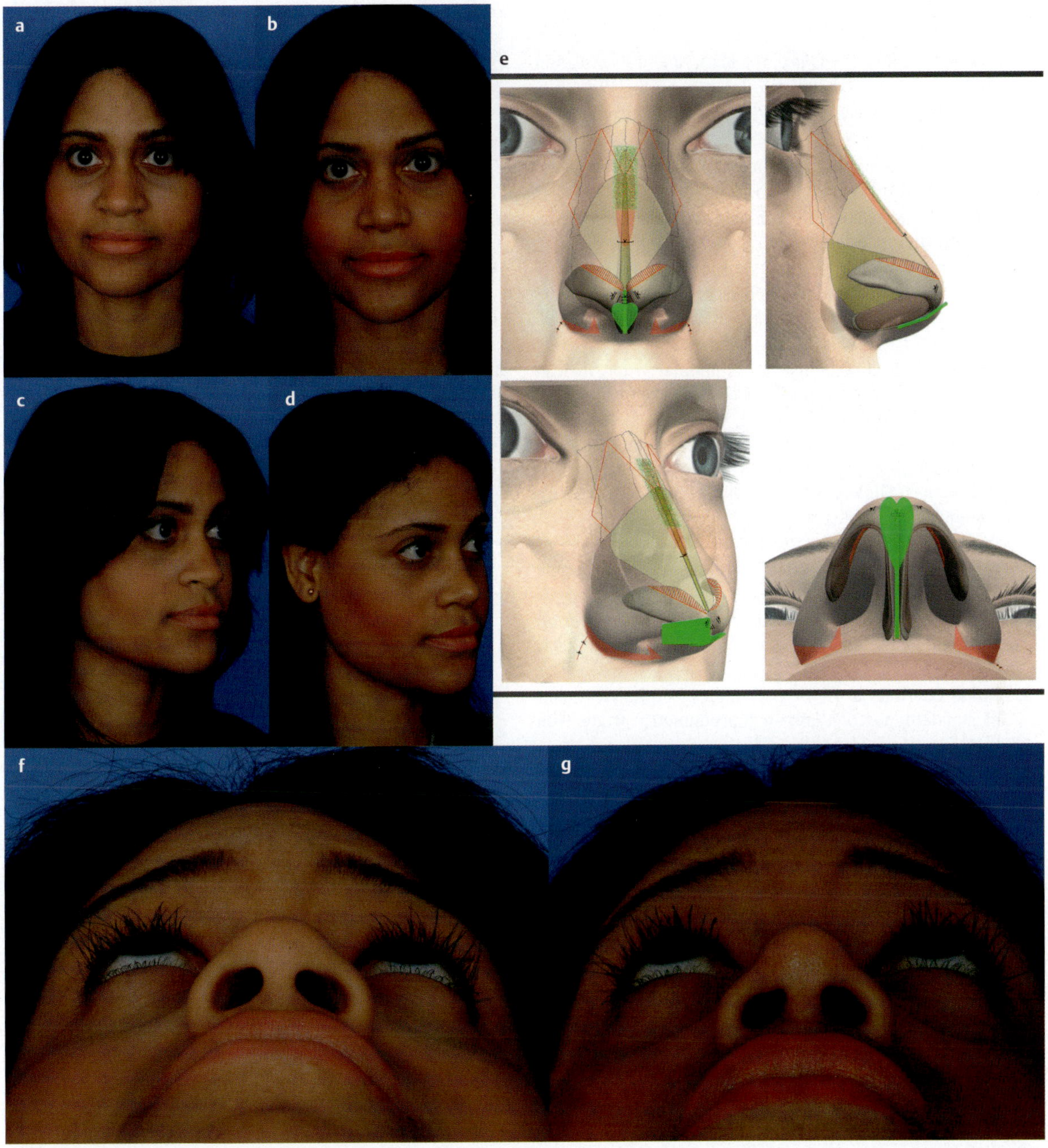

Fig. 14.18 (a,c,f) Preoperative views. **(b,d,g)** Postoperative views. **(e)** Nasal schematic depicting primary rhinoplasty in African American patient. Alar base correction performed using V-Y advancement with alar wedge and sill reduction. **(c,d)** Oblique views with minimal perceptible scarring at site of V-Y advancement. **(f,g)** Base views demonstrate tip refinement and reduction in interalar width, horizontal width of nasal sill, and alar flare.

References

1. Ofodile FA, Bokhari FJ, Ellis C. The Black American nose. Ann Plast Surg 1993;31(3):209–218, discussion 218–219
2. Patel AD, Kridel RW. African-American rhinoplasty. Facial Plast Surg 2010;26(2):131–141
3. Bernstein L. Rhinoplasty for the Negroid nose. Otolaryngol Clin North Am 1975;8(3):783–795
4. Kridel RW, Szachowicz EH II. Non-Caucasian rhinoplasty with the open approach. Facial Plast Surg 1988;5(2): 179–187
5. Rohrich RJ, Muzaffar AR. Rhinoplasty in the African-American patient. Plast Reconstr Surg 2003;111(3):1322–1339, discussion 1340–1341
6. Slupchynskyj O, Gieniusz M. Rhinoplasty for African American patients: a retrospective review of 75 cases. Arch Facial Plast Surg 2008;10(4):232–236
7. Calhoun KH, House W, Hokanson JA, Quinn FB. Normal nasal airway resistance in noses of different sizes and shapes. Otolaryngol Head Neck Surg 1990;103(4): 605–609
8. Ohki M, Naito K, Cole P. Dimensions and resistances of the human nose: racial differences. Laryngoscope 1991;101(3):276–278
9. Porter JP. The average African American male face: an anthropometric analysis. Arch Facial Plast Surg 2004; 6(2):78–81
10. Farkas LG, Hreczko TA, Deutsch CK. Objective assessment of standard nostril types—a morphometric study. Ann Plast Surg 1983;11(5):381–389
11. Ofodile FA, Bokhari F. The African-American nose: Part II. Ann Plast Surg 1995;34(2):123–129
12. Porter JP, Olson KL. Anthropometric facial analysis of the African American woman. Arch Facial Plast Surg 2001;3(3):191–197
13. Porter JP, Olson KL. Analysis of the African American female nose. Plast Reconstr Surg 2003;111(2):620–626, discussion 627–628
14. Topinard P. Elements d'anthropologie generale. Paris: Delahaye & Lacrosnier; 1885
15. Kridel RW, Castellano RD. A simplified approach to alar base reduction: a review of 124 patients over 20 years. Arch Facial Plast Surg 2005;7(2):81–93
16. Silver WE, Sajjadian A. Nasal base surgery. Otolaryngol Clin North Am 1999;32(4):653–668
17. Chike-Obi CJ, Boahene K, Bullocks JM, Brissett AE. Tip nuances for the nose of African descent. Facial Plast Surg 2012;28(2):194–201
18. Weir RF. On restoring sunken noses without scarring the face. 1892. Aesthetic Plast Surg 1988;12(4):203–206
19. Bernstein L. Esthetic anatomy of the nose. Laryngoscope 1972;82(7):1323–1330
20. Tebbetts JB. Primary Rhinoplasty: A New Approach to the Logic and the Techniques. St. Louis, MO: CV Mosby Company; 1998:481–492
21. Matory WE Jr, Falces E. Non-Caucasian rhinoplasty: a 16-year experience. Plast Reconstr Surg 1986;77(2):239–252
22. Bafaqeeh SA, Al-Qattan MM. Simultaneous open rhinoplasty and alar base excision: is there a problem with the blood supply of the nasal tip and columellar skin? Plast Reconstr Surg 2000;105(1):344–347, discussion 348–349
23. Tellioğlu AT, Vargel I, Cavuşoğlu T, Cimen K. Simultaneous open rhinoplasty and alar base excision for secondary cases. Aesthetic Plast Surg 2005;29(3):151–155
24. Rohrich RJ, Gunter JP, Friedman RM. Nasal tip blood supply: an anatomic study validating the safety of the transcolumellar incision in rhinoplasty. Plast Reconstr Surg 1995;95(5):795–799, discussion 800–801
25. Toriumi DM, Mueller RA, Grosch T, Bhattacharyya TK, Larrabee WF Jr. Vascular anatomy of the nose and the external rhinoplasty approach. Arch Otolaryngol Head Neck Surg 1996;122(1):24–34
26. Romo T III, Shapiro AL. Aesthetic reconstruction of the platyrrhine nose. Arch Otolaryngol Head Neck Surg 1992;118(8):837–841

15 Rhytidectomy in Dark-Skinned Patients

Satyen Undavia and Babak Azizzadeh

15.1 Introduction

Facial rejuvenation surgery has become increasingly popular over the past century due to the emphasis placed on beauty and youth in the media. Rhytidectomy, or facelift, is at the core of facial rejuvenation surgery, as it remains the most effective and reliable way to provide a more youthful appearance. The goals of rhytidectomy include tightening of the jawline, improving the cervicomental angle, and removing excess skin. While rhytidectomy literally means "removal of wrinkles," we now understand that facial aging is due to differences in skin quality and elasticity, alterations in the volume and distribution of facial fat, and changes in the facial skeleton.[1,2,3,4,5,6,7,8,9] These changes occur to a varying degree in all patients and it is critical that surgeons accurately assess them prior to performing any procedures. Dark-skinned patients differ from Caucasians in these areas due to different morphologic characteristics of their skin and craniofacial structure.[10,11,12,13] These characteristics lead to subtle differences in the aging process between the two groups. In this chapter, we first outline the differences between ethnic groups as they relate to facial rejuvenation surgery and then highlight changes in the surgical approach that are required to maximize cosmetic outcomes in these patients.

15.1.1 African Americans

Photodamage is known to play a critical role in the aging process.[14] Ultraviolet radiation accelerates this process by creating genetic mutations and damaging critical support structures of the skin. Melanin, which provides the pigment in skin, has been shown to be protective against the damaging effects of ultraviolet radiation.[15] Although there is no significant difference between the total numbers of melanosomes between the races, African American skin has larger melanosomes with significantly more pigment.[16] In addition, the melanosomes are more evenly distributed throughout the epidermis and are not confined to the stratum basale, as in Caucasians. While photodamage causes aging in all races, the effect is either less pronounced in African Americans or may present later in life. As a result, fine lines and wrinkles are less pronounced and are not a significant contributor to the aging process in this patient population.[10] In addition, the increased thickness of African American skin also protects against fine lines and wrinkles, due to the thicker stratum corneum and increased number of fibroblasts.[16] This quality is important in lower facial rejuvenation because the increased weight of the skin is the cause of jowling, as opposed to increased laxity, as in Caucasian populations.

The quality of the patient's hair is a critical factor in facial rejuvenation surgery because many of the scars are camouflaged in hair-bearing areas. An important consideration in African Americans is the high rate of traction alopecia, which occurs when tension is placed on the scalp for long periods of time. Hairstyles with tight braids and the use of chemical straighteners significantly increase the incidence of this condition in African Americans.[17]

Finally, structural differences in the craniofacial skeleton also affect the aging process in African Americans. The malar eminence is commonly hypoplastic and the orbit is slightly proptotic, which is known as a negative vector.[18] These two factors lead to a more concave appearance of the midface. In addition, the weight of the skin and lack of bony support lead to premature descent of the malar fat pads, which is a significant factor in African American facial aging.

15.1.2 Mestizo/Hispanic Patients

Mestizo skin is also thicker and contains more pigment than Caucasian skin; therefore, photoprotective effects of melanin apply. In general, Mestizo patients have fewer fine rhytids and their heavy skin is the contributing factor in jowling. In contrast, however, the malar eminence has slightly more projection, which protects against midface fat pad ptosis. In addition, the Mestizo chin is often slightly more retrusive, which contributes to the obtuse cervicomental angle.[13]

15.2 Historical Background

Early facelifts, described by German surgeons in the early twentieth century,[19] involved skin excision only, which resulted in excessive tension along suture lines and short-lived results. In the 1960s, Aufricht,[20] Webster,[21] and others described plication of the "deeper layers" to improve their results. Prior to the description of the superficial muscular aponeurotic system (SMAS), Skoog described using the platysma and superficial fascia of the face to support the tension of the lift.[22] In a landmark article by Mitz and Peyronie in 1976, the SMAS was characterized as the superficial fascia of the face and as the cephalad extension of the platysma.[23] Surgeons realized that tightening the SMAS provided an enhanced lift and increased the longevity of the results. This class of facelift became known as SMAS rhytidectomy. In general, SMAS facelifts produce substantial benefit in the neck and jowl but exert minimal effect on the midface or nasolabial fold (NLF).

The next major advancement in facial rejuvenation surgery came in 1990, when Hamra described the deep-plane facelift.[24] In this procedure, the SMAS is incised over the parotid gland and a plane is created beneath it and elevated toward the NLF. To achieve adequate midface and NLF elevation, the dense zygomaticocutaneous ligaments must be released. The theoretical drawbacks of this technique are prolonged recovery time and a potentially increased rate of facial nerve injury where the nerve is exposed at the anterior border of the parotid gland and lateral border of the zygomaticus major muscle. Proponents of this technique argue that, with careful and meticulous dissection, the branches of the facial nerve, which lie in the deeper parotimasseteric fascia, should be protected. Furthermore, they contend that elevation and suspension of the strong and resilient SMAS leads to increased lift with greater longevity and decreased tension on the suture line. Hamra later modified his technique to include elevation and suspension of the orbicularis oculi muscle to address laxity in the orbital region, and he termed the procedure a composite facelift.[25]

Owsley reported his facelift technique, the extended supra-SMAS rhytidectomy,[26] which seeks to achieve the lift and longevity of the deep plane facelift while reducing the risk of facial nerve injury.[27,28] In this procedure, first the SMAS is suspended to address the jowl and neck, as in a traditional facelift. In the second stage of the procedure, a supra-SMAS dissection is begun at the orbicularis oculi and zygomaticus major muscles and is continued medially beyond the NLF. The midface is then suspended superolaterally to the SMAS and temporalis fascia to elevate the midface and to efface the NLF. Another modification included a subperiosteal dissection to address the midface, which was described by Ramirez in 1991.[29] This deeper plane also provides a safer region to dissect while theoretically reducing injury to the facial nerve.

Facial rejuvenation surgery was also influenced by the growing popularity of minimally invasive techniques in the 1990s. Saylan was the first to describe a short-scar facelift, which he called the *S-lift* due to the S shape of the incision.[30] Today, Baker's SMASectomy[31] and Tonnard and Verpaele's minimal access cranial suspension (MACS) lift[32] are the short-scar facelifts that are most commonly performed. These facelifts do not have a postauricular component, and therefore they necessitate a more vertical vector of lift. While these approaches can be effective, patient selection is critical, as older patients or those with more advanced photoaging will likely benefit from more traditional approaches.

15.3 Anatomy

Facial anatomy is covered in detail elsewhere in this book, but a few key points are worth emphasizing. All surgeons should have a thorough understanding of facial nerve anatomy to safely and effectively perform rhytidectomy. The facial nerve trunk exits the stylomastoid foramen and enters the body of the parotid gland before splitting into five main branches (the temporal, zygomatic, buccal, marginal mandibular, and cervical).[33] It is critical to anticipate the variety of branching patterns that are possible from patient to patient. The most important concept to appreciate is that facial nerve branches are relatively unprotected between the anterior edge of the parotid gland and the lateral edge of the facial muscles. While the muscles around the eye and central face receive multiple inputs from numerous buccal and zygomatic facial nerve branches, the temporal (also known as the frontal) and marginal mandibular nerve are typically terminal branches. Because they are the sole innervation for these muscle groups, injury to these branches is more likely to result in facial asymmetry and to have more permanent effects.

Over the zygomatic arch, the temporal branch of the facial nerve is at increased risk in both traditional SMASectomy and deep-plane techniques. Typically, two to four rami pass over this region at the inferior border of the arch, ~ 8 mm medial to the external auditory canal and 17 mm posterior to the junction of the arch and the zygomatic body **(Fig. 15.1)**.[34] As the branches cross the arch, they are relatively deep within the parotidomasseteric fascia; however, as they pass above it, they become superficial.[35] The transition zone begins 15 mm superior to the zygomatic arch and 15 mm posterior to the lateral orbital rim. This is where the frontal branch enters the underside of the temporoparietal fascia. While dissecting in the temple, it is important to elevate either in the subperiosteal plane or just deep to hair follicles to help protect the nerve.

As the marginal mandibular branch of the facial nerve emerges from the parotid gland, near the angle of the mandible, it travels deep to the platysma muscle and parotidomasseteric fascia over the surface of the masseter muscle. It then passes superficial to the facial artery and vein before innervating the lip depressors. When elevating deep to the platysma, it is important to proceed cautiously and to use cautery sparingly, as the marginal nerve is long and thin and very susceptible to neuropraxia or inadvertent injury during cautery of small branches of the facial vessels.[36]

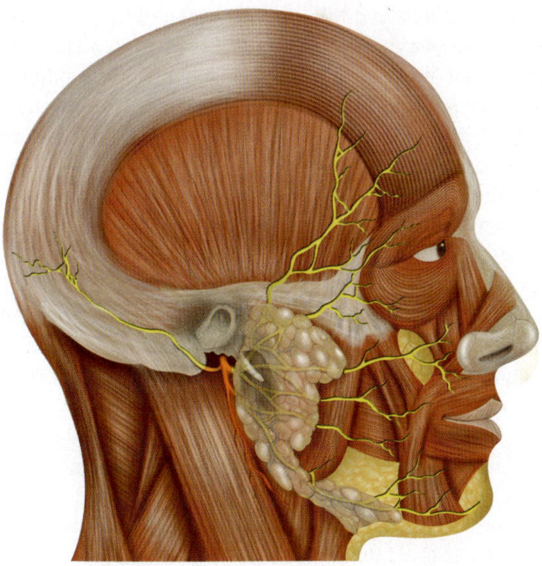

Fig. 15.1 Illustration of facial nerve anatomy. The temporal branch of the frontal nerve crosses over the zygomatic arch ~ 8 mm medial to the external auditory canal and 17 mm posterior to the junction of the arch and the zygomatic body.

15.4 Patient Evaluation and Preoperative Planning

During the initial facial rejuvenation consult, it is important to begin by eliciting the patient's desires and goals for treatment. It can be helpful to have the patient, while facing a mirror, point to the areas that they would like to have addressed. While patient's initial complaint may be aging-related changes in the lower third of the face, this is an important opportunity to evaluate the face as a whole. If patients have significant brow ptosis, upper lid dermatochalasia, pseudoherniated lower lid fat, or midface ptosis, facial rejuvenation of the lower face alone may not be adequate. Once lower facial rejuvenation has been decided upon, we prefer to have the patient look in a mirror while the surgeon uses his hands to lift both sides of the face to create an appearance that resembles an achievable postoperative result. When performing this technique, it is important not to over-correct the jowling in a manner that is not surgically attainable, because this could give the patient false expectations.

The submental and cervical areas deserve careful visual and tactile analysis to identify the precise anatomic components that need alteration. Aging in these areas can be due to any combination of increased skin laxity, excess submental and subplatysmal fat, poor hyoid position, platysmal banding, and/or microgenia. To create an effective surgical plan, it is important to identify the factors that are contributing to the patient's complaints. In ethnic patients, it is also important to evaluate the color changes in the skin. Rhytidectomy will usually involve some degree of skin advancement and excision, and significant color variation across the face can lead to color mismatch at the suture lines, making them more visible. As mentioned above, it is important to address skeletal structure as well, especially in ethnic patients. African Americans often have inadequate projection of the zygoma, leading to a hollowed look in this region. We often recommend multilevel fat grafting to address these areas.

As in all fields of medicine, a complete medical history must be obtained at the initial consultation. This is particularly important to ensure that the patient is healthy enough for elective cosmetic surgery. Chronic medical conditions like asthma, diabetes, and cardiovascular disease should be optimized before attempting any surgery. Any personal or family history of coagulopathy or problems with anesthesia must be carefully evaluated. All prior interventions that have been performed on the face should be discussed. This includes botulinum injections, facial fillers (specifically, type and location placed), laser treatment, and prior facial rejuvenation surgery. A history of herpes labialis warrants prophylactic treatment with valacyclovir 2 g twice daily the day before surgery to guard against reactivation. Patients on chemotherapeutic and immunomodulatory drug regimens, including oral steroids, should consult their prescribing physician prior to surgery. Tobacco use a critical component of the preoperative history. Active tobacco users are at higher risk of skin slough[37] and hematoma formation,[38] and they should be asked to quit for at least 2 to 4 weeks prior to surgery. Parikh and Jacono[39] examined 183 patients who underwent deep-plane facelift. In the 15 (8%) who were smokers, they found no increased risk of these complications. Their conclusion was that the deep-plane facelift, due to its minimal subcutaneous undermining and thick soft tissue flap, is a safe alternative in active smokers. Any significant psychiatric history, including anxiety and depression, should be elicited and addressed. Prior to surgery, all patients also have a set of photographs taken for documentation. Finally, it is important to obtain a detailed history of medication usage. Below is a list of medications that should be stopped 7 to 14 days before surgery:

- APC (aspirin, phenacetin, caffeine)
- Advil
- Alka-Seltzer
- Anadin
- Anaprox
- Arthritis Pain Formula
- Ascodeen-30
- Ascriptin
- Aspirin suppositories (all brands)

- Aspirin
- Bayer Aspirin
- Buff-a-comp
- Buffadyne
- Butalbatal
- Cama Arthritis Pain Reliever
- Cama-Inlay tabs
- Cheracol Capsules
- Congespirin
- Cope Coricidin
- Coricidin
- Darvon Compound
- Dristan
- Doan's Pills
- Duragesic
- Ecotrin
- Empirin
- Emprazil
- Equagesic
- Excedrin
- Fiorinol
- Four-Way Cold Tablets
- Indocin
- Measurin
- Midol
- Monacet with Codeine
- Motrin
- Naprosyn
- Norgesic
- Nuprin
- Os-Cal-Gone
- Pamprin

15.5 Techniques

Below is a detailed description of our technique for lower facial rejuvenation, the short-flap SMAS rhytidectomy. The technique is performed similarly among all races, but a few key points are mentioned. We also summarize the deep-plane facelift technique.

15.5.1 Incision Planning

The placement of incisions for a rhytidectomy is critical to maximize patient outcome and satisfaction. The incisions described below can be used in all skin types. In women, the starting point for the temporal aspect of the incision depends on the predicted amount of skin excision. If a significant amount of skin is to be excised, the incision should begin parallel to the hairline in a trichophytic manner. This will prevent significant displacement of the hairline. If a moderate skin excision is expected, the incision can simply pass obliquely within the hair down to the helical root **(Fig. 15.2a)**. From the helical root, the incision is continued inferiorly toward the tragus, with a gentle curve along the junction of the auricle and the face. Incisions are continued either in front of, or posterior to, the edge of the tragus. We prefer the posttragal incision in females as it camouflages the scar. The incision then continues in between the auricle and face and around the lobule of the ear. The incision over the concha is made several millimeters superior to the sulcus **(Fig. 15.2b)** to allow the healed scar to fall within the sulcus. At the point of maximal width of the auricle, the incision is angled toward the occipital hairline. To obtain adequate rotation while limiting dog-ear formation, the incision must either be carried into the hairline for 2 cm or along the occipital hairline. We prefer to carry the incision into the hairline, as incisions parallel to the hairline tend to be more visible.

The facelift incision in males must be tailored differently due to the differences in facial hair. Temporal incisions can be placed within the temporal tuft of hair because the skin that is pulled up to the incision following the lift will continue to grow hair and can become a new sideburn. The next major difference is in the pre-auricular incision. The incision should be placed ~ 8 mm in front of the auricular cartilage and should pass pretragally to avoid placing hair-bearing skin too close to the ear. If the expected skin excision is conservative, the postauricular incision can be made as described above. The challenge is when significant excision of skin is performed and redraping brings hair-bearing skin into the postauricular sulcus. To avoid this issue, the incision is made in the sulcus and not a few millimeters above it.

15.5.2 Submentoplasty

One of the main areas requiring attention in lower facial rejuvenation surgery is the submental area and cervicomental angle. The five visual criteria associated with a youthful neck profile, described by Ellenbogen and Karlin,[40] include: (1) distinct inferior mandibular border from mentum to angle, with no jowl overhang; (2) slight subhyoid depression at the cervicomental angle, which gives the impression of a long neck; (3) visible thyroid cartilage contour; (4) distinct, visible anterior border of the sternocleidomastoid muscle (SCM) from the sternum to retromandibular region; and (5) cervicomental angle between 105 and 120 degrees. Excess submental fat, a low and anterior hyoid, skin laxity, microgenia, platysmal banding, and abnormal occlusion are anatomical factors that contribute to an undesirable submental contour. The planned intervention must be tailored to address the above-mentioned factors to maximize patient satisfaction.

For thin-faced patients with minimal submental adiposity and limited platysmal banding, the lateral pull on

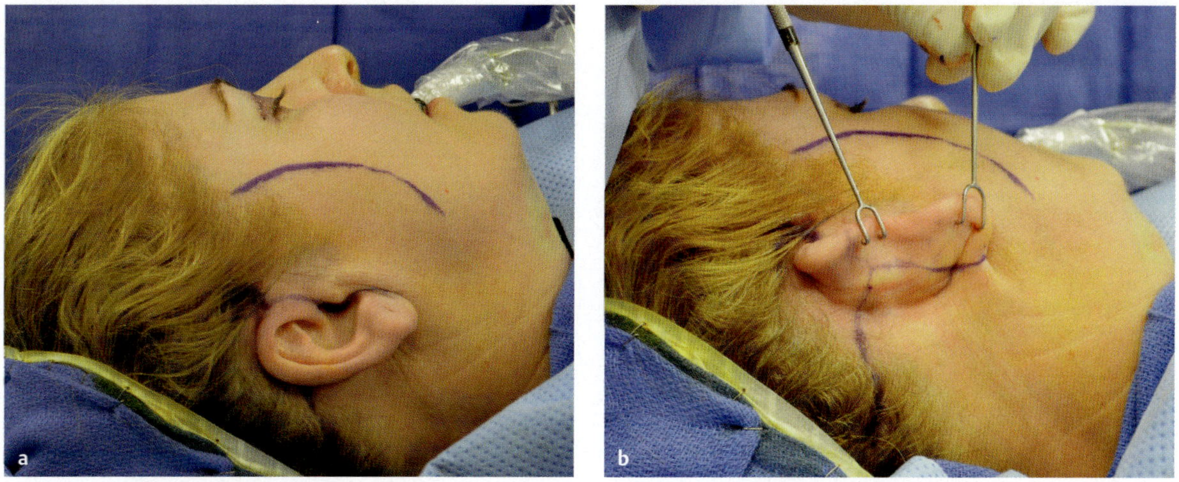

Fig. 15.2 **(a)** Representative markings for the incision in a female patient. Also demarcated is the planned area of maximal anterior dissection. **(b)** The postauricular incision locations.

the SMAS and skin excisions may be all that is required. Excess submental fat can be located either above (subcutaneously) or below the platysma. Failure to adequately address subplatysmal fat can lead to persistent submental fullness. Direct excision is the preferred modality, as submental cannula-assisted liposuction can lead to inadvertent marginal mandibular nerve injury. If a limited amount of subplatysmal adipose tissue is present, bipolar cautery can ablate the pad safely. Subcutaneous fat can be excised under direct visualization with scissors or with a liposuction cannula. Whichever technique is used, it is critical to maintain a uniform subcutaneous flap to avoid contour irregularities (**Fig. 15.3**).

While lateral manipulation of the SMAS will lead to some degree of platysmal elevation, patients with heavy platysmal banding require more aggressive interventions. A variety of methods are available to address laxity in the medial edge of the platysma. Techniques include placement of midline sutures, direct medial platysmal excision, lateral platysmal suspension, and platysmal transection. After placing a stab incision, the suction-assisted lipectomy is performed prior to the platysmaplasty, which aids in elevation of the subcutaneous flap. The incision is then extended in the submental crease for 2 to 3 cm, and a blunt and sharp dissection is performed with vertical spreading to complete the flap and to expose the medial borders of the platysma (**Fig. 15.4**). The platysma is exposed from the anterior border of the mandible down to the thyroid notch. The medial border of the platysma is then sutured together with interrupted 3–0 polydioxanone (PDS) sutures in a buried fashion.

Feldmen describes a modification of this technique in which a running suture is placed from the submentum down to the thyroid notch, back up to the submentum, and then finally the knot is tied at the thyroid notch.[41] This corset-like technique recruits the platysma laterally and overlaps the medial edges to create a smooth contour. Some authors have reported the creation of a single anterior band over time. Guyuron has described a vest-over-pants technique in which the medial borders of the platysma are overlapped to eliminate midline roll.[42] He found, in 88 patients over 26 years, that there was no recurrence of platysmal banding. Another modification of the traditional platysmaplasty involves performing a wedge resection of the medial border of the platysma near the hyoid bone. Proponents of the technique state that it allows for the cephalad portion of the muscle to migrate superiorly, which creates a sharper cervicomental angle. It also breaks the continuity of the anterior platysmal bands, which should prevent their recurrence. Most of these techniques recruit the skin and platysma more medially, which can lead to tethering of the skin laterally. This can be easily resolved by undermining the skin in these areas.

15.5.3 SMAS Techniques

Techniques for short-flap SMAS rhytidectomy (SFSR) and deep-plane rhytidectomy are described in detail below, followed by the potential complications.

SMAS Rhytidectomy

Our modification to the traditional rhytidectomy, performed as SFSR, involves conservative undermining of the skin in the facial region and a multivector SMAS imbrication. The anterior dermal-SMAS attachments, namely

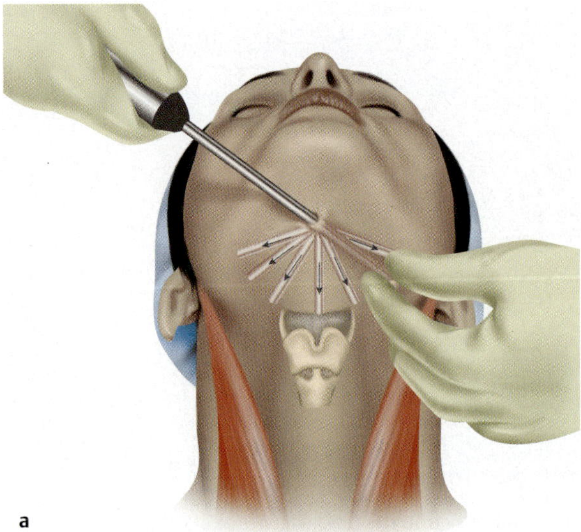

a

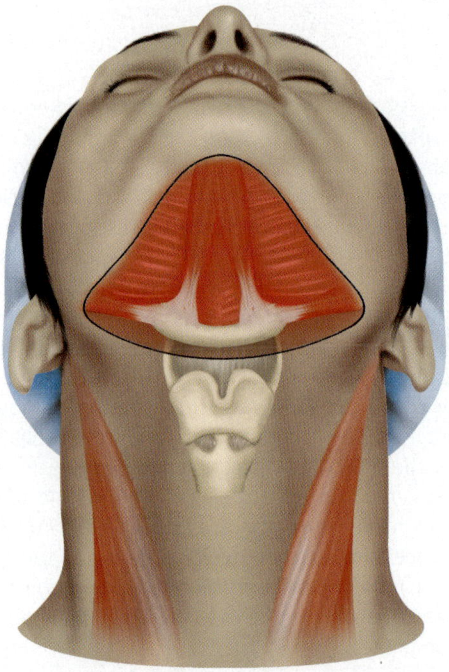

b

Fig. 15.3 (a,b) Illustration of technique used for submental liposuction.

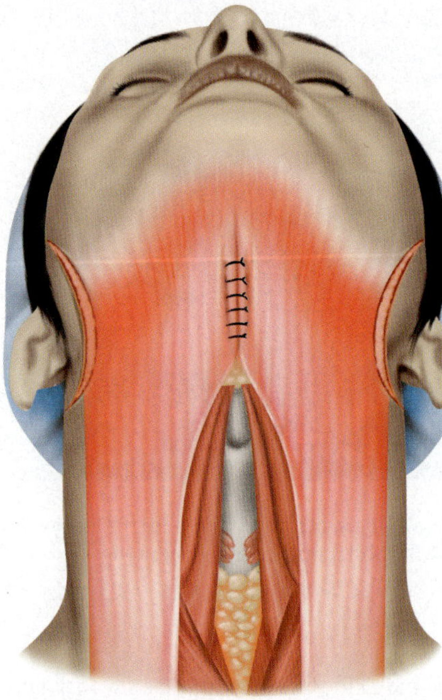

Fig. 15.4 Example of medial plication of the platysma for platysmaplasty in patients with significant banding.

zygomaticocutaneous and mandibulocutaneous ligaments, are undisturbed in this approach, which allows for aggressive SMAS suspension without applying significant tension on the wound. While some volume is added to the midface, we prefer using autologous fat grafting to restore volume and to establish a more youthful ogee curve. This is particularly important in African American patients who have under-projection of the malar eminence.

We prefer the SFSR because the limited cutaneous undermining minimizes the risk for facial nerve injury and for postoperative hematoma formation. Muzzafar and Mendelson demonstrated that releasing these ligaments in the prezygomatic space through extensive subcutaneous dissection can potentially cause injury to the facial nerve branches to the orbicularis oculi.[43,44] In addition, the likelihood of vascular compromise is also diminished, especially in smokers, diabetics, and elderly patients. Finally, we have found that patients undergoing this technique are able to resume normal activity within 7 to 10 days postoperatively.

This technique can be performed with either IV sedation or general anesthesia; however, we prefer the latter. We also routinely administer IV cefazolin and steroids and apply lower extremity intermittent compression devices. The incisions are marked preoperatively with the patient in the supine position. Lidocaine 1% with 1:100,000 epinephrine is infiltrated into one side of the face and the submental region if submentoplasty is planned. Our preferred method to secure hair away from the surgical field is to wrap autoclave tape circumferentially around the head 2 to 4 cm behind the hairline. After prepping the entire face, neck, and hair just beyond the tape, a sterile head drape is secured to the tape using surgical staples. The endotracheal tube and circuit are placed into a sterile, clear plastic sheath typically used for endoscopic sinus surgery, which allows for manipulation of the tube during the case (**Fig. 15.5**).

Once the adjunct procedures are completed, attention is directed toward performing the rhytidectomy. We use a ruler to mark out the planned distance of skin undermining prior to elevation, which is typically 4 to 6 cm depending on the patient's facial proportions (**Fig. 15.6**). The overhead lights are positioned so that one is directed at the incision from a posterior direction, and the other is directed at the skin flap from an anterior position. A gender-appropriate incision is made using a 15-blade scalpel as described above (**Fig. 15.3** and **Fig. 15.4**). A Brown-Adson forceps and the scalpel are used to begin the flap elevation in the subcutaneous plane in the preauricular region. After properly entering the plane and elevating for ~ 1.5 cm, the double-prong skin hooks or 4-prong cat-paws are engaged, and skin undermining proceeds with Metzenbaum scissors (**Fig. 15.7a**). Critical to maintaining the proper plane and uniform elevation is traction and countertraction on the skin flap. The surgeon pulls the skin hook in the posterior and superior vector while the assistant applies countertraction on the skin in the opposite direction. As mentioned above, overhead light positioning is critical, as transillumination through the flap helps to guide the surgeon in maintaining the plane.

The frontal nerve is at highest risk over the zygomatic arch and temple region, and subcutaneous elevation should be performed just deep to the hair follicles to minimize risk of injury. After elevation of the preauricular flap, a moist surgical sponge is placed under the flap to tamponade any bleeding. After the entire subcutaneous elevation has been performed, hemostasis will be obtained along the entire flap to maximize efficiency.

The posterior occipital area is elevated also initially with a no. 15 blade and forceps. The skin over the mastoid is very thin and easy to tear or perforate. Over the SCM, there is little subcutaneous fat and the skin tightly adheres to the underlying muscle and fascia. To avoid injury to the external jugular vein and great auricular nerve, the fascia overlying the muscle should be preserved. The inferior limit of the dissection is 4 to 5 cm below the auricle. If the patient has significant cervical skin laxity, undermining is performed toward the submental dissection and is connected to elevate this skin. A surgical sponge is placed under the postauricular flap.

The pre- and postauricular dissections are then connected (**Fig. 15.7b**). Flap elevation in this region should be performed judiciously or under direct visualization to avoid potentially entering the deep plane and inadvertently injuring the marginal mandibular branch of the facial nerve. Once the subcutaneous flap is completely elevated, hemostasis is meticulously achieved with bipolar cautery (**Fig. 15.7c**). An assistant always observes the face to identify any facial nerve stimulation and thereby to avoid inadvertent injury.

The SMAS imbrication is performed next. Starting ~ 15 mm anterior to the superior point of the tragus, a J-shaped strip of SMAS/plastysma 1 cm in width is excised anterior and inferior to the auricle with facelift scissors (**Fig. 15.8a**). Excision of the SMAS is safe in this region as the facial nerve

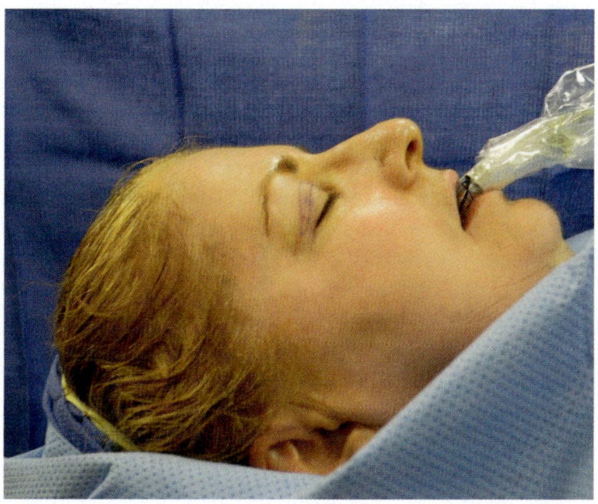

Fig. 15.5 Example of patient after the full face is prepped and a sterile head drape is applied. Prepping and draping the endotracheal tube and placing the ventilation tubing in a sterile camera bag allows for easy and safe manipulation of the head during the operation.

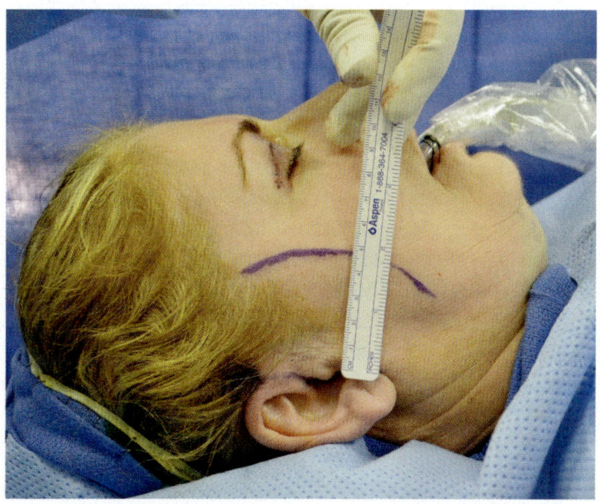

Fig. 15.6 Area of planned dissection, typically 5 cm.

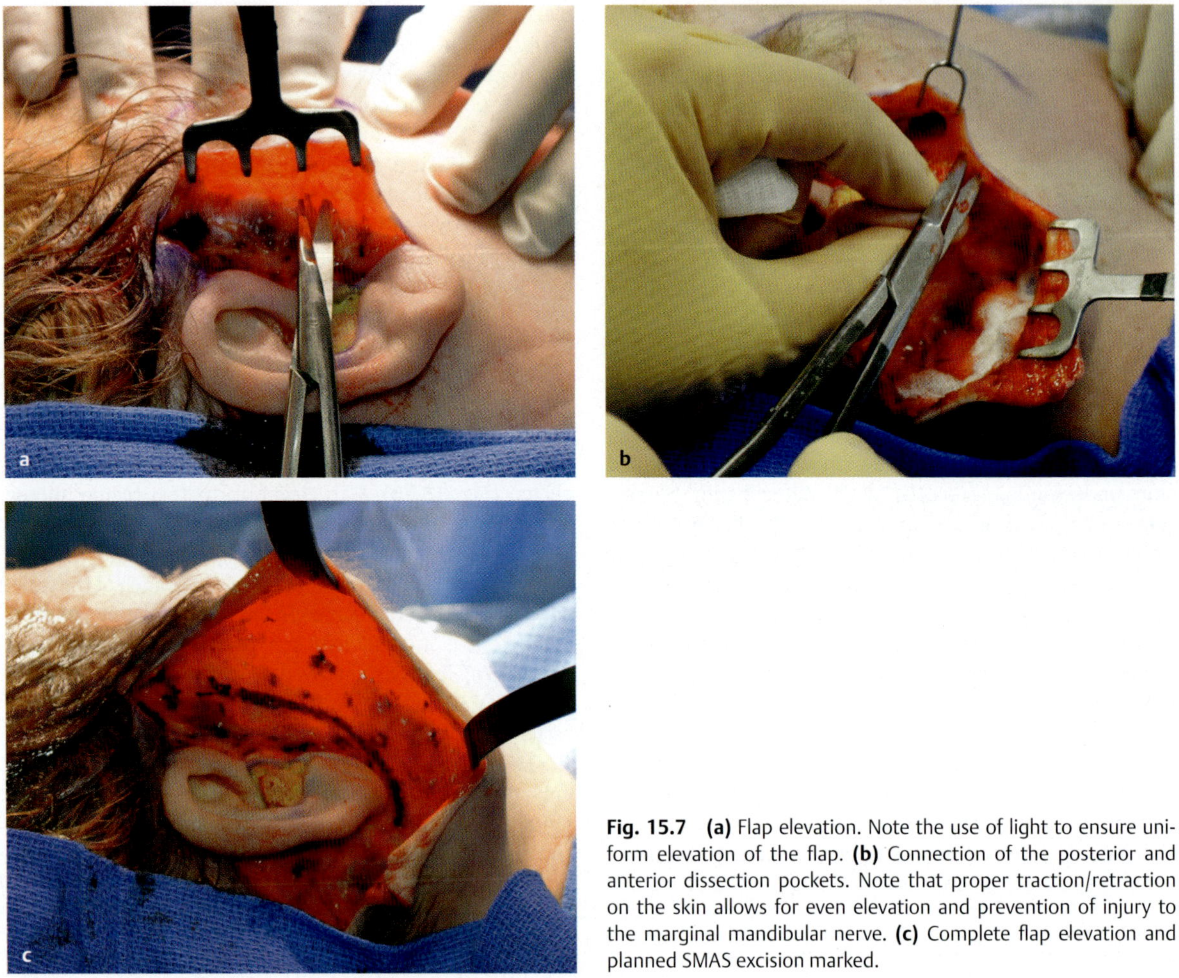

Fig. 15.7 **(a)** Flap elevation. Note the use of light to ensure uniform elevation of the flap. **(b)** Connection of the posterior and anterior dissection pockets. Note that proper traction/retraction on the skin allows for even elevation and prevention of injury to the marginal mandibular nerve. **(c)** Complete flap elevation and planned SMAS excision marked.

is well protected deep within the parotid gland. Sub-SMAS dissection can be performed if desired using this entry point **(Fig. 15.8b)**. The edges of the SMAS are then imbricated with multiple buried 3–0 PDS horizontal mattress sutures to suspend the soft tissue **(Fig. 15.8c)**. The upper portion of the SMAS is secured in a more vertical fashion by imbricating the tissue near the mandible to the tissue in front of the tragus. The lower SMAS/plastysma is secured in a more lateral vector by securing to the mastoid fascia. This vector of pull must be tailored to each patient, as it varies depending on the patient's age. Jacono and Ransom[45] recently described this concept. They found that younger patients required a more superior vector, whereas older patients needed a more lateral vector.

Any areas of SMAS fullness are oversewn using buried interrupted sutures. For individuals with cherubic faces and/or prominent parotid glands, gently cauterizing this region and also oversewing the SMAS can narrow the parotidomasseteric fascia just anterior to the auricle. This is a powerful technique that can further restore the triangle of youth.

Additional subcutaneous undermining is performed to release the tethering created after SMAS suspension. The wound is copiously irrigated and hemostasis is obtained one last time. A perforated 10-French Jackson-Pratt drain is placed in the wound and is immediately attached to suction drainage. The next step is skin redraping and excision to complete the rhytidectomy **(Fig. 15.9)**. The ideal redraping places minimal tension on the preauricular incision by distributing this tension posteriorly. This concept is critical to obtain a nearly invisible scar. There are multiple techniques for redraping and excising skin. We start by placing four key anchor points using 4–0 PDS buried sutures. We have found that a stepwise approach to skin redraping maximizes efficiency and reduces errors.

The first anchor point (AP1) is the helical root. A single-toothed forceps is used to calculate the excess skin to be excised, and a 15-blade scalpel is used to create a slit in the flap parallel to the orientation of the incision **(Fig. 15.10a)**. The incision is closed to the base of the slit with buried 4–0 PDS suture. A single-prong hook is then

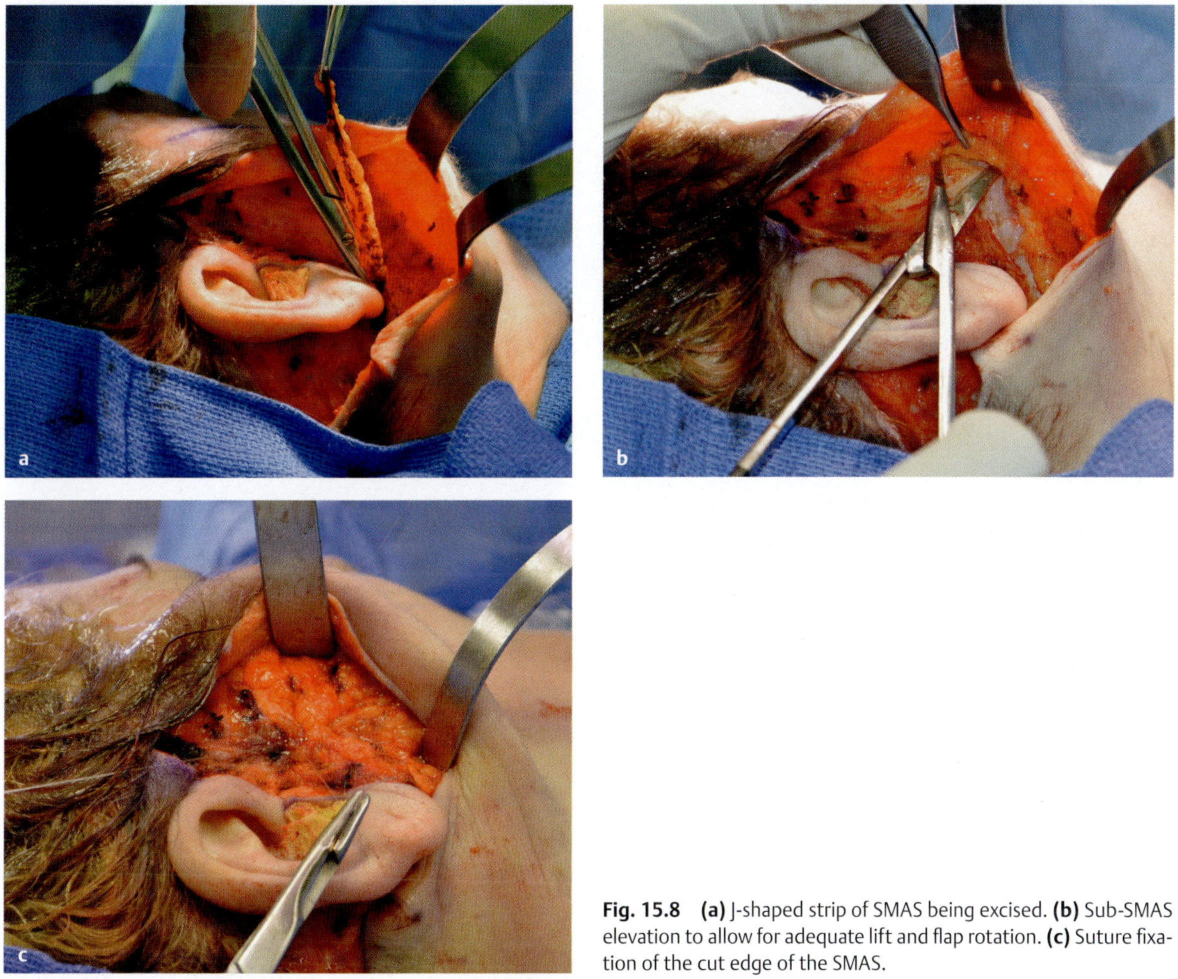

Fig. 15.8 **(a)** J-shaped strip of SMAS being excised. **(b)** Sub-SMAS elevation to allow for adequate lift and flap rotation. **(c)** Suture fixation of the cut edge of the SMAS.

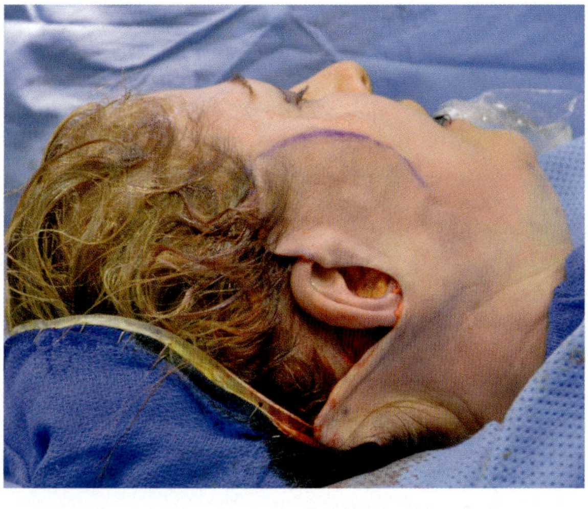

Fig. 15.9 Skin being redraped after SMAS suspension. Note the excess skin that now requires tailoring.

placed at the superior aspect of the temporal incision to elongate and straighten the wound. The excess skin superior to AP1 is excised using a gentle curve that allows for redraping without a significant dog-ear. The antitragus serves as the second anchor point (AP2), which is placed in a similar fashion to AP1 (**Fig. 15.10b**). Once AP2 has been placed, the intervening skin between AP1 and AP2 is excised. The skin is gently draped over the tragus in a manner that places no tension and then is marked along the planned excision. The skin is then stretched and excised along the marks. Because the new skin in this region is from a more anterior portion of the face, it must be defatted and thinned to create a natural contour. The third anchor point (AP3) is placed toward the apex of the postauricular region (**Fig. 15.10c**). It is critical to examine the neck contour to ensure that no significant redundancy was created in this region. Following this, a single hook is used to place traction at the lateral apex of the occipital incision, and the excess skin is excised in a similar manner to the temporal incision. Either a staple or

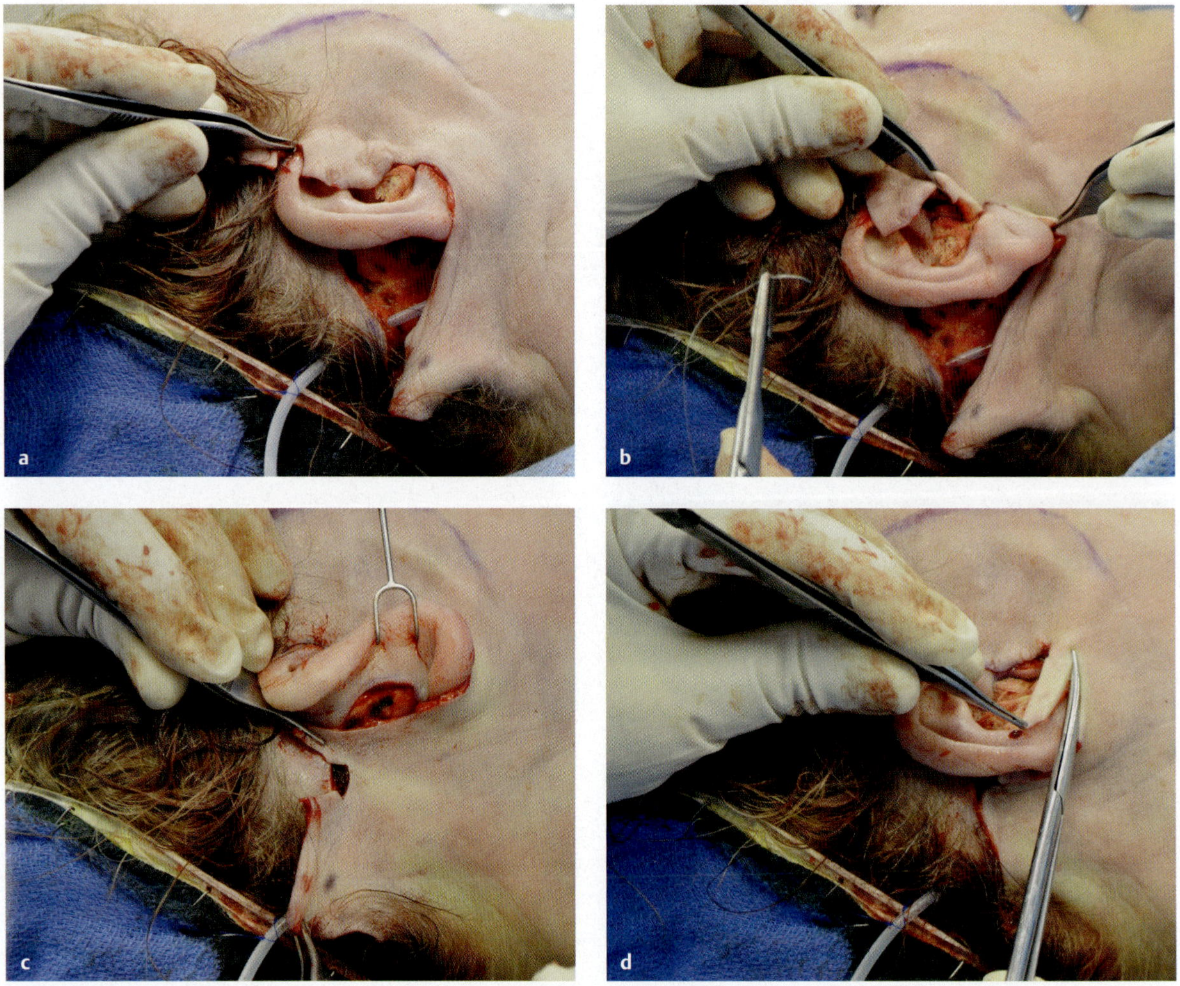

Fig. 15.10 **(a)** The first anchor point (AP1) at the root of the helix. **(b)** AP2 at the antitragus. **(c)** AP3 at the apex of the postauricular incisions. **(d)** Conservative excision of skin under the lobule to allow for proper ear position and prevention of the pixie ear deformity.

another deep suture is placed to perfectly align the occipital hairline and to avoid a step-off. The tissue between AP2 and AP3 is draped over the ear lobule to assess the amount of skin to excise. Facelift scissors are then used to carefully excise the postauricular excess skin, as the apex will become the anchor point of the lobule attachment (AP4). One must be careful to be very conservative in skin excision under the lobule **(Fig. 15.10d)**. If there is any tension in this location, a "pixie ear" deformity will result.

Skin excision is now complete and additional 4–0 PDS deep dermal sutures are placed as necessary. The preauricular incision is closed using a running locking 6–0 nylon or Prolene (Ethicon Inc.) suture between AP1 and AP4. A running 4–0 plain gut suture is used to close the skin in the postauricular region. Staples are used to close the hair-bearing areas to reduce the risk of alopecia **(Fig. 15.11)**. Ice is placed in a sterile glove and is applied on the first side while the facelift is performed on the second side. The cooling promotes vasoconstriction and limits perioperative ecchymosis.

As discussed earlier, volume restoration is a key component of facial rejuvenation and most patients at this point will undergo multilevel fat grafting, most commonly in the infraorbit, pyriform, buccal, and prejowl regions. At the conclusion of all the procedures, a light facial pressure dressing is applied and the patient is transported to the recovery room. **Fig. 15.12** shows a representative SFSR result in a Hispanic patient.

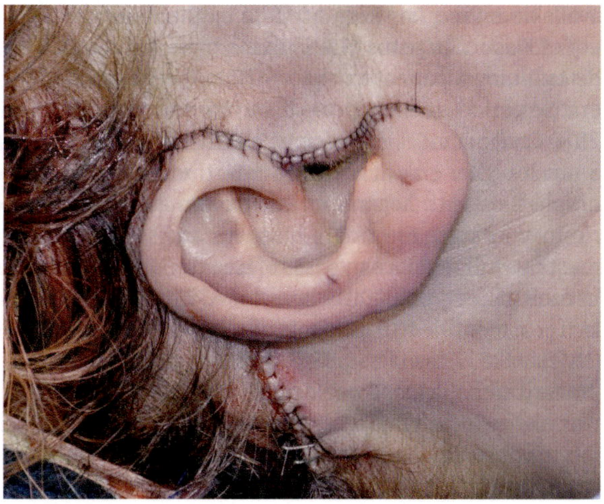

Fig. 15.11 Incisions after closure.

Deep-Plane Rhytidectomy

The first published description of the deep-plane rhytidectomy was in 1990 by Hamra, who developed the technique to achieve more effacement of the nasolabial fold than was possible with a SMAS facelift. In 1993, Hamra added the dissection of the orbicularis oculi to better address the nasojugal and palpebromalar grooves and termed the procedure a composite rhytidectomy. The rationale for the deep-plane and composite rhytidectomies was the belief that facial aging was due to descent of the platysma and orbicularis oculi muscles, as well as the "cheek fat." This concept and the terminology are now debated among aesthetic surgeons. Rohrich and Pessa have elegantly described in multiple studies the deep and superficial fat compartments in the midface,[7,46] and volume loss is now felt to be as important as tissue descent in causing the appearance of the nasolabial

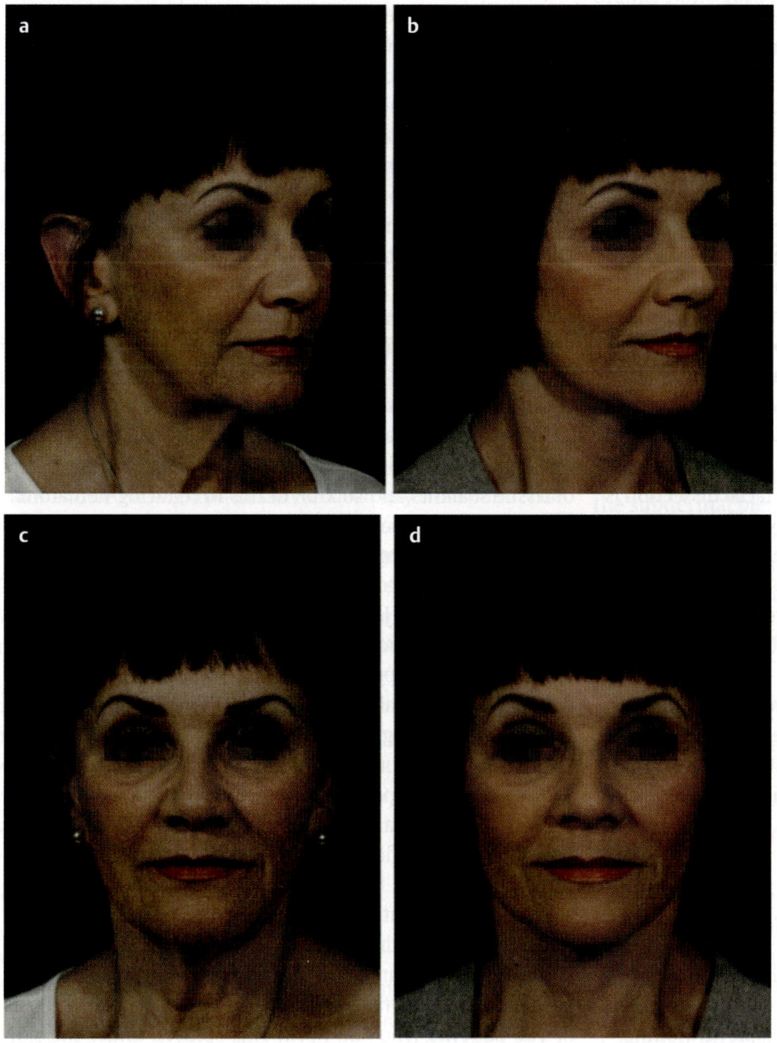

Fig. 15.12 **(a,b)** Oblique and **(c,d)** frontal views of a patient who underwent a rhytidectomy. Note the significant improvement in the jowls and platysmal banding.

Careful flap elevation under *direct visualization* is likely the best way to avoid injury to this nerve. If the nerve is transected, it should be repaired using 9–0 nylon suture under magnification, or with a nerve conduit to prevent neuromas.

The most feared complication of rhytidectomy is facial nerve injury. Theoretically, the facial nerve is at more risk during deep-plane and high SMAS and endoscopic subperiosteal facelifts, but no conclusive evidence of increased risk has been identified. This could be due to insufficient reporting of complications by some surgeons. Lidocaine can take up to 6 hours to wear off, and so a region of dense paresis should be observed initially. A dense paresis lasting longer than 24 hours can be due to either a stretch, cautery, or transection injury. The best treatment for a facial nerve transection involving the buccal and/or zygomatic branches is exploration and primary nerve repair. It is easier to find the injured nerve early on before significant scarring occurs. If a transection is judged to be unlikely, it is not unreasonable to observe the patient for 1 to 2 weeks for signs of recovery, but exploration should occur within 30 days if possible. Most studies suggest that open and honest communication of medical errors helps to prevent and to resolve malpractice claims.[65] If the facelift surgeon is uncomfortable performing facial nerve exploration, the patient should be referred to a facial nerve expert. Marginal and frontal branch injuries should probably just be observed, because the chance of meaningful reinnervation, even with successful exploration and repair, is low. Selective chemodenervation with injectable neurotoxins of the muscles on the contralateral face can create better facial symmetry.

15.7.4 Scars

Rhytidectomy incisions usually heal well in the absence of significant tension on the closure line. A tension-free closure is particularly important in dark-skinned individuals who are prone to hypertrophic scarring and keloid formation (**Fig. 15.13**). The portion of the incision between the auricle and occipital hairline is most at risk of this complication. Hypertrophic scarring typically responds to serial injections of triamcinolone, though this does carry some risk of skin atrophy and pigmentary changes in darker skin types. There is some recent evidence that 5-fluorouracil (5-FU) injections are similarly efficacious and have less risk of skin thinning and pigment change.[66,67] 5-FU is an antimetabolite that specifically targets synthetically active cells like fibroblasts, and it has been shown to specifically reduce type I collagen production in human fibroblasts.[68] We typically inject 0.1 to 0.5 mL of 5-FU in a 9:1 mixture with triamcinolone (10 mg/mL) every 2 to 4 weeks.

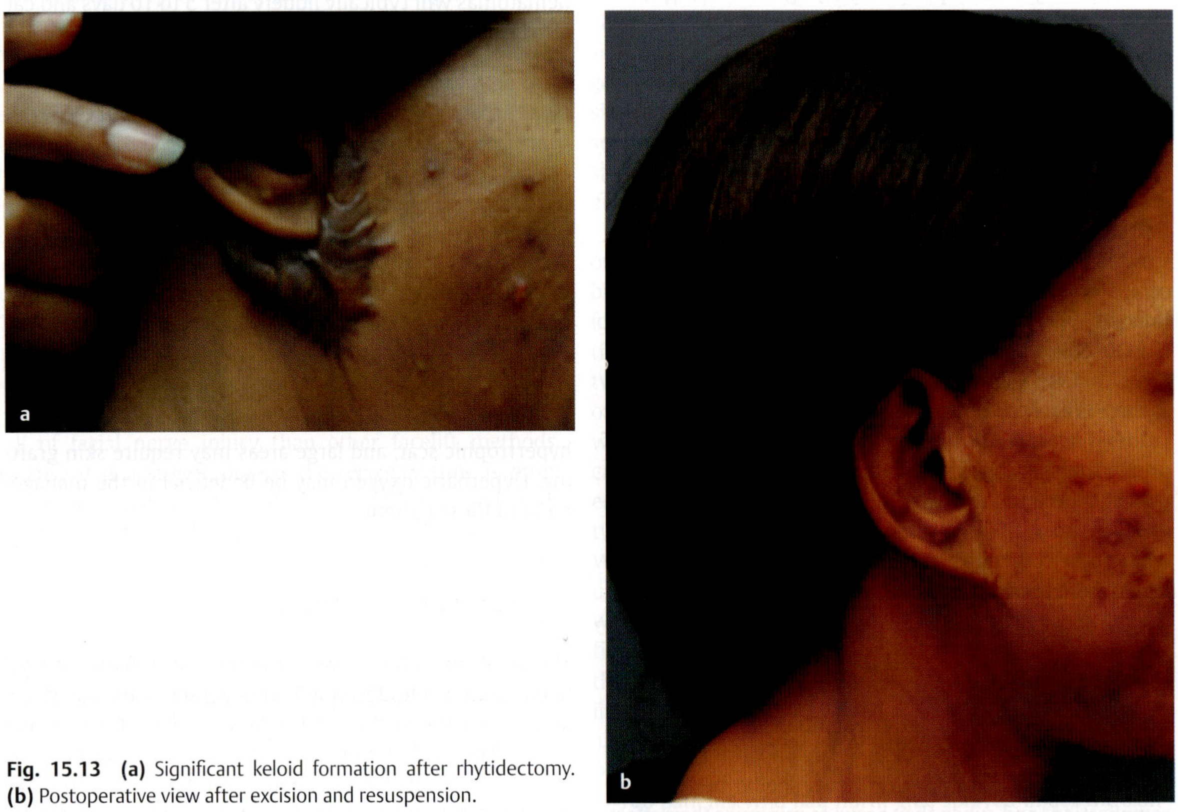

Fig. 15.13 **(a)** Significant keloid formation after rhytidectomy. **(b)** Postoperative view after excision and resuspension.

Tension on the skin closure around the ear lobule can cause a variety of deformities, including inferior displacement of the earlobe, obliteration of the sulcus between the auricle and face, or pixie ear deformity. These deformities can typically be repaired at 6 to 12 months after surgery with scar excision and a tension-free closure. A retracted or pixie ear lobule can be released with a V-Y superior advancement of the earlobe.

15.7.5 Hair Loss

Hair loss is most common in the sideburn and temple. Permanent hair loss can occur with poor surgical technique after transecting or cauterizing hair follicles. However, even dissection in the proper subfollicular plane can cause telogen effluvium, in which case the hair should return within 6 months. As discussed above, it is important to use a trichophytic incision inferior to the temporal tuft in women when planning significant skin excision to prevent excessive elevation of the preauricular hairline. Also, it is important to realign the occipital hairline after skin excision in the postauricular sulcus. In severe cases, micrograft hair transplantation is an option.

15.7.6 Parotid Injury

Sub-SMAS dissection risks injury to the parotid gland parenchyma and/or ductal system. This can result in a salivary accumulation beneath the superficial flap (sialocele), which may delay healing. If the parotid capsule is injured during facelifting, it should be repaired to prevent these complications. The SMAS can then be used to reinforce this area during SMAS suspension. If the injury is too large for primary closure, acellular dermis can be laid over the injury. Salivary pseudocysts should be treated with light pressure dressings and intermittent needle aspiration until resolution. Larger pseudocysts and fistulas through the skin may require closed suction dranage.[41]

15.7.7 Depression

Short-term depression occurs in up to 50% of women undergoing rhytidectomy.[69] This develops in the acute recovery period in response to the edema, bruising, and overall unnatural appearance. It typically resolves once the patient's appearance normalizes. In rare cases, a short course of antidepressant medication is necessary. For patients with a history of psychiatric illness currently on medication, the prescribing physician should be consulted prior to surgery. There is some association of selective serotonin reuptake inhibitors (SSRIs) with an increased risk of bleeding. However, a recent large retrospective analysis found no evidence that SSRI use increases the incidence of hematoma after rhytidectomy.[70]

15.8 Conclusion

Rhytidectomy continues to be one of the most powerful techniques for facial rejuvenation in our armamentarium. Most rhytidectomy techniques that employ SMAS suspension are very effective at improving the jawline and repositioning ptotic tissues. Rhytidectomy in dark-skinned individuals is similar to rhytidectomy in light-skinned individuals, with special attention paid to differences in skin color and thickness. In our practice, particularly in the African American population, complementary techniques, such as midface volume restoration, chin augmentation, and customized submentoplasty, have allowed more natural facial rejuvenation outcomes.

References

1. Uitto J. The role of elastin and collagen in cutaneous aging: intrinsic aging versus photoexposure. J Drugs Dermatol 2008;7(2, Suppl):s12–s16
2. Rohrich RJ, Pessa JE, Ristow B. The youthful cheek and the deep medial fat compartment. Plast Reconstr Surg 2008;121(6):2107–2112
3. Zadoo VP, Pessa JE. Biological arches and changes to the curvilinear form of the aging maxilla. Plast Reconstr Surg 2000;106(2):460–466, discussion 467–468
4. Pessa JE, Zadoo VP, Yuan C, et al. Concertina effect and facial aging: nonlinear aspects of youthfulness and skeletal remodeling, and why, perhaps, infants have jowls. Plast Reconstr Surg 1999;103(2):635–644
5. Pessa JE, Zadoo VP, Mutimer KL, et al. Relative maxillary retrusion as a natural consequence of aging: combining skeletal and soft-tissue changes into an integrated model of midfacial aging. Plast Reconstr Surg 1998;102(1):205–212
6. Pessa JE, Slice DE, Hanz KR, Broadbent TH Jr, Rohrich RJ. Aging and the shape of the mandible. Plast Reconstr Surg 2008;121(1):196–200
7. Gierloff M, Stöhring C, Buder T, Gassling V, Açil Y, Wiltfang J. Aging changes of the midfacial fat compartments: a computed tomographic study. Plast Reconstr Surg 2012;129(1):263–273
8. Shaw RB Jr, Katzel EB, Koltz PF, et al. Aging of the facial skeleton: aesthetic implications and rejuvenation strategies. Plast Reconstr Surg 2011;127(1):374–383
9. Richard MJ, Morris C, Deen BF, Gray L, Woodward JA. Analysis of the anatomic changes of the aging facial skeleton using computer-assisted tomography. Ophthal Plast Reconstr Surg 2009;25(5):382–386
10. Brissett AE, Naylor MC. The aging African-American face. Facial Plast Surg 2010;26(2):154–163
11. Munavalli GS, Weiss RA, Halder RM. Photoaging and nonablative photorejuvenation in ethnic skin. Dermatol Surg 2005;31(9 Pt 2):1250–1260, discussion 1261
12. Harris MO. The aging face in patients of color: minimally invasive surgical facial rejuvenation-a targeted approach. Dermatol Ther 2004;17(2):206–211

13. Cobo R, García CA. Aesthetic surgery for the Mestizo/Hispanic patient: special considerations. Facial Plast Surg 2010;26(2):164–173
14. Kligman LH, Kligman AM. The nature of photoaging: its prevention and repair. Photodermatol 1986;3(4):215–227
15. Pathak MA. The role of natural photoprotective agents in human skin. In: Fitzpatrick TB, Pathak MA, eds. Sunlight and Man. Tokyo, Japan: University of Tokyo Press; 1974
16. Taylor SC. Skin of color: biology, structure, function, and implications for dermatologic disease. J Am Acad Dermatol 2002; 46(2, Suppl):S41–S62
17. Fu JM, Price VH. Approach to hair loss in women of color. Semin Cutan Med Surg 2009;28(2):109–114
18. Brissett AE, Zevallos JP. Rejuvenation of the aging African face. In: Trustwell WH, ed. Surgical Facial Rejuvenation; A Road Map to Safe and Reliable Outcomes. New York, NY: Thieme Medical Publishers; 2009:146–152
19. Hollander E. Cosmetic surgery. In: Joseph M, ed. Hanbuch der Kosmetik. Leipzig, Germany: Veriag vot Velt; 1912
20. Aufricht G. Surgery for Excessive Skin of the Face. Transactions of the Second International Congress of Plastic Surgery. Edinburgh: Livingstone; 1960:495
21. Webster RC, Smith RC, Papsidero MJ, Karolow WW, Smith KF. Comparison of SMAS plication with SMAS imbrication in face lifting. Laryngoscope 1982;92(8 Pt 1):901–912
22. Skoog T. Plastic Surgery: New Methods and Refinements, Philadelphia, PA: Saunders; 1974
23. Mitz V, Peyronie M. The superficial musculo-aponeurotic system (SMAS) in the parotid and cheek area. Plast Reconstr Surg 1976;58(1):80–88
24. Hamra ST. The deep-plane rhytidectomy. Plast Reconstr Surg 1990;86(1):53–61, discussion 62–63
25. Hamra ST. Composite rhytidectomy. Plast Reconstr Surg 1992;90(1):1–13
26. Owsley JQ. Lifting the malar fat pad for correction of prominent nasolabial folds. Plast Reconstr Surg 1993; 91(3):463–474, discussion 475–476
27. Owsley JQ, Fiala TG. Update: lifting the malar fat pad for correction of prominent nasolabial folds. Plast Reconstr Surg 1997;100(3):715–722
28. Tessier P. Le lifting facial sous-périosté. Ann Chir Plast Esthet 1989;34(3):193–197
29. Ramirez OM, Maillard GF, Musolas A. The extended subperiosteal face lift: a definitive soft-tissue remodeling for facial rejuvenation. Plast Reconstr Surg 1991;88(2):227–236, discussion 237–238
30. Saylan Z. The S-lift for facial rejuvenation. Int J Cosmet Surg 1999;7:18–23
31. Baker DC. Minimal incision rhytidectomy (short scar face lift) with lateral SMASectomy. Aesthet Surg J 2001; 21(1):68–79
32. Tonnard P, Verpaele A, Monstrey S, et al. Minimal access cranial suspension lift: a modified S-lift. Plast Reconstr Surg 2002;109(6):2074–2086
33. Tzafetta K, Terzis JK. Essays on the facial nerve: Part I. Microanatomy. Plast Reconstr Surg 2010;125(3):879–889
34. Gosain AK, Sewall SR, Yousif NJ. The temporal branch of the facial nerve: how reliably can we predict its path? Plast Reconstr Surg 1997;99(5):1224–1233, discussion 1234–1236
35. Trussler AP, Stephan P, Hatef D, Schaverien M, Meade R, Barton FE. The frontal branch of the facial nerve across the zygomatic arch: anatomical relevance of the high-SMAS technique. Plast Reconstr Surg 2010;125(4):1221–1229
36. Janfaza P, Cheney ML. Superficial structures of the face, head and parotid region. In Janfaza P, Nadol JB, Galla R, Fabian RL, Montgomery WW, eds. Surgical Anatomy of the Head and Neck. Cambridge, MA: Harvard University Press; 2011
37. Rees TD, Liverett DM, Guy CL. The effect of cigarette smoking on skin-flap survival in the face lift patient. Plast Reconstr Surg 1984;73(6):911–915
38. Grover R, Jones BM, Waterhouse N. The prevention of haematoma following rhytidectomy: a review of 1078 consecutive facelifts. Br J Plast Surg 2001;54(6):481–486
39. Parikh SS, Jacono AA. Deep-plane face-lift as an alternative in the smoking patient. Arch Facial Plast Surg 2011;13(4):283–285
40. Ellenbogen R, Karlin JV. Visual criteria for success in restoring the youthful neck. Plast Reconstr Surg 1980;66(6):826–837
41. Feldman JJ. Corset platysmaplasty. Plast Reconstr Surg 1990;85(3):333–343
42. Guyuron B, Sadek EY, Ahmadian R. A 26-year experience with vest-over-pants technique platysmarrhaphy. Plast Reconstr Surg 2010;126(3):1027–1034
43. Mendelson BC, Muzaffar AR, Adams WP Jr. Surgical anatomy of the midcheek and malar mounds. Plast Reconstr Surg 2002;110(3):885–896, discussion 897–911
44. Muzaffar AR, Mendelson BC, Adams WP Jr. Surgical anatomy of the ligamentous attachments of the lower lid and lateral canthus. Plast Reconstr Surg 2002;110(3):873–884, discussion 897–911
45. Jacono AA, Ransom ER. Patient-specific rhytidectomy: finding the angle of maximal rejuvenation. Aesthet Surg J 2012;32(7):804–813
46. Rohrich RJ, Pessa JE. The retaining system of the face: histologic evaluation of the septal boundaries of the subcutaneous fat compartments. Plast Reconstr Surg 2008; 121(5):1804–1809
47. Lambros V. Observations on periorbital and midface aging. Plast Reconstr Surg 2007;120(5):1367–1376, discussion 1377
48. Hamra ST. A study of the long-term effect of malar fat repositioning in face lift surgery: short-term success but long-term failure. Plast Reconstr Surg 2002;110(3):940–951, discussion 952–959
49. Kamer FM, Frankel AS. SMAS rhytidectomy versus deep plane rhytidectomy: an objective comparison. Plast Reconstr Surg 1998;102(3):878–881
50. Becker FF, Bassichis BA. Deep-plane face-lift vs superficial musculoaponeurotic system plication face-lift: a comparative study. Arch Facial Plast Surg 2004;6(1):8–13

51. Litner JA, Adamson PA. Limited vs extended face-lift techniques: objective analysis of intraoperative results. Arch Facial Plast Surg 2006;8(3):186–190

52. Caprini JA. Thrombosis risk assessment as a guide to quality patient care. Dis Mon 2005;51(2-3):70–78

53. Pannucci CJ, Barta RJ, Portschy PR, et al. Assessment of postoperative venous thromboembolism risk in plastic surgery patients using the 2005 and 2010 Caprini risk score. Plast Reconstr Surg 2012;130(2):343–353

54. Reinisch JF, Bresnick SD, Walker JWT, Rosso RF. Deep venous thrombosis and pulmonary embolus after face lift: a study of incidence and prophylaxis. Plast Reconstr Surg 2001;107(6):1570–1575, discussion 1576–1577

55. Durnig P, Jungwirth W. Low-molecular-weight heparin and postoperative bleeding in rhytidectomy. Plast Reconstr Surg 2006;118(2):502–507, discussion 508–509

56. Jones BM, Grover R, Hamilton S. The efficacy of surgical drainage in cervicofacial rhytidectomy: a prospective, randomized, controlled trial. Plast Reconstr Surg 2007;120(1):263–270

57. Kamer FM, Nguyen DB. Experience with fibrin glue in rhytidectomy. Plast Reconstr Surg 2007;120(4): 1045–1051, discussion 1052

58. Zoumalan R, Rizk SS. Hematoma rates in drainless deep-plane face-lift surgery with and without the use of fibrin glue. Arch Facial Plast Surg 2008;10(2):103–107

59. Powell DM, Chang E, Farrior EH. Recovery from deep-plane rhytidectomy following unilateral wound treatment with autologous platelet gel: a pilot study. Arch Facial Plast Surg 2001;3(4):245–250

60. Farrior E, Ladner K. A retrospective review of the use of autologous platelet gels for rhytidectomy. Arch Facial Plast Surg 2012;14(2):83–84

61. Seeley BM, Denton AB, Ahn MS, Maas CS. Effect of homeopathic *Arnica montana* on bruising in face-lifts: results of a randomized, double-blind, placebo-controlled clinical trial. Arch Facial Plast Surg 2006;8(1):54–59

62. Pitanguy I, Machado BHB. Facial rejuvenation surgery: a retrospective study of 8788 cases. Aesthet Surg J 2012;32(4):393–412

63. Warren RJ, Aston SJ, Mendelson BC. Face lift. Plast Reconstr Surg 2011;128(6):747e–764e

64. Baker SR. Rhytidectomy. In: Cummings CW, Flint PW, Haughey BH, Robbins KT, Thomas JR, Harker LA, Richardson MA, Schuller DE, eds. Otolaryngology Head and Neck Surgery. Philadelphia, PA: Elsevier Mosby; 2005

65. Robbennolt JK. Apologies and legal settlement: an empirical examination. Mich Law Rev 2003;102:460–516

66. Fitzpatrick RE. Treatment of inflamed hypertrophic scars using intralesional 5-FU. Dermatol Surg 1999;25(3): 224–232

67. Manuskiatti W, Fitzpatrick RE. Treatment response of keloidal and hypertrophic sternotomy scars: comparison among intralesional corticosteroid, 5-fluorouracil, and 585-nm flashlamp-pumped pulsed-dye laser treatments. Arch Dermatol 2002;138(9):1149–1155

68. Bulstrode NW, Mudera V, McGrouther DA, Grobbelaar AO, Cambrey AD. 5-Fluorouracil selectively inhibits collagen synthesis. Plast Reconstr Surg 2005;116(1):209–221, discussion 222–223

69. Goin MK, Burgoyne RW, Goin JM, Staples FR. A prospective psychological study of 50 female face-lift patients. Plast Reconstr Surg 1980;65(4):436–442

70. Harirchian S, Zoumalan RA, Rosenberg DB. Antidepressants and bleeding risk after face-lift surgery. Arch Facial Plast Surg 2012;14(4):248–252

16 Lip Remodeling Surgical Techniques

Melissa Hu and Fred J. Stucker

16.1 Introduction

Cosmetic procedures for the lips largely focus on augmentation with fillers and autogenous materials. Perhaps the media and movies have directly influenced the concept that the ideal lip is fuller, more youthful, and sensual. It has also been suggested that the gradual internationalization of our society has influenced our cultural standards of ideal beauty. For Caucasian women, a more ethnic, fuller lip is now more desirable. However, for the ethnic female, a less protrusive, thinner lip may be more desirable. Whatever cultural preference the individual patient brings to the clinic, it is important that the surgeon not only understand cultural differences, but also master the surgical techniques that can assist our patients in achieving their desired cosmetic ideal.

16.2 Lip Anatomy

The lip serves important functional and aesthetic purposes. The sphincter formed by the orbicularis oris muscle is essential in maintaining oral competence to prevent the spillage and extrusion of food while eating. In speech, certain phonetic sounds require the approximation and tension formation of the lips. The lips not only play a vital role in verbal communication, but also communicate our emotions. When stretched in a smile, the lips connote happiness, pleasure, and contentedness. Frowning suggests anger, displeasure, and disgust, while tightened lips convey anxiety, stress, and uncertainty. The appearance of the lips may also suggest one's age, or even gender. Perioral wrinkles and the thinning of the red lip are signs associated with aging. A full, supple lip is often considered more feminine, while a thin, firmer lip may be considered more masculine.

The lip is a component of the lower face. It extends from the subnasale to the mental crease. The upper lip spans from the subnasale to the stomion superius, and horizontally between the nasolabial folds. The lower lip extends from stomion inferiorus to the mental crease, and lies between the oral commissures. Particular features of the upper lip consist of the philtrum, cupid's bow, and median tubercle. The philtral columns are paramedian, vertical prominences where orbicularis oris muscle fibers insert into skin after decussating in the depressed midline region of the upper lip.[1] The cupid's bow lies along the vermilion border or cutaneous-mucosal junction of the upper lip, at the base of the philtral columns. It is shaped like an M, or an archer's bow, with two apices divided by a central, median depression. The shape and definition of the cupid's bow often define an attractive lip. The median tubercle is a slight projection of the red lip that lies centrally, in line with, and inferior to, the philtrum. The absence of this tubercle is abnormal and may suggest lip pathology, such as cleft lip or a previously operated-on lip, for either reconstructive or cosmetic purposes.

The surface of the lip is composed of three histologically distinct regions: cutaneous, vermilion, and mucosal. The cutaneous region is composed of skin similar to the face. Here, there are hair follicles, eccrine glands, and sebaceous glands. This region ages similarly to the rest of the face, with development of rhytids along relaxed skin tension lines that radiate outward from the stomion from overuse of the orbicularis oris. The "white roll" consists of a pale line on the surface of the lip that marks the transition from the highly keratinized cutaneous skin to the thinner, less keratinized vermilion. The epithelium of the vermilion lacks hair follicles and apocrine sweat glands. The red color of the vermilion is due to the thin, transparent nature of the epithelium, and the superficial course of blood vessels in this region. The "red line" then marks the transition from the dry vermilion to the wet, intraoral lip mucosa. The mucosa consists of nonkeratinized squamous epithelium and multiple minor salivary glands in the submucosa.

The cross-sectional anatomy of the lip consists of epidermis, dermis, subcutaneous fat, orbicularis oris muscle, submucosa, and mucosa. The bulk of the lip is provided by the orbicularis oris. The orbicularis oris is composed of two divisions, superficial and deep. The superficial portion receives attachments from perioral muscles that contribute to fine movement of the lips. It consists of vertically and obliquely oriented fibers that curl outward at the free margin to form a slight protrusion of the lip.[2] The deep fibers of the orbicularis oris are oriented horizontally and provide the sphincteric action of the lips.

Sensory innervation of the upper and lower lip is supplied by the infraorbital nerve and mental nerve, respectively. The infraorbital nerve exits the infraorbital foramen 4 to 7 mm below the inferior orbital rim along a vertical from the medial limbus. The mental nerve exits its foramen ~ 6 to 10 mm inferior to the second mandibular bicuspid. These nerves may be blocked for procedures performed under local anesthesia. Motor innervation of the lips is provided by the buccal and marginal mandibular branches of the facial nerve.

The vascular supply of the lips is provided by the superior and inferior labial arteries, which divide from the facial artery. The labial arteries course between he orbicularis oris and the mucosa along the free edge of the lip. Venous drainage typically runs with the arterial supply and has additional pathways through the ophthalmic vein and cavernous sinus.

16.3 Facial Profile/Proportions

Analysis and evaluation of the lip is performed in both frontal and profile views. On frontal view, the horizontal width may be assessed, with the commissures ideally lying between the pupils. The upper and lower lip heights are assessed by subdividing the lower face into thirds. The upper third extends from the subnasale to the stomion, while the lower two-thirds measure from the stomion to the menton.[3] Thus, the ratio of upper lip height to lower lip height should be ~ 1:2. Additionally, the lower lip vermilion is slightly greater than the upper lip vermilion.

On profile, there are a few methods that may be used to evaluate the ideal lip position. Using a reference line extending from the subnasale through the inferior vermilion border and pogonion, the upper lip should ideally lie 3.5 mm anterior to this line, while the lower lip should lie 2.2 mm anterior.[4] Similarly, a line may be drawn from the subnasale through the upper lip. The inferior lip should lie 2 mm posterior to this line with the chin just posterior to the lower lip. Another method uses a line drawn tangentially from the nasal tip to the pogonion. The upper lip should lie 4 mm posterior and the lower lip 2 mm posterior to this line.

16.4 Differential Diagnosis

Macrocheilia, a larger than normal lip, has several etiologies, congenital and acquired. Congenital causes include ethnic variations of the lip, double lip, and labial pits. Acquired causes include inflammatory processes, such as cheilitis granulomatosa and angioedema; systemic disorders, such as Crohn disease; neoplasms, such as non-Hodgkin lymphoma and benign and malignant tumors; and infections, including tuberculosis and syphilis. Reduction cheiloplasty in a pediatric patient with congenital macrocheilia may have a profoundly positive psychological benefit (**Fig. 16.1**).

Double lip is a congenital anomaly caused by hyperplasia of the labial mucosa and accessory salivary glands. Due to redundant tissues, a fold develops within the red lip, thus creating the appearance of a second lip, which is particularly apparent with smiling. This occurs either in isolation or with

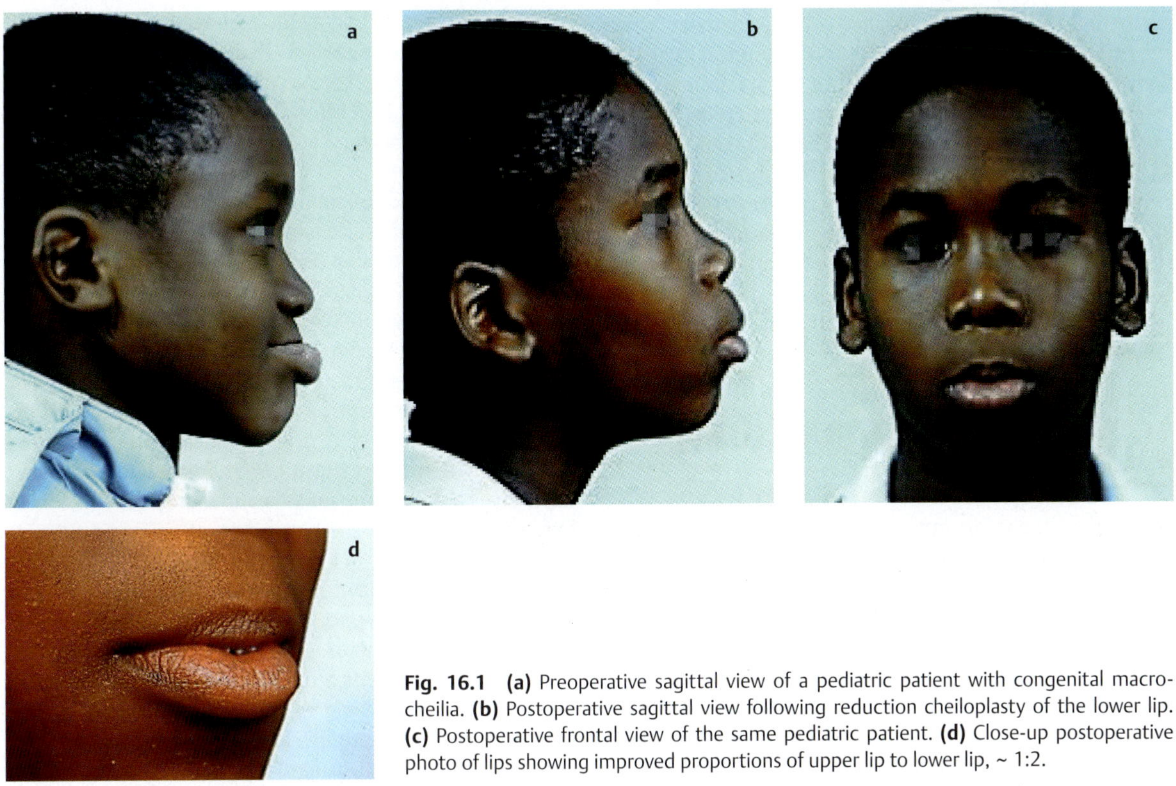

Fig. 16.1 **(a)** Preoperative sagittal view of a pediatric patient with congenital macrocheilia. **(b)** Postoperative sagittal view following reduction cheiloplasty of the lower lip. **(c)** Postoperative frontal view of the same pediatric patient. **(d)** Close-up postoperative photo of lips showing improved proportions of upper lip to lower lip, ~ 1:2.

other features, as seen in Ascher syndrome. Ascher syndrome is characterized by a double upper lip, blepharochalasis, and a nontoxic thyroid goiter.[5] Occasionally, double lip interferes with speech, mastication, and the ability to wear dentures.[6] Surgical management is considered for these cases but is more often performed for cosmetic reasons.

Labial pits are a congenital defect, often inherited in an autosomal dominant fashion, and are commonly associated with van der Woude syndrome. This syndrome presents variably with other traits, including cleft lip, cleft palate, and absent teeth. Labial pits usually present medially, on the vermilion portion of the lower lip. However, their presentation can be highly variable. They can occur singly or doubly and along the inner lip, outer lip, or margin between the inner and outer lip. Occasionally, a small mound of raised tissue is seen in place of a pit, as in the microform type.[7]

Cheilitis granulomatosa is an idiopathic, persistent swelling of the lip that is characterized histologically by a non-caseating granulomatous inflammation. It can occur in isolation or with other traits, as seen in Melkersson-Rosenthal syndrome, which also includes facial palsy and a plicated tongue.[8] Management includes dietary modifications, antibiotics, and systemic or intralesional corticosteroids for milder forms. Reduction cheiloplasty is performed when the swelling becomes cosmetically deforming and functionally debilitating.[9,10]

Pseudomacrocheilia has been used to describe the effect that underlying dento-alveolar abnormalities have on projecting lips, giving the appearance of abnormally enlarged and protuberant lips.[11] Thus, prior to any surgical intervention of macrocheilia, it is important to rule out other causes that may have other methods of management (**Fig. 16.2**).

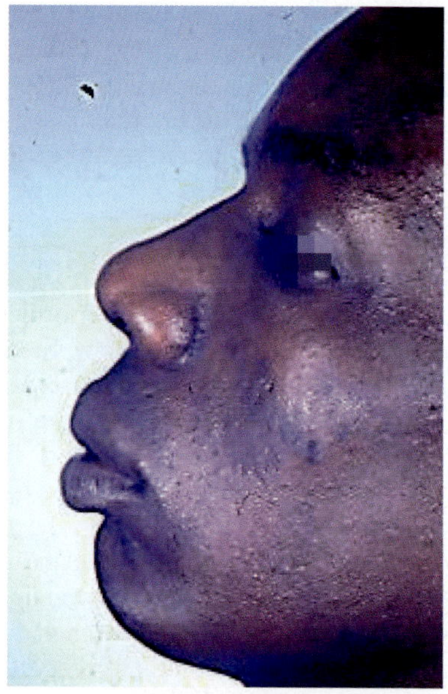

Fig. 16.2 Pseudomacrocheilia due to maxillary dento-alveolar abnormality and the subsequent appearance of enlarged, overly protrusive lips.

Lastly, macrostomia should not be mistaken for macrocheilia. The former may occur with branchial arch syndromes or in isolation. Macrostomia involves an expanded mouth and abnormal commissures displaced inferolaterally. Associated problems may include drooling, chronic skin irritation, and poor cosmesis, suggesting premature aging or neurological disorders. Repair of macrostomia typically involves reconstruction of the commissures (**Fig. 16.3**).

16.5 Characteristics of the Ethnic Lip

In general, ethnic lips appear larger than Caucasian lips. The ethnic lip has been described as diffusely enlarged, with thickening of the dermis, mucosa, submucosa, glands, and muscle.[12] More apparent is the contribution of redundant mucosa and hyperplastic minor salivary glands, which can measure between 2 and 4 mm.[13,14]

Recent studies have begun to quantify and describe the differences between ethnic lips and Caucasian lips. Farkas et al measured vermilion heights in male and female African Americans and Caucasians. The African American male was found to have an average upper lip height of 13.3 mm and an average lower lip height of 13.2 mm. The African American female had an average upper lip height of 13.6 mm and lower lip height of 13.8 mm. Caucasian males were found to have average vermilion heights of 8.0 and 8.7 mm for upper and lower lips, respectively, while Caucasian females averaged heights for upper and lower lip of 9.3 and 9.4 mm, respectively.[15]

The ethnic lip is also more protrusive. Anthropomorphic features of the ethnic face may contribute to the significant appearance of protrusion (**Fig. 16.2**). Sutter et al found that African Americans had greater midfacial height, which may enhance the perception of lip prominence.[16] Similarly, Chinese adults were found to have shorter midfaces and more convex facial profiles than Caucasians, which may further enhance their more protrusive upper and lower lips.[17] Cotton et al also found that African Americans often exhibited bimaxillary dental protrusion and larger anteroposterior differences between the maxilla and mandible, which may further contribute to the perception of upper lip fullness and protrusion.[18]

Several studies have shown that not only do the size and protrusion of lips vary among ethnicities, but aesthetic standards also vary across ethnic groups. Asians and Hispanic Americans prefer a more retrusive and thinner lip, while blacks prefer a more protrusive profile.[19,20,21,22] The preferred soft tissue profiles for African Americans do not fall within the normal values for whites. A more convex profile is preferred for African Americans.[23] Several studies

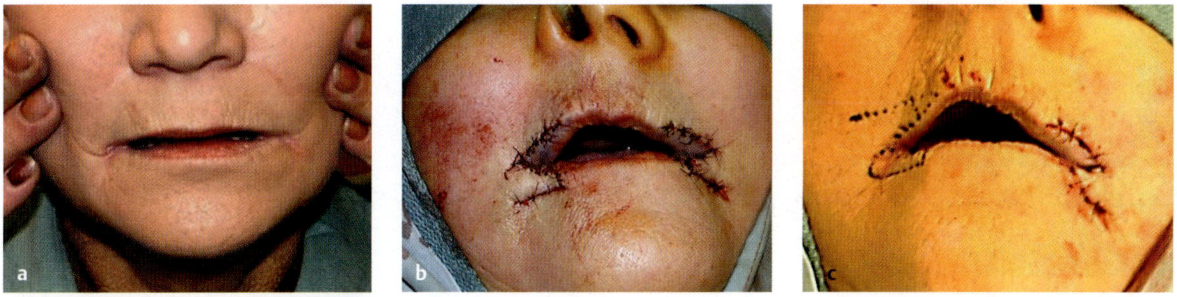

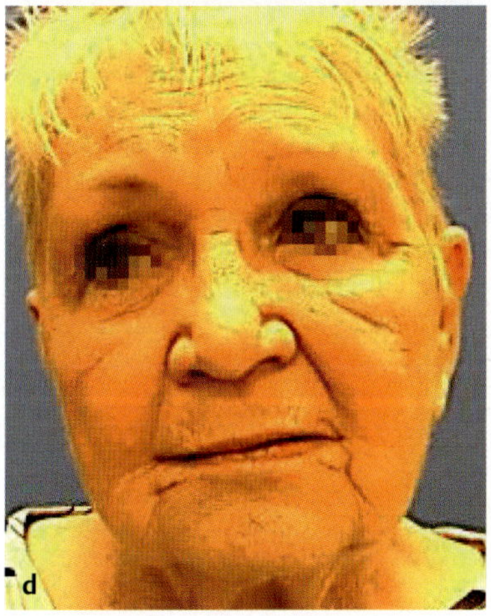

Fig. 16.3 **(a)** Preoperative photo of macrostomia. Patient has to elevate lateral commissures to prevent drooling. Chronic skin irritation from saliva is seen at the commissures. **(b)** Intraoperative view of macrostomia repair with Z-plasties. Left commissure is tighter and more elevated after Z-plasty. Right commissure shows the surgical markings for Z-plasty repair. **(c)** Intraoperative view of macrostomia repair with Z-plasties. **(d)** Postoperative photo of patient following commissure Z-plasties for repair of macrostomia. Drooling and skin irritation have been eliminated and patient has a more cosmetically pleasing appearance.

have attempted to describe the aesthetic standards of different ethnic groups.[15,24,25,26,27] Rather than trying to achieve a singly defined aesthetic ideal, the goals of aesthetic surgery have moved toward refining features based on patient preferences, the surgeon's aesthetic sense, and an ethnocentric balance for a more natural appearance.[22,28,29] Thus, to have a successful surgical outcome for lip reduction, not only should a thorough anatomic analysis of the lip be performed, but also detailed discussion of the individual's preference should occur.

16.6 Technique of Lip Reduction

Reduction cheiloplasty is a simple yet effective procedure. It involves the resection of mucous membrane and underlying minor salivary glands, followed by internal rotation and repositioning of the pouty lip. Due to intraoral contamination, reduction cheiloplasty should be reserved as the last procedure if it is done in sequence with other procedures, such as rhinoplasty and mentoplasty. Reduction cheiloplasty can easily be done under local anesthesia in the clinical setting.

The mucosa is marked along the wet line and carried slightly intraorally in the region of the commissure (**Fig. 16.4a**). The lip is then infiltrated with a minimum of 2 to 3 mL of 1% lidocaine with 1:100,000 epinephrine. Care should be taken not to inject in excess, which will balloon and distort the tissues. A 4 × 4 cm sponge is place in each buccal sulcus. The lip is then everted at the right and left commissure by placing a thumb and forefinger on opposite sides of the lip at the commissure and putting it under tension with lateral traction. At the junction of the wet line, a no. 15 blade is used to remove an ellipse of mucosa 1 to 2 cm wide, along with the underlying minor salivary glands (**Fig. 16.4b**). The entire resection must be internal to the wet line to camouflage the scar. If the muscularis is not violated, hemostasis is easily achieved with pressure (**Fig. 16.4c**). Electrocautery is avoided if possible, as postoperative edema and subsequent tissue trauma are directly related to thermal injury. Without undermining, the mucosa is reapproximated with a 4–0 silk suture (**Fig. 16.4d**). Silk suture is preferred because it lies flat when wet and is less detectable by the patient. When possible, a running suture is placed, because it better coapts mucosal vessels and markedly decreases any oozing.

The upper lip is more pouty and fuller, and the lower lip is usually less bulky but more greatly everted. The pattern of surgical excision must vary to take these differences into account. A bikini-shaped excision has been described to

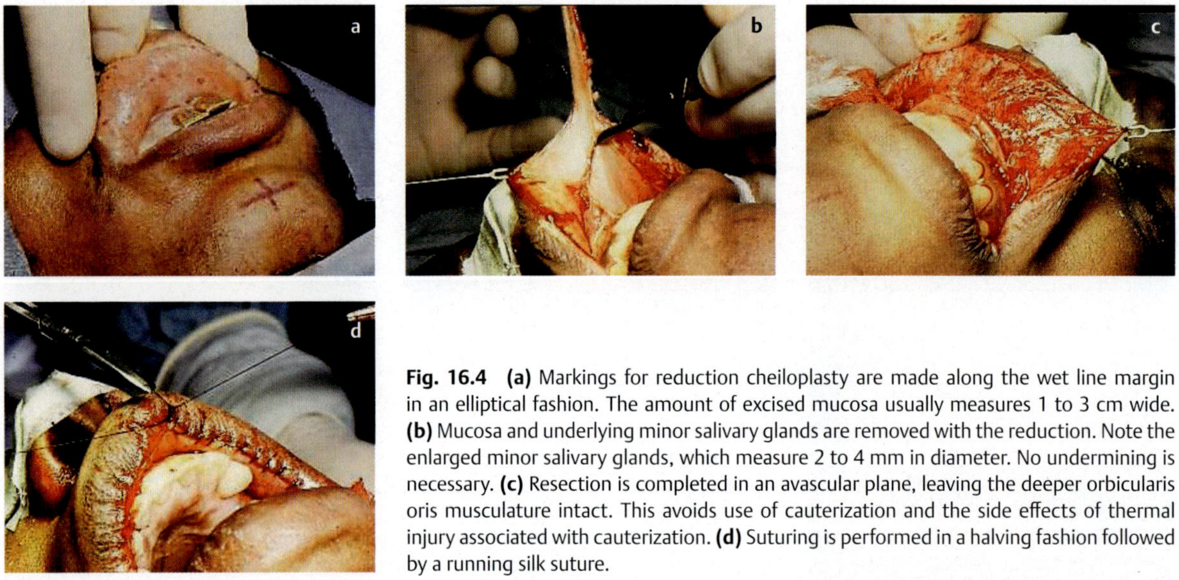

Fig. 16.4 **(a)** Markings for reduction cheiloplasty are made along the wet line margin in an elliptical fashion. The amount of excised mucosa usually measures 1 to 3 cm wide. **(b)** Mucosa and underlying minor salivary glands are removed with the reduction. Note the enlarged minor salivary glands, which measure 2 to 4 mm in diameter. No undermining is necessary. **(c)** Resection is completed in an avascular plane, leaving the deeper orbicularis oris musculature intact. This avoids use of cauterization and the side effects of thermal injury associated with cauterization. **(d)** Suturing is performed in a halving fashion followed by a running silk suture.

help preserve lip contour.[30] The excision may be interrupted at mid lip to maintain projection of the median tubercle.[12] A transverse W-plasty excision can be used to avoid dog ears and postoperative scar contracture.[31] This is usually not necessary if the halving technique is applied to close the upper and lower mucosal incisions. A vertically oriented wedge excision, typically performed for the grossly deformed lip with Melkersson-Rosenthal syndrome, may be considered to narrow the horizontal lip width.[32]

The patient is placed on a liquid to soft diet for 2 to 3 days and is instructed to keep oral activity to a minimum. Patients are also instructed to avoid acidic and salty food and drink for the first few postoperative days. Antibiotics are not usually prescribed for cheiloplasty but are employed if additional procedures are utilized. Some drooling and lip incompetency may be present postoperatively for up to 2 weeks. Application of iced saline sponges is routinely recommended to help decrease swelling. Sutures are removed on postoperative day 4 **(Fig. 16.5)**.

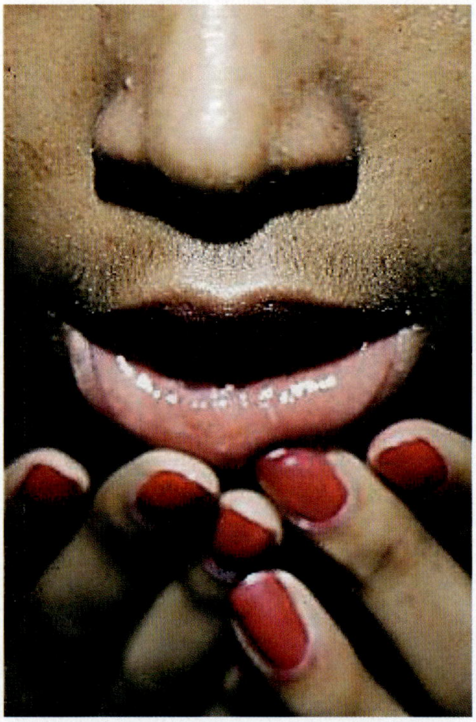

Fig. 16.5 Postoperative image of the incision after lower lip reduction cheiloplasty. The incision is barely perceptible.

16.7 Complications

Postoperative complications are rare. Hematoma may result from poor hemostasis and improperly closing dead space,[33] but hematoma is extremely unlikely if there has been no violation of the muscularis. Prolonged numbness may occur but is also very unlikely. Patients should be cautioned about smoking or eating hot foods until normal sensation returns. Granulation tissue formation occurs occasionally and can be treated with cauterization or injection of corticosteroids. Asymmetry, over-reduction, or under-reduction may result, particularly for the inexperienced surgeon.

16.8 Comment

Reduction cheiloplasty may offer a patient with ethnically full lips a more harmonious facial appearance. The procedure is simple and effective and is associated with few complications. Macrocheilia is often accompanied by other profile deformities, such as a depressed nasal dorsum or retracted chin. Reduction cheiloplasty can be conveniently performed as an adjunctive procedure alone or in conjunction with other cosmetic procedures, such as rhinoplasty and genioplasty, to achieve a more balanced profile (**Fig. 16.6** and **Fig. 16.7**). The technique described above may also be applied in other acquired or congenital disorders, such as chronic cheilitis (**Fig. 16.8**) or cleft lip/nasal deformity (**Fig. 16.9**). When applied in the appropriately selected patient, this simple technique can produce a cosmetically balanced, subtle, and natural-appearing lip.

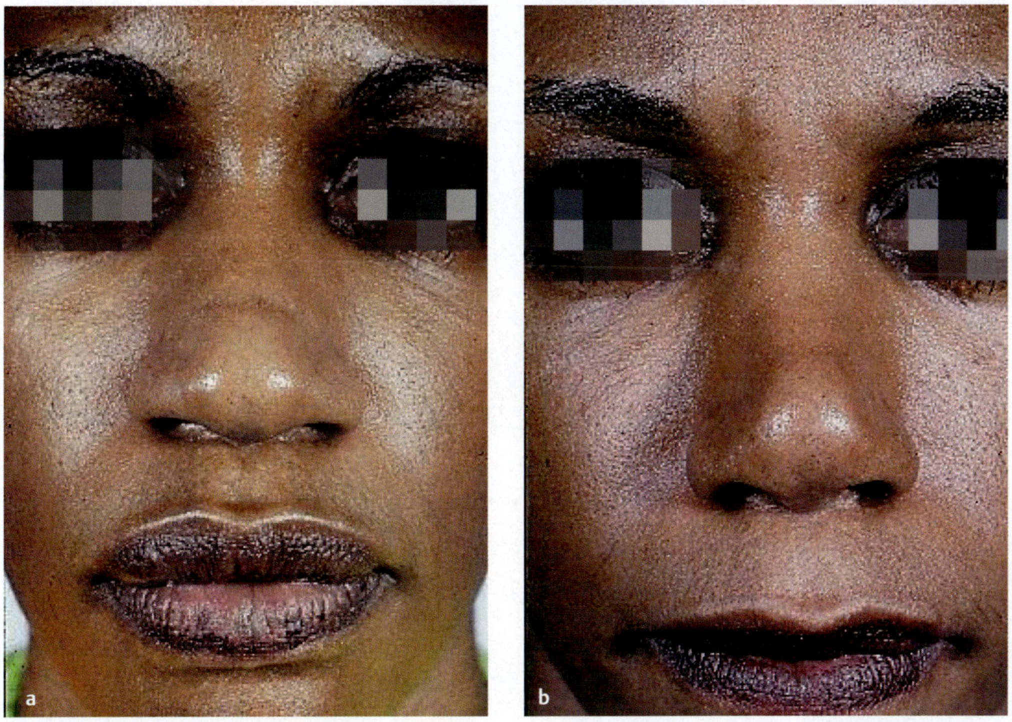

Fig. 16.6 **(a)** Preoperative frontal image of patient with ethnically enlarged lips and wide nose. **(b)** Postoperative image of the patient after rhinoplasty, alar base narrowing, and reduction cheiloplasty, which adjunctively restored harmony and femininity to her face.

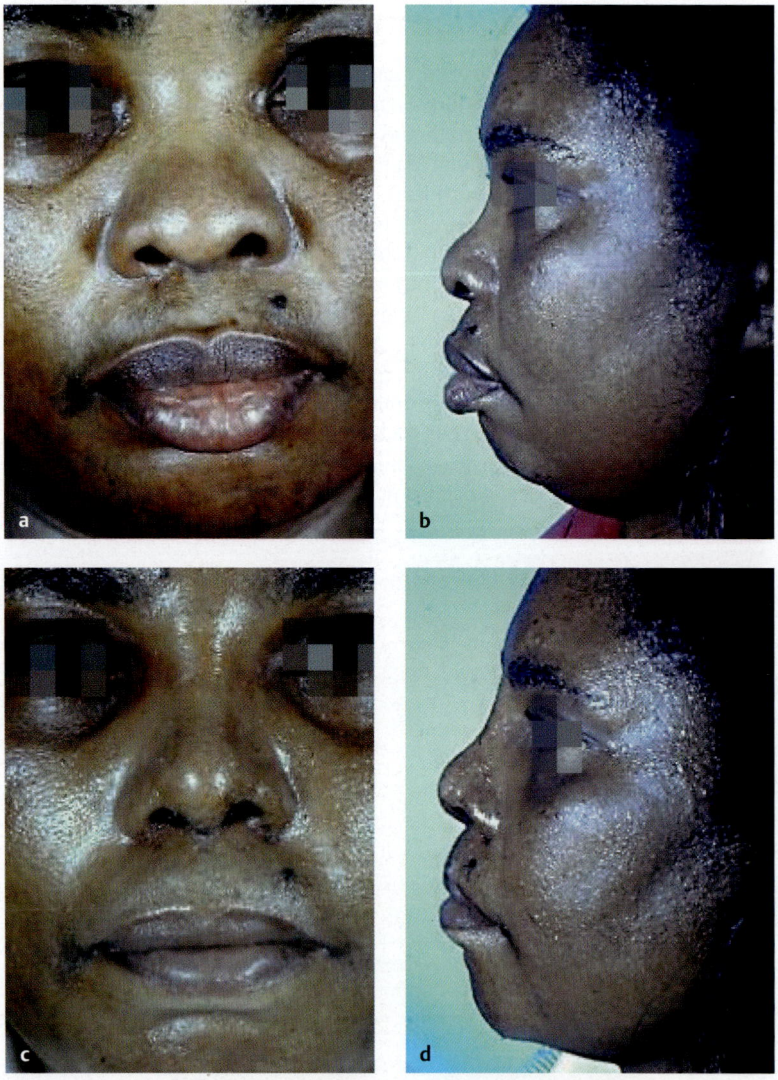

Fig. 16.7 **(a)** Preoperative photo of patient with ethnically enlarged lips and wide nose. **(b)** Preoperative sagittal view reveals a bulbous nasal tip, protrusive lips, and a retrusive chin. **(c)** Postoperative frontal view of patient after rhinoplasty, reduction cheiloplasty, and chin implant. **(d)** Postoperative sagittal view reveals a more balanced profile with less protrusive lips.

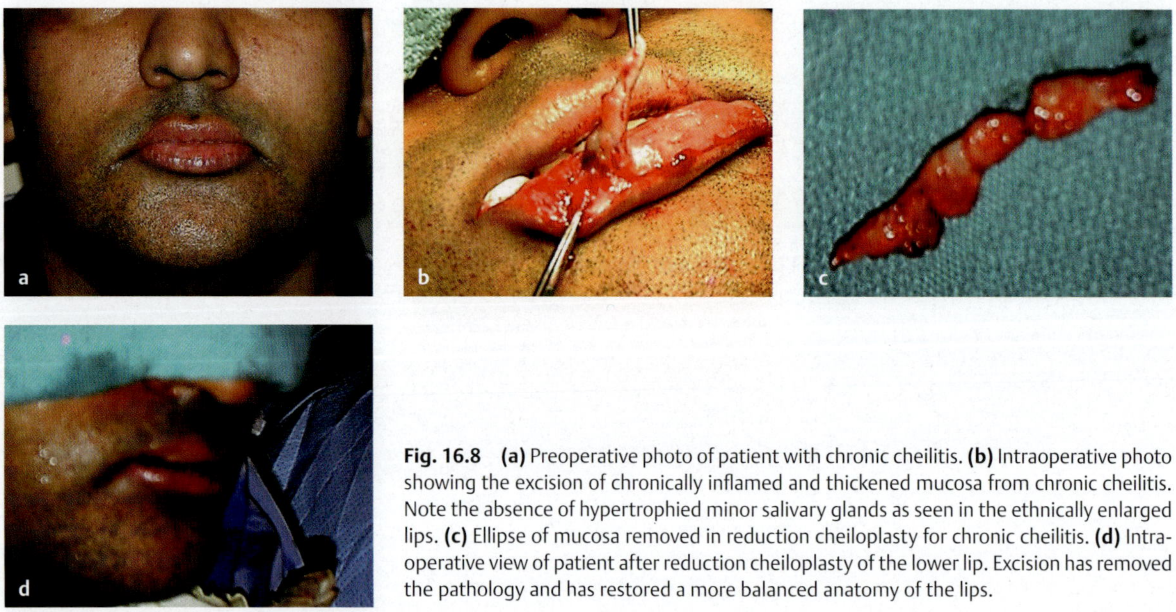

Fig. 16.8 **(a)** Preoperative photo of patient with chronic cheilitis. **(b)** Intraoperative photo showing the excision of chronically inflamed and thickened mucosa from chronic cheilitis. Note the absence of hypertrophied minor salivary glands as seen in the ethnically enlarged lips. **(c)** Ellipse of mucosa removed in reduction cheiloplasty for chronic cheilitis. **(d)** Intraoperative view of patient after reduction cheiloplasty of the lower lip. Excision has removed the pathology and has restored a more balanced anatomy of the lips.

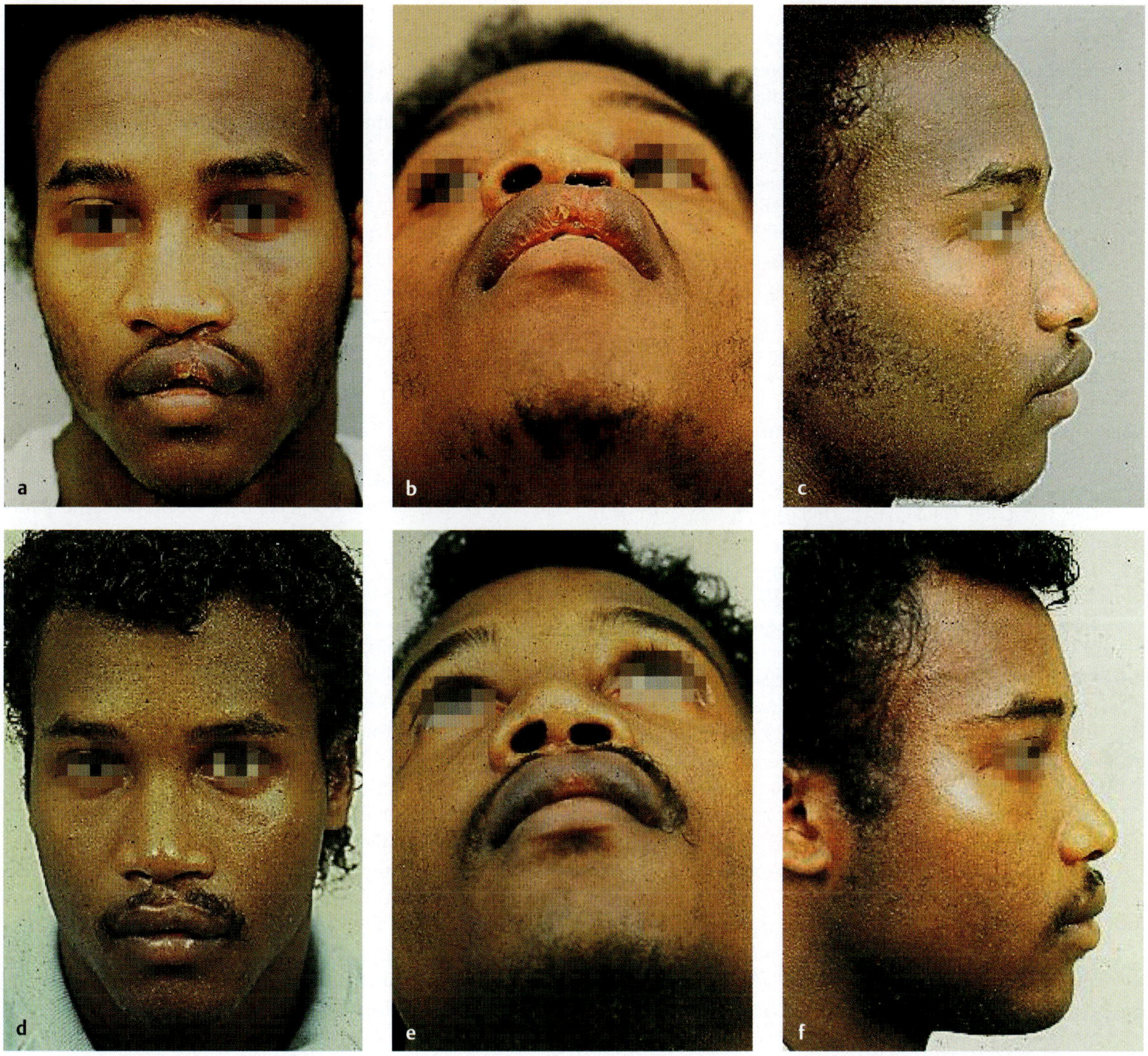

Fig. 16.9 (a) Preoperative frontal view of patient with unilateral cleft lip and nasal deformity following primary repair. **(b)** Base view of cleft lip and nasal deformity. The excessive width of the dry vermilion largely contributes to upper lip protrusion. **(c)** Preoperative profile of cleft lip and nasal deformity. Excessively protrusive upper lip creates the perception of chin retrusion. **(d)** Postoperative frontal view following upper lip reduction cheiloplasty and cleft nose rhinoplasty. **(e)** Postoperative base view shows significant de-projection of the upper lip. **(f)** Postoperative sagittal view reveals a more balanced profile and elimination of the appearance of a retruded chin.

References

1. Latham RA, Deaton TG. The structural basis of the philtrum and the contour of the vermilion border: a study of the musculature of the upper lip. J Anat 1976;121 (Pt 1):151–160
2. Alfen NV, Gilhuis HJ, Keijzers JP, Pillen S, Van Dijk JP. Quantitative facial muscle ultrasound: feasibility and reproducibility. Muscle Nerve 2013;48(3):375–380
3. Powell N, Humphries B. Proportions of the Aesthetic Face. New York, NY: Thieme-Stratton; 1984
4. Burstone CJ. Lip posture and its significance in treatment planning. Am J Orthod 1967;53(4):262–284
5. Ascher KW. Das syndrom blecharochalasis, struma, and doppellippe. Klin Wochenschr 1922;1:2287–2288
6. Palma MC, Taub DI. Recurrent double lip: literature review and report of a case. Oral Surg Oral Med Oral Pathol Oral Radiol Endod 2009;107(3):e20–e23
7. Souissi A, El Euch D, Mokni M, Badri T, Ben Osman Dhahri A. Congenital lower lip pits: a case report. Dermatol Online J 2004;10(2):10

8. Critchlow WA, Chang D. Cheilitis granulomatosa: a review. Head Neck Pathol 2014;8(2):209–213
9. Habel G, O'Regan B. Surgical management of macrocheilia of the lower lip. Br J Oral Maxillofac Surg 1990;28(5): 295–298
10. Kruse-Lösler B, Presser D, Metze D, Joos U. Surgical treatment of persistent macrocheilia in patients with Melkersson-Rosenthal syndrome and cheilitis granulomatosa. Arch Dermatol 2005;141(9):1085–1091
11. Epker BN, Wolford LM. Reduction cheiloplasty: its role in the correction of dentofacial deformities. J Maxillofac Surg 1977;5(2):134–141
12. Pitanguy I, Gonzalez R, Brentano J, Müller P, Moore T. Surgical treatment of macrocheilia. Head Neck Surg 1988;10(5):309–318
13. Stucker FJ Jr. Profile contouring including cheiloplasty. Arch Otolaryngol 1979;105(11):680–683
14. Stucker FJ Jr. Non-Caucasian rhinoplasty and adjunctive reduction cheiloplasty. Otolaryngol Clin North Am 1987;20(4):877–894
15. Farkas LG, Katic MJ, Forrest CR. Comparison of craniofacial measurements of young adult African-American and North American white males and females. Ann Plast Surg 2007;59(6):692–698
16. Sutter RE Jr, Turley PK. Soft tissue evaluation of contemporary Caucasian and African American female facial profiles. Angle Orthod 1998;68(6):487–496
17. Gu Y, McNamara JA Jr, Sigler LM, Baccetti T. Comparison of craniofacial characteristics of typical Chinese and Caucasian young adults. Eur J Orthod 2011;33(2):205–211
18. Cotton WN, Takano WS, Wong WM. The Downs analysis applied to three other ethnic groups. Angle Orthod 1951;21(4):213–220
19. Mejia-Maidl M, Evans CA, Viana G, Anderson NK, Giddon DB. Preferences for facial profiles between Mexican Americans and Caucasians. Angle Orthod 2005;75(6):953–958
20. Chong HT, Thea KW, Descallar J, et al. Comparison of White and Chinese perception of esthetic Chinese lip position. Angle Orthod 2014;84(2):246–253
21. Nomura M, Motegi E, Hatch JP, et al. Esthetic preferences of European American, Hispanic American, Japanese, and African judges for soft-tissue profiles. Am J Orthod Dentofacial Orthop 2009;135(4, Suppl):S87–S95
22. Wong WW, Davis DG, Camp MC, Gupta SC. Contribution of lip proportions to facial aesthetics in different ethnicities: a three-dimensional analysis. J Plast Reconstr Aesthet Surg 2010;63(12):2032–2039
23. Hall D, Taylor RW, Jacobson A, Sadowsky PL, Bartolucci A. The perception of optimal profile in African Americans versus white Americans as assessed by orthodontists and the lay public. Am J Orthod Dentofacial Orthop 2000;118(5):514–525
24. Farkas LG, Forrest CR, Litsas L. Revision of neoclassical facial canons in young adult Afro-Americans. Aesthetic Plast Surg 2000;24(3):179–184
25. Le TT, Farkas LG, Ngim RC, Levin LS, Forrest CR. Proportionality in Asian and North American Caucasian faces using neoclassical facial canons as criteria. Aesthetic Plast Surg 2002;26(1):64–69
26. Milgrim LM, Lawson W, Cohen AF. Anthropometric analysis of the female Latino nose. Revised aesthetic concepts and their surgical implications. Arch Otolaryngol Head Neck Surg 1996;122(10):1079–1086
27. Rhee SC, Kang SR, Park HS. Balanced angular profile analysis. Plast Reconstr Surg 2004;114(2):535–544
28. Porter JP, Lee JI. Facial analysis: maintaining ethnic balance. Facial Plast Surg Clin North Am 2002;10(4):343–349
29. Yellin SA. Aesthetics for the next millennium. Facial Plast Surg 1997;13(4):231–239
30. Fanous N, Brousseau VJ, Yoskovitch A. The "bikini" lip reduction: an approach to oversized lips. Plast Reconstr Surg 2008;122(1):23e–25e
31. Guerrero-Santos J, Altamirano JT. The use of W-plasty for the correction of double lip deformity. Plast Reconstr Surg 1967;39(5):478–481
32. Cederna PS, Smith DJ Jr, Newman MH; Fiala TGS. Melkersson-Rosenthal syndrome: reduction cheiloplasty utilizing a transmodiolar labial suspension suture. Aesthetic Plast Surg 1998;22(2):102–105
33. Pierce HE. Cheiloplasty for redundant lips. J Natl Med Assoc 1976;68(3):211–212

Section IV

The Asian Perspective

17 Aesthetic, Ethnic, and Cultural Considerations and Current Cosmetic Trends in the Asian Population

Gordon M. S. Soo, Choladhis Sinrachtanant, and Frederick T. C. Wong

17.1 Introduction

Asia is the world's largest continent, and includes the two most populous countries in the world and a vast trade-confederated region: China, India, and the southeast nations of ASEAN. In the discussion of ethnic Asian considerations in facial plastic surgery, one must keep in mind that Asian facial features vary considerably as one moves across the Asian continent from north to south as well as from east to west. Furthermore, with socioeconomic mobility and intermarriage over the centuries, Asia has become a melting pot of ethnicity and aesthetics. For the mixed Asian population, there still remain a few generalizations and rules that permit a discussion of the aesthetics of the Asian facial profile.

First, the Asian population includes essentially three different distinct ethnic types:

1. Asian-Oriental (Mongoloid)—from northern and southern China, Mongolia, Taiwan, the Korean Peninsula, and Japan
2. Asian-Malay—from Thailand, Vietnam, Myanmar, Indochina, the Philippines, the Malayan Peninsula, Borneo, and the Indonesian archipelago
3. Asian-Caucasian—from the Indian subcontinent, middle Asia, northern Asia to Russia, and western Asia toward Turkey

Naturally, these three facial types are now widely interspersed throughout the region as well as globally due to socioeconomic forces and migration over many centuries. For the purposes of this chapter, we concentrate on the more "politically correct" Asian-Oriental and Asian-Malay groups, as well as the current cultural preferences and cosmetic trends that form the common discussion of Asian facial aesthetics.

The chapter does not cover the parts of Asia where people have Western noses, which include the Middle Eastern regions, Russia to the north, and the Indian subcontinent to the south. These areas and the Middle Eastern nose are discussed elsewhere in this book; therefore, the Asian-Caucasian nose is not discussed in this chapter.

17.2 Asian Differences with the West

The Asian face can be very broadly categorized into two different facial groups: the Asian-Oriental (Mongoloid) features of the north, as seen among ethnicities from southern China to Japan, and the Asian-Malay features from Indochina and south to Indonesia (**Fig. 17.1**). A rough geographical and latitudinal division of ethnicity can be considered as north and south of the Tropic of Cancer. Anthropologically, this division would correlate with the Han Chinese origins of the north with the proto- and then deutero-Malays of the south.

The areas where Asian faces differ from their Western counterparts are mainly in the eyes, nose, and facial skeletal framework. Overall, Asian features are smaller.

17.2.1 The Forehead

The Asian forehead is broader and flatter, with less bossing. Eyebrows are usually level, as opposed to arched.

17.2.2 The Eyes

Asian eyes show the clearest difference from Western eyes. The differences can be analyzed metrically (anthropometry) and non-metrically (anthroposcopy). Classically, the Asian eye anthroposcopically consists of black eyebrows, black lashes, and brown irises.

Anthropometrically, Asian eyes have a lower index value than Western eyes for the interorbital width (distance between the medial canthi). The internal interorbital width is smaller in women than in men. Furthermore, if a line is drawn between the medial and lateral canthi of a Western eye, and the angle it makes with the horizontal is measured, the usual angle is 0 to 5 degrees. In the Asian eye, there is commonly an upward slant of the line, with a greater measured angle of 5 to 10 degrees, creating the stereotypical laterally upward-slanting Asian eye.

Phenotypically, the two most distinctive distinguishing features of an Asian eye are the superior tarsal fold and the medial epicanthal fold.

The Superior Tarsal Fold or Superior Eyelid Crease

About 50% of Asian-Orientals have a single eyelid, i.e., they do not have a superior eyelid crease. The superior eyelid crease is formed by the dermal attachments of fibrous strands from the levator fascia aponeurosis to the subcutaneous layer of the upper eyelids. During eye opening, the upward contraction of the levator aponeurotic fascia

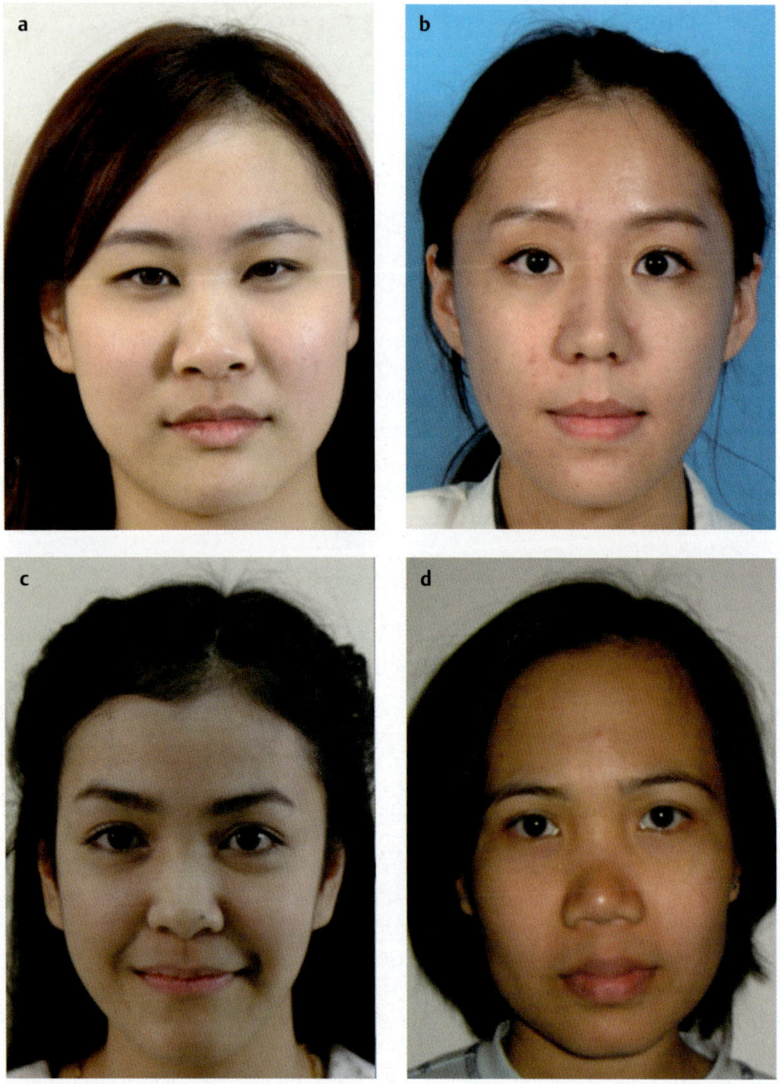

Fig. 17.1 Photographs of different East Asian peoples. **(a)** Northern Han Chinese. **(b)** Southern Han Chinese. **(c)** Thai. **(d)** Malaysian.

results in dermal pull and formation of a second supratarsal fold. This fold frames the eye and and can make the eye appear larger and more pleasing. The fold is dynamic and disappears on eye closure **(Fig. 17.2)**. The fold is present in 50% of Asians and, if present, varies in its height, depending on the attachment level of the levator fibers. Double eyelid surgery to create a fold, or to create a wider fold, is the most common aesthetic surgery undertaken in Asia. Many techniques have been described. They range from closed, nonincisional techniques to open surgical techniques.[1,2,3,4] The main difference in Asian patients' preference is differing goals for the height of the neo-fold created. North Asians tend to prefer a narrower width between the superior ciliary margin and fold: 4 to 6 mm, which is equal to the width of the tarsus.[4] Asians from the south, e.g., Thailand and Indochina, generally prefer a wider crease width: on average, 8 mm, with a range of 6 to 10 mm **(Fig. 17.3)**.

Another aesthetic feature of the superior crease is the medial crease configuration and the overall shape of the fold. The medial configuration of the superior crease can be either:

1. An innie, where the superior fold medially converges and merges with the medial fold angle, or
2. An outie, where the superior fold remains parallel and divergent from the medial fold angle.

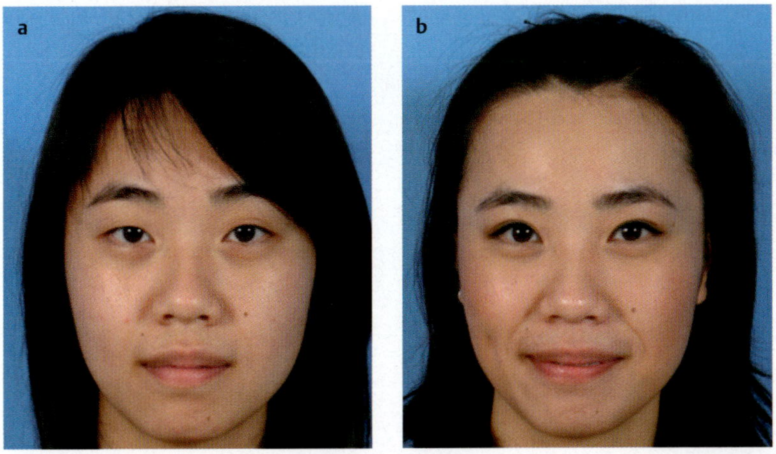

Fig. 17.2 **(a)** Single eyelids and **(b)** double eyelids after surgery in the same patient.

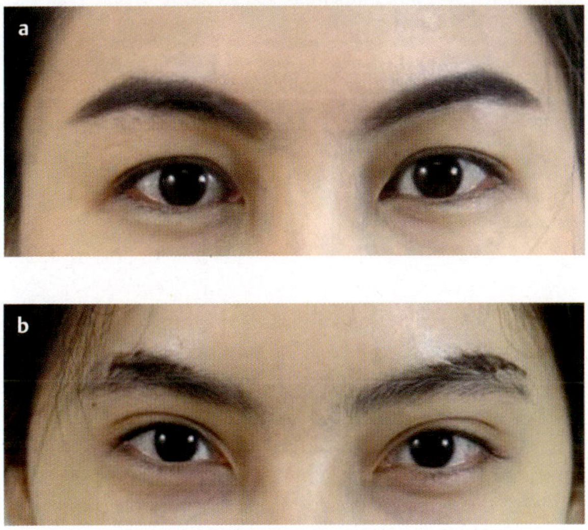

Fig. 17.3 **(a)** Narrow and **(b)** wide double eyelid crease.

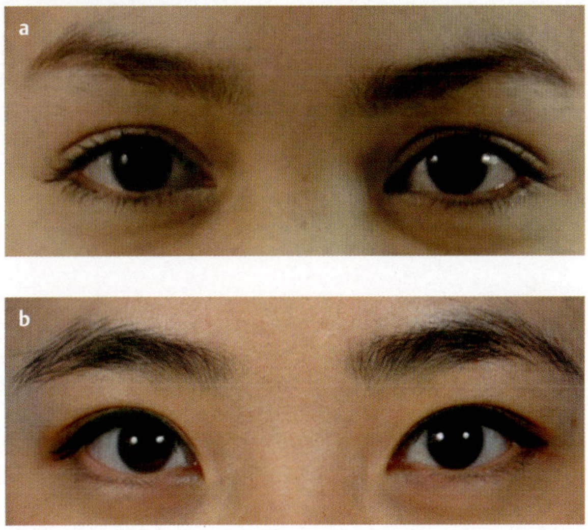

Fig. 17.4 Medial fold configurations. **(a)** Outie medial fold. **(b)** Innie medial fold.

An innie fold is associated with the Asian-Oriental eye, while an outie fold is associated with a Western appearance, because it is typically seen in the Western eye **(Fig. 17.4)**.

Another consideration is the overall shape of the superior crease, which can be:

1. Semilunar (half-moon) and rounded, more closely following the superior ciliary margin, or
2. Parallel and more closely following the shape of the brow.

The semilunar fold is associated with the Asian-Oriental eye, while the parallel fold is associated with the Western eye **(Fig. 17.5)**.

The Epicanthal Fold

The epicanthal fold is the fold of skin that is seen at the medial angle of the eye and that covers and hoods over the medial canthus. This fold is commonly seen in Asians and is a stereotype of the Asian face. It is associated with the lower development of the radix and the formation of a lower sweeping medial attachment of the orbicularis oculi.[5] The epicanthal fold **(Fig. 17.6)** may create the illusion of a pseudo-squint or a smaller eye; it also accentuates the laterally upward slant of the eye by increasing the intercanthal distance of the eyes while lowering the apparent medial canthal apex. To achieve a bigger and more

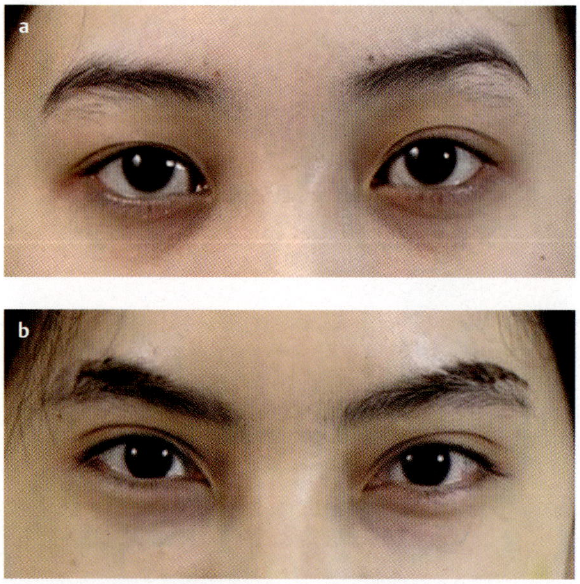

Fig. 17.5 **(a)** Semilunar folds and **(b)** parallel folds.

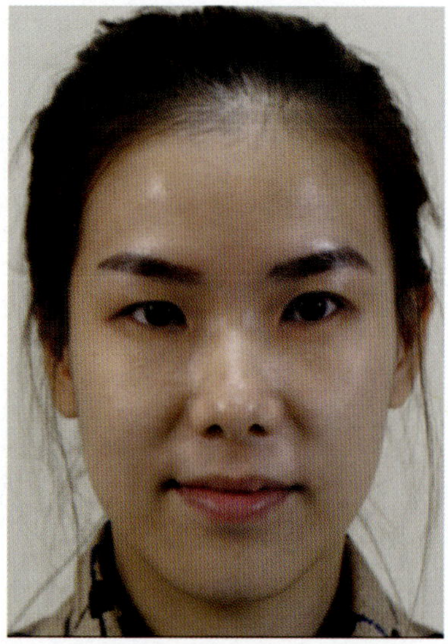

Fig. 17.6 Epicanthal folds hooding medial canthi.

balanced look, epicanthoplasty is often performed in addition to double eyelid surgery. Epicanthoplasty medializes the medial canthal angle, thereby removing the pseudo-squint illusion as well as creating a wider, less slanted palpebral fissure with an objectively measurable and subjectively bigger look to the eye. Different surgical techniques have been described, including correction by a medially placed subdermal-levator suture pexy technique; surgical flaps like z-plasty, w-plasty, or V-Y advancements; or direct medial division and repair.[1,2,3,4,5] Special care should be taken when correcting the epicanthal fold, as the medial skin of the eye is thicker in consistency than the superior and lower eyelid skin and hence prone to visible scarring in what is already a highly visible part of the face.

17.2.3 The Nose

The Asian nose is different from the Western nose and is developmentally smaller. While there is a wide spectrum of size, the archetypal Asian nose can be described as follows **(Fig. 17.7)**.

The nasal bone (and therefore radix) is lower. The nasion, if it can be seen, arises from a level more inferior than for the average Causcasian nose, anywhere from the level of the superior tarsal crease down to the mid-pupillary line. The septum of the nose is less projected and consequently the quadrilateral septal cartilage is small. The upper lateral cartilages (ULC) and the lower lateral cartilages (LLC) are also small and weak in comparison to those in Western noses. As a consequence, the nasal tip demonstrates less projection, with a more oblique cephalic-cephalad LLC axis and a thicker soft tissue envelope over the tip. The underlying anatomical findings and thicker nasal skin envelope translate into a rounder, less well-defined nasal tip with a higher incidence of nostril show on the frontal view. Alar base widths will also naturally vary.

17.2.4 The Radix

The radix is the most posterior soft tissue point of the root of the nose as seen on a lateral profile view. Asian radixes are either absent or present; if present, they are usually seen at a level congruent with the superior tarsal crease or lower to the mid-pupillary line. An observation is that lower radixes are often associated with an epicanthal fold and/or innie, semilunar superior crease, while higher radixes tend to be associated with a more outie and parallel superior crease.

The depth (or height) of the optimal Asian radix is not usually taught in Asian facial plastic surgical courses, unlike the extensive coverage of the Western radix in the literature. Yet dorsal augmentation is the most common request among Asians, and sometimes patients want to approximate the depth of the Western radix. However, one should ask: Is the optimal Asian radix synonymous with the Western radix reference, and is Westernization of the augmented Asian nose applicable and desirable today?

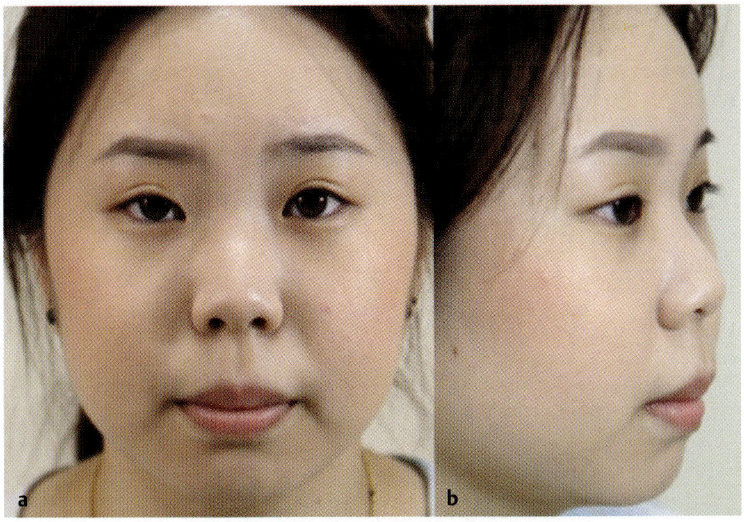

Fig. 17.7 (a,b) Asian nose.

The authors (GS and FW) undertook a comparative study in which desirable lateral radix profiles were digitally simulated for the study subjects, and then the simulated nasofrontal (NF) angle was measured after the digitally simulated augmentation **(Fig. 17.8)**. For the comparison, 10 independent judges were requested to undertake a similar task of digitally simulating the augmented radixes on lateral profile views of the same subjects; their measured NF angles were compared to the authors' findings.

The findings demonstrated that, within the same Asian community in Hong Kong, the study subjects and the independent male and female judges agreed on a similar NF angle of 140 degrees. Furthermore, this group preference was statistically different from the optimal Western NF (radix) angle of 113 to 120 degrees. This suggests that Asians prefer radixes that are not as high as their Western counterparts. Asian aesthetic preferences are definitely different.[6]

17.2.5 The Nasal Envelope and Nasal Tip

The dorsal soft tissue envelope of the Asian nose is notably thicker than that of the Western nose. The underlying framework is smaller and developmentally it stretches less. This is true especially for the Asian-Malay nose. The Asian-Oriental nose type tends to have a stronger, higher structural framework, with thinner skin in particular as the ethnic origin moves more to the north, e.g., northern China and Korea compared with southern China.

Augmentation rhinoplasty is the usual rule for the Asian nose. The aesthetic preference is for a higher nose, but usually the underlying donor tissue is insufficient. Augmentation with septal cartilage alone is usually insufficient, so alternative autologous tissue from the ear, rib, or fascia as well as implants and injectables are commonplace for the standard Asian augmentation rhinoplasty. These techniques are covered in other chapters of this book.

An interesting aspect of the Asian tip is its thicker soft tissue envelope. This gives it a softer and more "amorphous" look, especially when coupled to softer and weaker underlying LLCs. In most Western surgical courses, the prescribed tip aesthetic is a bi-tip with two high points, as seen with a two-point flash photo-documentation. Many surgical lectures discuss how to achieve this.

However, the bi-tip aesthetic should not be regarded as the Asian preference. Contemporary Asian cosmetic marketing and glossy magazine photographs show the majority of Asian models, celebrities, etc., with a smooth-contoured "mono-tip" with a straight dorsum and usually without a supra-tip break. The authors (GS and FW) undertook a comparative perceptual study that examined Asian nasal tip preferences among Asian observers. Two seemingly identical, frontal, two-point light-source photographs were shown to a group of Asian judges; the only difference between the photographs, unknown to the viewers, was the tip **(Fig. 17.9)**. One frontal image had a mono-tip (or amorphous tip), while the second image had a bi-tip. The alternative tip was simulated digitally but the photographs were identical in every other way. The study found that 91% of the Asian judges (Z test; p = 0.00003) demonstrated a preference for an Asian mono-tip nose **(Fig. 17.10)**.[7]

Possible reasons for the mono-tip preference include the subconscious recognition of the mono-tip as the general norm for the Asian nose, or the mono-tip confers a

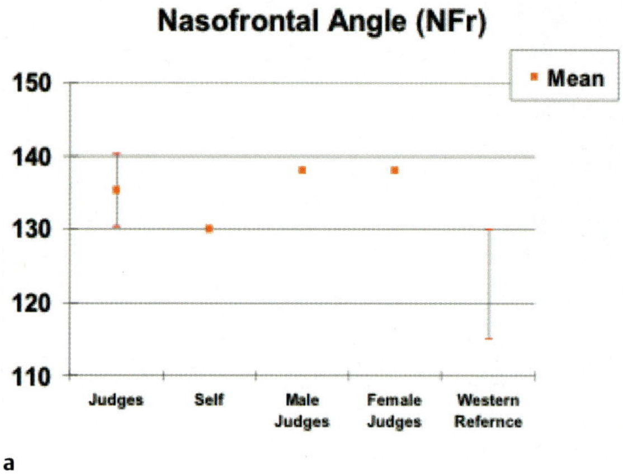

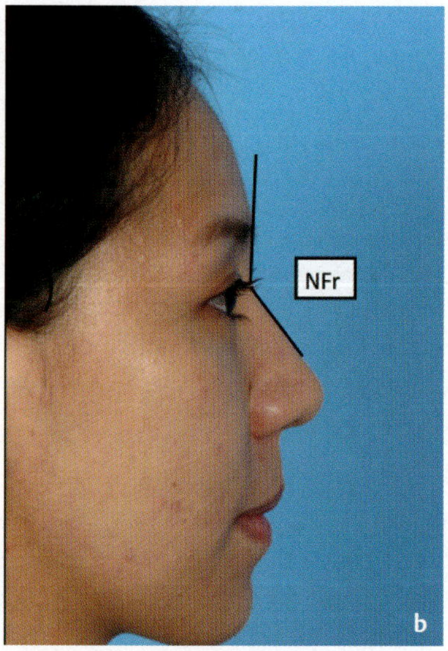

Fig. 17.8 (a,b) The Asian radix differs from Western norms.

softer, more demure and gentle appearance to the Asian face consistent with local values of beauty. In any case, the study's finding offers a further understanding about the allure of the injection rhinoplasty technique in terms of its aesthetics. No matter what product that is injected, whether temporary or permanent, injection rhinoplasty generally confers a more rounded and softer form to the radix, dorsum, or even nasal tip depots than is attained with harder, structured implants. The softer, rounded form is in part due to the "globular" subdermal injection resting upon a less firm nose with a thicker skin. Subsequent shrink-wrapping forces exerted on the injected depot also result in a more globular depot; this, in turn, can only impart a softer look **(Fig. 17.11)**.

17.2.6 The Mouth, Chin, and Mandible

Developmentally, the Asian mandible tends to be smaller and underdeveloped in comparison to the Western mandible.[8] Two notable mandibular conditions are commonly seen, especially in Asian-Orientals. One is a squarer and laterally displaced angle of the mandible, which gives a squarer jaw look. This is commonly seen in northern Asian-Orientals, e.g., in those of north China and Korean ethnicity. Mandibular contouring, which is requested for management of the square mandible,[9] is discussed in another chapter of this book.

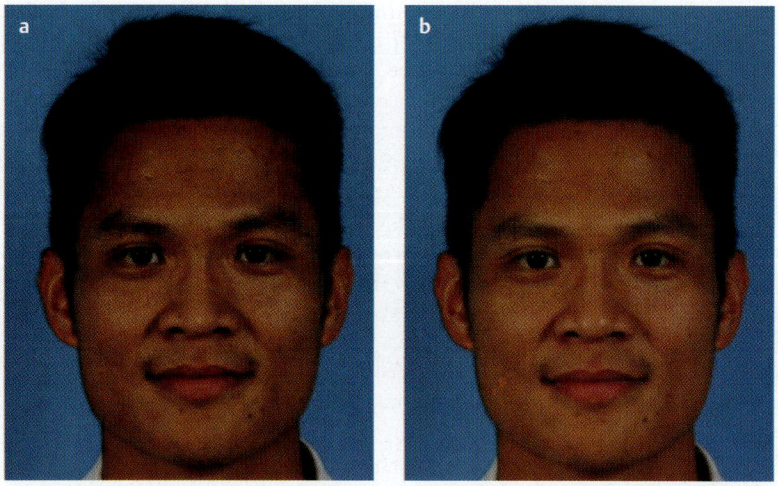

Fig. 17.9 Perceptual comparisons of **(a)** mono-tip and **(b)** bi-tip.

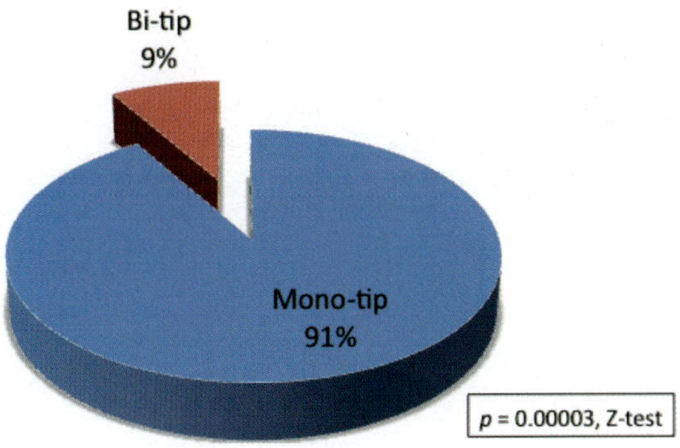

Fig. 17.10 Mono-tip versus bi-tip preference in Asian cohort.

In southern China, a smaller chin is more commonly seen; the *South China chin* is a well-known entity **(Fig. 17.12)**. The smaller mandible results in a crowded lower dental array and sometimes with chin "dimpling" due to mentalis overactivity as it tries to maintain lip closure by the lower lip. The frontal facial ratios are also notably changed, with the lower subnasale-mentum being proportionately less than the usual expected upper face and midface ratios of thirds. Patients may also have obstructive sleep apnea secondary to dynamic obstruction at the tongue base level.

Patients with this condition can be managed with a chin implant if the retrogenia is minimal. However, more significant retrogenia, especially with dental crowding and established obstructive sleep apnea, would best be managed with combination orthodontic and orthognathic care **(Fig. 17.13)**, which is optimal for improving the functional airway, the functional bite, and the desired aesthetics. In spite of this, the Asian female preference is for a slightly smaller, rounded chin, which is an acceptable Asian aesthetic feature. A strong, square jaw and strong and dimpled chin should be avoided.

17.3 Cultural Considerations in Asians

17.3.1 Ancient Chinese Face-Reading Philosophy

Throughout Asia, aesthetic considerations vary according to local and popular influences; however, this section discusses a specific aspect of Asian aesthetics that is based on the ancient art of Chinese face reading, which continues to affect the conscious desires or subconscious goals of Asian clients. It may come to the fore in aesthetic requests in consultations.

The art of face reading and its teachings have been documented in China since the Tang Dynasty (ca. 618–907 AD),[10] when China, or the Middle Kingdom, was vastly superior culturally and militarily in Asia. Many old kingdoms in Asia would provide tribute to, and trade with, China, and Chinese influence and ideas spread in Asia. In addition, historically, the spread of Chinese philosophy can be traced across Asia to Europe and the Americas. Hence, face reading continues to have effects outside of Asia today.

Chinese teachings are practiced among modern face and fortune readers, which keeps face reading in the consciousness of some Asian clients. It should be mentioned here that this ancient philosophy has not been rigorously tested scientifically but does form a large longitudinal, descriptive, and observational study of man over several centuries. For this reason, and because of the subtle implications of this philosophy for Asian practitioners, it is worth describing to readers, especially those with Asian-

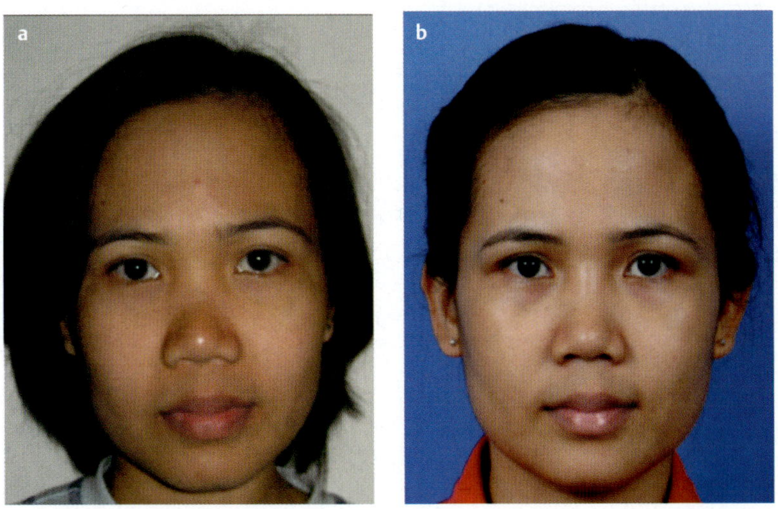

Fig. 17.11 NASHA injection rhinoplasty. **(a)** Before. **(b)** After.

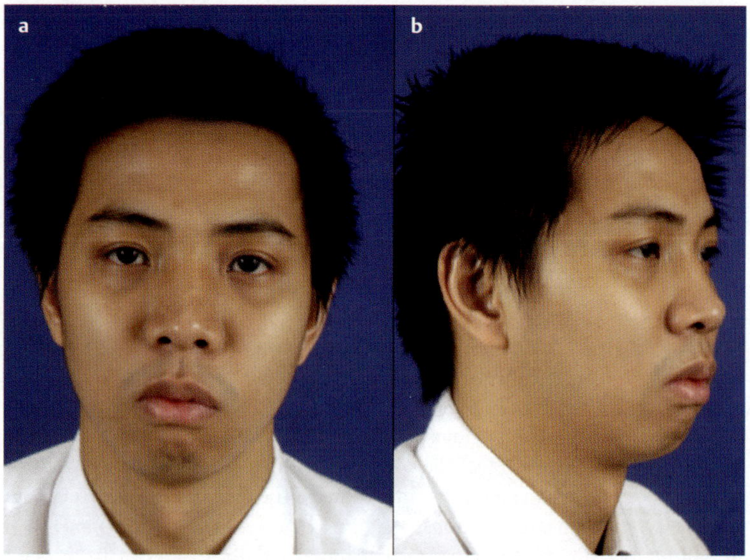

Fig. 17.12 (a,b) Retrogenic south China chin.

Oriental clients and those who may not be familiar with its concepts.

The basics are that the face is divided into 12 life palaces that signify different aspects of our lives **(Fig. 17.14)**. The face also is divided into different parts that represent different ages in one's life **(Fig. 17.15)**.[11] An example is that our nose represents our self and our ego, and thus we point to our nose in signifying "I" to others. So a high nose means high self- esteem in that individual, and vice versa. The life palaces for just the nose include the Life Palace (the radix), signifying luck and fame, and the Wealth Palace (the nasal tip), which governs wealth. A simple translation of this in practice today is that higher radixes are seen generally in successful Asians in the entertainment industry, which inspires patients' requests for dorsal augmentation. Also, a more bulbous nasal tip is acceptable in Asian men because it is regarded as a sign of fortune. What follows are some relevant Chinese face-reading philosophy considerations—the statements pertain only to face-reading philosophy.

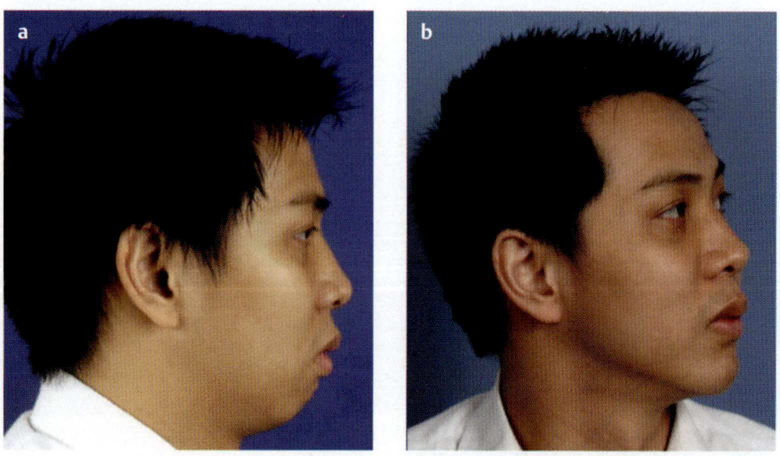

Fig. 17.13 Sliding genioplasty for retrogenia. **(a)** Before. **(b)** After.

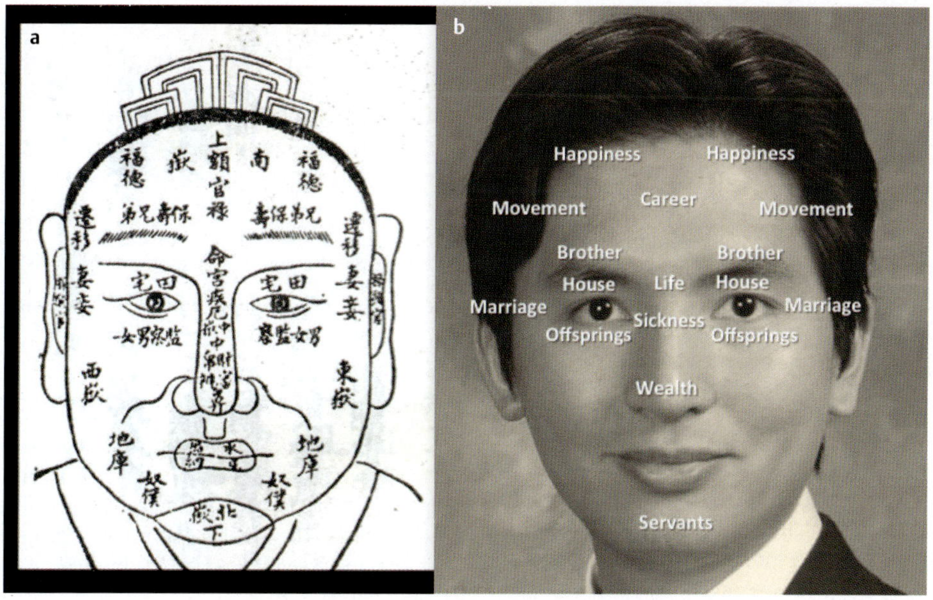

Fig. 17.14 (a,b) Pictorial representations of the 12 palaces of the face. (Courtesy of www.rhinoplastyarchive.com, Asian Rhinoplasty.)

Pigmented Lesions

There are no pigmented moles that are considered to be good. A pigmented lesion in an area like the Sickness Palace will denote ill health.

The Eyebrows

Laterally down-slanting brows are to be avoided, because they denote a pessimistic nature. Semi-circular brows are regarded as the best.

The Eyelids

Double eyelids, rather than single eyelids, are desirable. Double eyelids (and 50% of Orientals are double-creased) indicate the individual is more caring, passionate, and kind.

The Irises

Irises that are too large are associated with emotions (love). Interestingly, proprietary contact lenses for larger irises are widely used by females wanting a more attractive look.

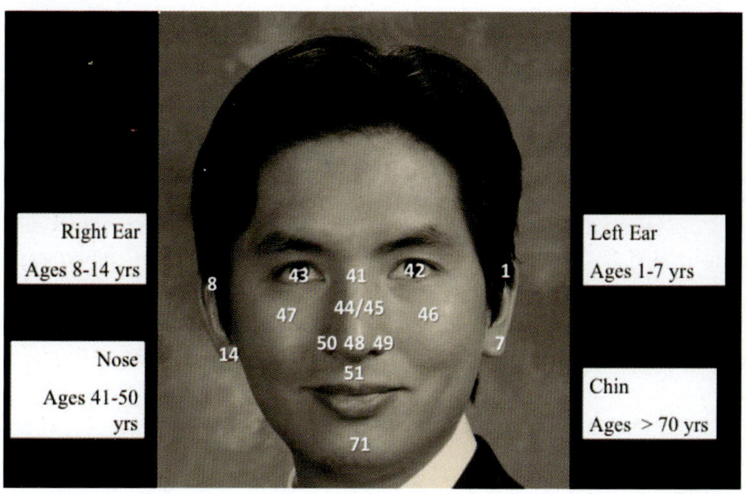

Fig. 17.15 Pictorial representation of age significance of the face. (Courtesy of www.rhinoplastyarchive.com, Asian Rhinoplasty.)

Small irises are regarded as cruel. The shinier the eyes, the more love affairs. Eversion of the upper eyelashes by use of eyelash curlers creates a more romantic (and shinier) eye.

The Lower Eyelids

Scleral show is to be avoided because it indicates a tendency toward risk taking, which could be dangerous. Bags under the eyes are not good, as they denote trouble with one's children. Neither are jugal festoons considered good. Hypertrophy of the lower orbicularis oculi muscle is regarded as good, producing a kinder-looking eye.

The Nose

The ideal nose is straight (denoting smooth life) without a hump or depression (which may suggest problems in life). Good tip support is ideal to show good fortune in one's later years. The nose should not have any nostril show, as nostril show is related to someone being generous or unable to save his or her money, and hence they become poor. The authors strongly recommend avoiding nostril show in Asian clients. A fleshy tip (usually a mono-tip due to the added soft tissue envelope) is desirable, especially for a man, as it is related to wealth. Surprisingly, a wider alar base is considered better, because it indicates the person can save more money.

The Lips

Thick lips are desirable, as they are more loving.

The Chin

A balanced chin is good for old age and a better retirement. A well-proportioned face, with the upper face, midface, and lower face each accounting for a facial third, is the ideal.

The Ears

Prominent ears typify a rebellious nature. The larger the ear lobule, the more kind hearted and empathetic is the individual.

The Hair

The hairline of an individual should sit normally or high. If it sits low, it may affect their youth.

17.4 Current Cosmetic Trends in Asian Facial Plastic Surgery

The cosmetic industry in Asia is on the rise. With the emergence of China, India, and the Asian tigers, increasing wealth and competition for service-sector positions have motivated Asian clients to seek facial improvement, maintenance, and rejuvenation.

Overall, the general cosmetic trend in Asia emphasizes:

- Minimally invasive surgery (MIS) with short downtime
- Painless procedures
- Economical procedures, due to cost sensitivity

The economic consideration is due to the relatively lower earning base in Asia in general among the masses. Also, the majority of clients are Asian women, who still earn less than their male counterparts. However, the growing demand is evidenced by the number of emerging cosmetic centers in Asia.

The MIS and painless procedures with short downtimes and immediate results are what most clients anywhere would prefer. Among Asians, however, undergoing surgery to achieve a result not possible with MIS poses a further psychological hurdle. The hurdle is more easily crossed in countries where cosmetic enhancement surgery appears to be more acceptable, e.g., South Korea.

Equally relevant to the cosmetic trend is the finding that the Asian face tends to age more slowly than same-age Western counterparts. Genetics surely play their part, but, in addition, Asians culturally value soft, smooth, white skin and avoid sun exposure. Thus, the cosmetic techniques required to enhance and rejuvenate the aging Asian face may not need to be as radical or invasive as a facelift.

For these reasons, cosmetic practice in Asia tends to lean toward acid peels, dermabrasion therapy, laser facials, radiofrequency and high-intensity ultrasound therapy for facial rejuvenation, and lasers for depigmentation and depilation. There is an increasing demand for polylactic acid injections, nonacidic synthetic hyaluronic acid, longer-term injectable calcium hydroxyapatite, and permanent polyacrylamide gel injectables for nasal augmentation and facial revolumizing.

If and when surgery is the only option, the southern Asian client tends to prefer the smaller procedure, e.g., silicone implant rhinoplasty instead of autologous rib reconstructive surgery. Procedural costs, as well as donor-site morbidity, are important in these instances. The areas of the Asian face where surgical procedures continue to be more prominent than MIS are aesthetic blepharoplasties for double eyelids, epicanthoplasty for bigger eyes, lower eye bag surgery, especially using the "scarless" transconjunctival approach, and reduction of the prominent square-angled jaw.[9]

By contrast, there are two areas that are not commonly corrected in Asia. The first is bilateral prominent ears. These are regarded as adorable by parents and there is no significant peer bullying and teasing (as seen as in the West) that would incentivize patients or parents to seek treatment. A more likely scenario for seeking surgery is when the ears are asymmetrical, e.g., there is a unilateral prominent ear.

The second area not corrected is the small (grade 1–2) retrogenic chin, which often is not obvious to the patient, and treatment is considered only after preoperative facial counseling for rhinoplasty or sleep apnea.

Another factor that has driven the current trend in Asian cosmetic surgery is local popular culture and media. Asian media celebrities with newfound fame after cosmetic surgery certainly play a part. This trend has been notable over the past few years, with the advent of Korean popular culture like K-pop and Korean films, which are now watched all over Asia. This has pushed the cosmetic industry toward Korean aesthetics, with requests not only from northern Asians with features similar to Korean ethnicity, but also among Southeast Asians, some with more Asian-Malay features. Naturally, cosmetic medical tourism, bringing clients to South Korea and Thailand, is also a booming industry.

17.5 Final Recommendations

Asian facial plastic surgery is very much the same as any other culturally specific facial plastic surgery. It consists of understanding the perceptual aesthetics of the individual in their community, coupled with the execution of the appropriate treatment technique. Today digital simulation software permits the practitioner and client to mutually understand and agree on desired outcomes before surgery. This technology is an invaluable tool, especially for ethnic clients whose aesthetic desires may be slightly different from the expected.

The technical aspects of Asian facial plastic surgery are a variation of techniques taught and encountered in training and courses. The main exceptions are aesthetic Asian eye surgery (for the creation of the double lid and epicanthoplasty) and augmentation surgery for the Asian nose. With the increasing popularity of Asian aesthetic surgery, the specific demand is best met by training in Asia to learn the nuances of the procedures.

17.6 Conclusion

The Asian nonsurgical and surgical cosmetic industry is increasing exponentially, in step with the growing economy in Asia. In some places, it is booming. Clients seek cosmetic improvements for a variety of reasons, including a higher disposable income, to remain competitive in their industry, and to conform to their society's increasing aesthetic expectations.

Asian aesthetics and the Asian perception of aesthetics differ from the Western perspective. Even when they are aligned, the technical challenges and chosen method can and do differ.

References

1. Chen WPD, ed. Asian Blepharoplasty and the Eyelid Crease. 2nd ed. Butterworth-Heinemann; 2006
2. Park JI. Modified Z-epicanthoplasty in the Asian eyelid. Arch Facial Plast Surg 2000;2(1):43–47
3. Sinrachtanant C, Soo G, eds. Asian Blepharoplasty—The Short Incision Technique. Singapore: Elsevier; 2014
4. Wong JK, Zhou X, Ai Y, Wang Z. A simple, minimally invasive method for creation of the superior palpebral fold in Asians with the modified continuous buried tarsal stitch: a joint assessment from Toronto, Ontario, Canada, and Chengdu, China. Arch Facial Plast Surg 2010;12(4): 269–273
5. Oh YW, Seul CH, Yoo WM. Medial epicanthoplasty using the skin redraping method. Plast Reconstr Surg 2007; 119(2):703–710
6. Soo G, Wong FTC, Sinrachtanant C. Asian Rhinoplasty. In: Becker D, Palma P, Rhinoplasty Archive, 2013. www.rhinoplastyarchive.com
7. Lai N, Soo G, Wong FTC, Chow J. Asian preferences for the nasal tip—A perceptual study of the mono-tip versus the bi-tip. Personal communication, 2013
8. Liu Y, Kau CH, Pan F, Zhou H, Zhang Q, Zacharopoulos GV. A 3-dimensional anthropometric evaluation of facial morphology among Chinese and Greek population. J Craniofac Surg 2013;24(4):e353–e358
9. Mu X. Experience in East Asian facial recontouring: reduction malarplasty and mandibular reshaping. Arch Facial Plast Surg 2010;12(4):222–229
10. Yap J, ed. Joey Yap's Art of Face Reading: Unmask the Secrets of Your Personality and Destiny. Cico; October 2009
11. Wong FTC, Soo G, Ng WP, van Hasselt CA, Tong MCF. Implications of Chinese face reading on the aesthetic sense. Arch Facial Plast Surg 2010;12(4):218–221

18 Primary Rhinoplasty Techniques: Use of Costal Cartilage

Dean M. Toriumi and Scott A. Asher

18.1 Introduction

Often the rhinoplasty surgeon will meet patients whose specific ethnicity may not be readily apparent. Generally, the principles of rhinoplasty are the same no matter what the patient's ethnicity: if the structures of the nose are surgically manipulated, they must be supported to prevent unwanted changes to shape over time secondary to scar contracture and the evolution of tissue healing. Adherence to these principles yields both a long-term aesthetic and functional result. Specifically in the Asian patient, primary rhinoplasty may require a significant amount of grafting material to adequately support the nasal structure or to offer meaningful augmentation. One successful method for achieving these goals is through the use of costal cartilage.

18.2 Preoperative Considerations

18.2.1 Patient Consultation

As with any consultation, a thorough history and physical exam are necessary to accurately diagnose the patient's condition and to determine options for treatment specific to each patient. Photographs should be obtained in a standardized fashion (frontal, lateral, three-quarter, and base views). Newer 3D stereophotogrammetry technology provides the surgeon an even more powerful tool for objectively quantifying the changes accomplished via rhinoplasty.[1,2] Digital image morphing software has made a dramatic impact on the surgeon's ability to communicate with patients preoperatively on prospective changes to the nose. Understanding the patient's desires is easier with photographic manipulation as opposed to verbal descriptions of potential alterations. By the same token, image morphing increases the pressure to perform surgically what can be a relatively simple task of modifying a picture on a computer screen. It is the authors' opinion that, although the patient may present by requesting changes to the profile, the surgeon should always keep the frontal view as the first priority. Profile changes must be secondary to the view in which individuals interact with others on a daily basis.

In consultation with a patient about primary rhinoplasty, it is very important when taking a history to ask if the patient has ever had any filler injected into the nose. Often patients will not consider it important, or simply forget to disclose the information. Filler techniques have become more and more common, especially in the Asian patient population, and encountering residual filler intraoperatively can wildly alter the surgical plan (**Fig. 18.1**).

Discussion with the patient should focus on what are realistic potential changes to the nose based on the structure of both the cartilaginous/bony framework and skin-soft tissue envelope (S-STE) found on physical exam. The surgeon should also understand the patient's aesthetic preferences for all parameters in appearance (dorsal line shape, nasal length, rotation, width, dorsal height, projection, tip refinement, etc.). "Normal" must be defined for certain parameters, such as radix location (Caucasian = superior palpebral fissure; Asian = mid-pupil).[3] During this conversation it may become apparent that the patient feels a social pressure to keep a small dorsal hump, or to leave the base wide, etc. Failure to preoperatively identify these feelings could ultimately lead to a dissatisfied patient, despite what the surgeon feels is an excellent result. For example, whereas one Asian female may feel the surgery is a failure if afterward she does not look Westernized, another may feel she looks unnatural and "operated" and may be embarrassed to allow her family and friends to see her new nose. Countless scenarios can be encountered, but the surgeon and patient absolutely must be on the same page before surgery is pursued.

The evolution of rhinoplasty from a primarily reductive procedure to one of more structural grafting requires that the surgeon have an adequate supply of material to be able to achieve surgical goals.[4] A lack of material should never be the limiting factor in obtaining the optimal result. In ethnic rhinoplasty in particular, the non-Caucasian nose often will have less septal cartilage and thinner/weaker upper and lower lateral cartilages. With weaker structural support to the nose, surgical trauma can have a more drastic effect on tissue healing; therefore, this emphasizes the importance of structural support for long-term results. For example, Asian rhinoplasty often involves dorsal augmentation or increasing the definition of an amorphous tip that has thick skin (**Fig. 18.2**). Accomplishing these changes will undoubtedly require a large amount of graft material. Thicker skin will often require making the nose significantly larger, to stretch the skin envelope and to allow underlying structure to provide definition. Such structural grafting will cause the nose to be much stiffer after surgery, and it behooves the surgeon to discuss this firmness and increase in nasal size with the patient so that postoperative expectations are appropriately set.

Other chapters discuss allografts and homografts versus autologous grafts in great detail. In the opinion of this

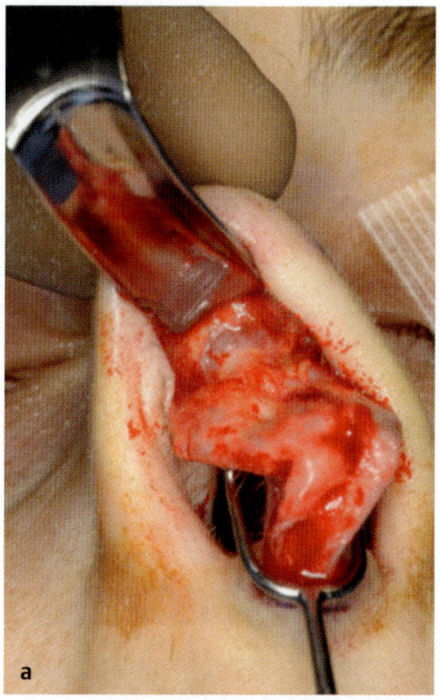

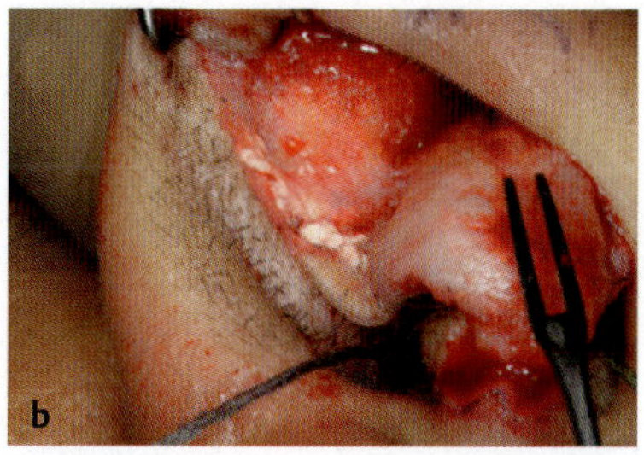

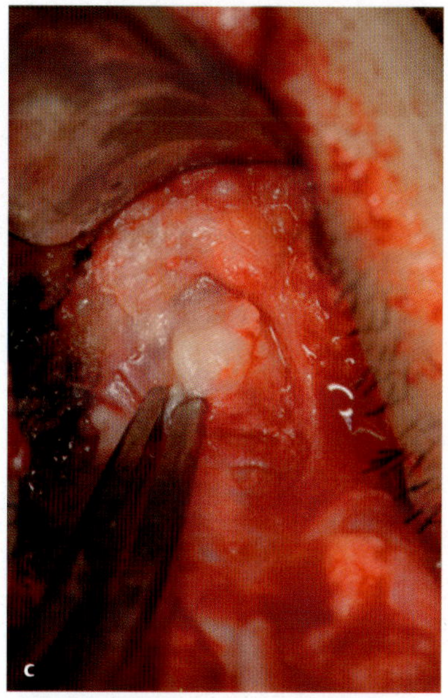

Fig. 18.1 Filler encountered during rhinoplasty. All filler should be removed intraoperatively to ensure that there will be no long-term contour irregularities. Filler was used by the previous surgeon in attempts **(a)** to straighten the dorsum, **(b)** to fill in the notching of the ala, and **(c)** for dorsal augmentation.

chapter's authors, if proper technique is learned, the use of autologous tissue can provide the best results both aesthetically and functionally. Septal, auricular, and costal cartilage all have specific uses in rhinoplasty, but this chapter focuses on costal cartilage grafting techniques. Overall, costal cartilage is much stronger than other autologous cartilage sources, and it can be cut thinner to avoid bulk in the nose. Costal cartilage has less vascular demand than auricular cartilage, and it is therefore less likely to be reabsorbed over time. It can be harvested in much larger volume than septal or auricular cartilage in cases requiring significant augmentation, such as primary rhinoplasty in the Asian patient. Donor-site pain is certainly a consideration.[5] Pain with costal cartilage harvest can be minimized by limiting wide dissection, avoiding cutting muscle, and by keeping the free margin of the chest wall intact. Unlike allografts, costal cartilage has little to no risk of harming the S-STE and is less likely to become infected or to extrude in the long term. Obvious disadvantages, which can be minimized through experience, are the extra time needed for harvest, the donor-site scar and/or pain, and the potential for graft warping.

18.2.2 Preoperative Chest Imaging

The authors do not obtain any preoperative imaging of the chest in preparation for costal cartilage harvest, but there are others who think that imaging is beneficial. Noncontrast computed tomography (CT)[6,7] or ultrasound[8] can be used if there is a concern about cartilage ossification based on age. Translation of the data provided by the scans to clinically applicable information about where to make one's incision and/or which rib to harvest is difficult. The surgeon must also keep in mind that many patients are undergoing elective cosmetic surgery and are paying for their care out of pocket (without help from insurance). The cost of imaging is not nominal.

18.3 Procedure

18.3.1 Costal Cartilage Harvest Technique

Although structures in the nose can vary dramatically among patients with different ethnic backgrounds, to our knowledge there are no data showing ethnic variation in costal cartilage. Gender may play a role in calcification pattern, but the patient's age is the most important factor when considering potential costal cartilage harvest in a rhinoplasty patient.[9,10,11] Younger patients are at much higher risk for warping of the cartilage. Older patients are at significantly higher risk for calcification of the cartilage, to a point where harvesting and carving become a challenge and grafts are prone to fracture with manipulation. In the authors' opinion, the ideal patient age for costal cartilage harvest is 30 to 50 years old. Gender and hair coverage of the area also play a role in morbidity of the donor site. A smaller breast in a female puts pressure on the surgeon to decrease the size of the incision to prevent a scar that cannot be hidden, but safety (through adequate visualization) should always be the primary concern. A history of keloids

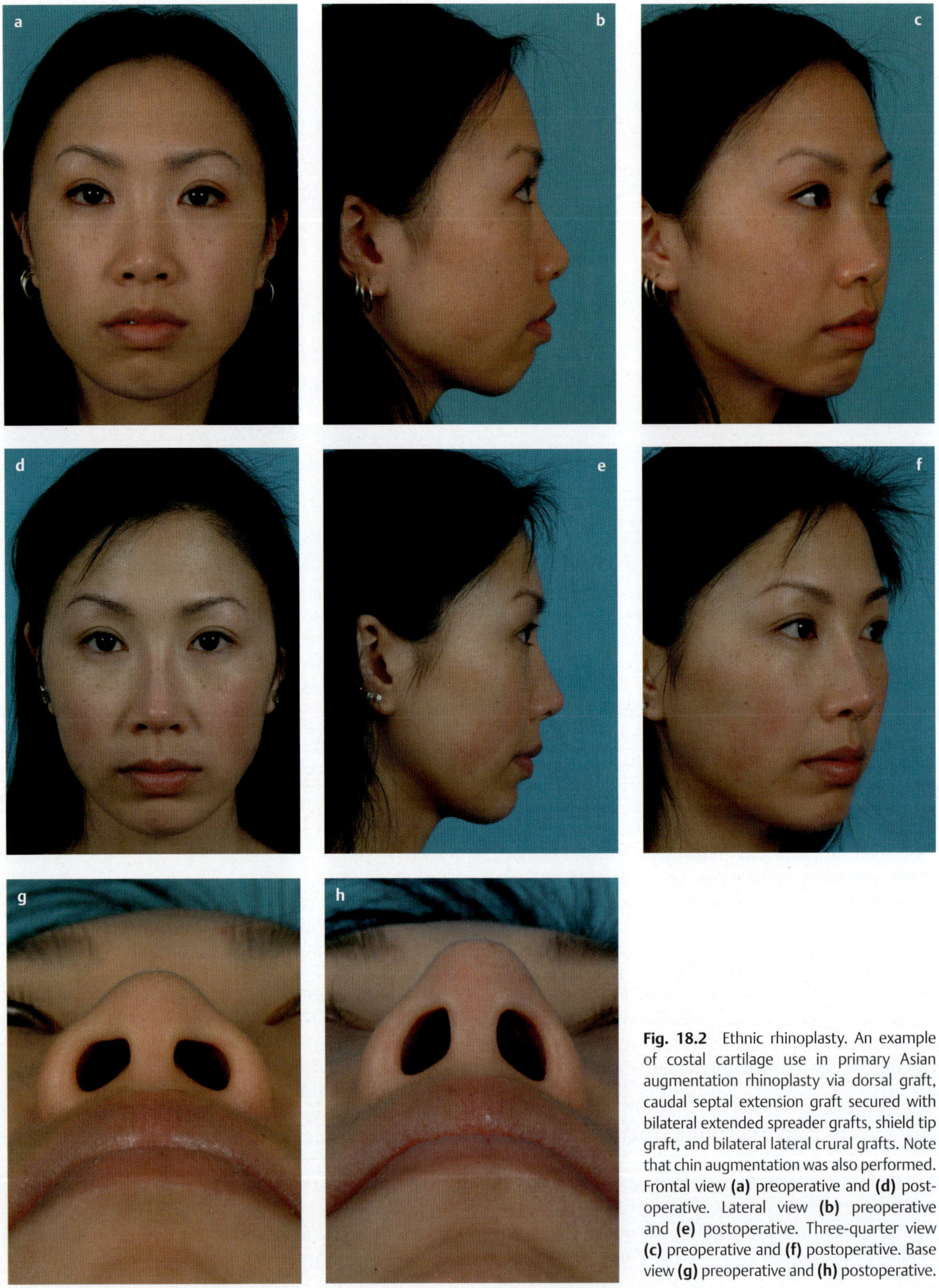

Fig. 18.2 Ethnic rhinoplasty. An example of costal cartilage use in primary Asian augmentation rhinoplasty via dorsal graft, caudal septal extension graft secured with bilateral extended spreader grafts, shield tip graft, and bilateral lateral crural grafts. Note that chin augmentation was also performed. Frontal view **(a)** preoperative and **(d)** postoperative. Lateral view **(b)** preoperative and **(e)** postoperative. Three-quarter view **(c)** preoperative and **(f)** postoperative. Base view **(g)** preoperative and **(h)** postoperative.

or hypertrophic scarring should also be taken into account, although the chest is less likely than the ear to be at risk for this complication.

Manual palpation up and down the chest wall should orient the surgeon to the options for costal cartilage harvest. Next, using a 1.5 inch 27 gauge needle, the degree of ossification in the cartilaginous portions of the rib and the location of the osseocartilaginous junction of the ribs can be determined for several potential donor sites (**Fig. 18.3**). Use of the needle is an advanced maneuver and should not be performed without extreme caution and supreme understanding of costal cartilage anatomy. A misguided needle could potentially injure the pleura and underlying lung parenchyma, causing what could develop into a tension pneumothorax. Use of the needle is, however, an important technique to master should the surgeon attempt to harvest costal cartilage through a limited incision.

The senior author prefers the donor site in the primary rhinoplasty patient to be on the right side. The incision is typically centered approximately one-third to one-half of the way from the sternum to a vertical line drawn down from the clavicle through the nipple. Attempt is made to hide the scar in the inframammary crease. Although the right side is typically chosen because it is closer to the primary (right-handed) surgeon's preferred side of the operating table, some centers use a double team approach where the right-handed surgeon opens the nose while a second surgeon simultaneously harvests costal cartilage from the left chest. Harvest from the right chest does have the advantage that inadvertent injury to the pericardium is impossible. Postoperatively, pain at the donor site on the right side of the chest also has less chance of being confused with angina.

Once potential sites for harvest have been determined and overlying skin is marked, the surrounding area is injected with 1% lidocaine with 1:100,000 epinephrine (more for vasoconstriction than analgesia). The chest and face can then be prepped in the usual fashion. Care should be taken throughout the operation not to contaminate the chest site with nasal flora; use separate gloves/gowns and cover the chest site with a blue towel when the surgeon is not actively engaged in the area.

Average harvest usually involves a single cartilaginous segment of 3 to 4 cm in length. The authors most commonly harvest the right sixth or seventh rib (the seventh rib is longer and straighter if major dorsal augmentation is planned), but consideration should also be given to the other ribs as options based on the particular grafts needed for each nasal operation. It is very important to realize that patients will experience significantly more pain if a segment of cartilage is removed from the free margin of the rib cage, as this area moves with every breath. Other factors affecting rib harvest are the anatomy of the breast/pectoralis muscle, very high body mass index (BMI), the presence of breast implants, or abnormal chest wall anatomy. Neither breast implants nor pectus excavatum is a contraindication to obtaining costal cartilage, but both increase the complexity of harvest.

Critical to safe costal cartilage harvest is thorough understanding of the anatomy. The fifth rib has a free superior and inferior margin. The sixth rib typically has a free superior margin, but separation of the joint with the seventh rib is usually required on its inferior margin. The seventh rib will usually have connections with surrounding ribs on both superior and inferior borders. The eighth and greater nonfloating ribs will also have significant connections to the surrounding ribs, and again harvest may result in greater pain due to involvement of the free margin of the rib cage. The fifth rib can lie underneath a significant amount of breast

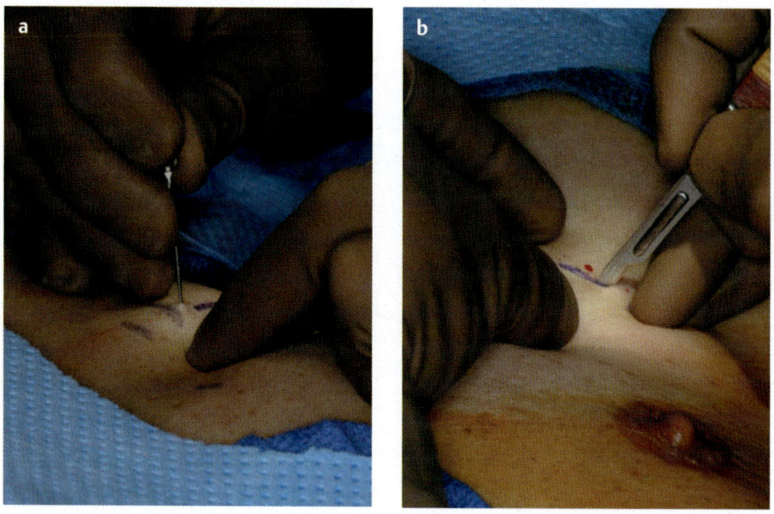

Fig.18.3 Optimizing incision site for rib harvest. **(a)** Careful palpation allows the surgeon to use a needle to probe for the osseocartilaginous junction, to estimate rib size and shape, and to determine any areas of ossification. **(b)** Smaller incisions can be utilized if this technique is employed.

tissue or pectoralis muscle, depending on the patient's body type. The sixth rib is usually at an ideal level, but the seventh and eighth ribs often are located deeper, away from the skin surface. The fifth rib is usually curved and, after carving, its cartilage may not be straight enough or of adequate size if significant dorsal augmentation is necessary. The sixth rib typically has a gentle genu that may also not be ideal if a long, straight segment is needed. The seventh rib is typically the longest and straightest rib so it provides the best rib for most major dorsal augmentations.

Incision is made sharply through the skin over the planned location. When first learning costal cartilage harvest, a generous 4 to 5 cm incision should be used. As the technique is mastered, it is possible to harvest more than adequate cartilage through as small as a 1 cm incision (**Fig. 18.4**). Sharp dissection down through the subcutaneous fat with lateral retraction is performed until the fascia overlying the muscular layer is encountered. Postoperative pain can be lessened by using bipolar cautery rather than monopolar cautery, and lessened even further by only using the minimal amount of energy necessary for hemostasis. If a small incision is to be utilized, a no. 15C scalpel should be used rather than the standard no. 15 blade. Three to four Ragnell retractors allow adequate visualization, but Senn or Army/Navy retractors can be substituted for larger incisions. Sharp incision should be made through the muscle fascia. The actual fibers of the muscle should then be spread, rather than cut, to decrease pain and bleeding. Once the muscle fibers have been retracted, the perichondrium of the underlying rib is visualized. The window of the skin incision can then be retracted medially and laterally to expose a much larger segment of rib than can be seen if dissection is simply carried straight down onto the rib only.

Once the rib is exposed, the surgeon can again very carefully use a needle to characterize the cartilage (**Fig. 18.5**). If the surgeon is pleased with the visible segment, the perichondrium on top of the rib is sharply elevated and harvested, exposing ~ 90 degrees of cartilage. For the safest method of costal cartilage harvest, the remaining 270 degrees of perichondrium should remain intact. The most reliable method to ensure the proper plane of dissection is to make a cut into the cartilage ~ 0.5 to 1.0 mm from both the superior and inferior margins to elevate a thin cuff of cartilage and to ensure the perichondrium is also elevating appropriately (**Fig. 18.6**). Cuts should also be made in the rib along the medial and lateral borders of the segment to be taken, but these cuts should be made with a scalpel only a minimal distance and the remaining dissection should be performed with a Freer elevator. Once dissection on all four sides slowly and progressively frees the rib, the undersurface should be dissected from the perichondrium in a pulling motion similar to the action of a shovel. Once the cartilage segment has been removed, care should then be taken to smooth the medial and lateral edges of remaining cartilage so that no rough edges remain. This can be accomplished with a Takahashi forceps.

The wound should next be thoroughly examined and then filled with saline. If the volume is constant and no bubbles are seen with a Valsalva maneuver, the chance of injury to the pleura or underlying lung parenchyma is low. The senior author recommends that less experienced surgeons obtain a postoperative chest X-ray to ensure no pneumothorax exists. They should also consider overnight prophylactic hospital observation, although the author performs surgery on an outpatient basis. If a tear in the perichondrium exposes a tear in the pleura, a red rubber catheter can be placed in the defect. The wound can be closed tightly with gentle suction on the red rubber catheter. Once the wound is closed, the red rubber catheter can be removed, because the lung is fully expanded. If the underlying lung parenchyma is injured, chest tube insertion will be necessary and placed to low wall suction.

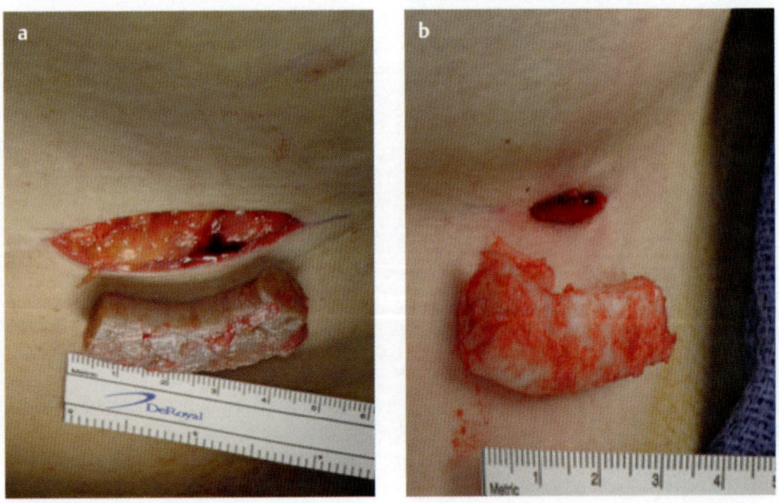

Fig. 18.4 Incision for costal cartilage harvest. **(a)** Novice surgeons should begin with a 4 to 5 cm incision to obtain a 3 to 4 cm segment of cartilage. **(b)** As one gains experience harvesting costal cartilage, one may be able to obtain the same size piece of cartilage through a 1 to 2 cm incision.

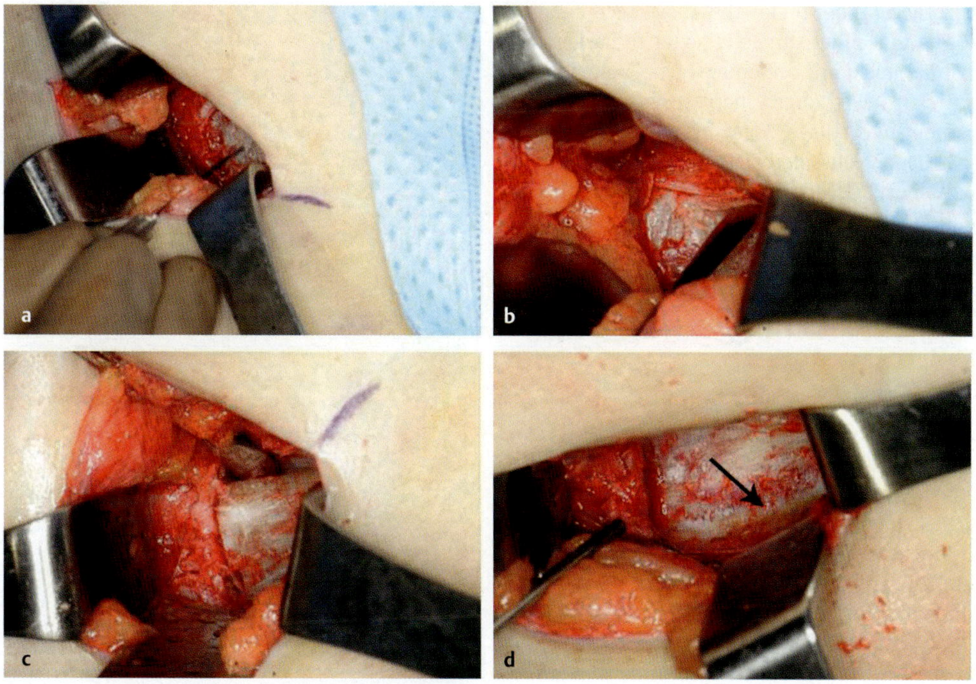

Fig. 18.5 Key steps in costal cartilage harvest. **(a)** A needle is used to further confirm the segment of cartilage to be harvested after skin, fat, and muscle have been retracted. **(b)** After the perichondrium has been harvested from the top side of the rib, the Freer elevator is used to cut into the rib to ensure the proper subperichondrial plane when dissection continues from the lateral edge onto the superior surface. **(c)** A side-to-side sweeping or lifting motion is used on the undersurface of the rib to carefully free it from the deep layer of perichondrium. **(d)** Deep layer of intact perichondrium can be visualized. Also note the thin rim of cartilage (*arrow*) along the inferior margin left behind to ensure a subperichondrial plane was maintained when transitioning from the inferior edge to the deep surface of the rib.

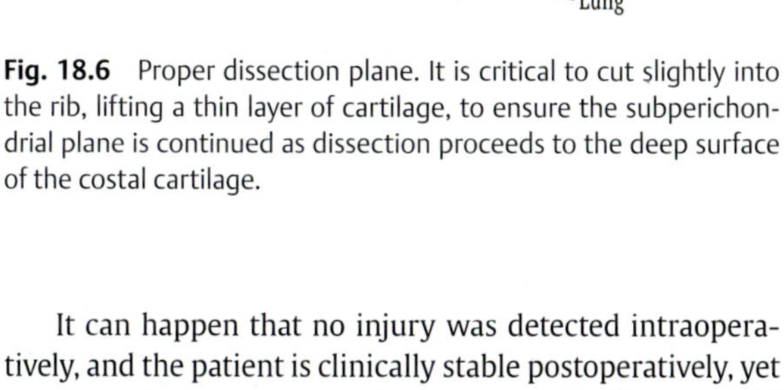

Fig. 18.6 Proper dissection plane. It is critical to cut slightly into the rib, lifting a thin layer of cartilage, to ensure the subperichondrial plane is continued as dissection proceeds to the deep surface of the costal cartilage.

It can happen that no injury was detected intraoperatively, and the patient is clinically stable postoperatively, yet a pneumothorax is seen on the postoperative film. It would be wise to consider consultation with a thoracic surgery or pulmonology team, but often such patients can be managed with supplemental oxygen and observation, as long as serial X-rays show improvement and the patient remains asymptomatic. Some surgeons have described intraoperative use of ultrasound to aid in detection of pneumothorax, but the senior author has not had experience with this technique.[12]

Antibiotic-soaked gauze is placed over the open chest wound and attention is turned to carving the cartilage and the nasal portion of the operation. The wound is left open in the event that more cartilage or more perichondrium is needed. Once the nasal portion of the operation is completed, the chest wound is again irrigated and closure is begun after the surgeon has changed gloves to avoid contamination of the chest with nasal flora. Next, 3–0 PDS suture is used to reapproximate the muscle edges and overlying fascia. Care is taken to repair the fascia separately to avoid an artificial tethering effect, because there is a natural glide plane between the fascia and overlying fat. The dead space in the subcutaneous fat is then reduced with several interrupted 4–0 PDS sutures. Interrupted 5–0 PDS deep dermal sutures approximate the wound edges and 5–0 fast-absorbing gut suture is then used to slightly evert the skin. A cyanoacrylate adhesive is routinely used to seal the wound and to provide extra strength to the mobile area while it is healing. Silastic sheeting is also utilized postoperatively, once the glue has fallen off, to further reduce the visibility of the scar.

Although the authors prefer the above techniques, it is worth noting that other surgeons prefer to harvest in a different manner, including obtaining partial anterior/posterior thickness using a gouge,[13] harvesting only a central isolated segment of cartilage,[14] leaving an inferior strip of preserved cartilage,[15] left-sided dissection using a rib stripper,[6] transumbilical endoscopic harvest of the eighth rib,[16] taking a floating (eleventh) rib,[17] or harvesting an osseocartilaginous graft.[18]

18.3.2 Costal Cartilage Carving and Grafting Techniques

The inexperienced surgeon may be primarily concerned about the harvest of the costal cartilage. The difficulty in mastering the use of costal cartilage however, is the preparation and placement of the grafts to avoid warping or deformity. Improper selection, carving, or fixation of the cartilage grafts could potentially create more unsightly deformity than any deficiency one is trying to repair.

Before any cuts are made in the harvested segment of cartilage, the surgeon should take the time to resurvey exactly what grafts may be needed. Most often it is advantageous to open the nose before harvesting the costal cartilage, to get a better idea of what type and size grafts will be necessary. If the costal cartilage was harvested first, it should be allowed to soak until the nasal cartilages are exposed. Allowing the cartilage to soak in saline, then partially air dry, and repeating this cycle several times throughout the operation will enable the cartilage to declare its tendency to warp. The surgeon is then able to use the bending to advantage, rather than quickly placing grafts inside the nose and discovering the warping tendency postoperatively.

Age should again factor into how the surgeon begins to carve the cartilage, keeping in mind that, although the perichondrium has been completely removed, there is still obvious heterogeneity in the cartilage segment. The outer portions of cartilage will have a much whiter appearance. This outer portion has a significant fibrous component and will be much more prone to warping in younger cartilage, and thus should be used with caution **(Fig. 18.7)**. In elderly, brittle cartilage, the outer whiter fibrous portion is quite valuable, however, as it has a more elastic quality and will be less prone to fracture when stress is applied to the graft. Overall, younger cartilage is much whiter than the yellow/brown cartilage seen as the patient ages **(Fig. 18.8)**.

One of the keys to successful costal cartilage grafting is to carve sequentially, allowing segments to declare the direction in which they are going to curve. The first step for typical grafting is to use a no. 10 blade to cut the harvested segment into three pieces along the two longest axes (an anterior superficial slice, a middle slice, and a posterior deep slice) **(Fig. 18.9)**. The three pieces can be further thinned and used for different grafts. The central piece will usually bend less than the peripheral pieces, but again may be weaker in older patients.[19,20] Other devices for cutting cartilage have been described, but can be ineffective if the cartilage is not symmetrical.[21]

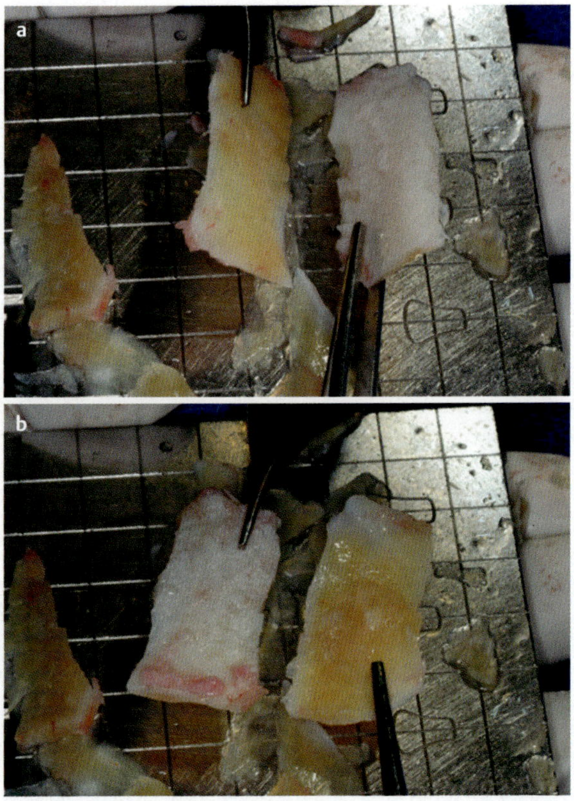

Fig. 18.7 Heterogeneity of costal cartilage grafts. **(a)** Two very nearly identical grafting segments with the outer fibrous component facing toward the surgeon in the right-most graft, and away from the surgeon in the left-most graft. **(b)** The grafts are both flipped to allow the reader to examine their opposite sides.

There are effective strategies to increase or decrease the degree of curvature in costal cartilage grafts **(Fig. 18.10)**. Curvature of a graft can be weakened/decreased by crosshatching its concave side. Two curved grafts can be manipulated in this manner, and then sewn together with their concave surfaces opposing one another to create a straight graft. Splinting grafts in this fashion can be a powerful technique. It cannot be overemphasized that sequential carving interrupted by soaking and drying segments of cartilage will, over the course of less than 1 hour, allow the bending of the cartilage to declare itself. In older patients, the cartilage is much less likely to warp, but it is unfortunately

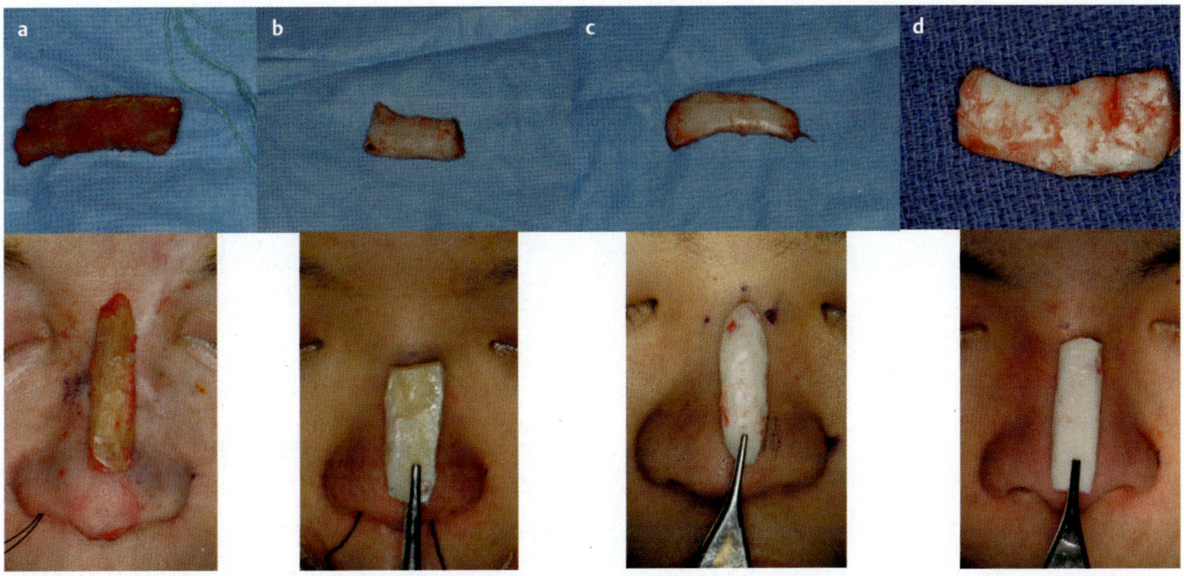

Fig. 18.8 Rib characterization correlated with age. Less yellow calcification can be seen as age decreases, as demonstrated with **(a)** 55-, **(b)** 33-, **(c)** 23-, and **(d)** 19-year-old cartilage.

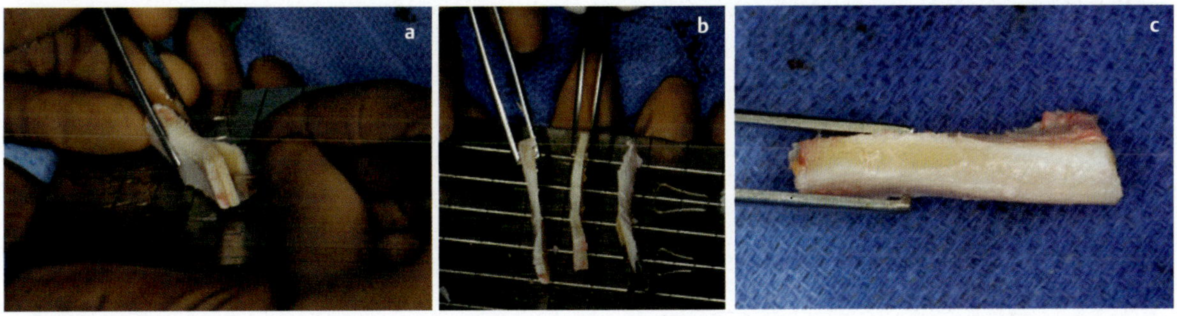

Fig. 18.9 Carving rib cartilage. **(a)** The segment should be divided into three pieces, based on the grafts needed. **(b)** The segments can be further carved for grafting. **(c)** This segment demonstrates why cookie-cutter type devices may not work well with the natural irregularities of costal cartilage.

less pliable and more likely to fracture if cut into thin segments due to brittleness and calcification. Cross-hatching and splinting are especially important in younger cartilage with a higher likelihood of warping. Similar to splinting, lamination of multiple thin grafts to form the required size of graft, rather than one single piece, can also be used to prevent warping.[22,23]

With an abundance of cartilage at the surgeon's disposal, the question often arises about how to adequately size the nose. The natural tendency with a large piece of cartilage is to make the nose too large or too wide. Over the last 10 years, the senior author has taken detailed measurements of all grafts placed in the nose.[24] This has allowed the development of a range of measurements to provide more objectivity to appropriately determine nasal size based on gender and skin thickness. It also allows confirmation of what visually and subjectively appears appropriate. The advantage of costal cartilage over other sources is that it can be cut thin, but grafts less than 1 mm thick can have a tendency to torque.

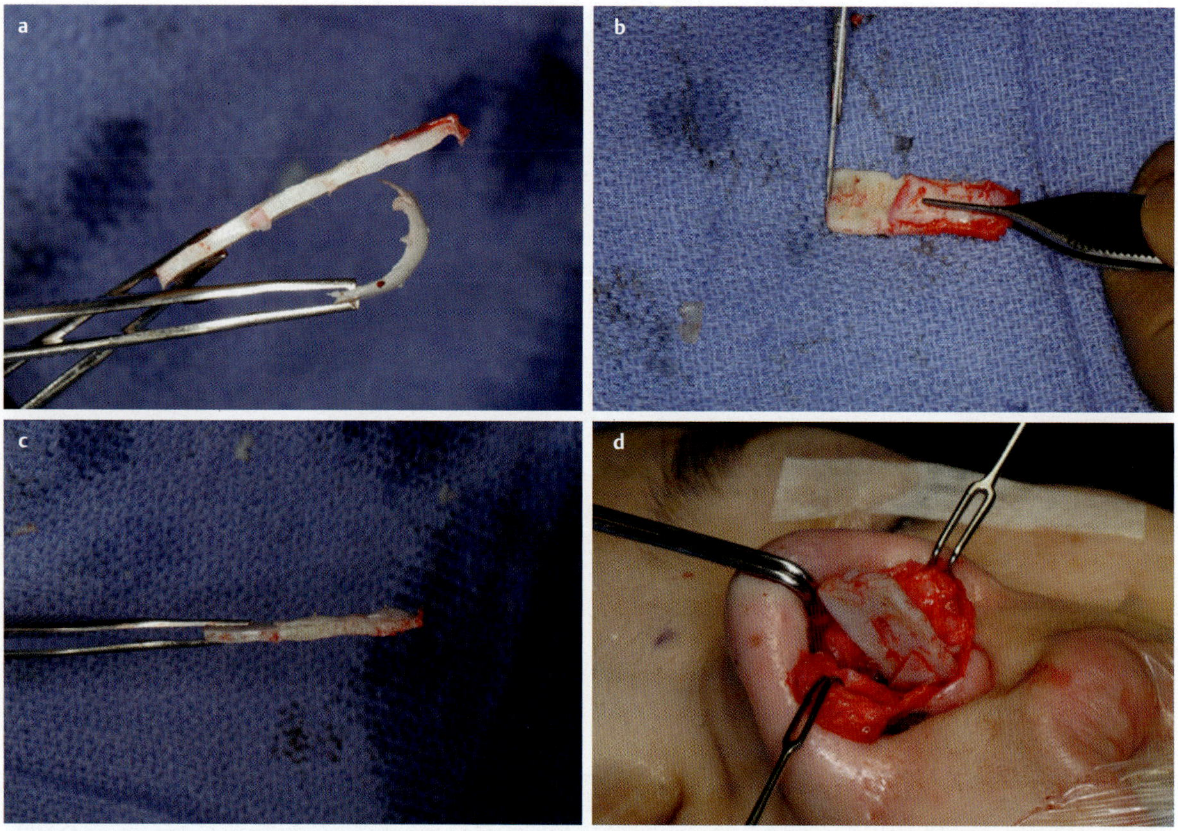

Fig. 18.10 Cartilage straightening techniques. **(a)** Slightly curved segment of costal cartilage with a sliver of cartilage to be used as a splinting graft. **(b)** The concave side of the graft is cross-hatched perpendicular to the direction of bending desired. **(c)** Splinting graft sewn in place against the concave/cross-hatched surface with PDS suture, now showing a straight graft. **(d)** Cartilage in place as a caudal septal replacement graft; this must be a straight graft or the nasal tip may deviate.

Opening the Nose

The authors find general anesthetic with endotracheal intubation most appropriate for cases involving rib harvest, time needed for autologous graft carving, and airway protection from blood and secretions with significant septal or turbinate work. Most often, structural rhinoplasty involving cartilage grafting is performed in the standard external approach. Preoperative injection of 1% lidocaine with 1:100,000 epinephrine in the standard fashion should be performed before prepping and draping in order for optimal vasoconstriction to take place. Rather than unmindful injection into the septum, as the surgeon uses hydrostatic dissection to begin elevating the mucoperichondrial flaps, he or she should be concomitantly sizing the cartilaginous versus bony components of the septum and begin formulating the amount of available cartilage for grafting.

Standard inverted-V incision is made across the columella (no. 11 blade), with special attention paid to where the incision will be located at the end of the operation (i.e., if the nose is de-projected by setting the base posteriorly, incise closer to the tip lobule, or, if the nose is to be projected, plan for an incision caudal to the standard midcolumellar incision). Bilateral marginal incisions should then be performed and connected to the extension of the columellar incision (no. 15 blade). Sharp dissection (Converse scissors) preserves the subdermal plexus to the delicate skin of the columella and tip, and may maximize vascularity and avoid the excessive swelling associated with broad spreading and tearing of the tissue with blunt dissection. Care should be taken to avoid injury to the soft tissue triangles, as damage to this area is difficult to repair. Three-point retraction by one or two assistants with sharp two-prongs aids significantly in dissection. Identification of the lower lateral cartilages is followed by exposure of the cartilaginous dorsum. Elevation of the periosteum over the nasal bones should then be performed (Joseph elevator) in a very calculated manner. When performing dorsal augmentation, it is critical to make a narrow, limited, midline subperiosteal dissection that will allow placement of the dorsal graft into a snug subperiosteal space that will hold the dorsal graft in midline position firmly against the bony dorsum. This is critical to enhancing fixation of the dorsal graft to the bone. Most often, septoplasty should be initiated next, either by a separate Killian incision, or with lateral retraction of the lower lateral cartilages and identification of the anterior septal angle. Bilateral mucoperichondrial flaps can be raised, leaving a strong cartilaginous L-strut to give long-term support.

Management of the Bony Vault

Creating a natural dorsum is one of the most difficult tasks in rhinoplasty. Management of the bony vault can be just as important as any dorsal augmentation. Although it is counterintuitive, if the surgeon's plan is to augment the nasal dorsum with an onlay graft, the nasal bones should not be narrowed with osteotomies unless they are deviated. This allows a wide-to-narrow tapering shape in the axial plane. If the bones are moved medially, it creates an unnatural narrow-to-narrow tubular look at the bridge of the nose. The tubular appearance creates unfavorable shadowing and obvious disruption of the brow–tip aesthetic lines.[25] If, however, no dorsal augmentation is planned, osteotomies may then be indicated to narrow the nose. The surgeon should always keep in mind his plans for changing the width of the tip and middle vault so that the nose remains in balance. Of course, certain osteotomies may be necessary to correct deviations in a crooked nose when comparing the upper third to the nasal base.

Management of the Nasal Base

After alignment of the bony vault, attention should be turned to the nasal base. Failure to recognize and discuss facial asymmetry with the patient preoperatively can often result in the surgeon's having to offer explanations for why a straight nose may still appear deviated postoperatively. Scrupulous physical examination and study of photographs can identify these and other deviations of the caudal septum, nasal spine, dentition, or lip contour in relation to the midline glabella. The primary surgeon should consider standing at the head of the bed for the best view to evaluate symmetry.

Often the nasal spine may need to be shifted, or a swinging-door maneuver performed to reset the midline. The nasal spine can be shifted by driving a 5-mm straight osteotome into the spine at a slight angle toward the new desired position. Once engaged in the bone, the osteotome can act as a lever to shift the spine. This will widen and move the notch. The septum or graft should be secured to the fibrous tissue lateral to the spine with two 4–0 PDS sutures. Of note, this maneuver can slightly shift the position of the septum, changing the projection and dorsal line.

Once the surgeon feels confident that the midline has been established, the next task is to stabilize the nasal base. According to alterations in projection, rotation, and length, a choice should be made among floating columellar strut, fixed/extended columellar strut, caudal septal extension graft, or caudal septal replacement graft. The authors prefer caudal septal extension or replacement grafts to prevent postoperative loss of projection, but more importantly to control rotation and length. Caudal septal extension grafts can be secured to the septum in an end-to-end fashion with extended spreader grafts and slivers of cartilage or rectangular segments of 0.25 mm PDS plate (**Fig. 18.11**). Although they are complex, caudal septal replacement grafts will often actually use less cartilage than attempting to straighten a severely damaged caudal portion of the L-strut (**Fig. 18.12**).[26] Care should be taken, because this technique requires mastery: it has the potential to simultaneously alter the tip rotation, length, and projection.

These grafts are the only cartilage segments in structural rhinoplasty that need to be completely straight.[27,28] Even if the surgeon is less worried about costal cartilage warping in an older patient, it may be wise to use any available septal cartilage for these grafts. If only curved segments of costal cartilage are available, they should be manipulated as previously described to ensure a final graft that will not warp.

If the nose is to be lengthened or the nasolabial angle is to be blunted, then the shape of the patient's smile becomes increasingly important. The changes in the nose can simultaneously alter the upper lip during the smile. Preoperative images should determine the degree to which the corners of the mouth turn up with full excursion, as this will limit the degree of change that is advisable. If the nose or nasolabial angle is moved down, as the smile goes up, the lip will likely be restricted in its upward movement and a horizontal crease may form. Even a small amount of change can create a feeling of stiffness, if not a crease, in the upper lip, and so honest preoperative discussion of this potential with the patient is necessary.

Management of the Middle Third

After the upper and lower thirds of the nose have been straightened and stabilized, the middle third can then be managed appropriate to the needs of the individual patient. The use of spreader grafts is a powerful technique to increase the area of the internal nasal valve. Spreader grafts can be placed in the traditional manner (between divided upper lateral cartilages and septum) or in a submucosal pocket without cartilage division to cantilever the upper lateral cartilage and to increase valve angle (**Fig. 18.13**). Preemptive division of the upper lateral cartilage from the septum may result in unnecessary operative

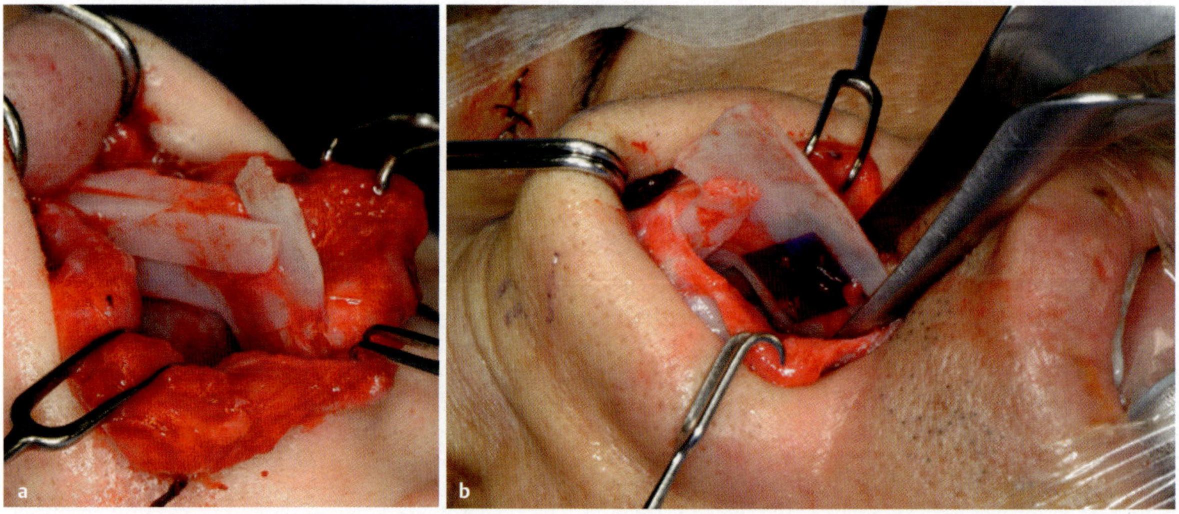

Fig. 18.11 Caudal septal extension grafts. Caudal septal extension grafts can be secured bilaterally with extended spreader grafts and **(a)** slivers of cartilage or **(b)** PDS plates in cartilage-deplete cases.

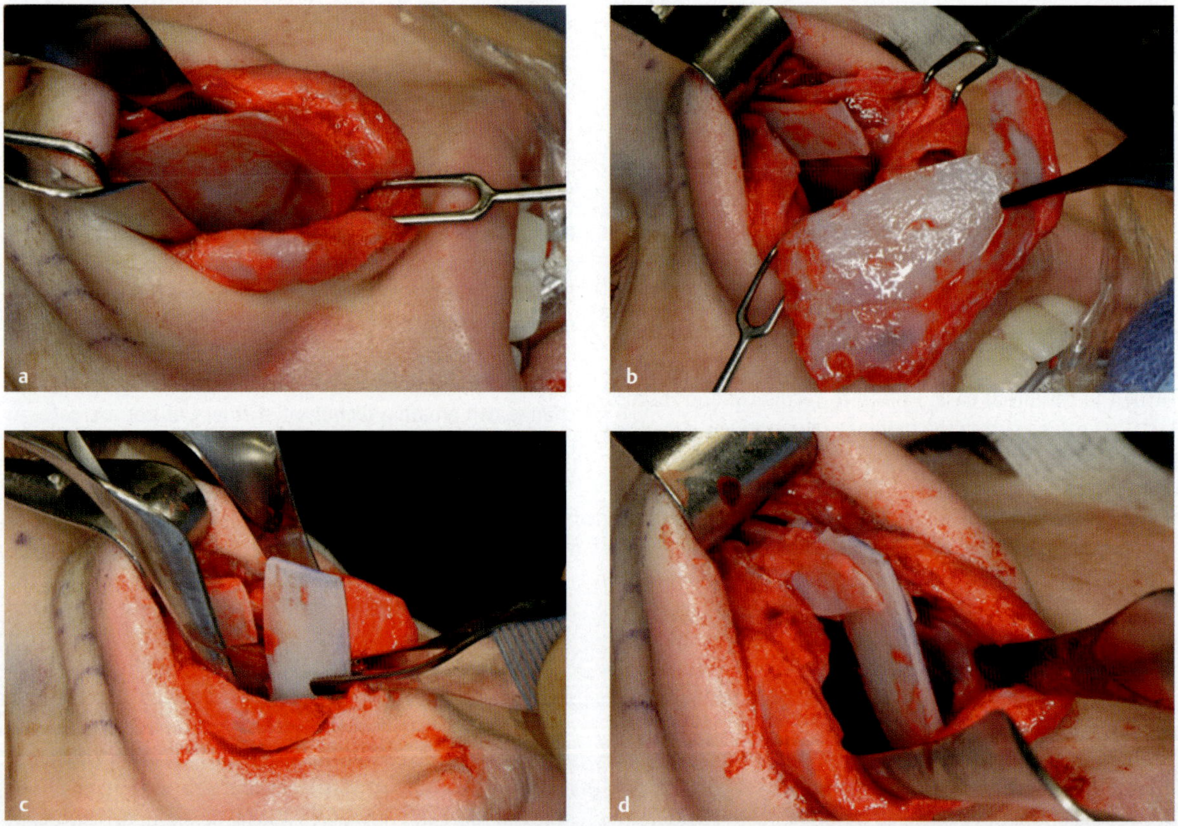

Fig. 18.12 Caudal septal replacement graft. **(a)** Severely deviated septum involving what would be the caudal segment of the L-strut. **(b)** Deviated septum removed, leaving only the dorsal strut. **(c)** Caudal septal replacement graft position determined. **(d)** Graft secured bilaterally with extended spreader grafts cephalically, and 4–0 PDS suture caudally to the nasal spine.

time in reconstructing the middle nasal vault to avoid palpable or visible deformity if onlay grafting is not to be utilized. Either method of spreader grafting can provide a robust foundation to prevent saddling and to prevent postoperative rotation/shortening. If an increase in projection is planned, postoperative rotation and shortening can be a real problem if not prevented.

Depending on the strength of the L-strut before spreader graft placement, spreader grafts can be fashioned from less desirable cartilage stock. If a saddle or weak dorsal septal strut is being reconstructed, then obviously significant emphasis must be placed on stronger, straighter grafts. If a strong L-strut exists, then spreader grafts can have some curvature because they are going to be buried in the nose. The best strategy in this situation is to use the concave sides medially; the opposing spreader grafts sutured to the septum should keep the nose straight.[29] Placing two curved spreader grafts with their concave sides parallel to one another to compensate for a crooked L-strut can be a dangerous strategy, should the curvature be accentuated by further warping postoperatively. However, there are some situations in which the configuration of the middle and lower thirds could make this strategy advantageous if it is carefully executed. The length of spreader grafts can vary considerably, depending on their function (20–40 mm). Often, extension cephalically underneath the caudal edge of an out-fractured nasal bone can stabilize the new position and prevent postoperative shift. Spreaders should be 4 to 6 mm wide in most situations. Thickness can also vary, but a standard range is 1 to 3 mm.

During the operation, the surgeon can expect to encounter some degree of swelling, no matter how smooth the dissection technique. Palpation up and down the lateral sidewalls of the nose can give a better indication of symmetry than relying on appearance alone. Often an additional or multiple additional unilateral spreader grafts may

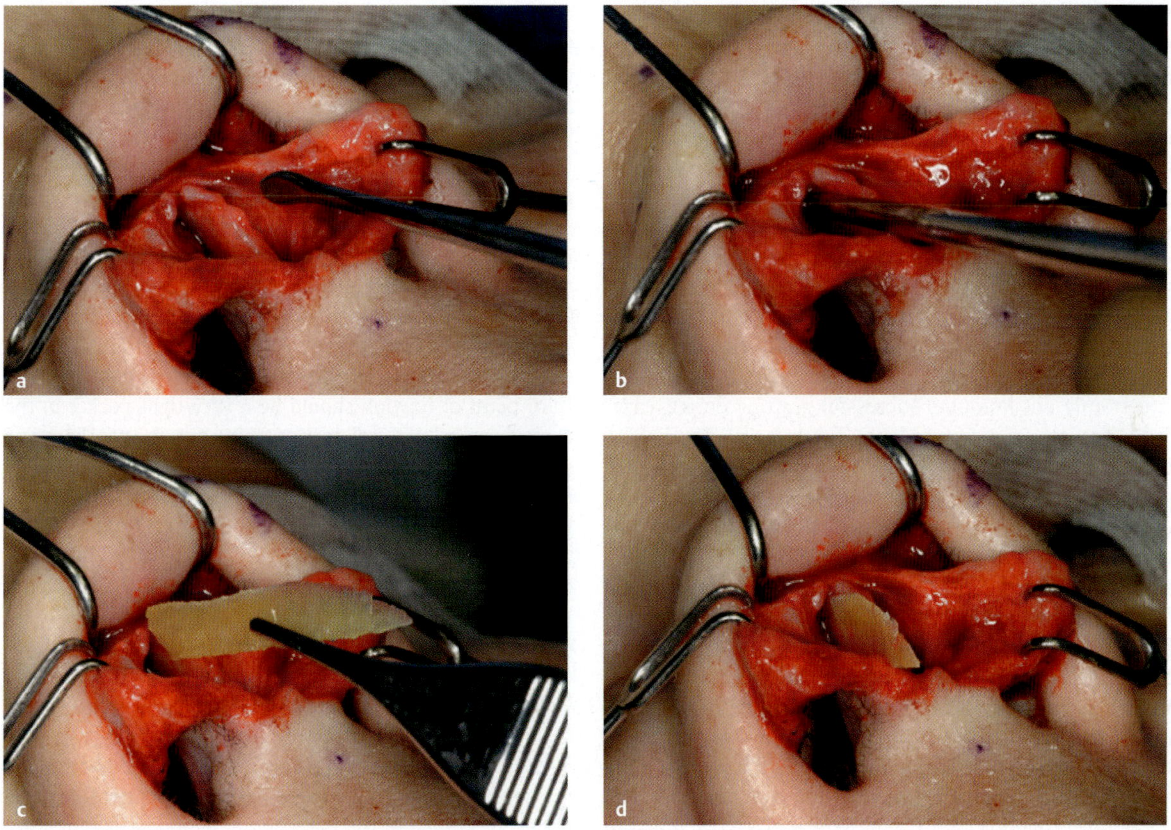

Fig. 18.13 Submucosal spreader technique. **(a)** When raising mucoperichondrial flaps during septoplasty, the surgeon must leave an undissected area along the dorsal strut. **(b)** Cottle elevator is then inserted in the subperichondrial space of the undissected region to form a tight pocket at the junction of the upper lateral cartilage and septal cartilage. **(c)** Cartilage graft is sized, and it can be lengthened to form an extended spreader graft if desired. **(d)** Extended spreader in place to cantilever the upper lateral cartilage and increase internal valve angle.

be necessary to straighten the nose. The surgeon should realize he is not limited with a spreader graft to widening the middle vault in its entirety. A spreader graft can span only a portion of the distance from the cephalic aspect of the upper lateral cartilage to the anterior septal angle, to create a favorable brow–tip aesthetic line. Care should also be given to preoperative recognition of a concave lateral sidewall, as often this should be augmented with an onlay graft or a batten graft. No matter what type of grafting is employed in the middle third, securing the upper lateral cartilages to the septum is a priority to avoid an inverted-V deformity or pinching of the internal valve over time. If there is still residual tilting of the nose and width has been properly determined, an asymmetrical clocking suture can align the crooked nose into a straight configuration.[30]

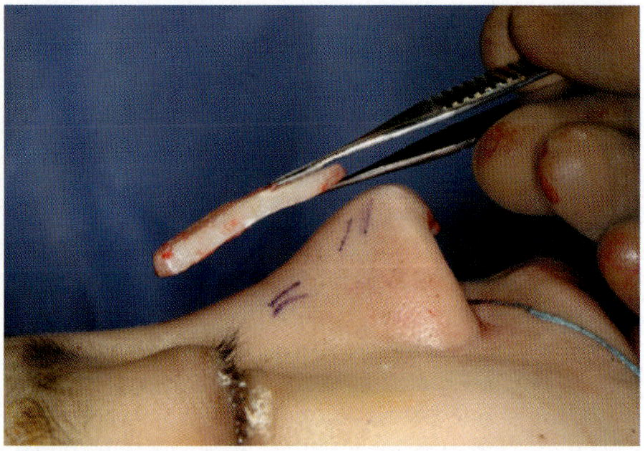

Fig. 18.14 Dorsal graft orientation. Surgeon should plan to place concave surface against the dorsum to allow contraction during the healing phases to oppose this force. If the graft is placed with the convex surface facing the dorsum, there can be continued warping of the cartilage, resulting in unwanted fullness in the radix and supratip.

Dorsal Grafting

Dorsal grafting is perhaps the most complex of any, due to its inability to tolerate any visible edges or even the slightest degree of warping postoperatively. Septal cartilage is an excellent choice if the degree of augmentation required is small, as this stock is the least likely to warp. Auricular cartilage is less desirable due to its inherent contour irregularities. It also has a tendency to resorb postoperatively if stacked, due to its increased vascular demand. If more augmentation is desired than there is septal cartilage available, costal cartilage should be used. If a longer dorsal graft is needed the seventh rib is preferred. The sixth rib has a genu and a long straight dorsal graft may not be possible. Long, rectangular sections of rib will have a natural curve, and the surgeon is foolish if he believes he will be able to carve it into a straight segment. Much has been written regarding strategies for successful carving.[19,20,31,32] Although the central core may be less prone to warping, it is certainly not immune. Successful grafting entails carving segments in a fashion that controls the bending to the advantage of the surgeon. The segment of costal cartilage chosen for a dorsal graft should be slowly carved over a period of time, taking down all sides until the cartilage has declared itself to curve in a definitive direction. Once the concave surface can be identified, the surgeon should plan to place this side against the nasal dorsum **(Fig. 18.14)**. Placement of the dorsal graft into the tight subperiosteal pocket will act against the tendency of the curved dorsal graft to lift away from the bone. Other maneuvers to enhance fixation will also counteract the tendency for the curved dorsal graft to lift away from the bone. The canoe-shaped graft can then be tapered to form a smooth transition into the radix/glabella as well as the supratip/tip. The width of the graft will vary according to the needs in creating a smooth brow–tip aesthetic line.

Another key to successfully using costal cartilage for dorsal augmentation is to rigidly fixate the graft.[33] If the graft has a tendency to warp and is not fixated, it will most certainly warp. If it is tightly fixated to the bony dorsum, however, these forces should outweigh the force needed to cause postoperative warping. Again, intraoperative cycling between incremental carving and soaking and drying of the cartilage is recommended. Attention can be turned back to the nose while waiting for the cartilage to soak/dry. The dorsal graft in the primary rhinoplasty patient should be secured with a three-point fixation strategy. Two lower/lateral points of fixation can be accomplished with interrupted 5–0 PDS sutures through the graft and through the edge of the upper lateral cartilage and/or spreader grafts. Care must be taken not to cut the sides of the graft with the cutting needles, as this is in effect cross-hatching. The third point of fixation should be a very tight pocket in the cephalic aspect of the dissection cavity over the nasal dorsum **(Fig. 18.15)**. Care must be taken to avoid wide subperiosteal dissection in this area to prevent a mobile graft. Mobility can be further inhibited by encouraging firm fixation/integration to the native bony dorsum. This can be achieved by one of two techniques. One way is to use a 2 mm straight osteotome to make 8 to 10 vertical perforations in the nasal bones **(Fig. 18.16)**. The second method would be to slightly lower the dorsum with a fine-toothed rasp. The key is to create a violation of the native cortical bone and to interpose a segment of perichondrium between it and the cartilage graft to form an osseous integration of graft to dorsum. Either method is a good choice in the primary rhinoplasty patient depending on the shape of the native dorsum and graft in respect to the final shape you wish to achieve. There is a need to underscore the importance of placing an interposed segment of perichondrium between the graft and the native dorsum to ensure firm integration of the graft and to prevent warping or mobility **(Fig. 18.17)**. Significant time should be taken

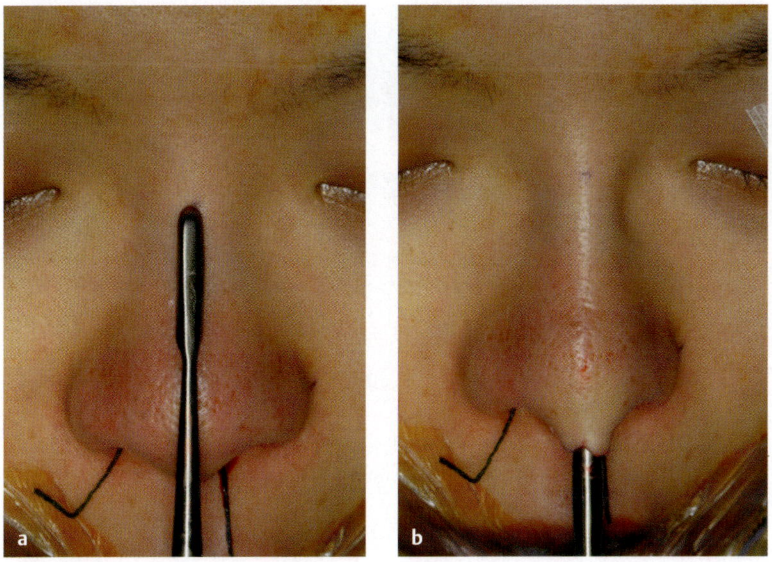

Fig. 18.15 Dissection for dorsal grafting. **(a)** When opening the nose in the external rhinoplasty approach, the surgeon will often use the Joseph periosteal elevator to dissect the upper third of the nose. **(b)** Anticipation of the potential need for a dorsal graft is necessary to avoid overly wide dissection at this level. If a tight subperiostial pocket is created, no suturing or K-wire is necessary to secure the cephalic aspect of cartilage graft.

to smooth all edges of the graft. Often if there is remaining perichondrium it should not be discarded, but consideration could be given to using it to help camouflage the transition of the sidewall of these or other grafts **(Fig. 18.18)**.

Although outside the scope of this chapter, in revision rhinoplasty where a misplaced, mobile, infected, extruded, or warped dorsal graft or implant requires removal, the surgeon will often find himself left with a large dissection pocket. If the rhinoplasty surgeon in the primary setting inadvertently dissects too widely across the upper dorsum, he may find himself in the same situation. Establishing the third point of fixation in these instances becomes much more complex, but it can also be accomplished with one of two techniques. The first is placing a temporary threaded 0.45 K-wire (Kirschner wire) drilled through the graft and nasal bones, to be removed on the seventh postoperative day with the nasal cast **(Fig. 18.19)**. The second method of fixation is to use a suture passed through tiny stab incisions on the dorsum over the graft, and under the graft through holes drilled in the nasal bones with a 16 gauge needle **(Fig. 18.20)**. If the dorsal graft is a thin graft, then it may not be amenable to K-wire fixation, as it must be thick enough for the threads of the wire to engage the graft.

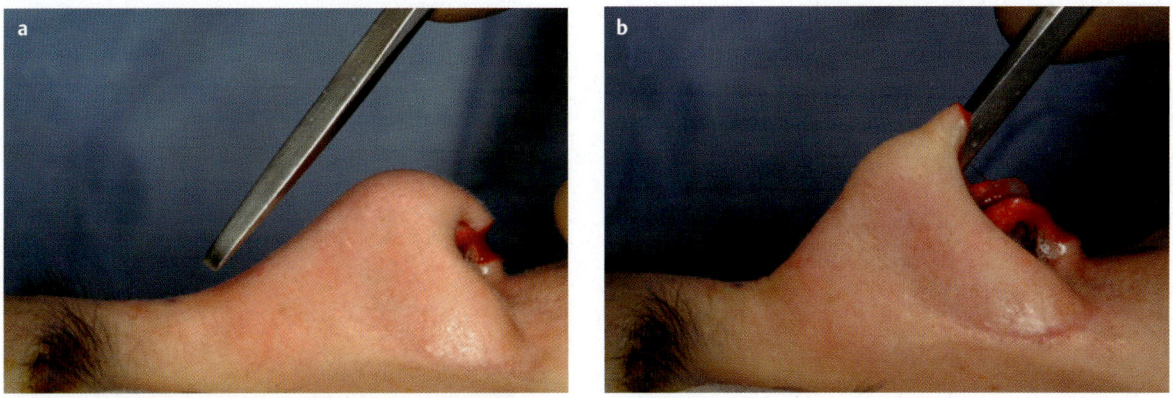

Fig. 18.16 Preparation for dorsal grafting. **(a)** Cephalic limit of dissection should be determined for graft placement. **(b)** Two millimeter osteotome can be used in a vertical fashion to violate the smooth cortical bone in 8–10 locations to create firm fixation of the interposed perichondrium graft to both the onlay cartilage graft and the native bony dorsum.

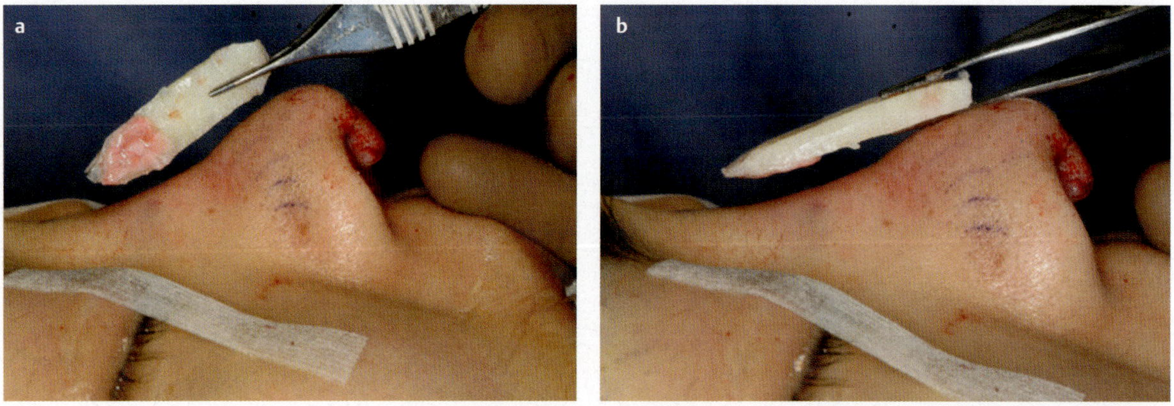

Fig. 18.17 Dorsal graft integration strategy. **(a)** Dorsal onlay cartilage graft rotated 90 degrees to visualize perichondrium sewn to cephalic undersurface. **(b)** Proper orientation of dorsal graft. The dorsal graft seen here will be firmly integrated as the perichondrial graft integrates to the cartilage graft and native dorsum.

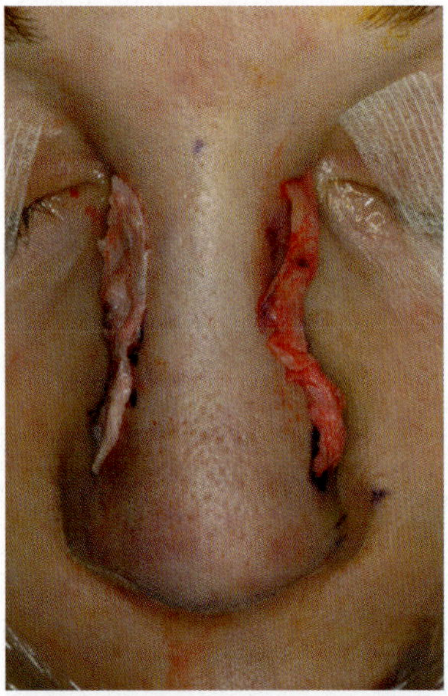

Fig. 18.18 Dorsal graft camouflage. Strips of perichondrium seen here prior to placement lateral to the edges of a dorsal onlay cartilage graft. This design may help smooth the transition between the graft and native lateral sidewall subunits.

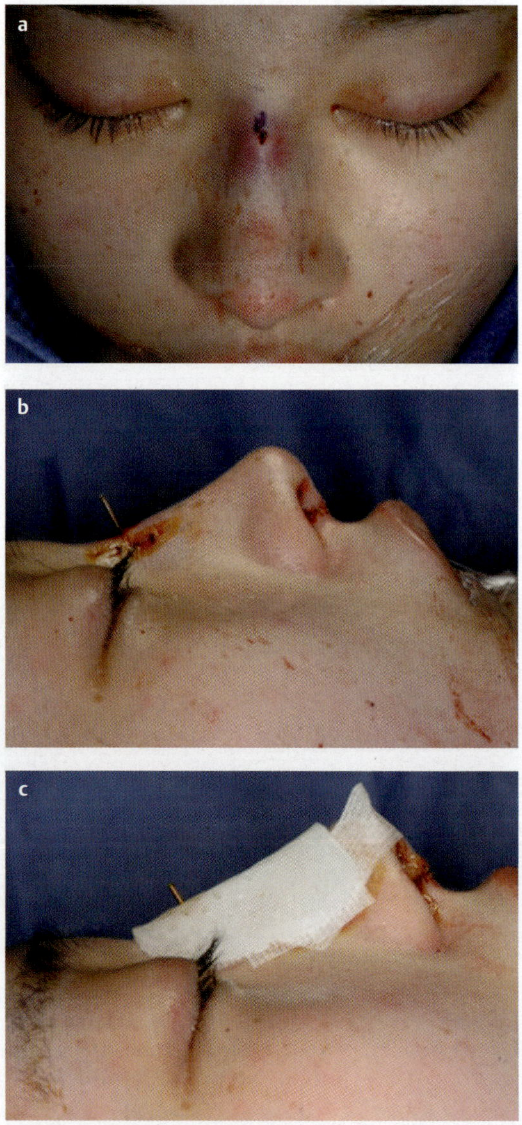

Fig. 18.19 Kirschner wire fixation. **(a)** Frontal and **(b)** lateral views of a temporary threaded K-wire placed at the completion of dorsal onlay cartilage grafting in a case where the creation of a tight cephalic soft tissue/skin pocket was not possible. **(c)** K-wire passed through existing perforation in cast.

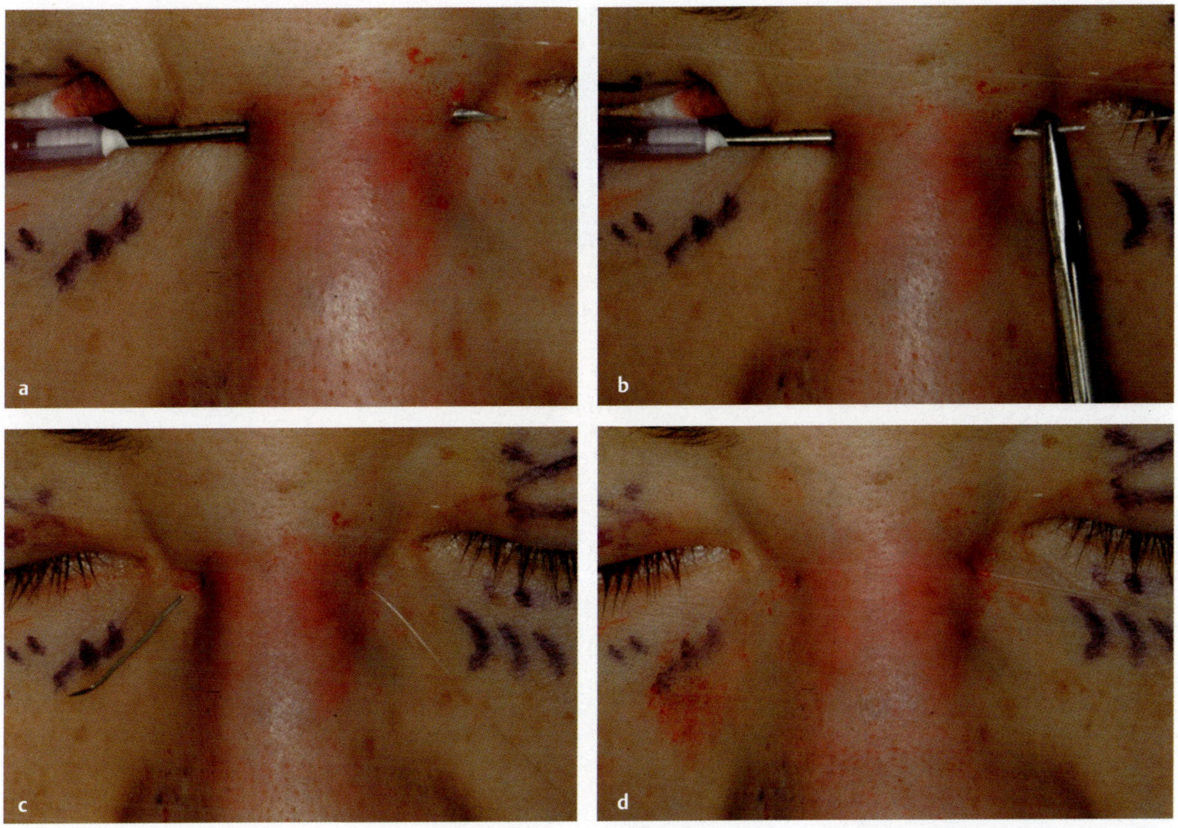

Fig. 18.20 Suture method for dorsal graft fixation. Thin dorsal onlay cartilage grafts may require elaborate suture techniques to adequately secure if a tight pocket does not exist. **(a)** Tiny stab incision made with no. 11 blade on bilateral dorsal skin, and 16 gauge needle drilled through skin, nasal bones, and septum. **(b)** PDS suture on a manually straightened P-3 sewing needle inserted into bore of 16 gauge needle. **(c)** Needles both pulled through in a retrograde fashion, thus looping suture below dorsal graft. **(d)** Second pass of suture initiated back through the existing skin incision, guided superficial to dorsal cartilage graft but deep to skin–soft tissue envelope (S-STE), and through opposite skin incision. The suture is then tied in an external manner, but the surgeon should ensure the knot is beneath the S-STE.

Tip Contouring

Extensive discussion regarding all the components of the nasal tip is beyond the scope of this chapter, but one of the key steps to completing a successful rhinoplasty is creating favorable tip contour.[34] Before successful manipulation of the lower lateral cartilages is undertaken, understanding the shape one is trying to achieve to attain desirable highlights and shadowing must first be mastered. Only then can the surgeon begin to correlate changes to the cartilage with changes to the appearance of the contour of the tip skin once it has been draped over these structures.

Beginning with a stable nasal base will allow the lower lateral cartilage to be secured in maneuvers that can alter length, rotation, and projection. A variety of techniques can then be used to alter tip shape, including grafting, excision, suturing, and repositioning. Most grafts in the lower third of the nose will tolerate, and actually benefit from, slight concavity/convexity. Tip work should begin by preliminarily securing the medial crura to the septal extension or replacement graft with a 4–0 plain gut suture on a Keith needle. If the surgeon is pleased with this position, several 5–0 PDS sutures should be used to further secure the medial and intermediate crura. The lateral crura of the lower lateral cartilages should next be examined, and the skin thickness should be considered to determine how aggressively projection should be increased to achieve the desired refinement in the tip.

Often in the Asian patient the lateral crura are small and weak, combined with thick, sebaceous skin and hanging alar lobules. In these patients, the tip can be augmented and strengthened with the combination of a shield graft and lateral crural grafts (**Fig. 18.21**). The shield graft can be positioned higher or lower to augment the infratip and variably increase projection. The medial edges of the lateral crural grafts should be beveled at ~ 45 degrees and attached to the posterior edge of the shield graft. They will help prevent alar collapse over time and help control over-rotation,

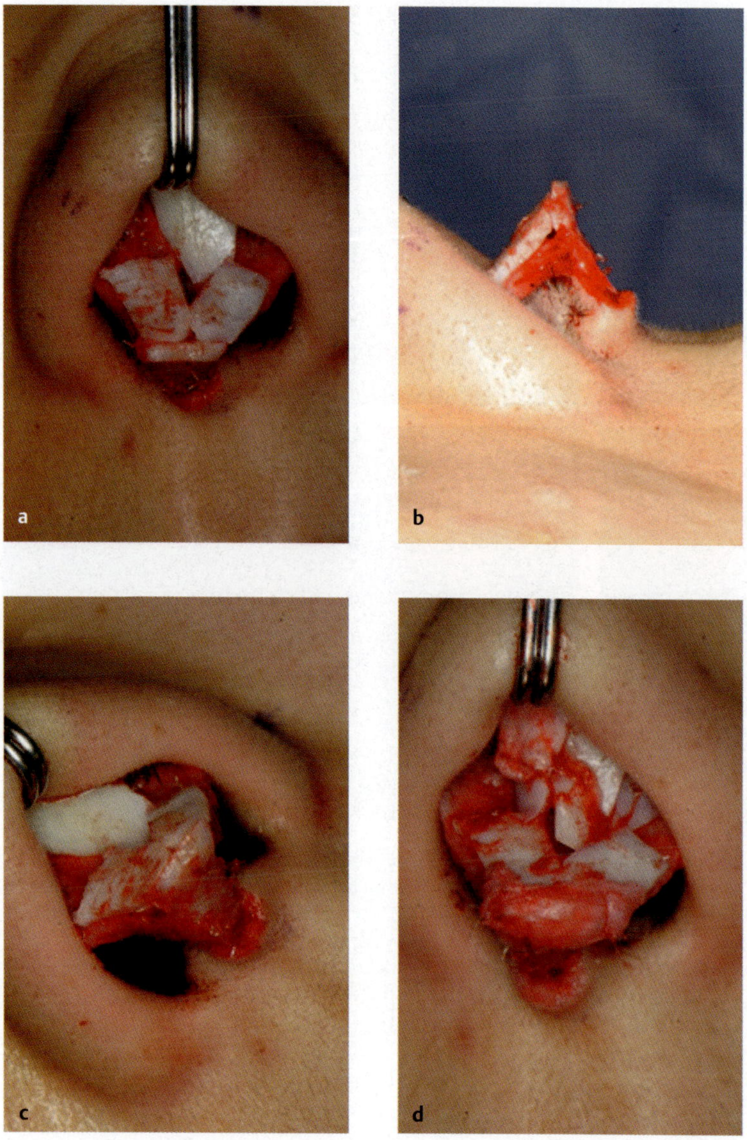

Fig. 18.21 Asian tip contouring. **(a)** Frontal, **(b)** lateral, and **(c)** three-quarter views of tip shield graft and lateral crural grafts. **(d)** Perichondrium is seen here serving to camouflage all edges of the grafts on the tip.

as the new projected shield/tip graft must overcome the contractile healing forces. They also prevent visibility of the shield graft. Even with thicker skin, it is advantageous to camouflage the leading edge of the shield graft with soft tissue, such as perichondrium. Both of these grafts can be carved from septal or costal cartilage.

If tip bulbosity is attributed to convex lateral crura, they can be flattened with lateral crural strut grafts **(Fig. 18.22)**. These grafts require the vestibular skin to be dissected from the undersurface of the native lateral crura. A pocket must then be created in the same vector as the lateral crura, extending toward the piriform aperture, long enough for the grafts to sit without bowing. This is much easier after hydrodissection by injection of 1% lidocaine with 1:100,000 epinephrine with the bevel of the needle flat against the undersurface of the cartilage. The grafts themselves should most often be carved between 25 and 30 mm × 4 to 5 mm × 1 to 2 mm. The medial edge of the graft should be beveled at a 45-degree angle and tucked as far medially into the dome as possible, with the cephalic edge close to, but not beyond, the cephalic edge of the native lateral crus. It is imperative that the graft be placed with the concavity facing the airway. If the graft is completely flat, the surgeon should beware, and either consider choosing an alternative graft or continue to carve, soak, and dry the graft until it declares the direction it is going to bend.

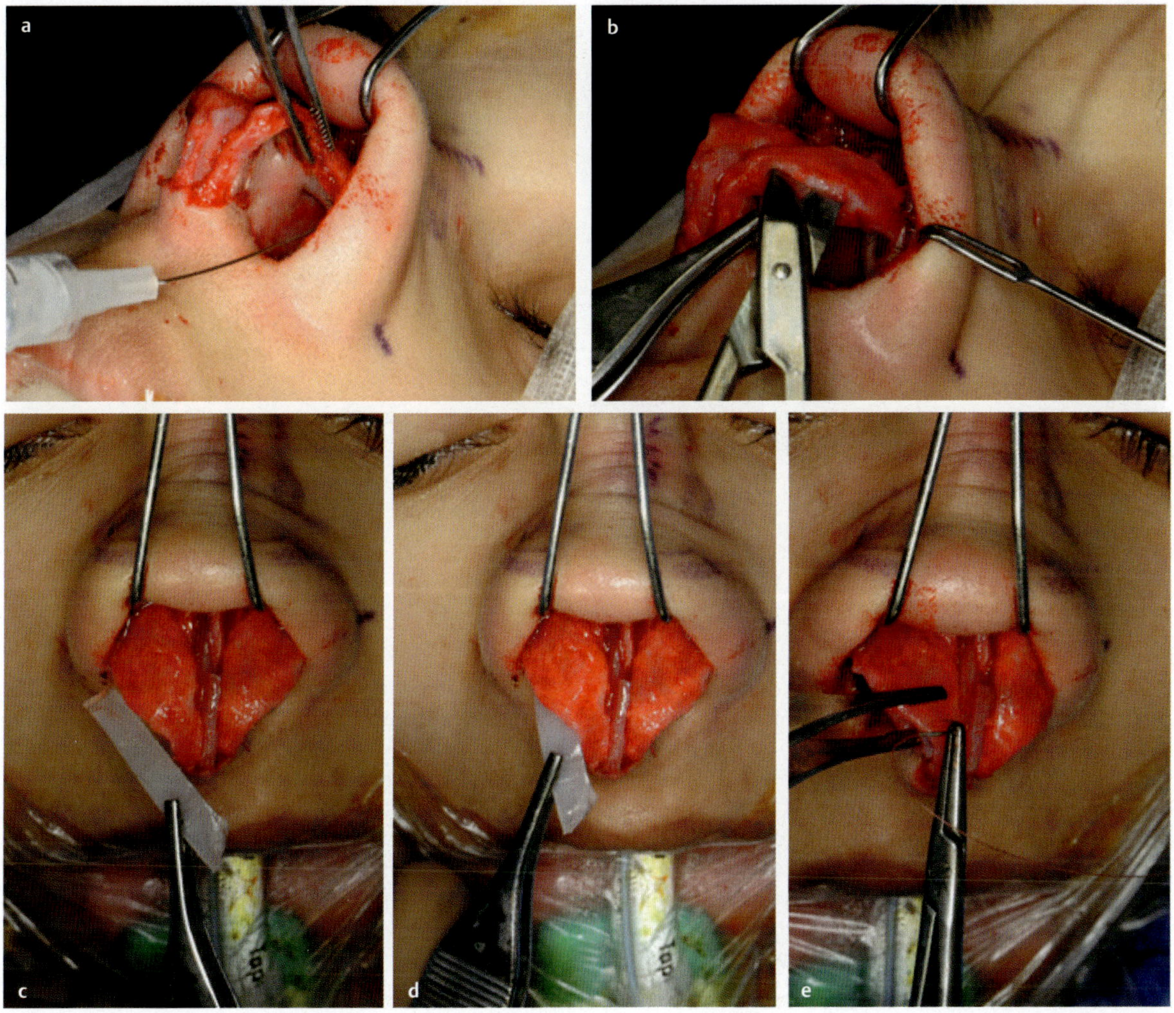

Fig. 18.22 Lateral crural strut grafts. **(a)** Hydrodissection of vestibular skin is performed with local anesthetic. **(b)** Vestibular skin is dissected free from the lateral crus of the lower lateral cartilage. **(c)** Lateral crural strut graft is carved with 45 degree bevel medially. **(d)** Graft is placed between lateral crura and vestibular skin. **(e)** Graft is sewn in place with 5–0 PDS suture.

If a straight segment is used that later warps to produce an internal convexity, it may block the airway. Grafts should be sutured to the native lateral crura with the knot placed away from the vestibular skin to avoid extrusion. The authors usually choose to also place a dome suture bilaterally to flatten the domes, and often an interdomal suture if more narrowing is required.

Depending on the ethnicity of the patient, more aggressive maneuvers may be necessary to change tip shape. Although Asian patients rarely require it, other ethnic patients may benefit from repositioning of the lateral crura (**Fig. 18.23**).[35] This can be accomplished in the same manner as placing lateral crural strut grafts described above, except once the lateral extent of the cartilage is dissected from the vestibular skin, it is divided from the soft tissue in the region of the sesamoid cartilage. The pockets for the lateral crural strut grafts can then be placed in whatever vector will be most favorable to change tip shape for that particular patient. Angling the pockets caudally can correct cephalic malposition of the lateral crura and arched or retracted alae, or bring down the lateral components of the nose to match central component lengthening. Asymmetric pockets can be created intentionally to result in symmetrical nostril final position. Repositioning can also be a powerful technique to allow change in the dome position when radical changes in tip projection are necessary.

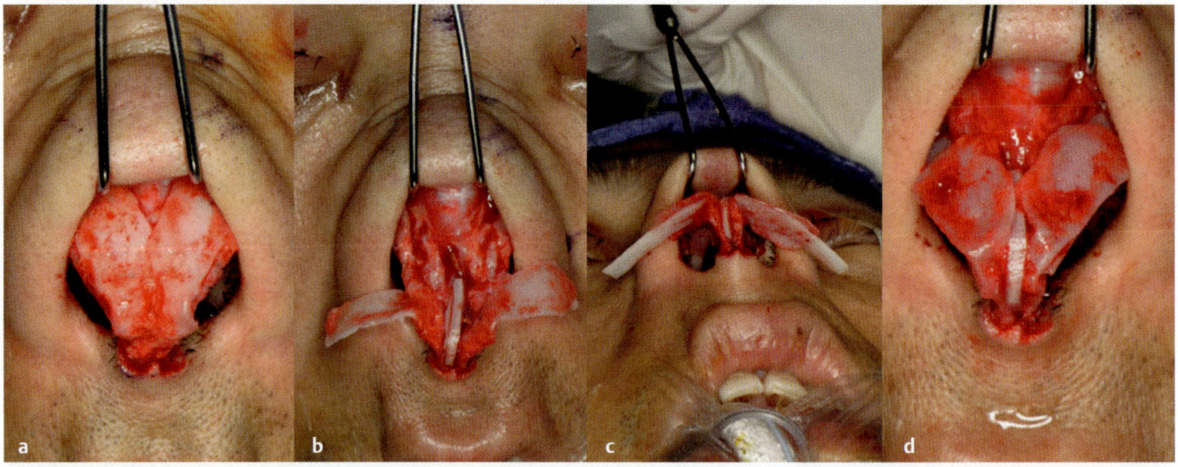

Fig. 18.23 Lateral crural strut grafts with repositioning. **(a)** Cephalic malpositioned cartilage. **(b)** Lateral crus of lower lateral cartilage has been dissected free from vestibular skin. **(c)** Lateral crural strut grafts sewn in place. **(d)** Grafts repositioned in pockets that are caudal to the original vectors of the lateral crura.

In Asian patients, this technique is most commonly used to correct alar retraction or notched ala. This technique, however, is rarely used in Asian patients because this maneuver can accentuate the hanging ala.

As an alternative to a shield graft, a rectangular tip onlay graft can be sutured horizontally across the domes if no infratip augmentation is necessary (**Fig. 18.24**). These grafts can be positioned higher or lower, with varying widths and thicknesses, to manipulate projection, tip width, and refinement, and to set supratip break. Although any cartilage can be used for this graft, often a soft piece functions best and will prevent tip bossae. An ideal piece is excess cephalic trim from the lateral crura.

Alar batten and rim grafts are usually the last grafts placed to tweak the contour of the tip complex. Alar battens can be necessary to strengthen the sidewall to avoid valve collapse if significant repositioning of the lateral crura is performed. They can also be placed to correct concavities seen on frontal view, to improve symmetry in the brow–tip aesthetic lines. They should be sutured into pockets created in precise locations. Alar rim grafts can be used to smooth the transition between tip lobule and alar lobule, to prevent dynamic external valve collapse, and to prevent pinching of the tip over time. They are especially important if the plane of the lateral crus of the lower lateral cartilages is in an unfavorable orientation (cephalic margin lies above the

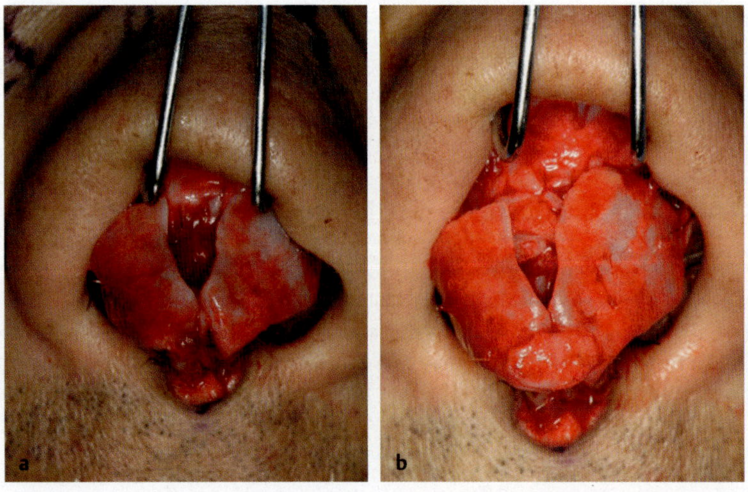

Fig. 18.24 Onlay tip grafting. **(a)** Tip structure after lateral crural strut grafts with repositioning of the lateral crura. **(b)** The tip is further refined and projection is slightly increased with rectangular tip onlay graft.

level of the caudal margin). These grafts can be placed by creating a tiny pocket just caudal to the marginal incision (**Fig. 18.25**). Both grafts can be carved from costal cartilage if necessary, but care should be taken to smooth/taper the ends to avoid graft visibility.

Keep in mind that, while it is unwise to employ a "cookie-cutter" technique to rhinoplasty in general, it is especially dangerous in the tip of the non-Caucasian nose. Powerful techniques, such as repositioning of the lateral crus of the lower lateral cartilages, may work for the flared nostril due to large, convex, cephalically oriented, lower lateral cartilages in the Middle Eastern patient, but may be contraindicated in the Asian patient with thin, weak, lower lateral cartilages and thick/fatty hanging alar lobules.

Closure

Closure should begin with a single 6–0 Monocryl suture (Ethicon, Inc.) in the midline to take the tension off the skin edges and to align the S-STE. When closing the incisions in a darker-skinned patient, absorbable sutures are not contraindicated, but they can result in prolonged erythema compared with the fair-skinned patient. Also, there is higher risk for suture tracking in these patients. Interrupted 7–0 nylon vertical mattress sutures are used to close and slightly evert the inverted-V columellar incision. The incision should be further reapproximated with additional 6–0 fast-absorbing gut interrupted simple sutures or more 7–0 nylon sutures. The marginal incisions should be closed with 5–0 chromic gut sutures in an interrupted fashion while the surgeon watches the nostril margin closely. If there is inadequate vestibular lining, this stitch can lead to notching, in which case a composite graft may be necessary.[36] The septum should be closed by reapproximating the mucoperichondrial flaps with a 4–0 plain gut suture on a Keith needle in a running mattress fashion.

Radiopaque 0.25 mm septal splints are sutured in place if turbinate and septal work was performed to prevent obstructive adhesions. Lateral wall splints should also be fashioned if lateral crural strut grafts were placed.[36] Vestibular splints can be used if there is asymmetry to the nostrils. The nose should be taped and a cast applied. Antibiotic ointment should be applied to all incisions and a "mustache" dressing applied to help with anterior dripping postoperatively.

Base Reductions

Often base reductions will be indicated at the end of a primary ethnic rhinoplasty after extensive costal cartilage grafting. Variation in the location of base reduction can narrow the nasal base or decrease base flaring with or without decreasing the size of the nostril. In most Asian noses, the authors prefer to use a lateral alar base reduction to reduce alar flare (**Fig. 18.26**). In these cases, the incision is made just above the alar groove to allow placement of vertical mattress sutures. If the surgeon is unsure whether base reduction should be performed, the best answer is likely to defer reduction. The surgeon can always come back at a later time and reduce the alar base. It is quite difficult to add tissue back once it has been removed. Of the techniques in the nasal surgeon's armamentarium, base reduction has the greatest potential to leave an obvious irreversible deformity and stigmata of previous rhinoplasty. Keys to successful reduction include planning the incision slightly adjacent to the alar/facial or alar/vestibular junction, avoiding all cautery, beveled incisions to promote eversion of the skin edges, and meticulous closure.

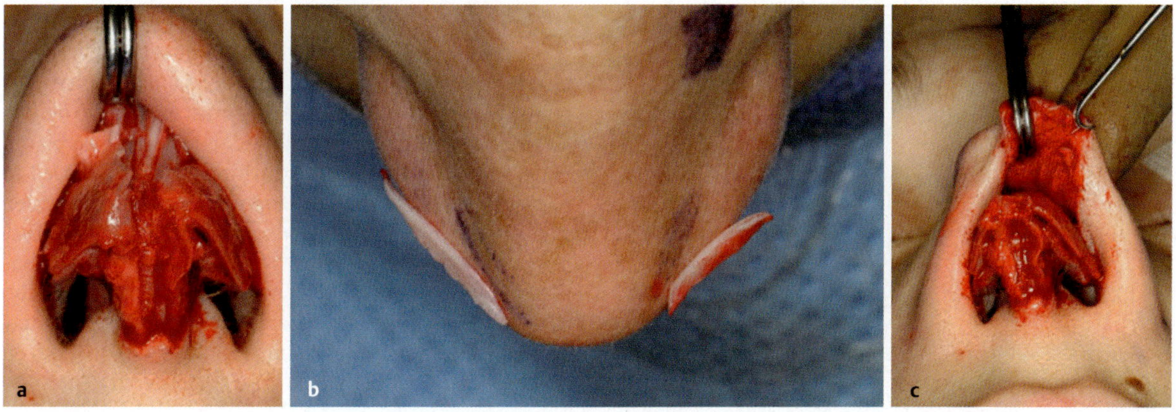

Fig. 18.25 Alar rim grafts. **(a)** Unfavorable orientation of the lateral crus of the lower lateral cartilages (cephalic margin lies above the level of the caudal margin). **(b)** Final rim graft location approximated overlying the skin–soft tissue envelope. **(c)** The end of the left rim graft can be seen in its pocket caudal to the marginal incision.

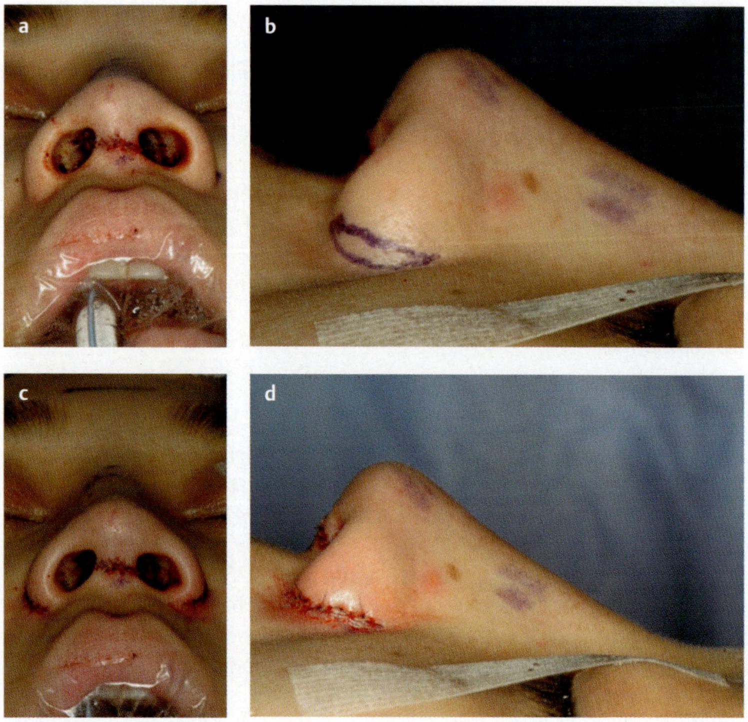

Fig. 18.26 Base reduction. Before and after base reduction seen on **(a,c)** base and **(b,d)** lateral views.

Postoperative Care

Patients undergoing costal cartilage grafting receive a prescription for an oral fluoroquinolone and perform antibiotic soaks in addition to routine prophylactic use of a second-generation cephalosporin. The cast, tape, splints, and sutures are removed at around 1 week postoperatively. If base reductions were performed, the sutures remain in place for 10 to 14 days. Patients are routinely given narcotic medication, but they are encouraged to try acetaminophen alone for pain. Aspirin and ibuprofen products are avoided to prevent epistaxis. Incentive spirometry and increased activity will decrease postoperative atelectasis, and they are important because the discomfort at the costal cartilage donor site will have a tendency to inhibit deep breathing.

18.4 Adjuvant Techniques in Ethnic Rhinoplasty

Although the authors do not employee the technique, there are many surgeons who use variations of crushed costal cartilage wrapped in some form of soft tissue envelope in a technique called the *Turkish delight*.[37,38,39,40,41] Unfortunately, these grafts often have a variable degree of resorption, giving an irregular, amorphous appearance to the dorsum, and rarely do they provide a well-defined brow–tip aesthetic line. Another somewhat popular technique includes placing a permanent K-wire through the long axis of dorsal grafts to prevent long-term warping.[42,43] This strategy has the disadvantages of potential extrusion and offering a false sense of security against warping. Permanent wires are also a foreign body that can be a potential nidus for infection.

Another adjuvant techniques often important to get good results in ethnic rhinoplasty is conservative thinning of a thick S-STE by removing fat from its undersurface. This is an advanced maneuver, and care must be taken to do it in a conservative fashion. A Converse retractor can be placed underneath the S-STE, and palpation can be employed to ensure uniformity to the envelope (distinguishing between irregularities and the underlying osseocartilaginous structure). Although this chapter focuses on primary rhinoplasty, this strategy should not be adopted for revision rhinoplasty in the ethnic patient. Revision rhinoplasty may involve removal of an implant (which tends to weaken and thin the skin), in which case opposite strategies are employed to thicken the S-STE.

18.5 Conclusion

Costal cartilage grafting is a powerful technique that extends the rhinoplasty surgeon's ability to improve many deformities that were previously not correctable. It is, however, complex and will require time to master.

18.6 Pearls for Costal Cartilage Use in Primary Ethnic Rhinoplasty

- Ensure the patient's aesthetic concerns and preferences are completely understood.
- Patient age is an important factor in the quality of costal cartilage.
- Subperichondrial dissection lowers risk of pneumothorax during rib harvest.
- Rib grafts must not be placed in the nose until the warping tendency has declared itself.
- Cross-hatching, splinting, and lamination can alter curvature of cartilage grafts.
- Proper fixation of costal cartilage grafts can inhibit postoperative warping.
- Osteotomies are rarely indicated when significant dorsal augmentation is planned.
- A stable foundation is required to increase projection while controlling length/rotation.
- Ethnic tip contour changes require different techniques from those for the Caucasian nose.

References

1. Dixon TK, Caughlin BP, Munaretto N, Toriumi DM. Three-dimensional evaluation of unilateral cleft rhinoplasty results. Facial Plast Surg 2013;29(2):106–115
2. Toriumi DM, Dixon TK. Assessment of rhinoplasty techniques by overlay of before-and-after 3D images. Facial Plast Surg Clin North Am 2011;19(4):711–723, ix
3. Toriumi DM, Swartout B. Asian rhinoplasty. Facial Plast Surg Clin North Am 2007;15(3):293–307
4. Toriumi DM. Structure approach in rhinoplasty. Facial Plast Surg Clin North Am 2002;10(1):1–22
5. Anantanarayanan P, Raja DK, Kumar JN, et al. Catheter-based donor site analgesia after rib grafting: a prospective, randomized, double-blinded clinical trial comparing ropivacaine and bupivacaine. J Oral Maxillofac Surg 2013;71(1):29–34
6. Marin VP, Landecker A, Gunter JP. Harvesting rib cartilage grafts for secondary rhinoplasty. Plast Reconstr Surg 2008;121(4):1442–1448
7. Windfuhr JP, Chen YS, Güldner C, Neukirch D. Rib cartilage harvesting in rhinoplasty procedures based on CT radiological data. Acta Otolaryngol 2011;131(1):67–71
8. Bozzato A, Bumm K, Hertel V, Wurm J. Ultrasonographic evaluation of calcification patterns in costal cartilage: implications for rib graft harvesting. JAMA Facial Plast Surg 2013;15(6):457–460
9. Rejtarová O, Slízová D, Smoranc P, Rejtar P, Bukac J. Costal cartilages—a clue for determination of sex. Biomed Pap Med Fac Univ Palacky Olomouc Czech Repub 2004; 148(2):241–243
10. Balaji SM. Costal cartilage nasal augmentation rhinoplasty: study on warping. Ann Maxillofac Surg 2013;3(1): 20–24
11. Sunwoo WS, Choi HG, Kim DW, Jin HR. Characteristics of rib cartilage calcification in Asian patients. JAMA Facial Plast Surg 2014;16(2):102–106
12. McCarn KE, Weber SM. Ultrasonography for rapid detection of pneumothorax after costal cartilage harvest. Arch Facial Plast Surg 2011;13(1):57–59
13. Ağaoğlu G, Erol OO. In situ split costal cartilage graft harvesting through a small incision using a gouge. Plast Reconstr Surg 2000;106(4):932–935, discussion 936–937
14. Lee M, Inman J, Ducic Y. Central segment harvest of costal cartilage in rhinoplasty. Laryngoscope 2011; 121(10):2155–2158
15. Chauhan N, Sepehr A, Gantous A. Costal cartilage autograft harvest: inferior strip preservation technique. Plast Reconstr Surg 2010;125(5):214e–215e
16. Ching WC, Hsiao YC. Transumbilical endoscopic costal cartilage harvesting: a new technique. Ann Plast Surg 2014; 72(4): 423–427
17. Gentile P, Cervelli V. Nasal dorsum reconstruction with 11th rib cartilage and auricular cartilage grafts. Ann Plast Surg 2009;62(1):63–66
18. Christophel JJ, Hilger PA. Osseocartilaginous rib graft rhinoplasty: a stable, predictable technique for major dorsal reconstruction. Arch Facial Plast Surg 2011;13(2):78–83
19. Lopez MA, Shah AR, Westine JG, O'Grady K, Toriumi DM. Analysis of the physical properties of costal cartilage in a porcine model. Arch Facial Plast Surg 2007;9(1):35–39
20. Kim DW, Shah AR, Toriumi DM. Concentric and eccentric carved costal cartilage: a comparison of warping. Arch Facial Plast Surg 2006;8(1):42–46
21. Foulad A, Manuel C, Wong BJ. Practical device for precise cutting of costal cartilage grafts to uniform thickness. Arch Facial Plast Surg 2011;13(4):259–265
22. Park JH, Jin HR. Use of autologous costal cartilage in Asian rhinoplasty. Plast Reconstr Surg 2012;130(6): 1338–1348
23. Swanepoel PF, Fysh R. Laminated dorsal beam graft to eliminate postoperative twisting complications. Arch Facial Plast Surg 2007;9(4):285–289
24. Toriumi DM. Intraoperative measurements. http://deantoriumi.com/new_methods.asp Accessed February 1, 2014
25. Toriumi DM, Pero CD. Asian rhinoplasty. Clin Plast Surg 2010;37(2):335–352
26. Toriumi DM. Subtotal septal reconstruction: an update. Facial Plast Surg 2013;29(6):492–501
27. Toriumi DM, Bared A. Revision of the surgically overshortened nose. Facial Plast Surg 2012;28(4):407–416
28. Suh MK, Ahn ES, Kim HR, Dhong ES. A 2-year follow-up of irradiated homologous costal cartilage used as a septal

extension graft for the correction of contracted nose in Asians. Ann Plast Surg 2013;71(1):45–49

29. Ahmed A, Imani P, Vuyk HD. Reconstruction of significant saddle nose deformity using autogenous costal cartilage graft with incorporated mirror image spreader grafts. Laryngoscope 2010;120(3):491–494

30. Guyuron B, Uzzo CD, Scull H. A practical classification of septonasal deviation and an effective guide to septal surgery. Plast Reconstr Surg 1999;104(7):2202–2209, discussion 2210–2212

31. Taştan E, Yücel OT, Aydin E, Aydoğan F, Beriat K, Ulusoy MG. The oblique split method: a novel technique for carving costal cartilage grafts. JAMA Facial Plast Surg 2013; 15(3):198–203

32. Farkas JP, Lee MR, Lakianhi C, Rohrich RJ. Effects of carving plane, level of harvest, and oppositional suturing techniques on costal cartilage warping. Plast Reconstr Surg 2013;132(2):319–325

33. Toriumi DM. Discussion: Use of autologous costal cartilage in Asian rhinoplasty. Plast Reconstr Surg 2012;130(6):1349–1350

34. Toriumi DM. New concepts in nasal tip contouring. Arch Facial Plast Surg 2006;8(3):156–185

35. Gunter JP, Friedman RM. Lateral crural strut graft: technique and clinical applications in rhinoplasty. Plast Reconstr Surg 1997;99(4):943–952, discussion 953–955

36. Losquadro WD, Bared A, Toriumi DM. Correction of the retracted alar base. Facial Plast Surg 2012;28(2): 218–224

37. Erol OO. The Turkish delight: a pliable graft for rhinoplasty. Plast Reconstr Surg 2000;105(6):2229–2241, discussion 2242–2243

38. Daniel RK. The role of diced cartilage grafts in rhinoplasty. Aesthet Surg J 2006;26(2):209–213

39. Harel M, Margulis A. Dorsal augmentation with diced cartilage enclosed with temporal fascia in secondary endonasal rhinoplasty. Aesthet Surg J 2013;33(6):809–816

40. Jang YJ, Song HM, Yoon YJ, Sykes JM. Combined use of crushed cartilage and processed fascia lata for dorsal augmentation in rhinoplasty for Asians. Laryngoscope 2009;119(6):1088–1092

41. Kim YH, Kim JT. Nasal reconstruction with double-layer tensor fascia lata-wrapped diced rib cartilage in a patient with severe dorsal collapse. J Craniofac Surg 2011; 22(2):628–630

42. Gunter JP, Clark CP, Friedman RM. Internal stabilization of autogenous rib cartilage grafts in rhinoplasty: a barrier to cartilage warping. Plast Reconstr Surg 1997;100(1): 161–169

43. Sarifakioglu N, Cigsar B, Aslan G. K-wire: a simple and safe method for internal stabilization of costal cartilage in L-strut grafts. Ann Plast Surg 2002;49(4):444

19 Implants in Rhinoplasty

Yong Ju Jang and Min Joo Kim

19.1 Introduction

Dorsal augmentation is the most important part of rhinoplasty for Asians. It is critically important not only in simple cosmetic rhinoplasty but also in all types of rhinoplasty for their aesthetic perfection. Aesthetic perfection of the nose is determined by the height and shape of the nasal dorsum seen from the side and front, and by harmonious alignment with the nasal tip. Thus, to create a beautiful nose, one must possess an aesthetic understanding of what kind of dorsum constitutes a beautiful dorsum. In this chapter, characteristics of various dorsal implant materials are discussed.

19.2 Aesthetic Considerations

The beauty of the nasal dorsum viewed from the front is primarily determined by the dorsal aesthetic line. This line must be adequately formed in all rhinoplasty procedures. The dorsal aesthetic lines start from the supraorbital ridges, passing the corrugators, and converge at the medial canthal ligaments. Then, they diverge a little at the keystone area, descend parallel to each other, and reach the tip-defining points. In males, it is acceptable for the lines to connect almost parallel to the tip without the width between them changing. For female patients, however, a gentle slope from the supraorbital ridge to the tip is preferable. If the dorsal implant is too wide, the risk of displacement or implant visibility is relatively lower, but the dorsal line looks masculine, creating an aesthetically less pleasing dorsal appearance in females. If the dorsal implant is too narrow in the radix area, the risk of implant visibility or deviation increases. Therefore, the implant should be designed with an appropriate width. Female dorsal lines, as seen from the side, may preferably be placed a little lower than the line connecting the nasofrontal angle and the tip, in a slightly concave shape. In male patients, to avoid a feminine appearance, the dorsal line should be placed on or a little above the nasofrontal angle–tip line. In female East Asian patients, the nasion or nasal starting point's level should be placed between the mid-pupillary line and the double-eyelid line, also taking into consideration the patient's preferred nose shape. For male patients, it may be preferable to place the nasion a little higher. The nasofrontal angle should have a gentle curvature. But for patients who have a sunken radix, showing relatively sharp nasofrontal angles, if beveling of the implant's upper end was not performed well, the implant's cephalic margin can be conspicuous when viewed from the front. To satisfy the aforementioned aesthetic elements, the surgeon must design a dorsal implant or graft of appropriate width, length, and shape. This is a difficult process that requires experience and immense effort. An implant's base should be wide, the area placed near the surface should be narrow, and it should be in good contact with the nasal dorsum to prevent implant movement. Normally, implants required for dorsal augmentation should be ~ 3 to 5 cm long and 0.7 to 1.0 cm wide.[1]

19.3 Selection of Dorsal Implant

To raise the height of the nasal dorsum, the appropriate augmentation material must be chosen. Augmentation material can be classified into biologic implants and alloplastic implants **(Table 19.1)**.[2] Biologic implants include autologous cartilage, fascia, and dermofat. Homologous tissues, such as costal cartilage, fascia, and dermis obtained from cadaver donors, also are biologic implants. Biologic implants obtained from other species are also included in this category. Alloplastic implants include silicone, Gore-Tex, and Medpor. Determining the material of choice for dorsal augmentation depends on the surgeon's experience, surgical proficiency/mastery, philosophy, treatment methods, and rhinoplasty patient groups' characteristics. So far, there is no ideal dorsal implant material that can satisfy all criteria. Inserting a foreign material between the nasal skin–soft tissue envelope (S-STE) and the nasal framework is a procedure bound to involve unexpected complications. The surgeon must adequately explain the risks to patients and must be able to handle problems appropriately when they occur.

19.3.1 Biologic Implants

Cartilage

Septal Cartilage

In rhinoplasty, septoplasty is frequently undertaken to solve nasal obstruction, and it calls for removal of the middle part of cartilage as a part of the procedure. The removed cartilage is an important graft material used preciously in rhinoplasty. According to the author's research, the dimension of the average septal cartilage harvested during external rhinoplasty, leaving an L-strut of 1 cm, has caudal length, dorsal length, and area of 15.1 mm, 18.2 mm,

Table 19.1 Dorsal augmentation materials

Dorsal augmentation materials
Biologic implants
Cartilage
Septal cartilage
Conchal cartilage
Costal cartilage
Homologous costal cartilage
Bone
Iliac bone
Calvarial bone
Dermofat
Fascia
Alloplastic implants
Silicone
Gore-Tex
Medpor

and 520.9 mm², respectively. The thickness of the septal cartilage differs greatly from patient to patient. Cartilage harvested from patients with thin septal cartilage is difficult to use for grafting purposes. Thin cartilage is commonly seen in female patients with a poorly developed nasal skeleton. The author believes that the use of septal cartilage for dorsal augmentation is not an ideal surgical option. First, it is difficult to obtain a long enough piece of septal cartilage (3–4 cm) for dorsal augmentation.[3] Second, using septal cartilage with an angled margin for dorsal augmentation is less aesthetically suitable than alloplastic implants. Thus it is uncommon to use septal cartilage as a one-piece dorsal augmentation material. Usually, the piece of cartilage remaining after structural grafting or tip grafting is crushed using a cartilage crusher and is used as volume filler to correct focal depressions or uneven areas in the nasal dorsum or tip.

Conchal Cartilage

Conchal cartilage, unlike septal cartilage, has the disadvantage of leaving an additional scar during cartilage harvest, but its elasticity and softness, as well as its having the most histological similarity to the lower lateral cartilage, make it popular as graft material for the nasal tip. However, due to its intrinsic curvature and limitations in length, conchal cartilage has clear limitations as dorsal augmentation material. For full-length nasal augmentation using conchal cartilage alone, from the radix to the tip, one must harvest a big piece of cartilage. In such cases, its natural curvature can be eliminated by cutting it in a convex shape and stacking it into multiple layers.[4] However, dorsal augmentation using such methods increases the possibility of contour visibility of the graft through the skin over time. Conchal cartilage can be used as dorsal implant in the form of fascia-wrapped diced cartilage, a method that became popular among many rhinoplasty surgeons.[5] When there is only a partial depression or a minor saddle in the nasal dorsum, partial dorsal augmentation can be nicely achieved through making cuts in the cartilage with the perichondrium of the harvested conchal cartilage intact and still attached, making the divided pieces maintain a state of attachment with each other through the perichondrium (**Fig. 19.1** and **Fig. 19.2**).

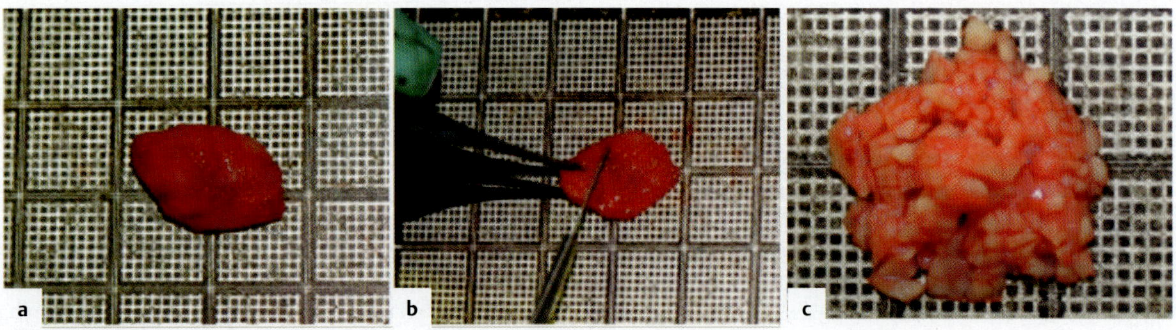

Fig.19.1 **(a–c)** Diced conchal cartilage with the perichondrium intact and still attached.

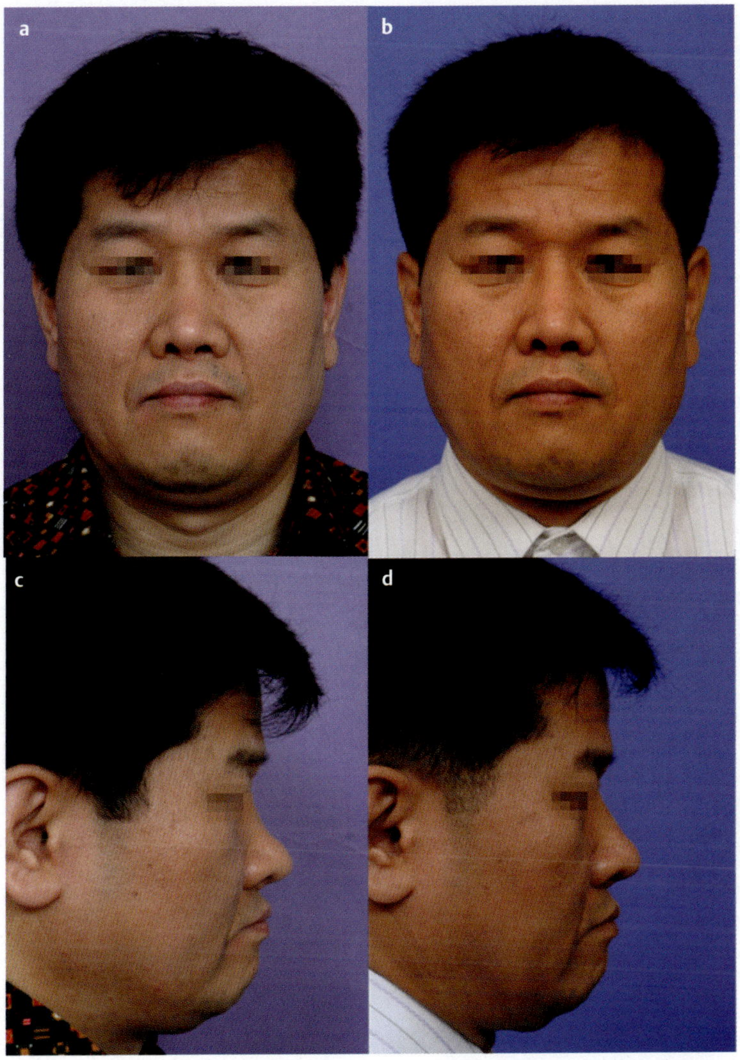

Fig. 19.2 **(a,c)** Preoperative and **(b,d)** postoperative frontal and lateral views of a patient whose dorsum was augmented using diced conchal cartilage with perichondrium attached.

Costal Cartilage

Autologous Costal Cartilage

Costal cartilage is an important graft material for rhinoplasty in that it provides large amounts of quality cartilage. Like septal cartilage, costal cartilage is a hard hyaline cartilage useful for structural grafting. Carving and trimming it well makes it applicable for both the nasal dorsum and nasal tip, justifying its value as a versatile graft material.

The author uses costal cartilage for:

- Reconstructive rhinoplasty that requires large amounts of sturdy cartilage for nasal septal reconstruction and grafting due to severe deformation
- Saddle nose
- Short nose **(Fig. 19.3)**
- A patient who has small nose and wants major changes **(Fig. 19.4)**
- A patient with very thick skin who wants well-defined and well-projected nasal tips with distinct contour

The sixth costal cartilage, in most cases, has a round cross section and has a bent shape in the part fused with the seventh costal cartilage. The seventh costal cartilage has a flatter cross section than the sixth costal cartilage and has a more linear shape, and thus it is more appropriate for dorsal augmentation.[1] However, for a successful one-piece dorsal augmentation using rib cartilage for the entire dorsum, it is very difficult to create a natural-looking smooth dorsum and it requires a lot of experience. Aesthetic complications, such as warping, implant visibility, contour irregularity, graft mobility, and resorption of the dorsal implant, are common.[6] Because of the shrink-wrap

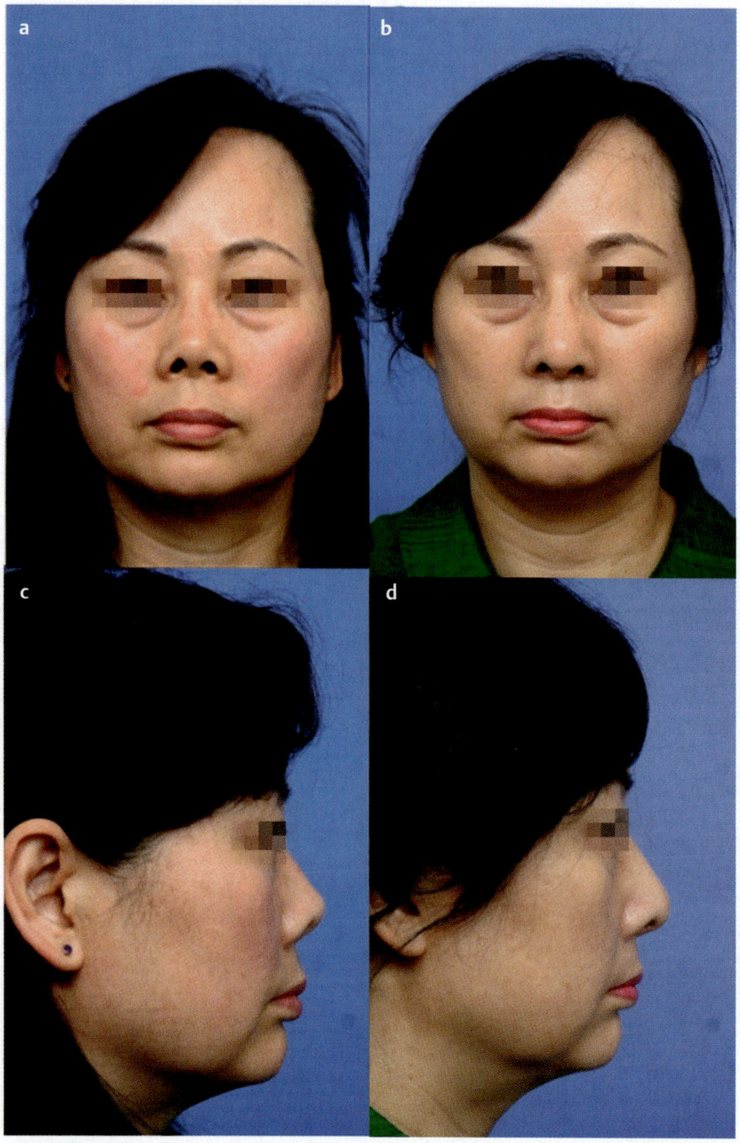

Fig. 19.3 **(a,c)** Preoperative and **(b,d)** postoperative facial photo of short-nose deformity treated using costal cartilage.

phenomenon, in the long-term follow-up of the patient, especially the thin-skinned individual, there is high risk of development of a prominent contour of the cartilage graft. The author, therefore, does not recommend using costal cartilage as a nasal dorsal implant unless there are no other choices. Methods like using a core of cartilage or K-wire to prevent warping of costal cartilage have been introduced, but applying such methods does not ensure freedom from the risk of warping. Other methods to prevent warping include stacking prepared long pieces of cartilage. This method is called laminated cartilage grafting.[7] In the author's experience, applying this technique moderately lowers the risk of warping.

Homologous Costal Cartilage

Processing methods for harvested costal cartilage may differ in each tissue bank, but most methods include gamma irradiation processing (15–24 kGy for 1.5–2.0 hours), osmotic destruction, and freeze drying. Reports frequently indicate that homologous cartilage is often more easily absorbed than autologous cartilage, and the author has had similar experience (**Fig. 19.5**). Furthermore, since cartilage differs in physical characteristics based on tissue-processing methods, and the cadavers who provide the cartilage are of different age groups, it is hard to expect consistent quality of cartilage from these implants. In the author's experience using Tutoplast-processed costal cartilage, complications like resorption, fracturing, and deformation were somewhat frequent.

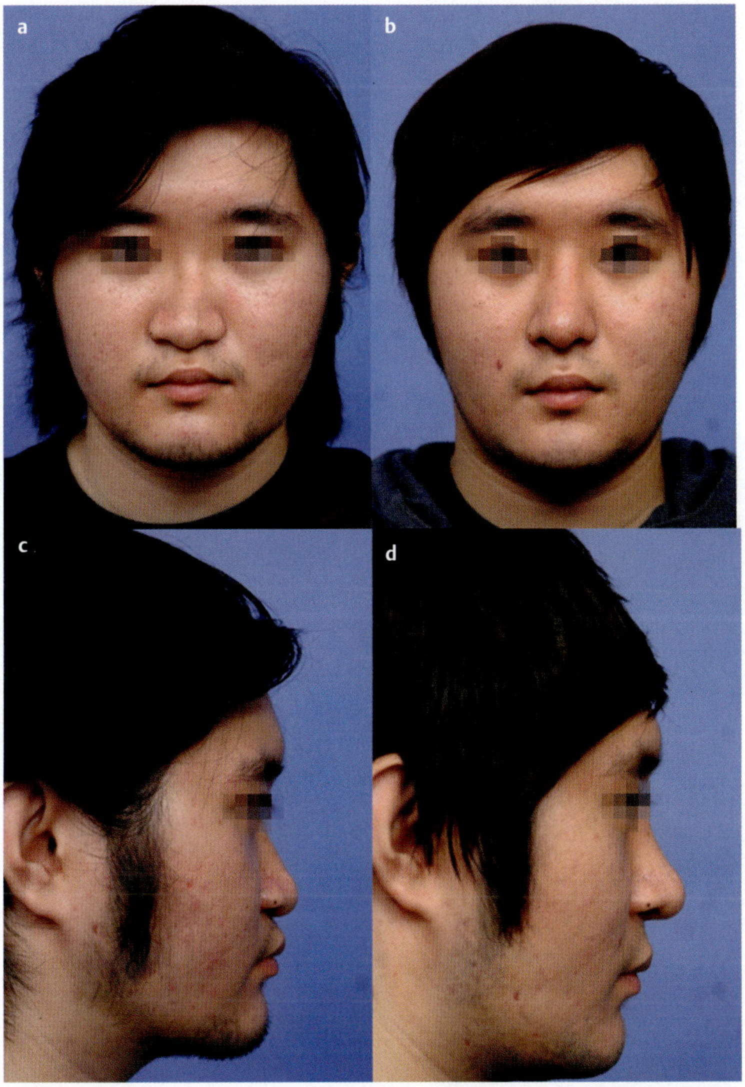

Fig. 19.4 **(a,c)** Preoperative and **(b,d)** postoperative frontal and lateral views of a patient with a very small nose. Costal cartilage was used as a dorsal augmentation material.

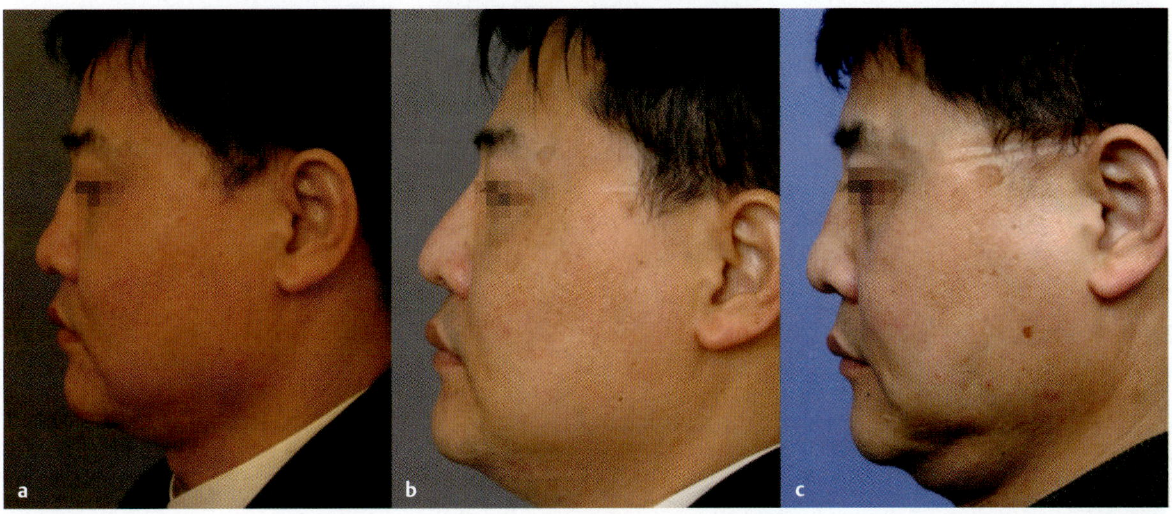

Fig. 19.5 **(a)** Preoperative and **(b,c)** 10-month postoperative lateral view of patient who showed a resorption of homologous cartilage 8 years after surgery.

Dermofat

Dermofat is easy to harvest and has low donor-site morbidity. It is resistant to infection, and it is flexible enough to be made into various shapes easily. The most commonly used donor site is the sacral area (**Fig. 19.6**).[8] The advantage of sacral dermofat is its low absorption rate, due to its thick dermis, and the low scar visibility; the disadvantage of dermofat in general as dorsal augmentation material is resorption. Use of dermofat as dorsal augmentation material is recommended when the patient strongly prefers autologous tissue (**Fig. 19.7**). Dermofat is particularly useful when:

- The skin is in bad condition due to multiple revisions
- The nasal bridge requires smoothening after osteotomy or humpectomy
- Alloplastic implants cannot be used due to the thin nasal dorsal skin

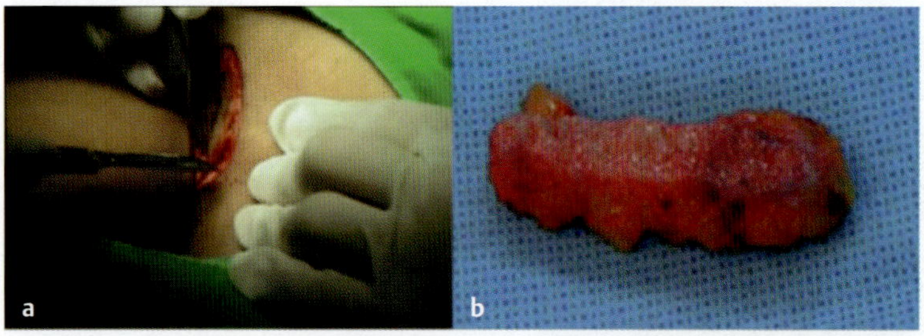

Fig. 19.6 (a,b) Harvesting of dermofat from sacral area.

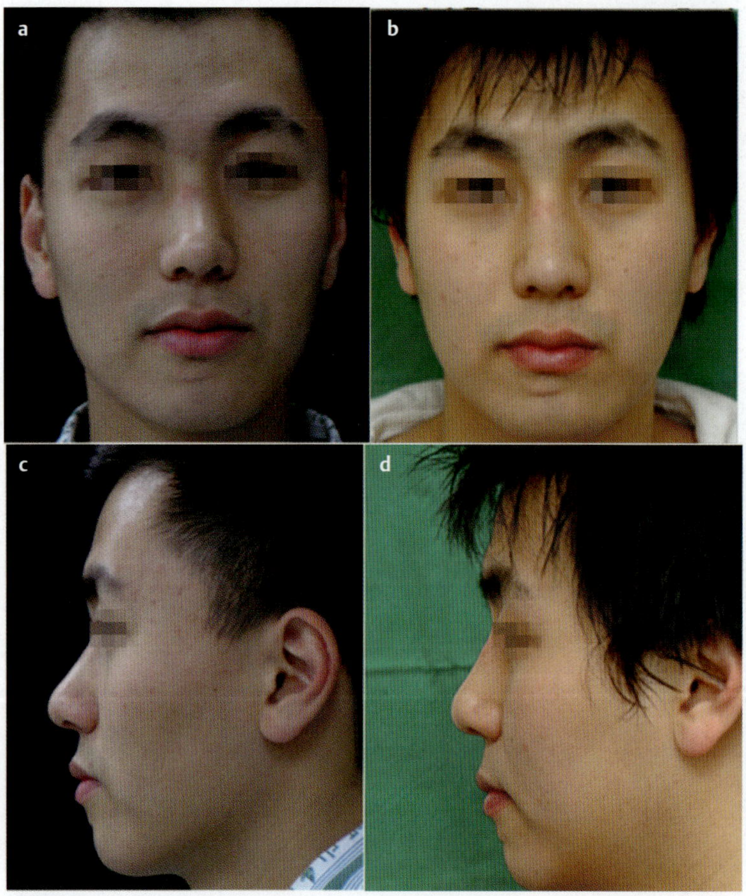

Fig.19.7 (a,c) Preoperative and **(b,d)** 2-year postoperative frontal and lateral views of a patient who had revision rhinoplasty using dermofat.

Fascia

Autologous fascia, such as temporalis fascia and fascia lata, is an appropriate graft material for use in rhinoplasty to increase the volume of the nasal soft tissue. Fascia is especially beneficial because it creates a smooth dorsal contour, free of problems like graft visibility and dorsal irregularities that can arise after dorsal augmentation using cartilage. Another advantage is its considerably low risk of infection and reduced inflammation in comparison to alloplastic implants. Fascia is known to be absorbed steadily into the body, being substituted with the individual's own fibrous tissue. Homologous fascia can also serve as dorsal implant material, which can reduce harvest-induced donor-site morbidity.[9] The most critical point when using fascia in rhinoplasty is the unpredictability of surgical results, due to postoperative absorption of the implant. Several techniques are available when using fascia on the nasal dorsum. The methods that can be used for both autologous and processed fascia are:

- Using fascia only **(Fig. 19.8)**
- Overlapping fascia with cartilage[5]
- Fascia-wrapped diced cartilage.[10] This method involves dicing conchal or septal cartilage and wrapping the cartilage with fascia to be implanted in the dorsum. Conchal cartilage is most suitable for this. Fascia-wrapped diced cartilage can be made to cover the entire nasal dorsum, and reducing its size makes it appropriate for insertion in cartilaginous dorsum.

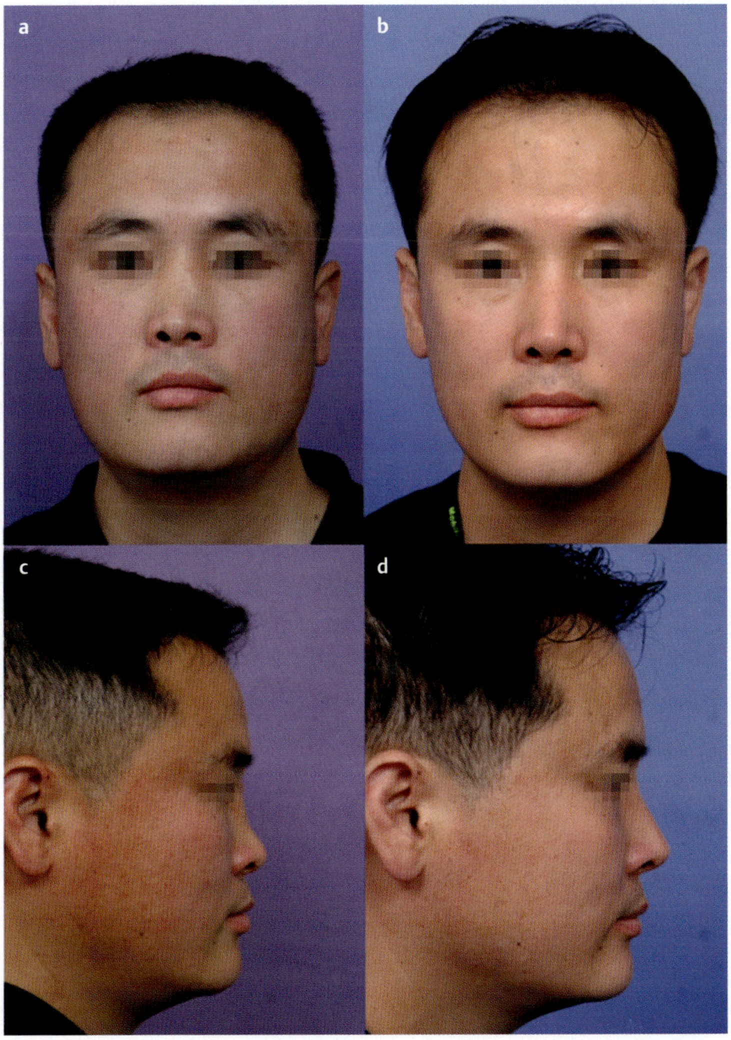

Fig. 19.8 **(a,c)** Preoperative and **(b,d)** postoperative frontal and lateral views of a patient whose dorsum was augmented by combined use of fascia lata and crushed cartilage.

19.3.2 Alloplastic Implants

Silicone

A silicone implant has a smooth surface, is easy to design, and brings excellent aesthetic results; therefore, silicone is the most commonly used implant material in Asia **(Fig. 19.9)**. The reason for this is that Asians have thicker skin than Caucasians, and thus have lower risk of complications like implant extrusion.[11]

Silicone has the following advantages:

- Excellent biocompatibility
- Stable to heat and withstands a wide range of temperature (−60–260°C)
- Cannot be dissolved by enzymes
- A smooth surface and can be carved very precisely
- Various levels of hardness
- Easy to remove when problems occur
- Less costly

Silicone implants can be carved during surgery by using a no. 15 surgical blade, surgical scissors, carving knives, or sterilized razors. It is also possible to shape the implant before surgery using a milling machine and then to sterilize the implant before usage. In order for silicone to be used as a dorsal implant, a canoe-shaped implant is designed; the caudal end of the implant is carved in a sharp, angulated shape to fit the cephalic divergence of the alar cartilages; and the implant is fixed to the surrounding cartilage tissue using sutures **(Fig. 19.10)**. The implant can be placed so that the caudal end of the implant connects directly to the tip onlay graft **(Fig. 19.11)**. A simpler type of implant placement would be to make the implant reach the caudal end of the nasal tip and to place one or two layers of autologous cartilage in the form of an onlay or shield graft over the caudal or upper part of the caudal end of the silicone implant **(Fig. 19.12)**. L-shaped silicone is used to raise both the nasal tip and dorsum.[1] When using the L-shaped implant, if the surgeon gives the tip too much tension in hope of achieving a tent-pole effect, the skin of the nasal tip

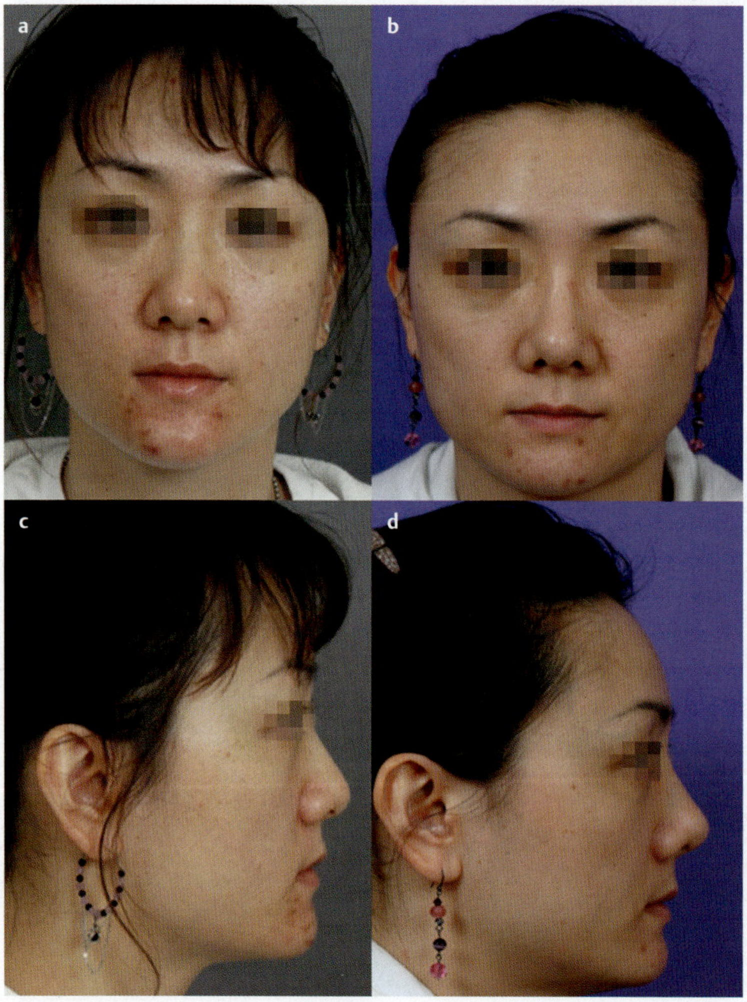

Fig. 19.9 **(a,c)** Preoperative and **(b,d)** postoperative frontal and lateral views of a patient with silicone implant for dorsal augmentation.

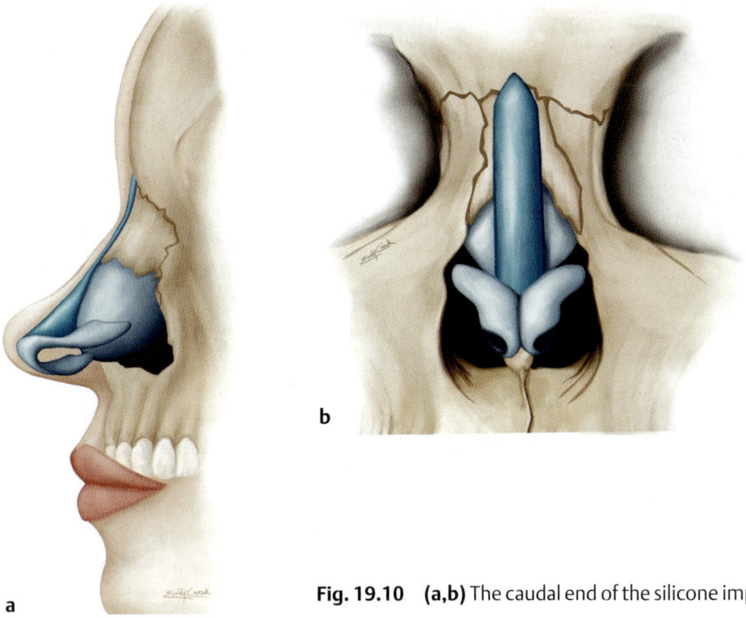

Fig. 19.10 (a,b) The caudal end of the silicone implant fits the cephalic divergence of alar cartilage.

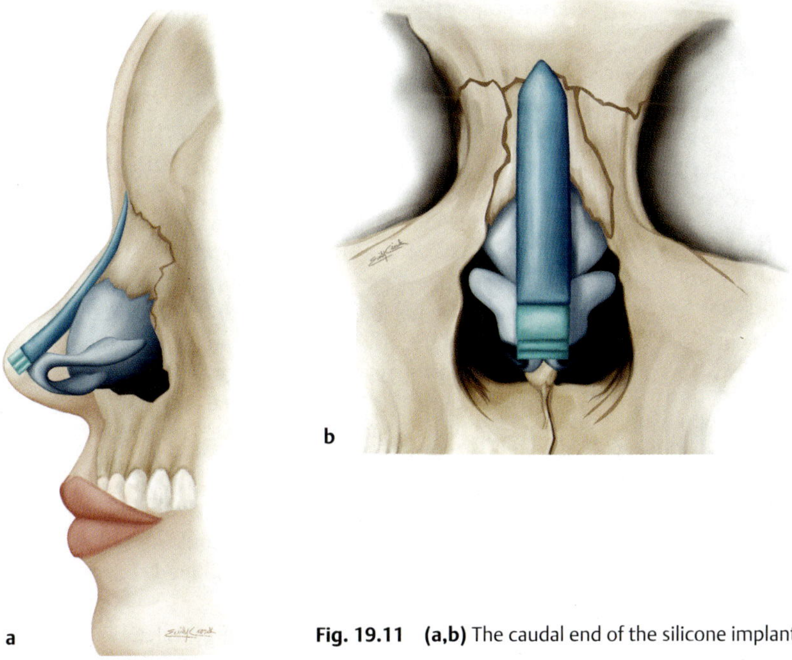

Fig. 19.11 (a,b) The caudal end of the silicone implant connects directly to the tip onlay graft.

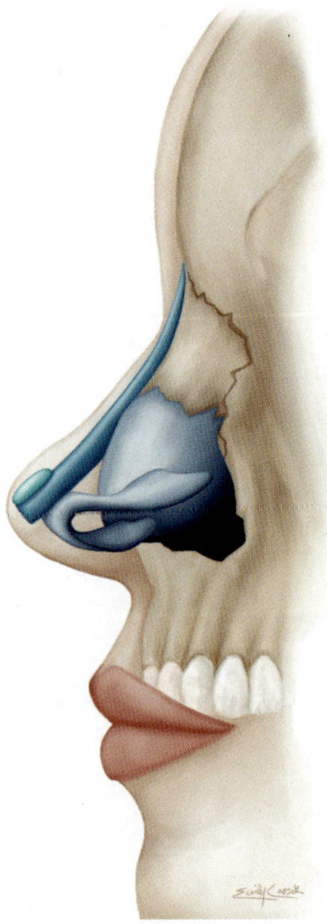

Fig. 19.12 The caudal end of the silicone implant reaches the caudal end of the nasal tip, and one or two layers of onlay or shield graft are placed over the caudal or upper part of the caudal end of the silicone implant.

could become too thin in the long term. This method causes many complications, such as tip skin necrosis and columellar deformity, and is not recommended. Despite the ease of using silicone in creating a smooth dorsal contour, there are problems related to its use in dorsal augmentation. Capsule formation, skin contraction, telangiectasia, chronic recurrent inflammation, and partial calcification of the silicone, resulting in an irregular surface showing through the skin, are not uncommon complications. More common complications include extrusion, implant displacement, movable implant, and infection.[12] Alloplastic implants are susceptible to infection and, when infected, exhibit typical signs, such as erythema, swelling, and purulent secretions. In addition, temporary erythema and swelling from subclinical infections can also occur recurrently.

Thorough sterilization of the surgical field is necessary for reducing infection, especially in the nasal vestibule and the nasal cavity. Inserting gauze soaked in antiseptic solution further inside the nasal cavity to separate the already sterilized nasal inlet area from the inner nasal cavity space during surgery is also helpful. It is also advisable to isolate the area around the mouth from the surgical field using a mask or sterilized gauze. During surgery, it is important to prevent breakage of natural barriers, such as a mucous membrane injury. In cases that involve a significant modification of the normal anatomical structure, like osteotomies, infection should be a chief concern. Aesthetically improper implant design is also a common complication. Dorsal augmentation using silicone is an essential part of Asian rhinoplasty, and can bring about excellent aesthetic outcomes with relative ease. To obtain the best results with silicone implants, meticulous surgical planning and aesthetically appropriate implant design are crucial, along with mastery of the various tip surgery techniques.

Expanded Polytetrafluoroethylene (ePTFE)

The ePTFE compound cannot be chemically degraded due to its strong bonds between carbon and fluorine, and it is biologically inert; it therefore maintains a high level of physical stability once inserted in the human body. ePTFE has numerous micropores, and the porous structure of ePTFE affects the interaction between the implant and the surrounding tissue. Fibroblasts and many other cells can penetrate through the micropores, and connective tissue can grow into the implant over time. Such bonding keeps the graft firmly fixed to the surrounding tissue after it has been inserted into the nasal dorsum. ePTFE is not hard like silicone; thus it is not as uncomfortable when inserted into the nasal dorsum, it cannot be easily palpated through the skin, and it can be carved and stacked into desired shapes and sizes due to the relative ease in handling.[13] The most widely used ePTFE product for dorsal augmentation was the Gore-Tex subcutaneous augmentation material (SAM). However, Gore-Tex SAM is very soft, is difficult to handle, and can decrease in thickness after insertion. Recently, ePTFE materials other than Gore-Tex SAM have been developed and used. Surgiform is a facial plastic surgery material composed of 100% ePTFE. Surgiform is harder than the original Gore-Tex and it has a denser structure that makes it easier to handle and carve.

Precautions for handling e-PTFE are:

- Use a new pair of surgical gloves with the powder completely removed.
- Surgical tools used to shape the implant, such as scissors, knife, and caliper, should also be new, and free of contamination by blood or secretions (no-hands technique).
- Put the implant inside a syringe filled with antibiotic or povidone-iodine solution and induce permeation of the solution into the pores by exerting negative pressure, or immerse the implant in povidone-iodine solution before surgery.
- Unpack the ePTFE right before implantation to minimize the implant's exposure to the outside environment.

Although prefabricated implants are commonly used, the sheet-type ePTFE implant is more commonly used (**Fig. 19.13**). This implant is very adaptable because the surgeon can modify its shape freely based on the need. Since the thickness of commonly used ePTFE is usually 1 to 2 mm, multiple sheets should be stacked to increase dorsal height. When using ePTFE sheet, good beveling of the sheet's margins is essential, especially for sheets over 2 mm thick (**Fig. 19.14**).[1] When ePTFE is used in the nasal dorsum, infection or inflammation can occur months, even years, after surgery, requiring implant removal. Although delayed inflammation can be treated easily if detected early, if untreated, it could cause irreversible damage to the skin covering. Therefore, it is important that symptoms and signs of delayed inflammation are explained thoroughly to patients who undergo rhinoplasty with ePTFE. These patients should be advised to visit the hospital immediately if erythema, swelling, or tenderness occurs in the nasal dorsum. Infection could manifest in various forms after surgery. Intermittent erythema or pain can initially be managed by antibiotics and anti-inflammatory agents. However, if the inflammation progresses into a purulent lesion, the implant must be removed immediately. Other common complications are implant displacement, deviation, and bending.

Medpor

Medpor (Porex Surgical, College Park, GA) is a biocompatible material composed of porous high-density polyethylene (PHDPE). Its hardness is similar to cancellous bone, yet it is quite flexible. The pores provide space for blood

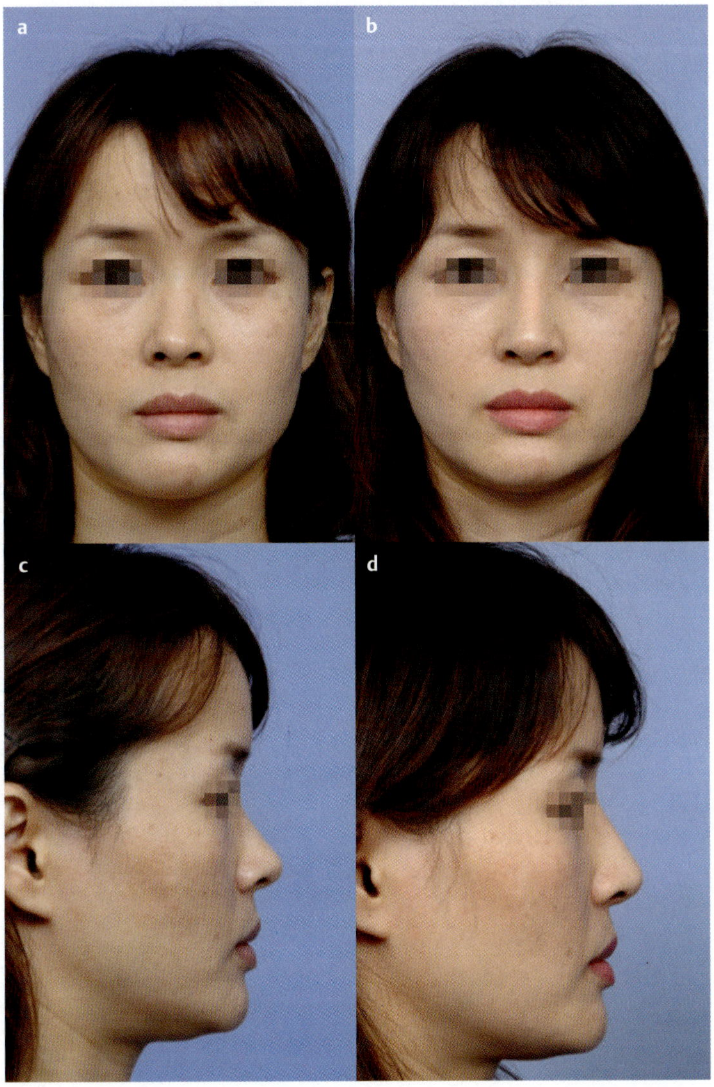

Fig. 19.13 **(a,c)** Preoperative and **(b,d)** postoperative frontal and lateral views of a patient with ePTFE implant for dorsal augmentation.

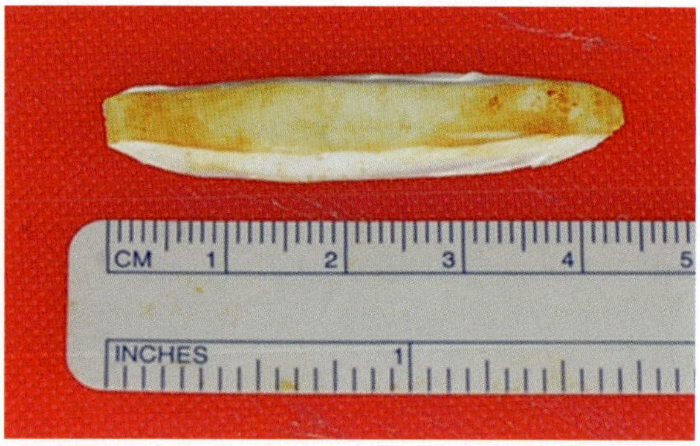

Fig. 19.14 Good beveling of the sheet's margins is essential in order not to show the graft contour.

vessels and fibrous tissue to grow inward and for collagen to embed, thus ensuring proper bonding with the implant site and high integration and stability. Medpor implants can be considered for patients when autogenous materials are unavailable or insufficient for multiple grafts. However, patients who have undergone multiple revisions or who have a history of external injuries have a higher risk of extrusion due to the compromised circulation and altered wound-healing process.[14] Unlike Gore-Tex, Medpor can be used not only for dorsal augmentation but also for structural grafting, since it possesses flexibility, firmness, and the ability to fuse well with the surrounding tissues.[15] However, risks of implant extrusion and secondary infection should always be kept in mind. In all rhinoplasties in which Medpor is used, the surgeon should sterilize the surgical field meticulously. Before insertion, the implant should be soaked in antibiotic or sterilizing solution and should be rinsed well before actual insertion. For dorsal augmentation, a pocket should be created ~ 10% larger than the implant itself.[1] Placing the Medpor implant close to the incision line, which increases the risk of wound breakdown, infection, and extrusion, should be avoided. Covering the surface of the implant with autologous tissue, such as fascia or cartilage, can be helpful in preventing implant extrusion through the skin or nasal mucosa. The common complications are infection and implant extrusion.[14]

19.4 Final Recommendation and Conclusion

Dorsal augmentation is a key rhinoplasty procedure, and the importance of dorsal implant selection cannot be overemphasized. The ideal implant should be biocompatible, biointegrated, and nonabsorbable, and it should not cause an inflammatory response. However, every material has advantages and disadvantages, and there is no single ideal implant or graft for dorsal augmentation. Thus, when surgeons choose a dorsal implant material, they should consider the merits and drawbacks of each material, anatomical characteristics of the patient, and their own level of expertise in using each material.

References

1. Jang YJ. Rhinoplasty and Septoplasty. Seoul, Korea: Koonja; 2014
2. Bullocks JM, Echo A, Guerra G, Stal S, Yuksel E. A novel autologous scaffold for diced-cartilage grafts in dorsal augmentation rhinoplasty. Aesthetic Plast Surg 2011; 35(4):569–579
3. Kim JS, Khan NA, Song HM, Jang YJ. Intraoperative measurements of harvestable septal cartilage in rhinoplasty. Ann Plast Surg 2010;65(6):519–523
4. Hagerty RC, Mittelstaedt S, Vu P, Harmatz AS, Harvey TS. Countercurve placement of conchal cartilage grafts used for correction of nasal tip deformities. Ann Plast Surg 2007;59(5):566–568
5. Jang YJ, Song HM, Yoon YJ, Sykes JM. Combined use of crushed cartilage and processed fascia lata for dorsal augmentation in rhinoplasty for Asians. Laryngoscope 2009;119(6):1088–1092
6. Moon BJ, Lee HJ, Jang YJ. Outcomes following rhinoplasty using autologous costal cartilage. Arch Facial Plast Surg 2012;14(3):175–180
7. Swanepoel PF, Fysh R. Laminated dorsal beam graft to eliminate postoperative twisting complications. Arch Facial Plast Surg 2007;9(4):285–289
8. Na DS, Jung SW, Kook KS, et al. Augmentation rhinoplasty with dermofat graft and fat injection. J Korean Soc Plast Reconst Surg 2011;38:53–62
9. Jang YJ, Wang JH, Sinha V, et al. Tutoplast processed fascia lata for dorsal augmentation in rhinoplasty. Otolaryngol Head Neck Surg 2011;144:528–532
10. Velidedeoğlu H, Demir Z, Sahin U, Kurtay A, Erol OO. Block and Surgicel-wrapped diced solvent-preserved costal cartilage homograft application for nasal augmentation. Plast Reconstr Surg 2005;115(7):2081–2093, discussion 2094–2097
11. Jang YJ, Yu MS. Rhinoplasty for the Asian nose. Facial Plast Surg 2010;26(2):93–101
12. Jang YJ, Wang JH, Lee BJ, et al. Use of silicone sheets for dorsal augmentation in rhinoplasty for Asian nose. Acta Otolaryngol Suppl 2007;588:115–120
13. Godin MS, Waldman SR, Johnson CM Jr. Nasal augmentation using Gore-Tex. A 10-year experience. Arch Facial Plast Surg 1999;1(2):118–121, discussion 122
14. Skouras A, Skouras G, Karypidis D, Asimakopoulou FA. The use of Medpor© alloplastic material in rhinoplasty: experience and outcomes. J Plast Reconstr Aesthet Surg 2012;65(1):35–42
15. Kim YH, Kim BJ, Jang TY. Use of porous high-density polyethylene (Medpor) for spreader or extended septal graft in rhinoplasty: aesthetics, functional outcomes, and long-term complications. Ann Plast Surg 2011;67(5):464–468

20 Rhinoplasty in Patients from South Asia

Santdeep Paun

20.1 Demographics of the South Asian Population

This chapter covers rhinoplasty in the diverse group of patients from the region of South Asia (often also termed the Indian subcontinent) representing India, Pakistan, Bangladesh, and Sri Lanka.

With an estimated one-quarter of the world's population, the Indian subcontinent represents a vast diversity of ethnicity. While the national census of India, for example, does not officially recognize ethnic groups, there are approximately 2,000 such groups known, thereby giving a rich diversity of facial features. Within India alone, approximately one-third of the population is under the age of 40, and interest in rhinoplasty is increasing in this enormous cohort of patients.

South Asians comprise four major overlapping ethnoracial groups: Caucasoids, Australoids, Negritos, and Mongoloids. The Caucasoids generally originate from the northern and central parts of the subcontinent, and Australoids from the south. Negritos are a cohort originating specifically in the Andaman Islands. Mongoloids are from the northeastern region of the subcontintent.

According to a 2009 study published by Reich et al,[1] the modern Indian population is composed of two genetically divergent and heterogeneous populations that mixed in ancient times (~ 1200–3500 BC), known as Ancestral North Indians (ANI) and Ancestral South Indians (ASI).

Internationally, there has been a huge emigration of people of South Asian descent across the globe, with large population bases in Europe (including the United Kingdom, where the author is based), North America, Southeast Asia, and East Africa in particular. With interracial relationships, the boundaries of what represents typical facial features in this group have further been changed and will continue to change over generations to come.

20.2 Nasal and Facial Characteristics

With such a varied population, it is difficult to typify the characteristics of the South Asian nose. Despite the varied backgrounds, facial features share more Caucasoid than Mongoloid features, other than in patients from the northeastern region. Caucasoid skull features are defined as having limited prognathism and retreat of the zygomatic area, giving rise to a more pointed face and more vertically positioned nasal apertures. Skin tone in this population varies from the fairer skin of the population in Pakistan and Northern India to the significantly darker skin of the Southern Indian, Bangladeshi, and Sri Lankan population.

Nasal skin is generally a little thicker than in a typical Anglo-Saxon patient, but varies significantly across the population. The majority of patients have a nose with a generally less projected tip and often a prominent dorsum, so reduction rhinoplasty tends to be their aim. There are, of course, some regional variances in features, but a typical rhinoplasty in a South Asian patient will involve addressing the usual issues of a dorsal hump and a ptotic and poorly defined tip, as well as the patient's wish to accentuate a Western appearance.

To have an aesthetically pleasing, acceptable, and normal look is undoubtedly a universal wish, and the South Asian population has always embraced beauty as an overwhelming desire. Formerly, social stigma detracted from the use of cosmetic procedures, but, with the ever-increasing popularity of all aspects of media, attitudes have changed significantly within a generation. From the glamor of Bollywood, the world's most prolific movie industry, to increasing Western influences through the Internet and television exposure, and with the pervasiveness of social media now linking a global audience, cosmetic surgery in this population has grown exponentially. A burgeoning middle class, as a result of increasing socioeconomic prosperity in the region, has further fueled this popularity.

In the United Kingdom, rhinoplasty surgery is by far the most common aesthetic procedure requested by South Asian patients, with surgery for the aging face still not as popular within this group.

20.3 Analysis

20.3.1 History and Examination

The importance of preoperative assessment in patients seeking rhinoplasty cannot be over-emphasized. It is beyond the scope of this chapter to discuss full facial analysis in detail, and it is assumed that the rhinoplasty surgeon has a comprehensive knowledge of the relevant concepts.

A complete and discerning history includes original cosmesis and function, as well as prior procedures and accurate chronological detailing of postoperative changes. Photographs may assist in relating to the patient's ongoing concerns. Patient anxieties and expectations should be elucidated early in the consultation to ensure that they are specific, rather than a general dissatisfaction with a prior surgical result. The evaluating specialist needs to ensure that the patient's expectations are realistic and in keeping with predictable postoperative outcomes. Where any doubt exists, sensitive counseling of the patient and referral for psychiatric review are always prudent, and surgery may be deferred.[2,3] Pertinent decisions about indications for surgery and potential improvements can then be made. Approach and technique planning are then discussed with the patient and documented in the notes.

Diagnosis of the underlying anatomical deformity is essential prior to embarking upon the surgical plan. Inspection and palpation are equally important, particularly when assessing the skin–soft tissue envelope (S-STE) and minor dorsal irregularities. The main pillars for documenting the analysis are the length, projection, and rotation of the nose. Specifically, the nose can conveniently be divided into thirds for analysis, and deformities can be evaluated and documented in each area separately. Within these areas, a further analysis of underlying skeletal support, soft tissue thickness, scarring, and overlying skin texture will help elucidate anatomical and structural deformities. Intranasal examination may be complemented with endoscopic evaluation to identify the presence of residual septal deviations, adhesions, nasal valve problems, and mucosal disease. It is important to check if there is alar collapse on inspiration, but, even in its absence, valve collapse cannot be excluded. Assessment with the Cottle maneuver (**Fig. 20.1**) is often advocated but can be nonspecific; lateralizing the alar cartilage with a probe or cotton bud may be a better evaluation technique (**Fig. 20.2**).

20.3.2 Documentation

Documentation should include accurate assessment of all the nasal thirds in turn. The osseocartilaginous structure is assessed for asymmetry, deviations are noted, and irregularities sought. Over- or under-resection of the dorsum should be checked. Any tip abnormalities, including alar pathology, are recorded. The nasal turbinates are examined and nasal valve narrowing is assessed. Skin quality and scarring are also noted. A surgical plan is formulated to correct the specific deformities. The plan should be discussed with, and agreed upon by, the patient. Preoperative photography is an absolute requirement for analysis and medicolegal purposes. Standard photographic views form a useful way of communicating deformities and potential changes to the patient. They also assist in operative planning and are invaluable for reference during surgery. In combination with postoperative images, they are essential for self- and peer-reviewed assessment of results. Standardization of the photographic views and lighting and background conditions are critical. Digital SLR photography lends itself well to computer archiving.

Digital Imaging

Digital imaging has evolved immensely over the past few years, and morphing is possible with even the simplest photo-imaging software both on computers and tablet/ mobile devices. Indeed, patients are becoming increasingly adept at creating their own ideal digitally morphed photographs. With the ubiquitous selfie, there has never been more emphasis on personal satisfaction with photographs.

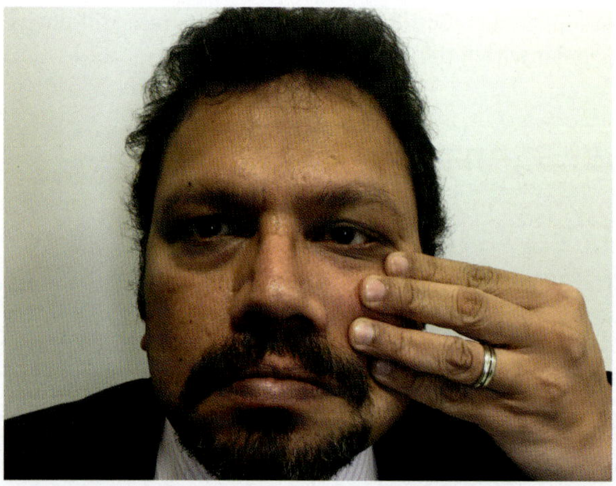

Fig. 20.1 Cottle maneuver.

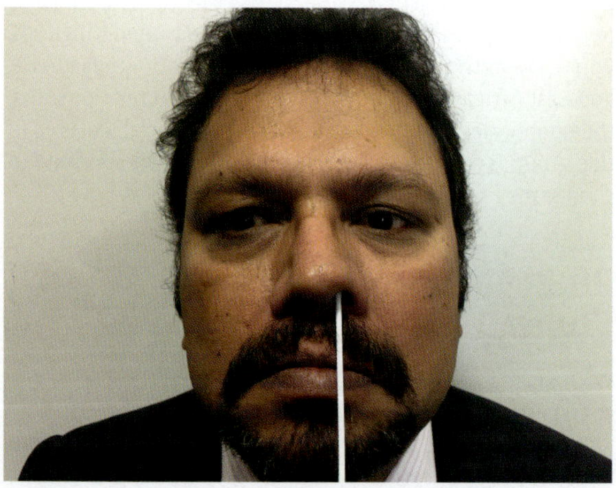

Fig. 20.2 Alar lateralization with a cotton bud.

More complex programs are readily available, with or without archiving capability, and have purpose-made user interfaces and allow more advanced digital manipulation of the images. They can be very useful in showing patients potential changes and postoperative outcomes. Detailing profile changes in the lateral view is always relatively straightforward with any 2D digital software, but showing the patient the frontal view they would see in a mirror was challenging. Now, latest-generation 3D image manipulation (Vectra, Canfield Imaging) is becoming increasingly popular; it provides the patient with a more complete picture of the potential postoperative result, including changes in the frontal view and refinement in the nasal tip area (**Fig. 20.3**). Dedicated programs have measurement abilities and so can be extremely helpful in operative planning. It is important not to convey unrealistic changes to the patient and indeed to point out such on any digitally morphed photos of themselves they may bring. As a rule, slightly underestimating the postoperative result is preferable to an unrealistic, unachievable simulation. Most surgeons choose not to give the patient printed images of the predicted changes, but if the surgeon elects to do so, a printed waiver should make clear that the image is only an indication of the likely result.

It is essential to ensure that the patient is given realistic expectations for the intended surgery, and that the surgeon and patient discuss both the limitations and the potential complications of the surgical procedure. It is important to ensure that improvement is indeed possible, and a risk-benefit profile may need to be detailed to the patient prior to obtaining consent.

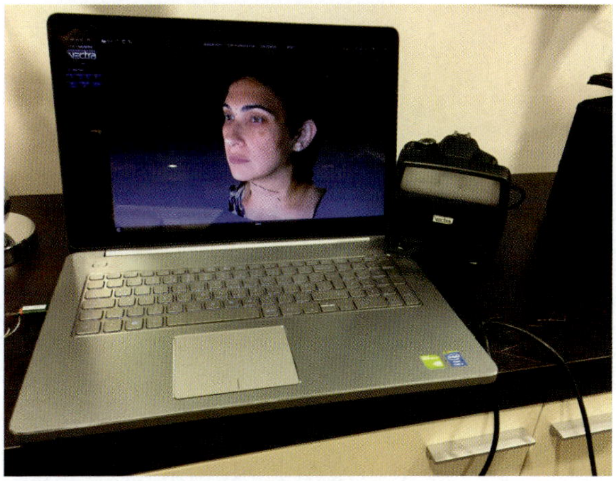

Fig. 20.3 Use of 3D imaging and digital manipulation software.

20.3.3 Preoperative Counseling

Cosmetic surgery in the South Asian patient is still subject to social stigma. Despite the increasing number of patients undergoing rhinoplasty, many patients choose not to tell close friends and family of any potential surgical choices, a decision that can create issues with regard to support for the individual.

The nose can provide cultural, ethnic, and symbolic identities, and their psychological significance should not be underestimated.[4] Indeed, in the South Asian male patient in particular, a somewhat prominent nasal hump may be seen as desirable. Western influences, however, have changed long-standing perceptions, and it is now the accepted norm for individuals to seek a less culturally sensitive appearance. Because the nose occupies the central aspect of the face and is its most prominent feature, it has a unique place in facial identity. Relatively minor changes in nasal appearance can give rise to more profound overall effects on the face and any discussion with patients seeking rhinoplasty should highlight this.

Motivations for surgery are complex and are generally intricately related to the patient's self-esteem and persona. It is important to ensure that the patient's expectations of surgery are realistic, not only for postoperative outcome, but also for how a favorable result could affect the patient's life and psyche.

The revision rhinoplasty patient may further present with psychological issues relating to the original surgery, and these must be both recognized and addressed during any preliminary consultation.[3,4] In doing so, it is important to distinguish between a truly inadequate result and a patient-perceived unfavorable result. While the former scenario may be easier to manage, assuming realistic expectations, it is particularly important in the latter case not to convey false expectations regarding the revision procedure. Doctor–patient rapport and trust must be built, to lay the foundation for conveying realistic expectations for outcome of revision surgery. If the surgeon feels an improvement cannot be predictably achieved, the patient is best not operated on, irrespective of the patient's desires or pressure on the surgeon. The potential difficulty in dealing with male patients has been widely reported,[5] and this may also extend to postoperative dissatisfaction.

20.4 Nasal Anatomy

It is important to emphasize salient aspects of the nasal anatomy. **Fig. 20.4** shows the anatomical subunits of the nose, which are conveniently divided into thirds. The bony pyramid, consisting of the nasal bones with their articulation to the ascending processes of the maxilla and the bony septum, constitutes the upper third. The paired upper lateral cartilages insert just under the caudal end of the nasal bones, and their fusion with the midline cartilaginous septum in a T configuration forms the middle third (vault). The internal nasal valve gives physiological resistance to

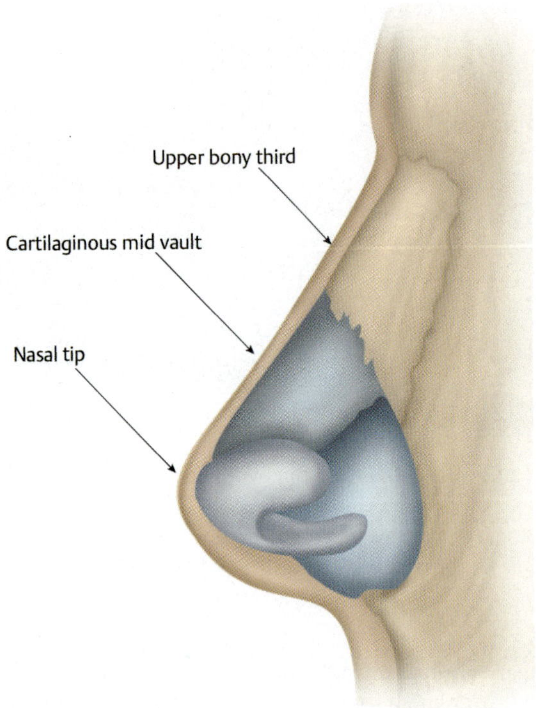

Fig. 20.4 The nasal thirds.

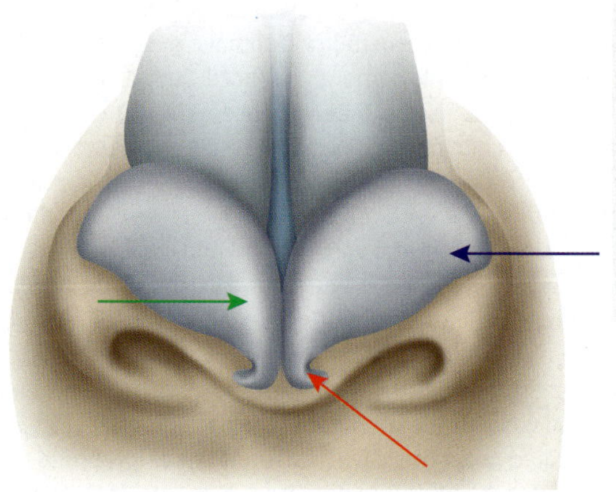

Fig. 20.5 Lower lateral cartilage crurae (*blue arrow*, lateral crus; *green arrow*, intermediate crus; *red arrow*, medial crus).

breathing and is bounded by the nasal septal cartilage's articulation with the upper lateral cartilages, inferior turbinates, and soft tissue, with accessory cartilages providing lateral boundaries. The scroll attachment of the caudal aspect of the upper lateral cartilages to the cephalic aspect of lower lateral cartilages forms the boundary of the lower third of the nose. The paired lower lateral cartilages form the nasal tip and are traditionally divided into the lateral, intermediate, and medial crurae **(Fig. 20.5)**. The domes and tip-defining points lie within the intermediate crus. The medial crural footplates extend to the lower aspect of the columella and lie just anterior but form an attachment to the caudal aspect of the nasal septum. The superficial muscular aponeurotic system (SMAS) provides a rich vascular covering to the underlying skeleton, with arterial supply derived from the superior labial and facial artery branches and their accompanying venous and lymphatic vessels.

20.5 Surgical Planning

Accurate notation of the deformities and intended corrective procedures should be made for all rhinoplasty patients. Some deformities, particularly if not related to the underlying structure, may not be evident until after elevation of the soft tissue envelope. The surgical approach, be it endonasal or external, should be discussed with the patient and incisions outlined and documented. The surgical plan should be decided at the time of consultation and should be clearly written into the notes; the plan is used as a framework for performance of the surgery, although potential irregularity of the findings in revision surgery means that the plan may need to be flexibly altered.

20.5.1 Approaches

The author uses both endonasal and external approaches for rhinoplasties in the South Asian patient. The adage of limiting the surgical dissection to a minimum dependent on the needs of each individual case remains the foremost consideration. Minimizing the risk of vascular compromise of the skin–soft tissue envelope (S-STE) is achieved by careful dissection in ideal surgical planes. In this way, scarring is prevented and subsequent healing is more predictable. The S-STE may be thin and adherent to the underlying structures, particularly in revision cases and in cases where prior grafts were used over the dorsum. Augmentation of specific areas is best performed in precise pockets, and limited dissection makes it easier to judge the ideal position for placing a graft. An endonasal approach with minimal soft tissue dissection is thus preferable for minor deformities and is ideal for correcting minimal bony dorsal irregularities.

The external approach's requirement for more soft tissue dissection is balanced by the unparalleled view of the nasal structural components it affords. It facilitates accurate diagnosis in cases where the underlying anatomy is not obvious. Binocular vision, bimanual tissue handling, and the ability to precisely place and suture cartilaginous grafts, as well as its use as a teaching tool, are further advantages.[6] The author personally favors this approach for most reconstructive revisions and particularly where the nasal tip needs addressing. Because intercartilaginous incisions are not used, the valve area is preserved. It is important to appreciate that, while the major tip support mechanisms are respected in the external approach, the disruption of the S-STE from the lower lateral cartilages and the division of the medial intercrural ligamentous tissue lead to loss of some of the minor tip support mechanisms, and therefore some ptosis of the nasal tip should be anticipated in all cases. Any loss of tip projection can be countered by placement of a columellar strut to maintain support. However, with the open approach, it may be difficult to assess the dorsum, supratip, and the desired tip projection due to the lack of traction of the soft tissue prior to closure of the columellar incision, with final assessment of these areas made after preliminary closure.[6]

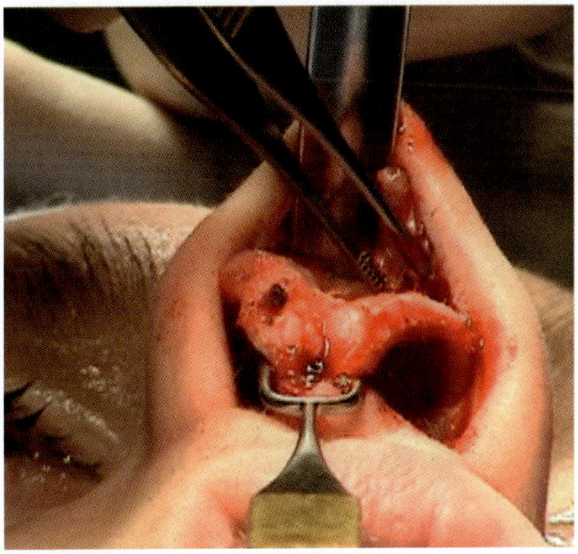

Fig. 20.6 Brown-Adson forcep used to pluck soft tissue in the thick-skinned nose.

20.5.2 Skin Considerations

The basic surgical principle of respecting the S-STE is relevant even with thicker skin types. Neglecting to evaluate the S-STE when other, more marked deformities are visible is done at the surgeon's peril. Accurate documentation and marking of specific irregularities are critical because perioperative injection of local anesthesia may mask such deformities. Dissection in the correct surgical planes, during both primary and revision rhinoplasty, prevents postoperative scarring and differential thickness of the soft tissues. Circumspect resection of such irregularities during revision rhinoplasty may be required, but caution is advised, because S-STE changes are largely permanent and correction can prove troublesome.

Thicker skin has the problem of hiding underlying structural change. Patients with very thick skin may be disappointed by the lack of definition of the nasal contour postoperatively and should thus be appropriately counseled preoperatively to temper their expectations. The underlying soft tissue can be gently trimmed by judicious plucking of the subdermal area using a multi-toothed Brown-Adson forcep, removing only what easily comes away (**Fig. 20.6**). Sharp dissection using scissors in the region is best avoided as it risks damage to the subdermal plexus. Postoperative steroid (triamcinolone) injections to the subdermal area to reduce the risk of pollybeak formation are performed 2, 6, and 16 weeks after surgery (**Fig. 20.7**). It is important to ensure that the steroid is not injected directly into the dermis itself, as necrosis is a risk in this scenario. If any blanching of the skin occurs, the injection should be stopped immediately.

Thinner-skinned patients may be prone to redness postoperatively, and minor irregularities are easily seen through thin skin. Underlay soft tissue camouflage grafts may be required. Temporalis fascia is excellent for this purpose, although alloplasts may be used as alternatives.

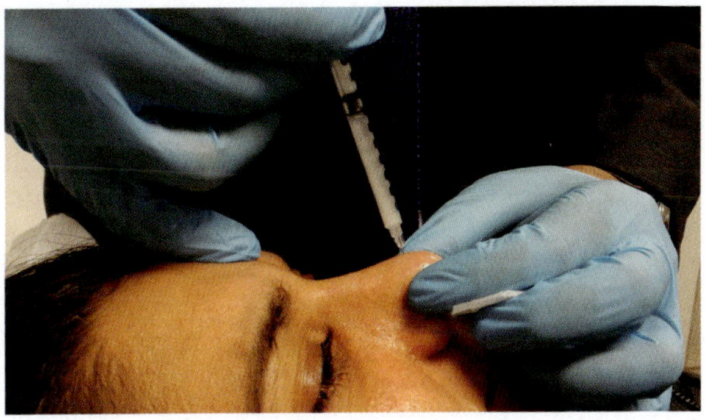

Fig. 20.7 Injection of triamcinolone into the supratip area.

20.5.3 Dorsal Deformities

The majority of South Asian patients are concerned with prominence of the dorsal hump, with only those from northeastern India having more Mongoloid features and a dorsum that may need augmentation.

Dorsal reduction is performed with sequential reduction of the cartilaginous hump initially. The quadrilateral cartilage of the septum is divided extramucosally from the upper lateral cartilages and lowered to the relevant level. The upper laterals may be reduced to match, but, where possible, are scored and the cartilage is inverted medially to create an autospreader graft or spreader flap (**Fig. 20.8**),[7] thereby providing stability to the mid third of the nose and

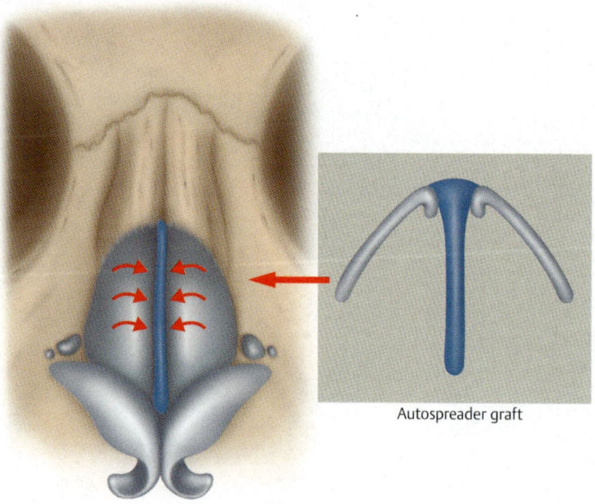

Fig. 20.8 Spreader flap technique.

internal nasal valve region. This is particularly important in the patient with a long cartilaginous dorsum and short nasal bones, who may be prone to developing a typical inverted-V deformity.

The inverted-V deformity is a consequence of either excessive resection of, or collapse of, the upper lateral cartilages inferomedially due to inadequate support after removal of a dorsal hump. The nose displays a washed out appearance, with prominence of the caudal edge of the nasal bones. There may be associated internal nasal valve collapse, giving rise to nasal obstruction. Spreader grafts are an effective way of resolving this deformity and can improve nasal valve dysfunction. The spreader graft uses cartilaginous strips placed longitudinally between the upper lateral cartilage and septum (**Fig. 20.9** and **Fig. 20.10**). While the mucosa between the cartilages is often divided, in accord with Sheen's original work,[8] this should be avoided; rather, the spreader graft should be placed extramucosally. Functional improvement has been difficult to quantify objectively but subjective improvement is to be anticipated. Placement via an external approach allows for accurate visualization and fixation, but, when required, placement can be accomplished equally well endonasally[9] into tight submucoperichondrial pockets, and the graft can be held with tissue glue or with percutaneous trans-septal sutures if required. Unilateral placement of spreader grafts may also correct asymmetries of the dorsum. Autospreader/spreader flaps can be an effective and simple alternative and negate the need for a separate cartilaginous source (**Fig. 20.8**).

Dorsal bony reduction is then performed using a rasp or, if the hump is excessive, with an osteotome. Irregularities may then be minimized by careful palpation with a wet finger, followed by final bony reduction with a fine rasp to ensure a smooth profile. It is important that any bony fragments are cleared because they may form further visual or palpable irregularities with time. Acellular dermis (Alloderm, Lifecell), temperoparietal free fascia grafts,[10] SMAS autografts,[11] and lightly bruised septal cartilage[12] have variously been described as being useful cover for any potential residual unevenness.

Under-resection of the cartilaginous middle third of the nose can lead to the pollybeak deformity, which is one of the most common reasons for revision rhinoplasty. This supratip prominence is most often a consequence of inadequate lowering of the dorsal septal–upper lateral cartilage complex comprising this area. There is often a combination of a lowered bony dorsum, a relatively high septal angle, and postoperative loss of tip support, with resultant tip de-projection.

Soft tissue thickening after rhinoplasty in the thick-skinned patient can also give rise to this complication. It is minimized by interval steroid injections (10 mg/mL triamcinolone)[13] into the subcutaneous region of the supratip early after revision surgery. Injection can be repeated

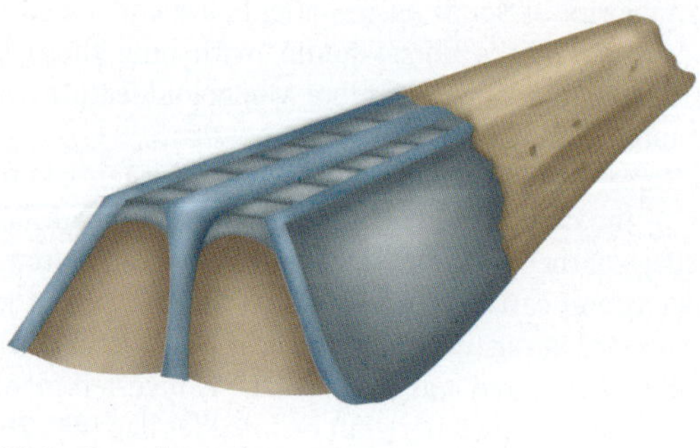

Fig. 20.9 Spreader grafts.

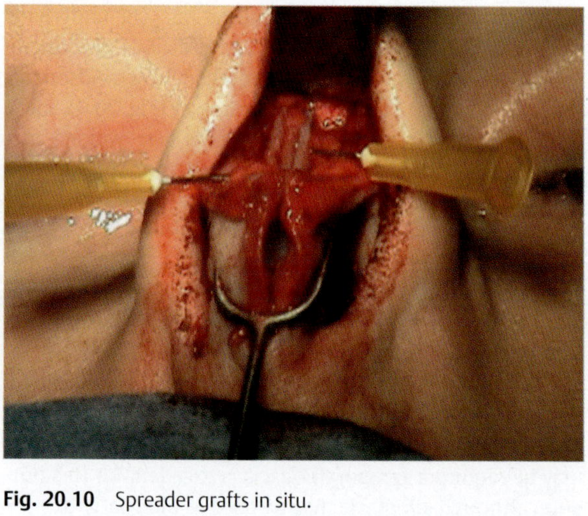

Fig. 20.10 Spreader grafts in situ.

monthly if required. Nighttime taping of the supratip area may help reduce recurrence by limiting the dead space into which tissue thickening can occur.

Overall, over-resection of the dorsum may be a failure of recognition of the anatomical basis of the hump and its overlying S-STE. The rhinoplasty surgeon should recognize the bony/cartilaginous contributions to the dorsum and the fact that the S-STE thickness varies along it, being thicker in the nasofrontal region and in the supratip and at its thinnest overlying the rhinion.

Osteotomies

Osteotomies are performed with a standard technique. A medial fading osteotomy is performed routinely even if a large dorsal hump has been resected to ensure accurate bony back fracture in this area. High, low, and high lateral osteotomies may be performed endonasally but also externally percutaneously, and this can provide accurate correction. Inadequate, asymmetric, improperly placed, or lateralized osteotomies may give a residual deviation of the bony bridge or an open roof deformity. A step deformity can persist where original osteotomies are placed too high on the nasal bones. Persistence of the open roof despite osteotomies can be adequately managed by insertion of an extended spreader graft obliterating the potential space. A rocker deformity occurs when the osteotomies are taken too high into thick frontal bone, causing the superior part of the nasal bone to rock laterally when infractured. Rocker deformity can be prevented and corrected by percutaneous superior osteotomies to allow a controlled fracture in a favorable position.

Intermediate osteotomies may be required in the markedly deviated nose where one nasal bone is significantly longer than the other. They are performed endonasally or percutaneously and are placed parallel to, and are done before, the lateral osteotomy, because once the nasal bone is mobilized, intermediate fractures are challenging to make. Sequential osteotomies may then be required to deal with the deviation. These have been likened to opening the pages of a book[14] and comprise initial mobilization of the nasal bone opposite to the deviation, followed by the bony septum and then finally the other nasal bone.

20.5.4 Tip Deformities

The main problems identified in the tip region of the South Asian patient relate to projection, with a bulbous, ptotic tip being the usual complaint. Thickness of the overlying skin predictably gives rise to poor definition in this area. Over-projection and over-rotation are unusual in this group of patients.

Correction relies on knowledge of the tripod theory of the nasal tip **(Fig. 20.11)**. According to this theory, the conjoint medial crura are considered one part of the tripod, with each lateral crus representing a separate lateral limb. Manipulation of any part of the tripod normally leads to predictable changes in both the projection and rotation of the nasal tip (some examples are described below).

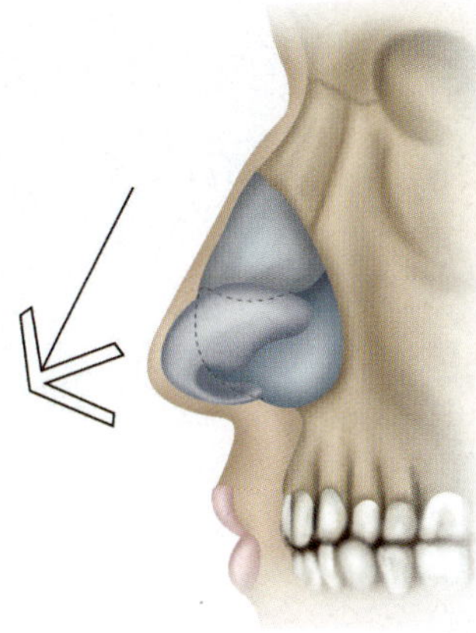

Fig. 20.11 Tripod theory.

Management of the Poorly Projected Tip

An under-rotated, poorly projected tip can be corrected with a variety of maneuvers, based on the tripod theory. It should be noted that rotation changes are usually linked with some projection change, and knowledge of what will happen in both aspects is required. The simplest maneuvers involve suturing of the domes with inter- and transdomal sutures, placed cephalically in a newly created domal area. This will narrow a bulbous, poorly defined tip displaying a boxy plateau externally, often accentuated by a thicker skin type. The sutures may also give a small degree of additional projection that can be aided by a strong columellar strut to straighten and strengthen otherwise weak medial crurae. If further projection is required, a lateral crural steal technique with recruitment of the lateral crura medially using domal suturing can also be usefully employed.[15] The lateral crus can be separated from the underlying vestibular skin and then mobilized medially. The medial crus is thus lengthened at the expense of (by stealing from) the lateral crus **(Fig. 20.12)**. The maneuver can also rotate the tip, and caution is advised in this regard. It is also important not to over-tighten sutures, which can create a pinching effect.

Cephalic resection of the lower lateral cartilages or resection of the anterior septal angle can also create a degree of rotation, but these approaches are neither predictable nor powerful rotators of the nasal tip and should only be employed as a sole measure in patients requir-

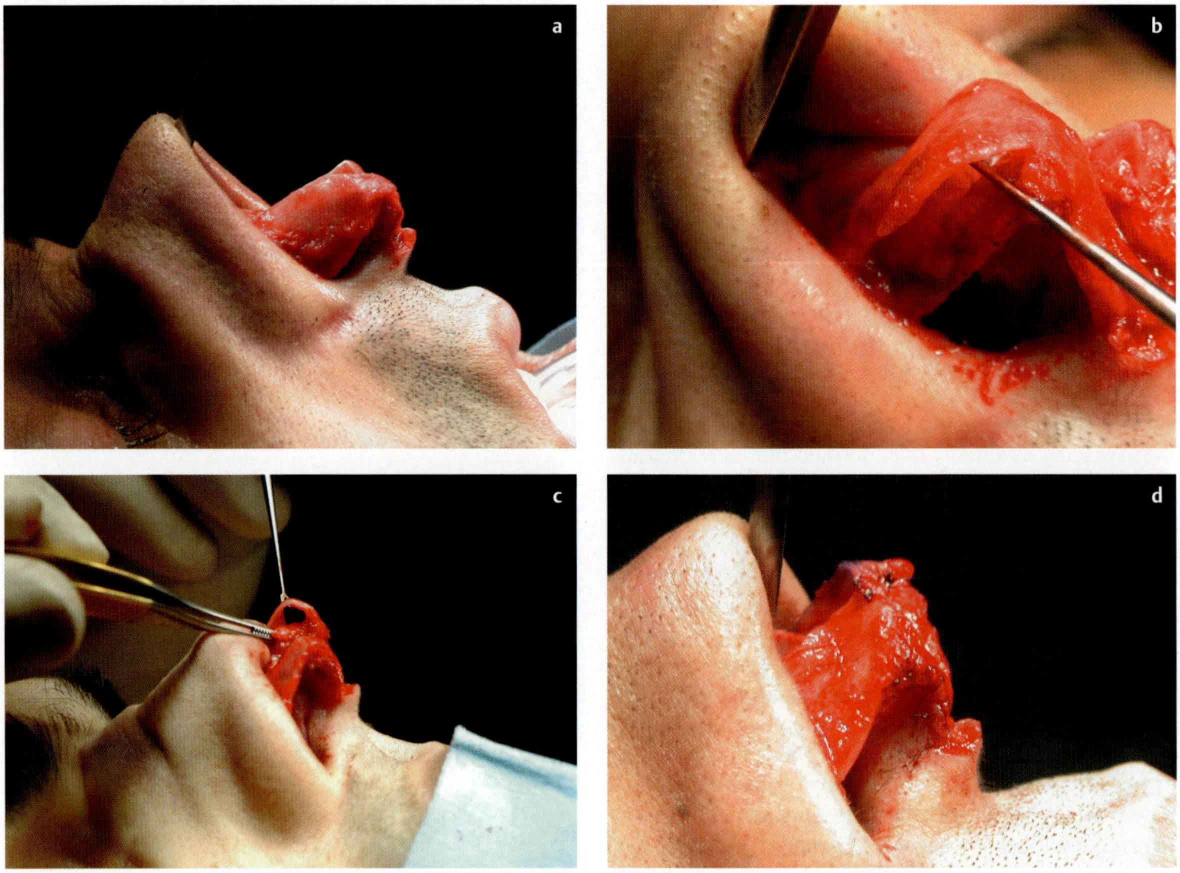

Fig. 20.12 Lateral crural steal procedure. **(a)** Under-projected tip. **(b)** Mobilization of vestibular skin. **(c)** Recruitment of lateral crus to lengthen medial crus. **(d)** Left dome projected and rotated due to steal.

ing minimal rotation changes. Care needs to be employed in cephalic strip reduction, however, and the author has become far more conservative in this regard. Over-resection of the cephalic edge of the lower lateral cartilages creates weakening of the intact rim strip of the lower lateral cartilages. The useful edict of leaving behind more cartilage than was resected should always be remembered, although it is recommended that an absolute minimum of 6 mm of cartilaginous support be left. Following patients over many years suggests that leaving more may be more favorable in many cases. Aggressive domal suturing, with its resultant alteration in tip orientation and dynamics, can also cause notching in the dome region, particularly after aggressive cephalic reduction, predisposing to a pinched tip effect. Knuckling of the lower lateral cartilages in the domal area can form so-called bossae. The triad of thin skin, strong alar cartilages, and bifid tip can predispose to bossa formation when there is an excess cephalic strip reduction and inadequate narrowing of the domes.[16] Postoperative scar contracture in this area causes the deformity.

The ideal aesthetics of the basal view of the nasal tip is that of an equilateral triangle. The lateral crurae should exhibit a slight outward convexity and gentle rounding in the dome region; specifically, there should be no pinching of the lateral alar walls.

The lower lateral cartilages can be strengthened, if required, with lateral crural strut grafts, which can prevent postoperative concavity but equally can help flatten the appearance of the lateral crurae in patients with overt convexity of the alar rims. Another effective solution in patients undergoing cephalic reduction is not to excise the cartilage but to score and bend it backward into a pocket created between the lateral crus and underlying vestibular skin—the so-called lateral crural flap or auto lateral crural strut. Once again, this negates the need for an additional cartilaginous source, and it allows a more significant cephalic reduction to be performed, if required, as strength is maintained in the area, protecting against eventual collapse. A useful tip for elevating the vestibular skin below the lateral crus is to inject it first with local anesthesia, thereby creating hydrodissection in an area that can otherwise be difficult to dissect without damage. Alar rim grafts can also recreate convexity and rounding of the nasal tip contour as assessed on the frontal and basal views.

Plumping grafts and columellar struts can be also used to create an illusion of rotation. Resection and overlay of the lateral crura (lateral crural flap technique) can produce rotation, especially when the overlap occurs toward the most lateral part of the alar cartilage. Such a technique is generally used to shorten the nose as well when over-projection is problematic.

The tongue-in-groove technique of septocolumellar suturing[17] is another option and is a useful way of setting both projection and rotation of the nasal tip. A disadvantage of the technique is the rigidity and lack of mobility it imparts to the tip, but they are generally well tolerated in most patients. The technique does cause a degree of columellar retraction, which may be favorable in the presence of a hanging columella. If such retraction occurs, a septal extension graft is employed to provide a stable base on which to project the tip complex. Such grafts are versatile and are generally secured in an end-to-end fashion to the caudal septum. Septocolumellar sutures can be a powerful rotator of the tip and it is important to guard against excessive rotation.

Shield and tip grafts work well in thicker-skinned patients and can finesse a poorly projected tip. They are reserved for when other tip suture techniques do not produce the desired degree of tip projection. Grafts are beveled at the edges to avoid their showing through the skin in the long term. They are generally secured into position using fine 6–0 permanent sutures. Crushed cartilage is also useful to help camouflage minor deformities over the dorsum or tip region.

An overly rotated nasal tip ("piggy nose") is as unaesthetic in the South Asian patient as in most population groups. Over-rotation is most often due to a combination of factors in the original surgery, such as resection of the anterior septal angle, the visoring effect of excessive cephalic strip excision of the lower lateral cartilages, and perhaps other maneuvers involving the lateral crurae. Options for correction can be limited in this situation; therefore, caution needs to be exercised to avoid its occurrence in primary surgery. The mainstay of management is placement of a caudal septal extension graft to effectively lengthen the nose. Extended spreader grafts are then used to stabilize the septal complex (**Fig. 20.13**), and the lower lateral cartilages are then rotated downward and are fixed to the extension graft.[12]

20.5.5 Alar Base Widening

Alar base widening is often requested by South Asian patients. The techniques of alar base reduction reflect whether there is excess alar flare, excess nostril sill size, or, most commonly, a combination of the two.[6] If the sill alone needs narrowing, the incision is limited to this area alone and need not extend into the lateral aspect of the alar base. If a lateral extension is required to deal with alar flare, the incision is made just above, rather than within, the alar crease. Symmetry is challenging in alar base surgery, so accurate measurement with calipers can be helpful.

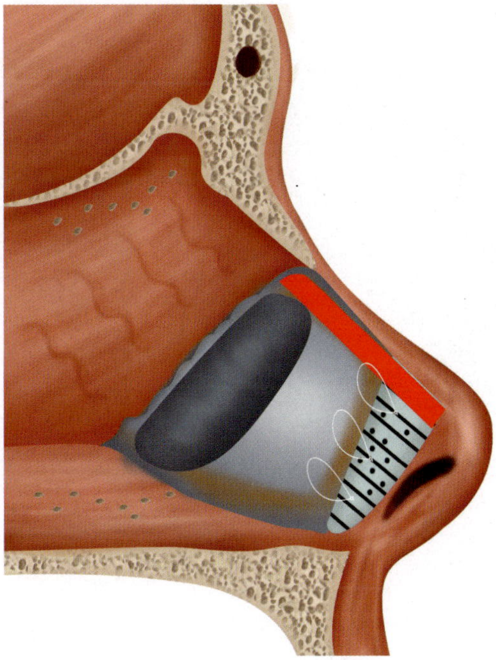

Fig. 20.13 Septal extension graft with extended spreader grafts (*red*) to derotate the nasal tip.

20.6 Case Studies

Fig. 20.14, Fig. 20.15, Fig. 20.16, Fig. 20.17, and **Fig. 20.18** illustrate South Asian patients who underwent rhinoplasty. Typical findings of a moderate dorsal hump, ptosis of the nasal tip, and moderately thick skin are illustrated, and management is detailed for each case.

20.7 Conclusion

The vast South Asian population will inevitably have regional variations in facial features, and skin tone in particular varies significantly. Caucasoid features, however, predominate, and rhinoplasty techniques reflect this, with reduction by far the most common procedure performed. Western features remain a perceived ideal for many patients from this population. While established techniques are used, care must be taken to maintain ethnicity in this complex population. Traditionally, social stigma limited the number of patients seeking pure cosmetic surgery, but increasing socioeconomic conditions and powerful media influence both within the countries and beyond have fueled an exponential rise in patients seeking rhinoplasty.

Within the United Kingdom's South Asian population, rhinoplasty is the most commonly requested facial cosmetic operation, and it is usually requested by younger, Westernized patients.

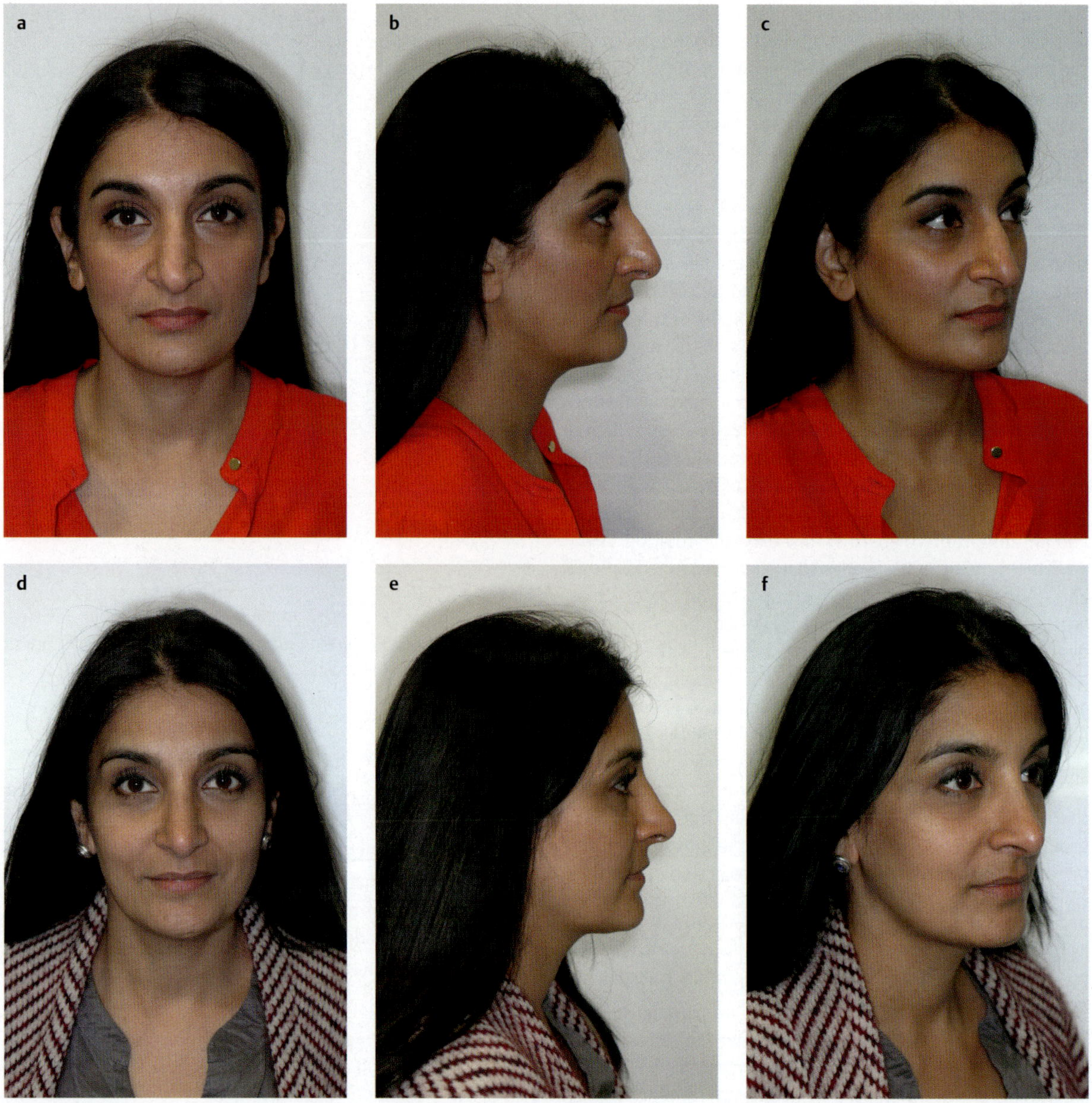

Fig. 20.14 (a–f) Over-projected nose with dorsal hump and excess columellar show. Management with an open approach, septal correction, dorsal reduction with medial and lateral osteotomies, tongue-in-groove to de-project the nose and reduce the columellar show, dome sutures.

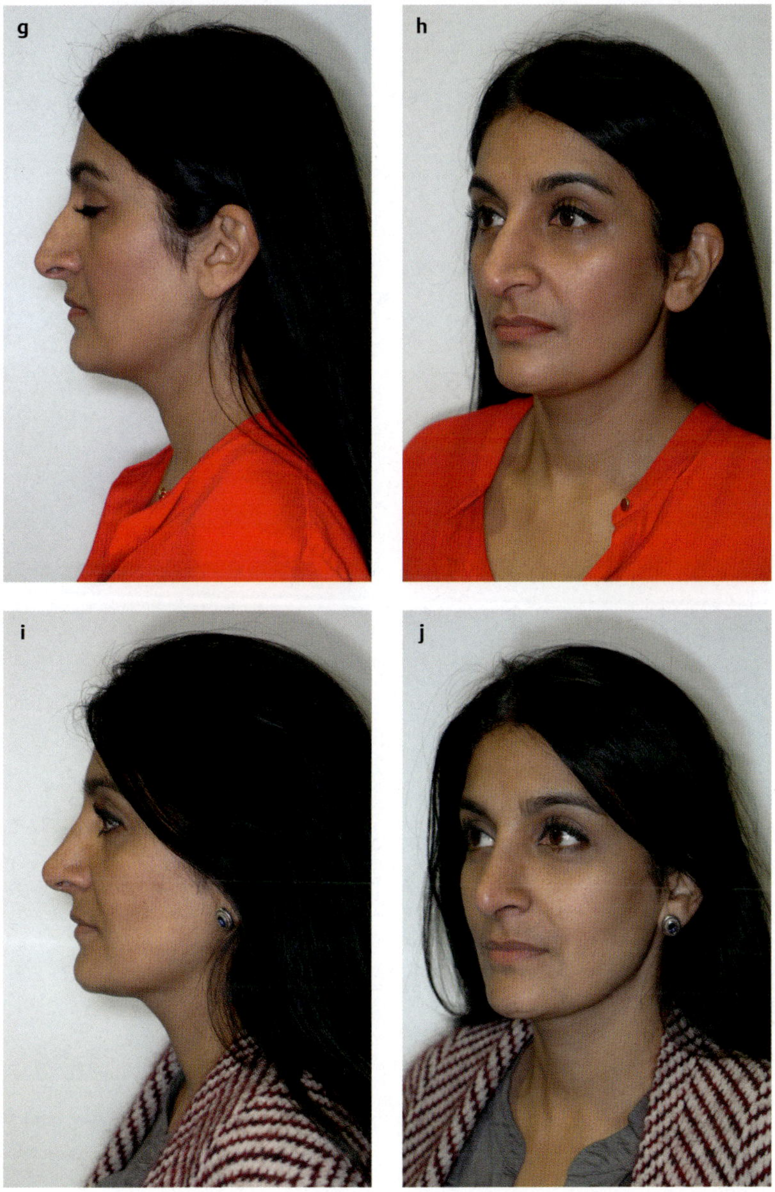

Fig. 20.14 *(Continued)* **(g–j)** Over-projected nose with dorsal hump and excess columellar show. Management with an open approach, septal correction, dorsal reduction with medial and lateral osteotomies, tongue-in-groove to de-project the nose and reduce the columellar show, dome sutures.

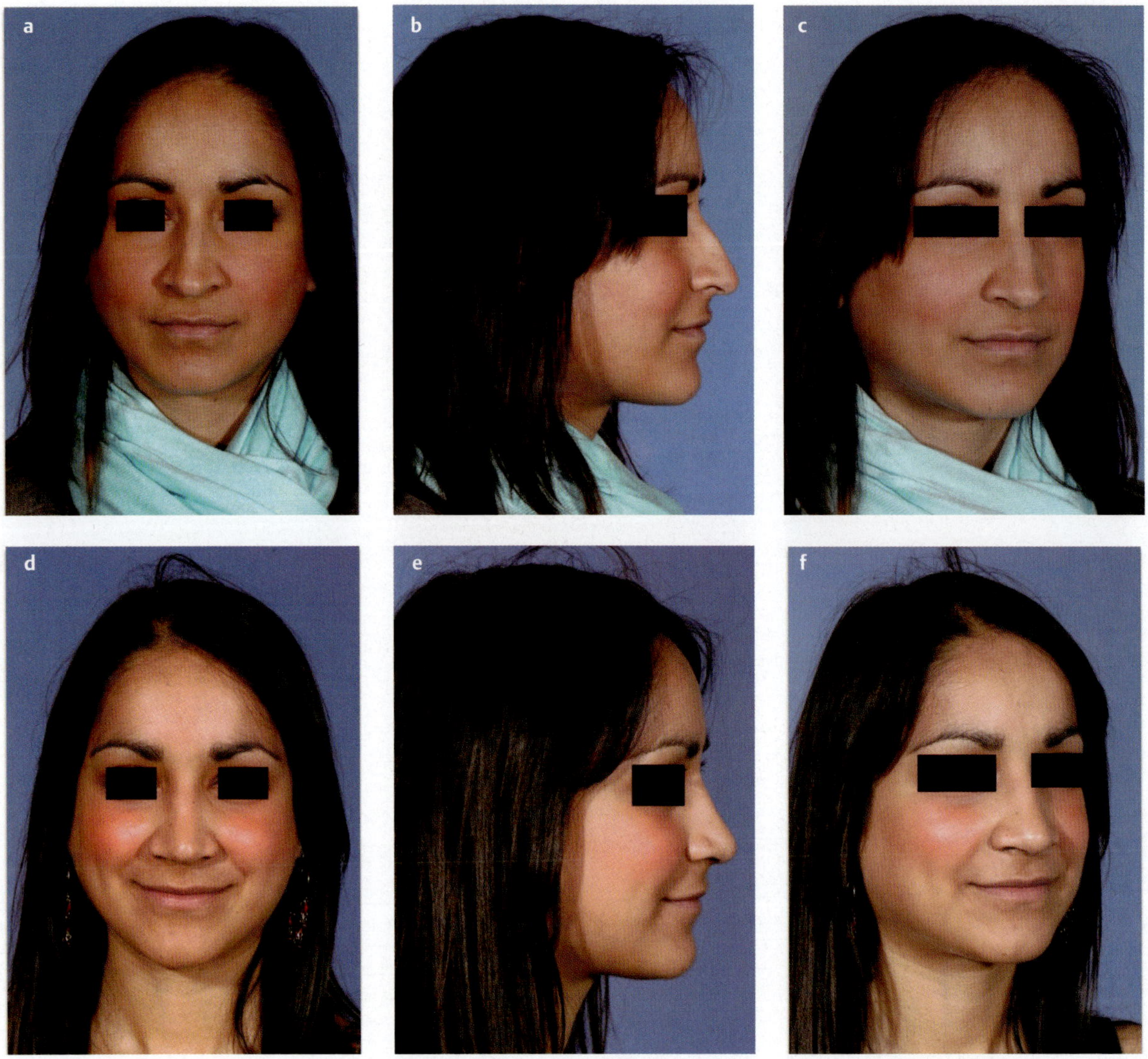

Fig. 20.15 (a–f) Dorsal hump with nasal tip ptosis. Management with an open approach, septal correction, dorsal reduction with medial and lateral osteotomies, lateral crural overlay, dome sutures, columellar strut.

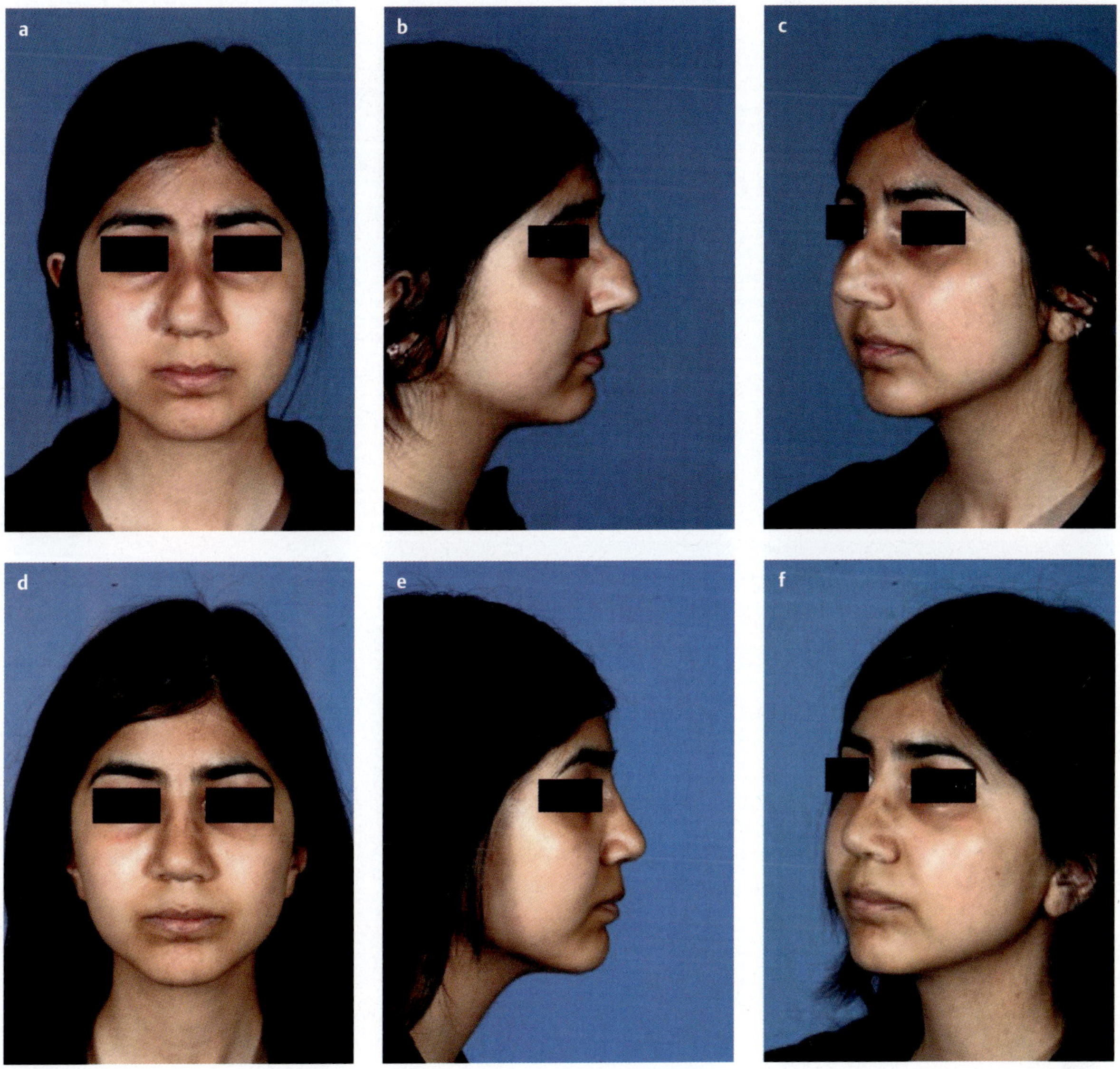

Fig. 20.16 (a–f) Large dorsal hump with excess cartilaginous dorsum. Management with an open approach for extracorporeal septoplasty; dorsal reduction; medial, lateral, and intermediate osteotomies; dome sutures; and defatting of tip skin. *(Continued on page 244)*

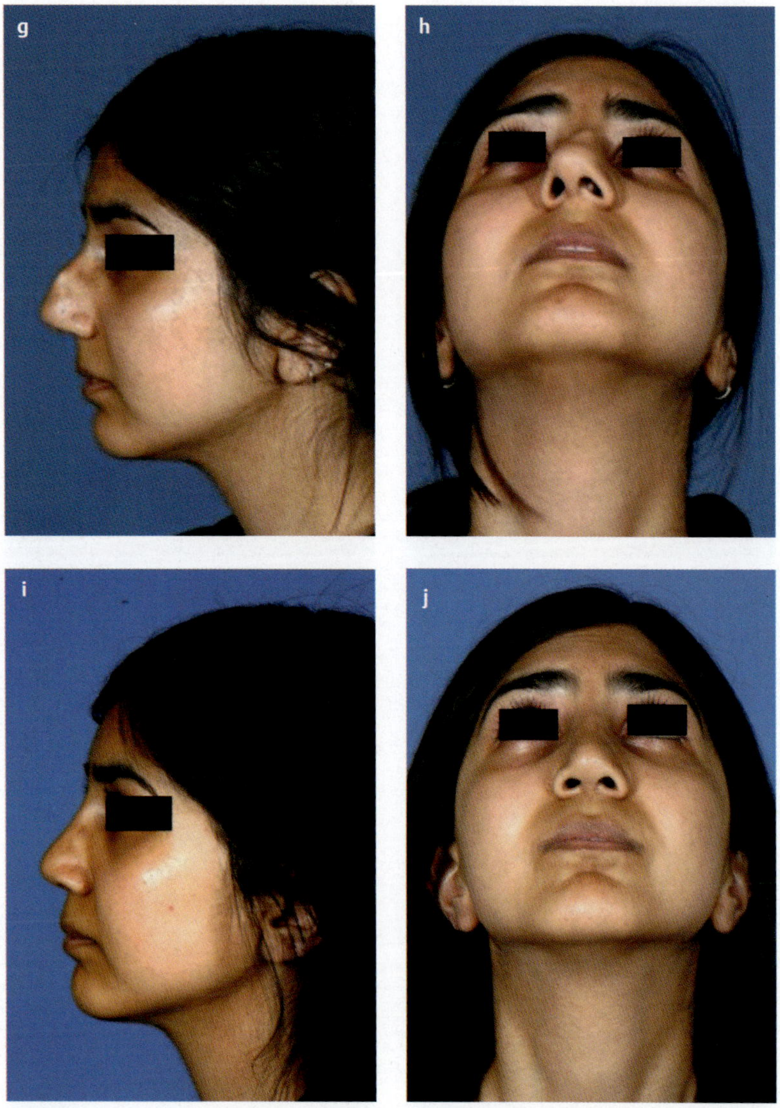

Fig. 20.16 *(Continued)* **(g–j)** Large dorsal hump with excess cartilaginous dorsum. Management with an open approach for extracorporeal septoplasty; dorsal reduction; medial, lateral, and intermediate osteotomies; dome sutures; and defatting of tip skin.

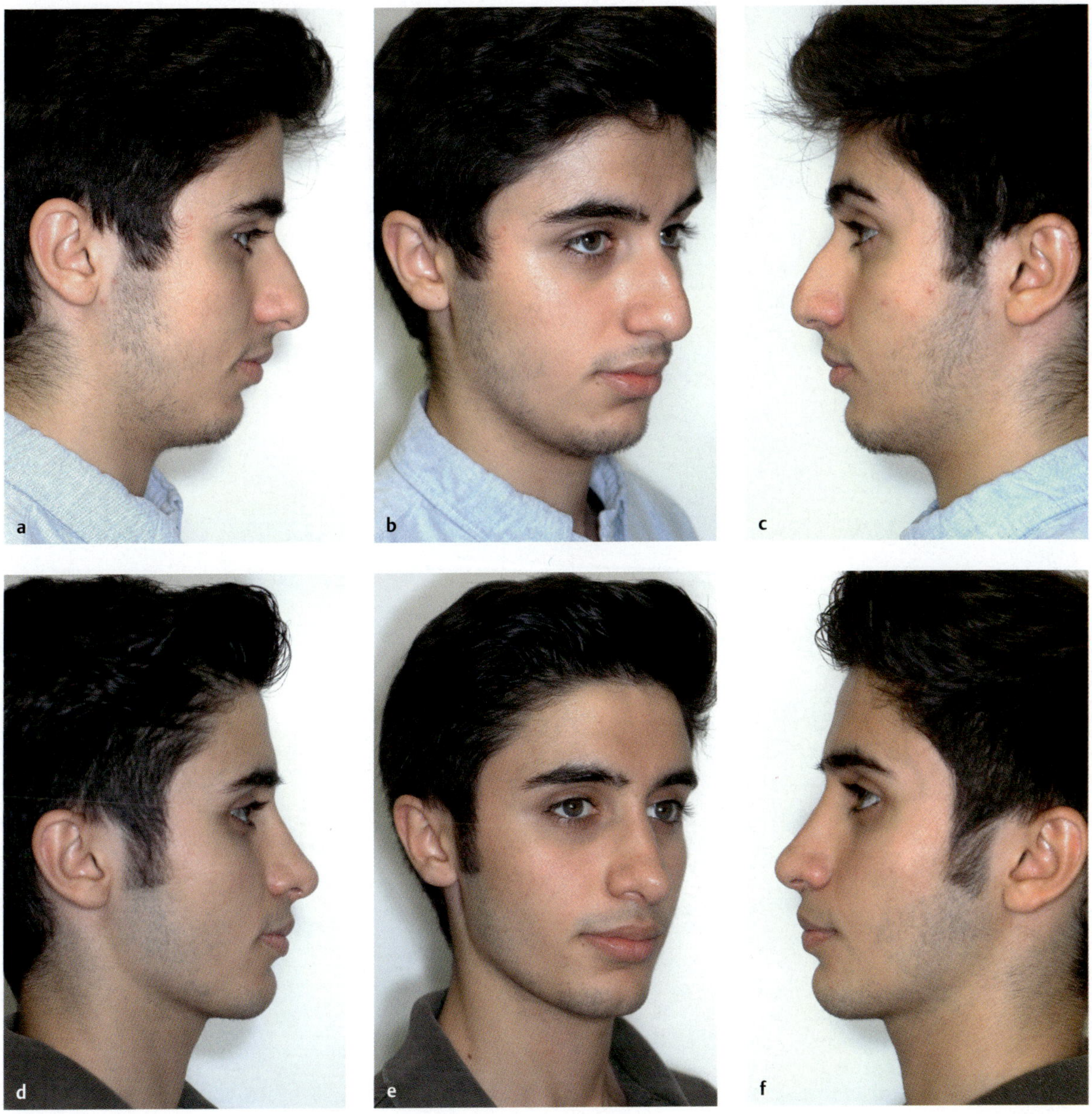

Fig. 20.17 (a–f) Thick-skinned male with dorsal hump and ptotic nasal tip. Management with an open approach, dorsal reduction, medial and lateral osteotomies, tongue-in-groove, dome sutures, and defatting of nasal tip.

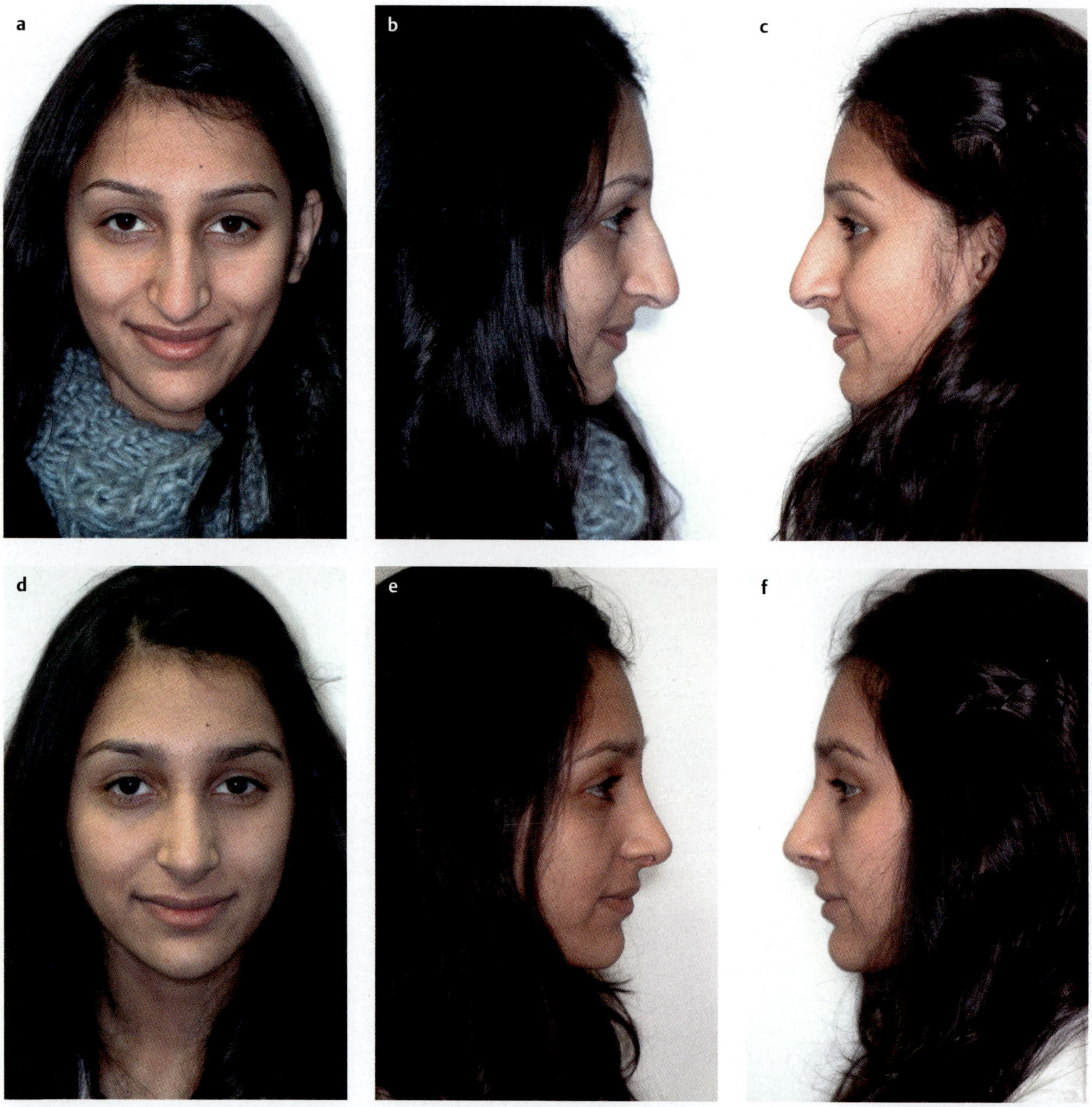

Fig. 20.18 (a–f) Moderately thick-skinned female with large dorsal hump and tip ptosis. Management with lateral crural overlay, dome suturing, dorsal reduction with medial and lateral osteotomies, and spreader grafts.

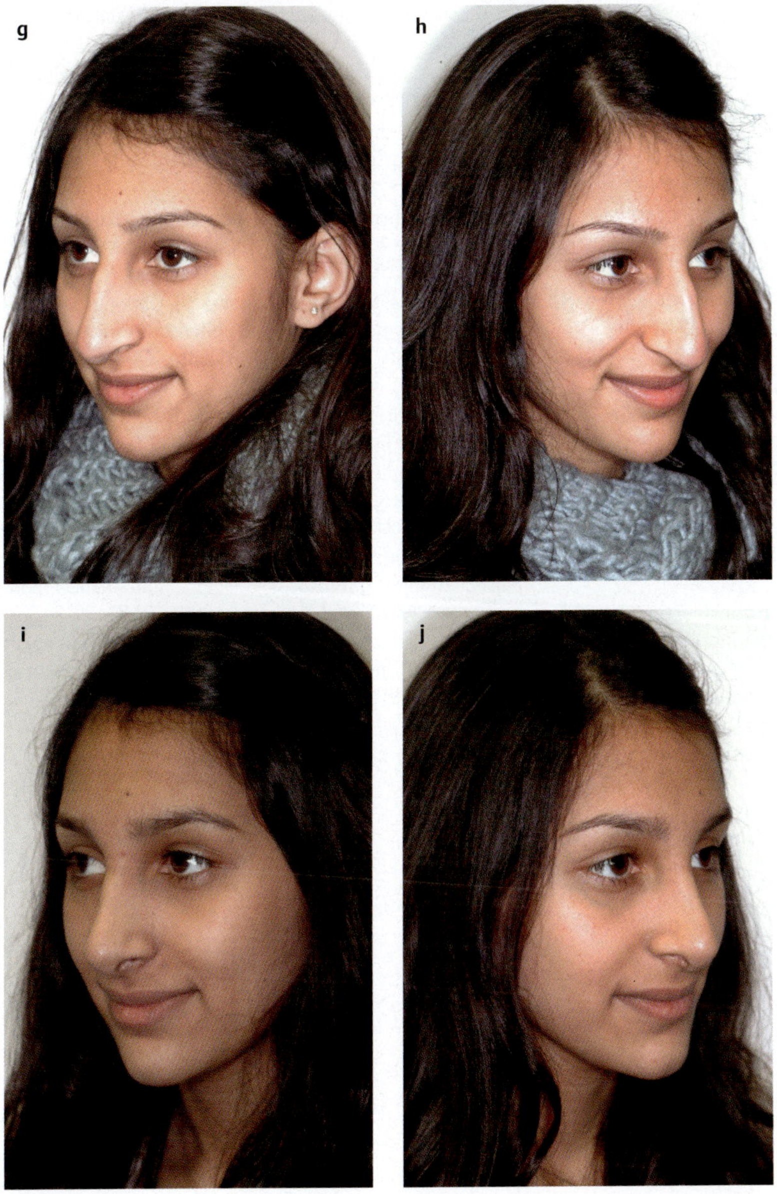

Fig. 20.18 *(Continued)* **(g–j)** Moderately thick-skinned female with large dorsal hump and tip ptosis. Management with lateral crural overlay, dome suturing, dorsal reduction with medial and lateral osteotomies, and spreader grafts.

References

1. Reich D, Thangaraj K, Patterson N, Price AL, Singh L. Reconstructing Indian population history. Nature 2009; 461(7263):489–494
2. Ambro BT, Wright RJ. Psychological considerations in revision rhinoplasty. Facial Plast Surg 2008;24(3):288–292
3. Vuyk HD, Zijlker TD. Psychosocial aspects of patient counseling and selection: a surgeon's perspective. Facial Plast Surg 1995;11(2):55–60
4. Paun SH, Nolst Trenité GJ. Revision rhinoplasty: an overview of deformities and techniques. Facial Plast Surg 2008;24(3):271–287
5. Rohrich RJ, Janis JE, Kenkel JM. Male rhinoplasty. Plast Reconstr Surg 2003;112(4):1071–1085, quiz 1086
6. Nolst Trenite GJ, Paun S. External rhinoplasty. In: Gleeson M, ed. Scott Brown's Otolaryngology, 7th ed. London: Arnold; 2004:2959–2969
7. Gruber RP, Park E, Newman J, Berkowitz L, Oneal R. The spreader flap in primary rhinoplasty. Plast Reconstr Surg 2007;119(6):1903–1910
8. Sheen JH. Spreader graft: a method of reconstructing the roof of the middle nasal vault following rhinoplasty. Plast Reconstr Surg 1984;73(2):230–239
9. André RF, Paun S, Vuyk H. Endonasal spreader grafts placement. The use of endonasal spreader grafts as a treatment for internal nasal valve insufficiency. Arch Facial Plast Surg 2004;6:36–40
10. Daniel RK, Calvert JW. Diced cartilage grafts in rhinoplasty surgery. Plast Reconstr Surg 2004;113(7):2156–2171
11. Tardy ME Jr, Schwartz M, Parras G. Saddle nose deformity: autogenous graft repair. Facial Plast Surg 1989;6(2): 121–134
12. Gunter JP, Rohrich RJ. Augmentation rhinoplasty: dorsal onlay grafting using shaped autogenous septal cartilage. Plast Reconstr Surg 1990;86(1):39–45
13. Hanasono MM, Kridel RW, Pastorek NJ, Glasgold MJ, Koch RJ. Correction of the soft tissue pollybeak using triamcinolone injection. Arch Facial Plast Surg 2002;4(1):26–30, discussion 31
14. Larrabee WF Jr. Open rhinoplasty and the upper third of the nose. Fac Plast Clin N Am 1993;1(1):23–28
15. Kridel RW, Konior RJ, Shumrick KA, Wright WK. Advances in nasal tip surgery. The lateral crural steal. Arch Otolaryngol Head Neck Surg 1989;115(10):1206–1212
16. Gillman GS, Simons RL, Lee DJ. Nasal tip bossae in rhinoplasty. Etiology, predisposing factors, and management techniques. Arch Facial Plast Surg 1999;1(2):83–89
17. Kridel RW, Scott BA, Foda HM. The tongue-in-groove technique in septorhinoplasty. A 10-year experience. Arch Facial Plast Surg 1999;1(4):246–256, discussion 257–258

21 Upper Eyelid Blepharoplasty Techniques in East Asian Patients

Sufan Wu and Hangyan Shi

21.1 Introduction

Asian people have typical Mongolian eyes, with a narrow optic fissure, a wide orbital distance, and puffy upper eyelids without a fold but with an epicanthus.[1] These characteristics are even found in Terra Cotta Warriors **(Fig. 21.1a–c)**, who resemble ancient Chinese of the second century BC, and they are distinctly different from the characteristics of Caucasian eyes **(Fig. 21.1d,e)**. In China, upper eyelids with no fold are called single eyelids, whereas folded eyelids are called double eyelids. It is estimated that half the population in China have single eyelids, and most so-called double eyelids are narrow or half folds of the upper eyelids **(Fig. 21.2)**, so that a full and wide double eyelid has to be created by means of plastic surgery.[2] Patients want to have larger and brighter eyes with an appropriate crease in the eyelids, and they hope to remove the puffy and excess skin of their upper eyelids. Therefore, *upper eyelid blepharoplasty* basically means *double eyelid surgery* in China and other parts of East Asia, and it is the most common plastic surgery procedure in these countries. The purpose of upper eyelid blepharoplasty in East Asian patients is basically to create a pretarsal crease on creaseless upper eyelids (whereas it is used in rejuvenation in Western countries).[3] In this chapter, the surgical techniques of double eyelid surgery are discussed in detail, including epicanthoplasty.

21.2 Anatomical Differences between Asians and Caucasians

The basic anatomy of the human eyelid is identical among various races, including the sequence and structure of the tissues of the eyelids: skin, subcutaneous tissue, orbicularis oculi muscle, levator muscle, tarsus, nerves, and blood vessels. The structure and anatomy of these tissues are not discussed in detail in this chapter, but the anatomical differences between Asians and Caucasians are focused on. Asian eyelids differ from those of Caucasians in several anatomical features: (1) the width of the upper tarsus in Asians is around 6 to 8 mm, whereas it is 10 mm in Caucasians; (2) the orbital septum fuses with the levator aponeuroses at a lower point in Asians than in Caucasians, and the terminals of the levator aponeurosis attached to the dermis are fewer in Asians; (3) more subcutaneous and suborbicularis fat is present in Asian eyelids, and there is a pretarsal fat pad in the Asian eyelid; 4) the distance between brow and eyelids is wider in Asians **(Fig. 21.3, Table 21.1)**.[4,5]

The possible reasons that the majority of Caucasians have an upper eyelid crease while few Asians have one are:

1. Insertion of the levator into the skin **(Fig. 21.4a)**. Research showed that, in the double eyelid, the levator aponeuroses penetrate through the orbicularis muscle to fuse with the skin in the palpebral sulcus, which is not the case in the creaseless eyelid. It was concluded that a fiber-linked structure between eyelid skin and levator aponeurosis is essential for the formation of the double eyelid. If the levator aponeurosis inserts into the pretarsal skin, the skin will be elevated when the levator contracts (the eyes open), creating the crease on the eyelids termed double eyelids **(Fig. 21.4b)**. Compared with Caucasians, Asian people have less or even no levator muscle inserting into the pretarsal skin **(Fig. 21.4c)**, leading to narrow or partial double eyelids or no double eyelids when the eyes are open **(Fig. 21.4d)**.[6]
2. Connection of pretarsal skin to the tarsus. The closer the pretarsal skin connects to the tarsus, the higher the possibility for double eyelids. In Caucasians, there is less and thinner tissue between skin and tarsus, and the septo-aponeurotic sling is located higher, which allows the pretarsal skin to move up with the tarsus and produce the crease. In Asians, in contrast, more fat and thicker connective tissue in their puffy eyelids separate the skin and tarsus, and, moreover, the septo-aponeurotic sling is located lower, which means that the skin cannot follow the movement of the tarsus and produce a crease.[7]

The aesthetic criteria for upper eyelid creases are also different between Asians and Caucasians. Asian people prefer a narrow fold (2–3 mm on forward gaze, 6–8 mm with the eyes closed) and an arch-shaped fold, so that the eyelid fold gradually widens from the medial canthus to the external canthus. The fold starts from the lash line of the medial canthus, gradually widens to a maximum height at the midline of the pupil, and then keeps the height until the last point of the fold at the lateral orbital rim. In Caucasians, the folds are wider, have a parallel shape, and have similar heights at the medial canthus and external canthus. Surgeons should be aware of the different aesthetic criteria of different races and should give patients appropriate recommendations.

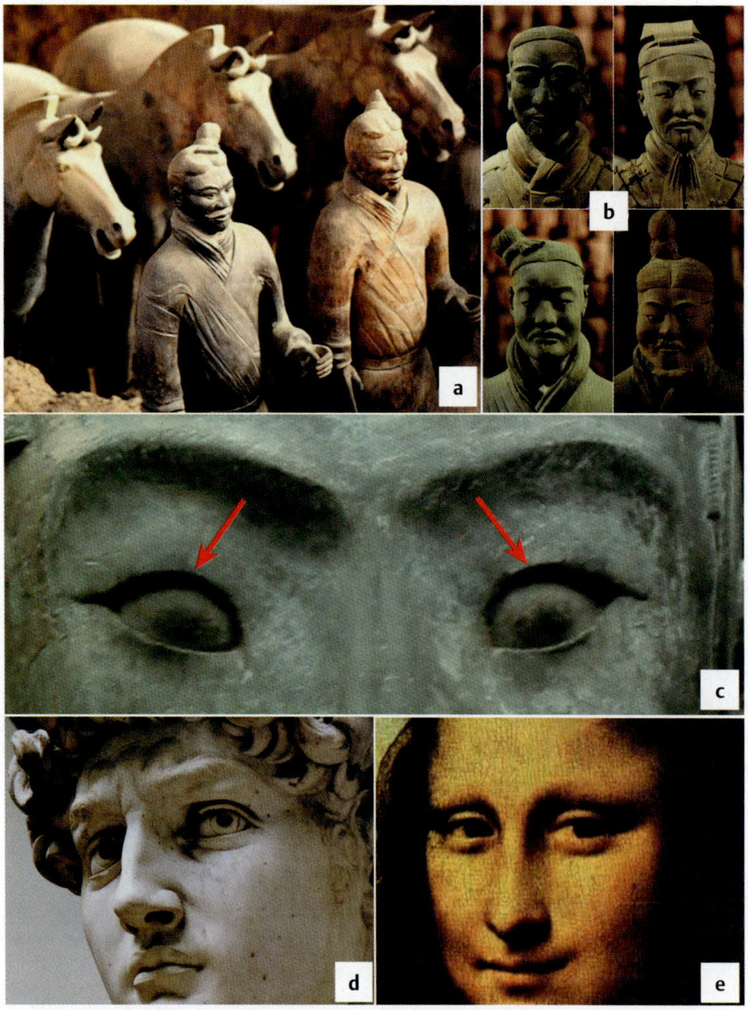

Fig. 21.1 Typical Asian eyes compared with Caucasian eyes. **(a)** Terra Cotta Warriors, made in the Qin Dynasty, represent ancient Chinese from the second century BC. **(b,c)** Typical Mongolian eyes have a narrow optic fissure, a wide orbital distance, puffy upper eyelids with no fold (*red arrows*), and a wide distance between brow and eyelids, **(d,e)** which are distinctly different from Caucasian eyes.

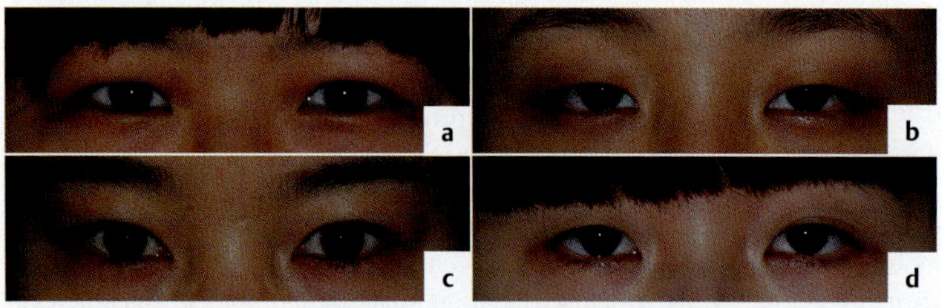

Fig. 21.2 **(a,b)** Typical eyes of young Chinese females. An estimated 50% of the Chinese population have no upper eyelid fold, while **(c)** some have narrow folds or **(d)** half folds.

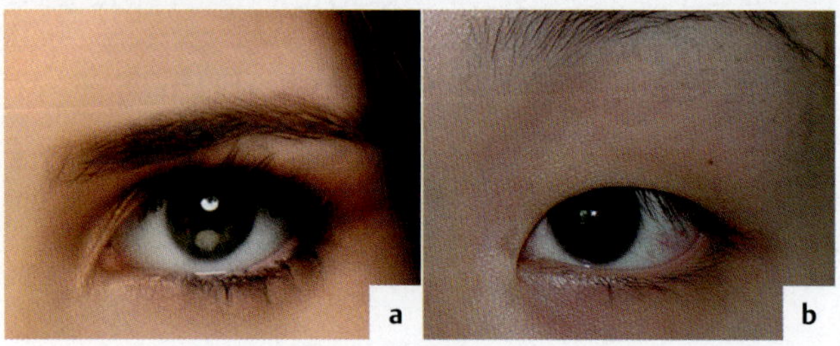

Fig. 21.3 Differences between **(a)** Caucasian and **(b)** Asian eyes. Compared with Caucasians, Asians have a narrow upper tarsus, no crease on the eyelid, more fat, a wider distance between brow and eyelids, and a concealed caruncle due to the epicanthal fold.

Table 21.1 Major anatomical differences between Asian and Caucasian upper eyelids

	Caucasian	Asian
Upper eyelid fold (crease) prevalence	Almost 100%	Less than 50%
Width of crease with eyes closed	10–12 mm	6–8 mm
Width of crease on forward gaze	5–10 mm	2–3 mm
Width of tarsus	10–12 mm	6–8 mm
Length of tarsus	30–34 mm	27–30 mm
Pretarsal tissues (skin, subcutaneous tissues, orbicularis oculi)	Thin	Thick
Fat (subcutaneous fat, septal fat, pretarsal fat)	Less	More
Height of septo-aponeurotic sling	Higher	Lower
Insertion point of levator	Tarsus and pretarsal skin	Tarsus only
Epicanthus	Almost none	More than 50%
Distance from eyebrow to eyelid	Narrow	Wide

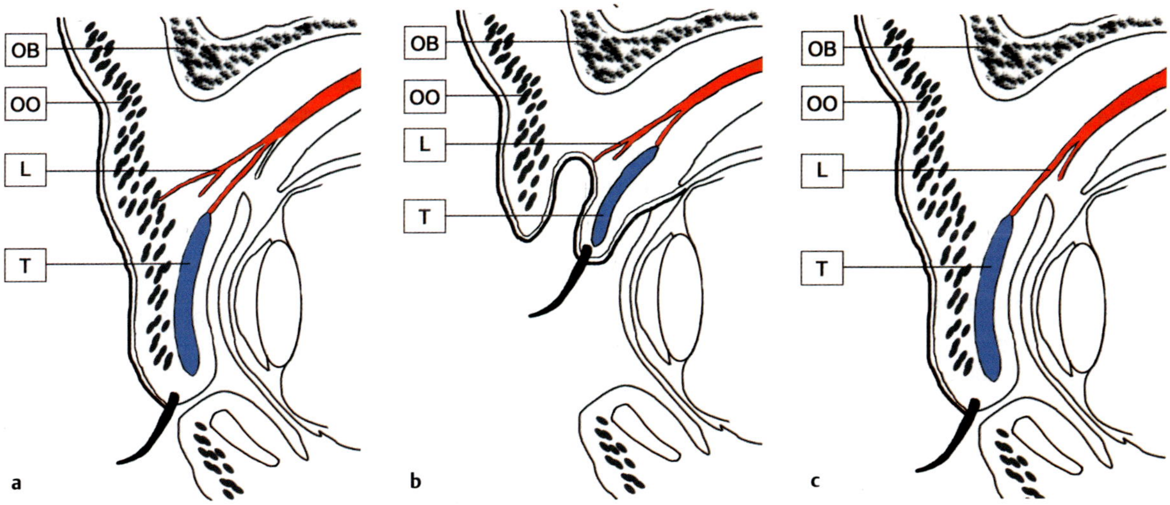

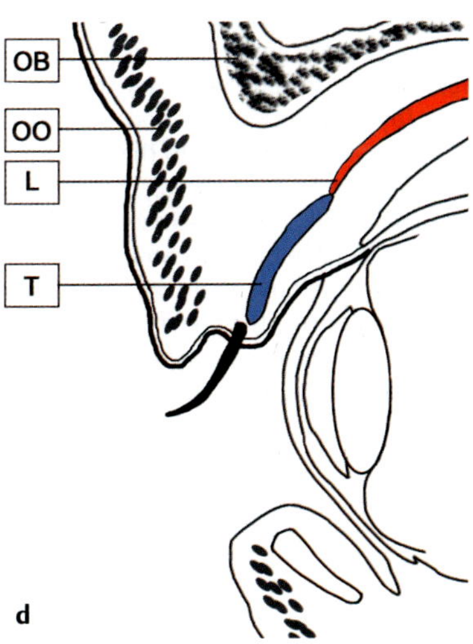

Fig. 21.4 Anatomical mechanism of upper eyelids with and without creases. **(a,c)** In creased eyelids, the levator aponeuroses (*red*) penetrate through the orbicularis oculi muscle to fuse with the pretarsal skin, which will be elevated along with the tarsus (*blue*) to form a crease when the eyes are open. **(b,d)** In creaseless eyelids, no levator aponeurosis fuses with the pretarsal skin, leading to a narrow or partial double eyelid or no double eyelid when the eyes are open. OB, orbicularis bone; OO, orbicularis oculi; L, levator; T, tarsus.

preferable for a patient with tight skin and excess fat tissue, whereas the full incision method is advisable for puffy eyelids with excess skin and fat. Clinically, the correct procedure should be chosen for the patient based on his or her conditions and requirements.

21.6.1 No Incision (Thread Embedding) Blepharoplasty

Indications

The no incision method is indicated for patients with tight and thin skin without excess septal fat, who are usually young, or patients who need a relatively short recovery time, or patients who do not want any surgical marks remaining on the eyelids.

Advantages

This method is a relatively simple surgical procedure, has a rapid recovery time, and leaves no scar on the eyelid.

Disadvantages

Surgical results are sometimes not reliable due to loosening of the connection between skin and tarsus.

Design

The embedding lines of the upper eyelid are designed and marked while the patient lies supine on the operating table. It is recommended that the width of the embedding lines be equal to the height of the tarsus (6–8 mm), so that the suture point is set just in the upper edge of the tarsal plate, which can make the pretarsal skin stretch flat and turn up the eyelashes. While the eyes are closed, the lines are marked at a height of 6.5 to 7.5 mm from the margin of the upper eyelids, starting from the medial canthus and ending with a similar width at the endpoint of the crease between the upper eyelid and lower eyelid (~ 0.5 mm laterally to the lateral canthus). At this height, when the skin at the midpoint of the pupil (key point) is pushed up with a tiny stick while the eyes are open in a straight gaze, the exposed pretarsal skin should be 2 to 3 mm. The line is

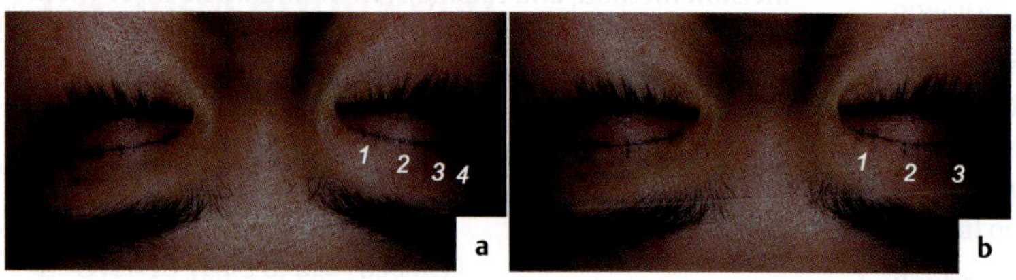

Fig. 21.7 Design of a nonincision (thread embedding) blepharoplasty. The embedding lines are marked in a height of 6.5 to 7.5 mm from the margin of the upper eyelids. On the embedding lines, the suture points are marked based on the embedding methods: **(a)** 8 points fo 4 stitches of running embedding method; **(b)** 6 points for 3 stitches of interrupted embedding method.

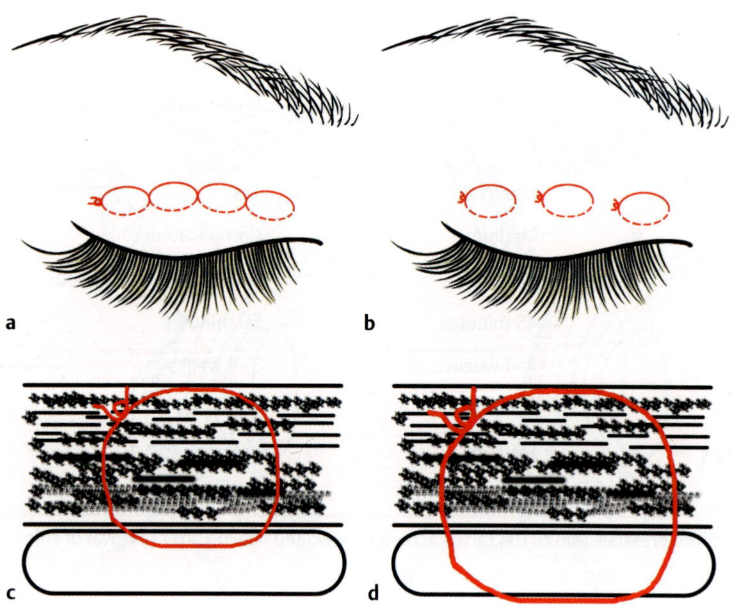

Fig. 21.8 Schematic diagram of nonincision (thread embedding) blepharoplasty. **(a)** Running embedding suture method with 4 stitches. **(b)** Interrupted embedding suture method with 3 stitches. **(c)** Suturing to the superficial layer of tarsus. **(d)** Sutures penetrating full-thickness tarsus.

arch-shaped, so that its highest point is located at the junction of the medial third and central third (located at the pupillary line). Medially, the line can have two shapes: it can cross to the eyelash line or it can parallel the eyelash line, depending on whether the marking line is set medially and stopped ~ 2 mm or 4 mm away from the medial canthus, respectively. On marked embedding lines, the suture points are indicated based on the embedding methods: 6 or 8 points for the interrupted embedding method, 8 or 10 points for the running embedding method **(Fig. 21.7)**.[11]

Surgical Procedures

- Disinfection and surgical draping are performed routinely on the exposed whole face.
- Local anesthesia is achieved by injection of 1 mL of 2% lidocaine with 1:100,000 epinephrine under the embedding lines and by waiting 15 minutes until the epinephrine takes effect.
- Insert the corneal protection plate between the tarsus and cornea to protect the cornea from the needle injury.
- Make small holes using a no. 11 blade on the skin at the marked points along with the designed embedding lines; the holes that will hold the knots need to be made deeper than the others.
- Two suture methods can be used: a running suture with three to four stitches **(Fig. 21.8a)**, or three to four interrupted stitches on the tarsus **(Fig. 21.8b)**. Two depths of sutured points in the tarsus can be used: suturing to the superficial layer of the tarsus **(Fig. 21.8c)**, or penetrating the full thickness of the tarsus **(Fig. 21.8d)**.
- Running method: The needle goes in the most lateral hole, out from the next hole, and then enters the third hole, so that there is one stitch on the dermis and another stitch on the tarsus. After the needle reaches the most medial hole, it is returned to the lateral hole one stitch by one stitch, and the suture is knotted in the most lateral hole **(Fig. 21.8a)**.
- Interrupted method: The needle goes in one hole to the tarsus, out from the next hole, and enters this hole again out from first hole, by which a loop is made within the two holes. Suture dermis of pretarsal skin to the upper edge of tarsal plate using 6–0 nylon or Prolene through each closed two holes **(Fig. 21.8b)**. The suture is knotted and the knot is inserted into the hole.
- Have the patient open and close the eyes to confirm that: (1) the heights of the creases on both sides of the upper eyelids are identical and symmetrical (otherwise, the sutures need to be removed and adjusted to obtain symmetrical creases); (2) all sutures and knots are buried within the skin (the knots need to be inserted into the deep layer beneath the skin at the holes using a syringe needle); (3) the sutures tightly combine the skin with the tarsus by retracting the sutures to hang on the tarsus separated from cornea.
- The holes are sealed with chlortetracycline ointment and the operation is finished.
- All of the above steps are usually completed within 30 minutes.

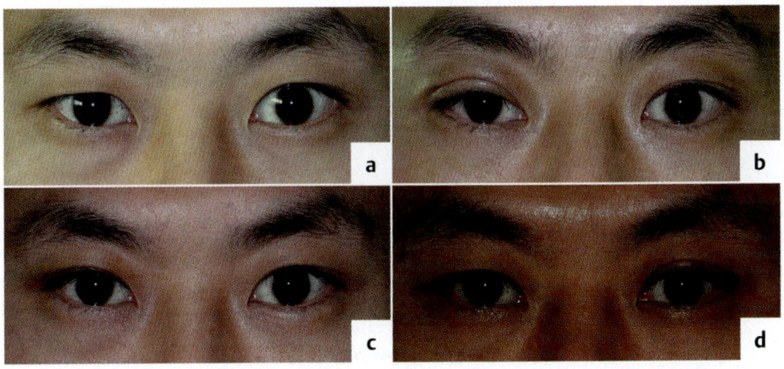

Fig. 21.9 Gradually narrowed creases after nonincision (thread embedding) blepharoplasty. **(a)** A 31-year-old male patient with asymmetrical upper eyelids, one side no crease and the other side partial crease. **(b)** Appearance immediately after thread embedding (interrupted superficial tarsus method); blepharoplasty only on the right side. **(c)** One month postsurgery. Two sides of eyelids are well symmetrical. **(d)** After 8 years, The crease of the right side has narrowed.

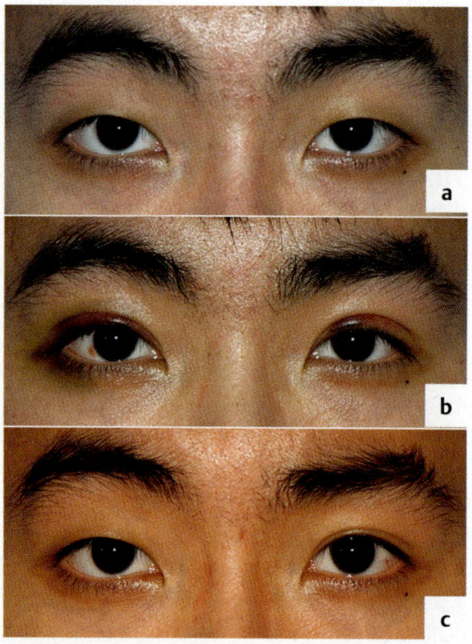

Fig. 21.10 An unreliable result of nonincision (thread embedding) blepharoplasty. **(a)** A 19-year-old male patient with noncrease upper eyelids. **(b)** One week after thread embedding (interrupted superficial tarsus method) blepharoplasty. The shapes of the creases on both sides are symmetrical and smooth. **(c)** Six months after the operation. The crease on the left side has narrowed, and the crease on the right side has disappeared.

Outcomes

No incision (thread embedding) blepharoplasty can create natural creases on the upper eyelids and has a short recovery time of 1 to 2 weeks. The disadvantage of this method is that the results are shorter-lasting than those of the incision method, and the increase of the upper eyelid will become narrow **(Fig. 21.9)** or even disappear **(Fig. 21.10)**.

21.6.2 Full Incision Blepharoplasty

Indications

Full incision blepharoplasty is indicated in young patients with puffy eyelids, thick skin, and septal fat tissue, and in older patients with excess skin for the purpose of rejuvenation.

Advantages

Surgical results are very reliable and permanent due to the tight connection of pretarsal skin to the tarsus. The creases created on the upper eyelid do not narrow or disappear.

Disadvantages

Compared with the no incision method, full incision blepharoplasty involves more complicated and skillful surgical procedures, a relatively longer recovery time, and an operative scar on the skin of the upper eyelid.

Design

The incision lines on the upper eyelid are designed and marked while the patient lies supine on the operating table. While the eyes are closed, the lines are marked at a height of 6.5 to 7.5 mm from the margin of the upper eyelids, starting from the medial canthus and ending with a similar width at the endpoint of the crease between the upper and lower eyelids (~ 0.5 mm laterally to the lateral canthus). The line is arch-shaped, so that the highest point is located at the junction of the medial third and central third (almost at the pupil line). The lines should be drawn twice: (1) in the natural situation, with skin of the upper eyelid relaxed; (2) while gently stretching the skin upward for a tight state of the upper eyelid skin **(Fig. 21.11)**. If the upper eyelid skin is loose, two lines can be drawn in each of the two states of the skin. The skin between the two lines is removed during surgery **(Fig. 21.12)**. In young patients with tight skin, the two lines are partially or totally overlapped, and only partial or no excess skin needs to be removed.

Surgical Procedures

- Disinfection and surgical draping are performed routinely on the exposed whole face.
- Local anesthesia is attained by injection of 1 mL of 2% lidocaine with 1:100,000 epinephrine in each side of the upper eyelid beneath the incision lines and by waiting 15 minutes until the epinephrine takes effect.
- The incisions are made with a no. 11 blade along the designed lines, cutting in the full thickness of the skin. In cases with two lines on one side of the upper eyelid, the skin between the two incisions, including a piece of the orbicularis oculi beneath it, is excised using tissue scissors.
- Pretarsal skin is sharply elevated from the orbicularis oculi muscle.
- Total tarsal plates and levator aponeurosis are exposed after removal of pretarsal tissues, including orbicularis oculi muscle, connective tissues, and pretarsal fat. Attention should be paid to keeping the levator aponeurosis intact on the tarsal plate.[12]
- In cases with puffy eyelids, the orbital septum is opened with a small incision, and the excess prelevator fat tissue is gently pressed out and is excised.[13]

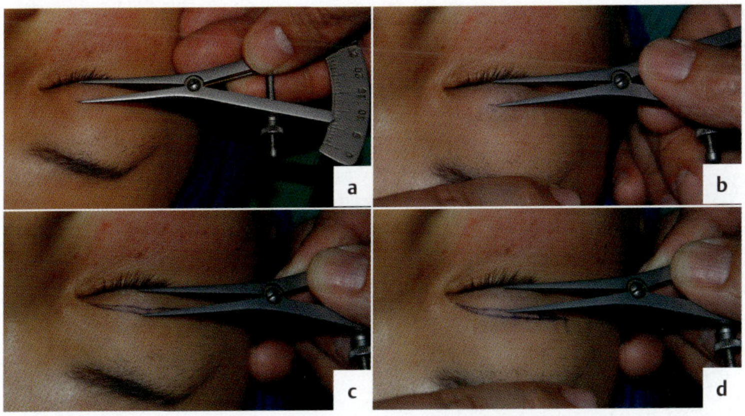

Fig. 21.11 Design of the incision lines for blepharoplasty. **(a,c)** Designed dots and the incision line are marked in the natural state of the upper eyelid skin with the eyes closed. **(b,d)** Designed dots and the incision line are marked in a tight state by gently stretching the pretarsal skin upward. The dots and lines are at different heights in the two states, and the line closer to the eyelashes is the one drawn in a tight state.

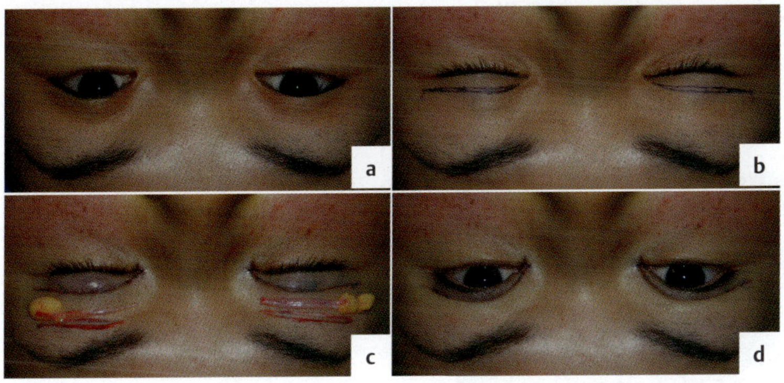

Fig. 21.12 Preoperative and postoperative views of a full incision blepharoplasty. **(a)** Patient without creases is in a supine position during design. **(b)** Two incision lines have been marked in the tight and relaxed states of the upper eyelid skin. **(c)** Operation is completed. A piece of pretarsal skin (between two designed lines), pretarsal tissue, and excess prelevator fat have been removed. **(d)** With the patient's eyes open, the shape and height of the creases on the two sides are checked and compared; they should be identical and symmetrical.

- Bipolar cautery is always used to control bleeding in each step.
- Incisions are closed by interrupted sutures in a skin-tarsus-skin way using 7–0 Prolene, which bite both sides' skins of incision and attach to the up edge of tarsus. Usually, six to seven stitches are necessary to close one incision: the central four stitches are clearly anchored to the tarsus, whereas the bilateral two stitches are sutured to the deep tissue beside the levator aponeurosis.
- Have the patient open and close the eyes to check and compare the shape and height of the creases on the two sides, which should be identical and symmetrical. Otherwise, one or several stitches at wrong positions need to be removed and sutured again, to adjust the bite position of the stitch on the tarsus until a symmetrical result is achieved.[14]
- Sutured incisions are cleaned and sealed with chlortetracycline ointment and are kept open or slightly covered with a piece of gauze.
- All of the above steps are usually completed within 60 minutes.

Outcomes

The full incision method can create very reliable and permanent surgical results due to the tight connection of the pretarsal skin to the tarsus. The creases created on the upper eyelid seldom narrow or disappear (**Fig. 21.13** and **Fig. 21.14**).

21.6.3 Incision and Anchor Suture

In the full incision blepharoplasty, adherence between the skin and tarsus results from natural wound healing. In some cases, however, the attachment is not stable enough to suspend the pretarsal skin on the tarsus and the crease fades away or is even lost. The main explanations for this are that soft tissue remained between the skin and tarsal plate and/or in some puffy eyelids the tissues are relatively heavy (**Fig. 21.15**). To resolve this problem, modified methods for enhancing the attachment of pretarsal skin and tarsus should be considered. The author prefers to use a hybrid method of full incision combined with anchor suture, which is a conventional external incision procedure plus anchor sutures to join the dermal and tarsal plates.[15]

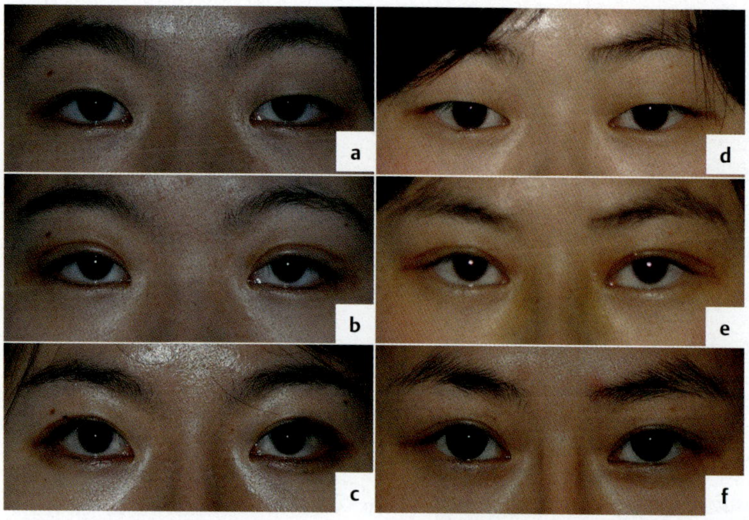

Fig. 21.13 Outcomes of full incision upper eyelid blepharoplasty. Patient 1 was a 22-year-old female with a right side partial crease and a left side creaseless eyelid. **(a)** She underwent full incision blepharoplasty and was followed up at **(b)** 7 days and **(c)** 3 years. Patient 2 was a 25-year-old female with creaseless eyelids on both sides. **(d)** She underwent full incision blepharoplasty and was followed up at **(e)** 7 days and **(f)** 4 years. It can be seen that her creases narrowed after 3 to 4 years.

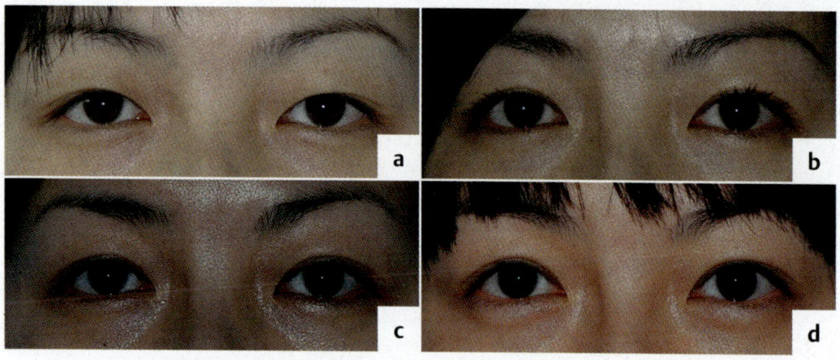

Fig. 21.14 **(a–d)** Long-term follow-up after full incision blepharoplasty. A 27-year-old female with partial creases on both eyelids underwent full incision blepharoplasty and was followed up at 3.5 years, 4.5 years, and 8 years. The shapes and height of the crease on the eyelids were durable and reliable.

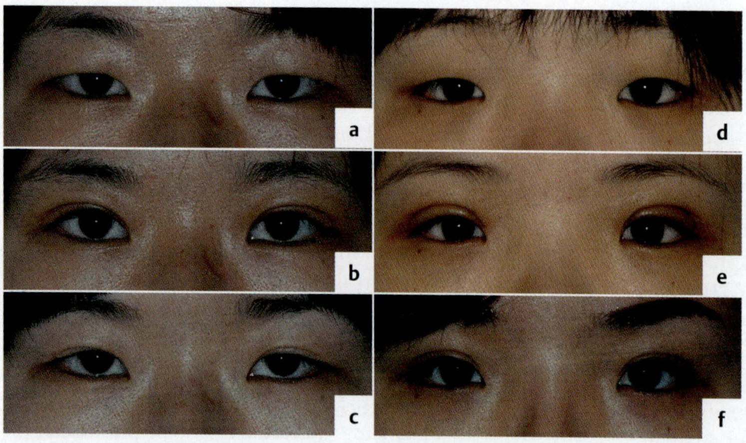

Fig. 21.15 Narrowing and loss of creases after full incision blepharoplasty. **(a)** Patient 1 was a 20-year-old female with creaseless eyelids on both sides. She underwentfull incision blepharoplasty, and was followed up at 7 days and 10 months. **(b)** The initial heights of her creases were narrower than normal, and **(c)** the creases disappeared after 10 months. **(d)** Patient 2 was a 25-year-old female with creaseless eyelids and epicanthus. She underwent full incision blepharoplasty, and was followed up at **(e)** 7 days and **(f)** 39 months. Her creases significantly narrowed. It is noteworthy that she had puffy eyelids with thick skin and pretarsal tissues.

Indications

The indications are the same as for full incision blepharoplasty, especially for Asian patients with puffy eyelids. The modified method can be performed in both young, creaseless eyes and in aging eyes. The anchor suture can be used routinely during full incision Asian blepharoplasty, especially in cases with a relatively small tarsus and puffy upper eyelids.

Advantages

The anchor suture can join the tarsal plate to the pretarsal dermis more firmly,[16] the sutures are buried under the skin, which yields a more reliable and long-lasting adherence of upper eyelid skin to tarsus, and the created creases will not narrow or disappear.

Disadvantages

Anchor sutures take a little longer time for the operation, and the sutures are sometimes visible if they are located too superficially.

Design

Design is the same as for the full incision method.

Surgical Procedures

- Disinfection, draping, anesthesia, incision making, undermining, skin removal, muscle removal, and fat removal are the same as for the full incision method.
- Before suturing, one additional anchor stitch between dermis and the upper edge of the tarsus is made in the key point using 7–0 Prolene, which can join the skin to the tarsal plate tightly **(Fig. 21.16)**. Attention should be paid that the stitch to the tarsal plate does not penetrate the medial of the tarsus and the position of the stitch was not too high to the levator aponeurosis. Usually, one stitch on each side is enough, but several stitches can be used in very puffy cases.
- After the anchor sutures are completed on both sides, the patient is asked to open the eyes to confirm the folds' shape and symmetry. The anchor stitches can be adjusted until the folds on the two sides are symmetrical.
- The skin incisions are then closed with 7–0 Prolene using interrupted sutures in six equidistant positions. The stitches are performed skin-tarsus-skin, except for one lateral stitch that is sutured skin-aponeurosis-skin due to the tarsal plate's decreasing laterally.

Outcomes

The full incision method combined with anchor suture can create more reliable results than the full incision method alone, and it is more suitable for puffy eyelids. Also, the tension on the incision is decreased due to the anchor suture, so the incision can heal better, with less scar **(Fig. 21.17)**.

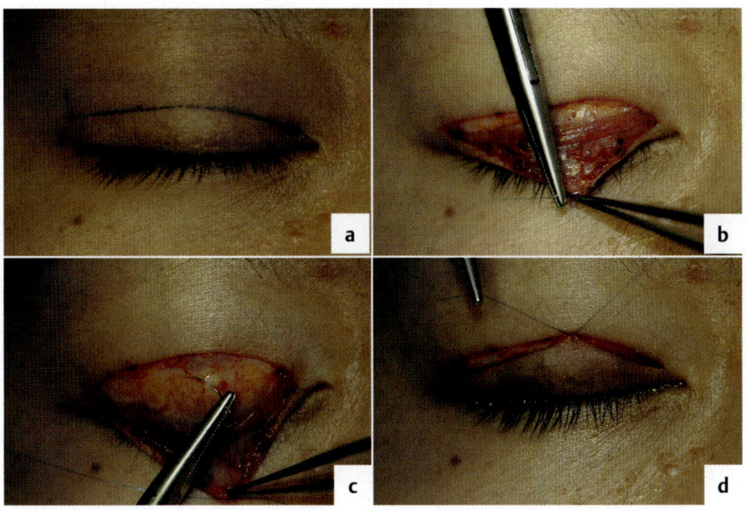

Fig. 21.16 The incision plus anchor suture method of upper eyelid blepharoplasty. **(a)** The incision line is designed to be arch-shaped, with the top in the key point at the mid pupil, 7 mm above the eyelashes. After conventional external incision blepharoplasty, **(b)** an additional anchor stitch was set from the dermis of the pretarsal skin to **(c)** the upper edge of tarsal plate, so that **(d)** it joined the pretarsal skin to the tarsus tightly after ligation.

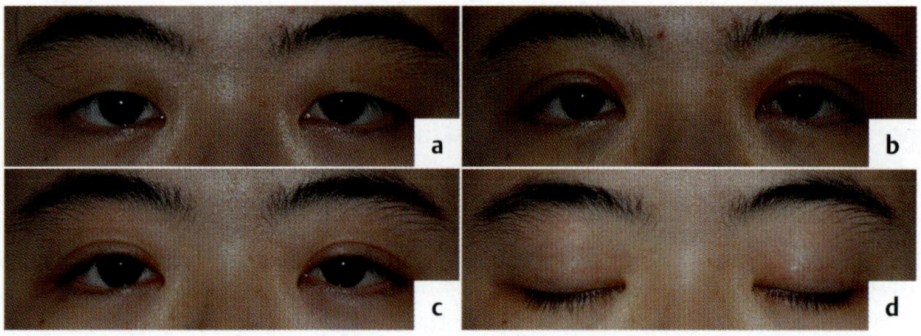

Fig. 21.17 Surgical results of full incision combined with anchor suture. **(a)** A 23-year-old female with creaseless eyelids underwent full incision blepharoplasty combined with anchor suture. She was followed up at **(b)** 7 days and 6 months. **(c)** The creases were not narrower after 6 months, and **(d)** the surgical scar was minimal.

21.6.3 Partial Incision Blepharoplasty

Indications

Partial incision blepharoplasty is indicated for the patient who has puffy upper eyelids without excess skin, and whose excess fat and some orbicularis oculi could be removed through short incisions.

Advantages

The scar is shorter than that with the full incision method. It is possible that almost no surgical marks will remain on the eyelid skin if the incisions are shorter than 5 mm, which is the most important advantage of this method. The results are usually more reliable and permanent than those of the no incision method.

Disadvantages

Compared with the full incision method, the surgical procedures are more difficult, due to the limited exposure through the short incisions.

Design

The design of crease lines is same as that for the no incision method. In each side of the upper eyelid, a line is designed and marked at a height of 6.5 to 7.5 mm, starting from the medial canthus and ending at the point above the lateral canthus. The line is arch-shaped, so that the highest point is located at the junction of the medial third and central third (almost at the pupil line). One to three short incisions are marked on the designed lines—the number depends on the condition of the eyelids and the surgeon's technique.[2,17]

Surgical Procedures

- Disinfection and surgical draping are performed routinely on the exposed whole face.
- Local anesthesia is attained by injection of 1 mL of 2% lidocaine with 1:100,000 epinephrine in each side of the upper eyelid beneath the incision lines, and by waiting 15 minutes until the epinephrine takes effect.
- Short incisions are made with a no. 11 blade along the designed lines, cutting the full thickness of the skin.
- A piece of orbicularis oculi beneath the incisions is excised using tissue scissors.
- The orbital septum is opened through a small incision, and excess prelevator fat tissue is gently pressed out and is excised.
- Tarsal plates and levator aponeurosis are exposed after removal of pretarsal tissues.
- Incisions are closed by one stitch in a skin-tarsus-skin way using 7–0 Prolene, which joins both sides of the incision and the upper edge of the tarsus.
- The height and shape of the upper eyelid creases on the two sides are checked and compared carefully—they should be identical and symmetrical. Otherwise, the stitches need to be removed and sutured again, to adjust the position of the stitch on the tarsus until symmetrical results are achieved.
- Sutured incisions are cleaned and sealed with chlortetracycline ointment and are kept uncovered or slightly covered with a piece of gauze.
- All of the above steps are usually completed within 45 minutes.

21.7 Procedures of Epicanthoplasty

An epicanthal fold is a characteristic of Asians; the epicanthal fold is vertical excess skin located at the medial canthus. In patients with epicanthal folds, the caruncle is partially obscured or even not visible due to coverage by the fold. Epicanthal folds extend the distance between the medial canthi of the two eyes and decrease the width of the eyes, so that epicanthal folds severely change the ratio of the eyes to the face. Furthermore, epicanthal folds shorten the upper eyelid crease and affect the results of upper eyelid blepharoplasty. So, removal of the epicanthal folds, epicanthoplasty, is usually performed along with the upper eyelid blepharoplasty in Asians.

Many scholars believe that the epicanthal fold is not a problem of excess skin, but a disorder of skin distribution: the skin is excessive in the horizontal direction, but inadequate in the vertical direction. In accord with this hypothesis, the author prefers to use the modified z-plasty to correct epicanthal folds.

21.7.1 Design

A new medial canthus point, point 1, is marked first, just above the original medial canthus point. Point 1 is usually located 2 to 5 mm medially from the inner edge of the epicanthal fold, so that the distance between the canthus points of the two eyes is equal to the width of the eye. The fold line is marked along with the inner edge of the epicanthal fold. A horizontal line starting from the new medial canthus point crosses to the fold line and creates point 2. The end of the epicanthal fold is marked as point 3. The original medial canthus point is point 4. A triangle flap is designed with the base line at points 2 and 4 and the apex at point 3. The triangle flap will be inserted into the gap caused by opening an incision between points 1 and 2. The line from 3 to 2 is usually located at the extension of the incision line of upper eyelid blepharoplasty, which could be either connected through each other or separated by a piece of intact skin **(Fig. 21.18)**.[18]

21.7.2 Surgical Procedures

- Epicanthoplasty is usually performed simultaneously with upper eyelid blepharoplasty. Disinfection and anesthesia procedures are the same as those for blepharoplasty described above.
- Three incisions are made: from point 1 to 2, from point 2 to 3, and from point 4 to 3. A sharp no. 11 blade with an acute angle is essential for the procedure. Magnified surgical eyeglasses are helpful.
- After the incisions are made, extensive undermining is performed in the medial canthus area using a sharp microscissors. Some connective tissue and orbicularis oculi between the skin and medial canthal ligament should be released or dissected. The ligament can be shortened using sutures if necessary.
- After extensive undermining and dissection, a triangle flap is elevated with the base line at points 2 and 4 and the apex at point 3, and a triangle defect area is created in the incision from 1 to 2.
- The triangle flap is turned ~ 90 degrees to cover the triangle defect, and the apex point of the flap at point 3 is sutured to the new medial canthus point at point 1.
- The donor site of the triangle flap is sutured by close two side of incision line 2 to 3 to incision line 4 to 3.
- The sutures should be made using 7–0 Prolene without any tension on the flap or skin; if there is tension, more undermining and dissection should be done.

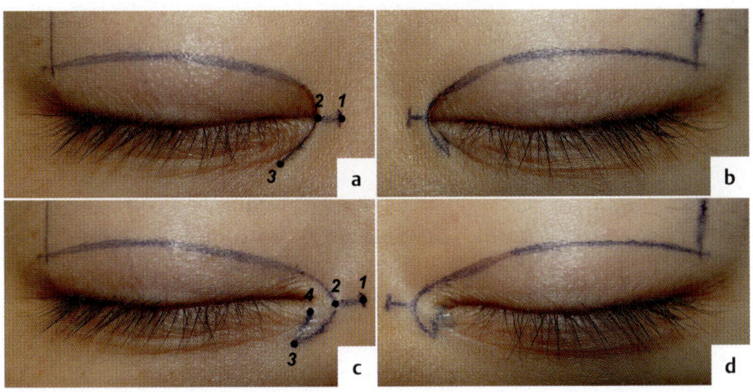

Fig. 21.18 (a–d) Design of an epicanthoplasty with the modified z-plasty method. Point 1 is the new medial canthus point, located at the fold of skin just above the original medial canthus point; point 2 is created by the horizontal line that starts from point 1 and crosses to the fold line; point 3 is the end of the epicanthal fold; point 4 is the original medial canthus point. The lines between points 1 and 3, points 3 and 2, and points 2 and 4 are shown and are connected to the crease lines.

- It should be confirmed that most or all of the caruncle is visible when the eyes are open, and that the two sides are symmetrical and identically shaped.
- Sutured incisions are cleaned and sealed with chlortetracycline ointment and are kept uncovered without dressing.
- Epicanthoplasty of both sides is usually completed within 30 minutes.

21.7.3 Outcomes

The modified z-plasty epicanthoplasty is a reliable method that adjusts the distribution of the skin with no excess skin removal and by which the epicanthal fold can be corrected remarkably with only a subtle scar (**Fig. 21.19** and **Fig. 21.20**).

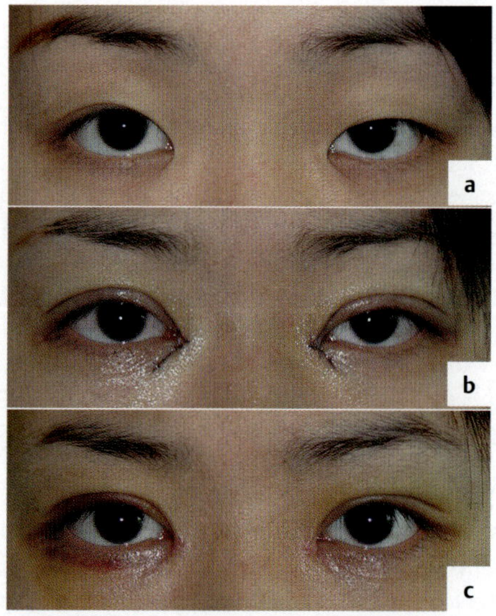

Fig. 21.19 Outcomes of epicanthoplasty. **(a)** A 17-year-old female with severe epicanthus and left pseudoptosis underwent modified z-plasty epicanthoplasty. **(b)** The triangle flap was turned to the new medial canthal point and was inserted into the gap created by cutting a line from the new medial canthal point. **(c)** Sutures were removed 7 days after surgery. The epicanthal folds are almost completely removed, and the distance between the medial canthi has been narrowed remarkably. The caruncles are visible when the eyes are open.

21.8 Postoperative Care

After the operation, the incision is covered with eye ointment. The operated region is left exposed, without any dressing or bandage. Patients are encouraged to open and close their eyes as usual. The operative areas are cleaned on the second day after surgery. Swelling and bruising are common and usually disappear within 2 weeks (**Fig. 21.21**), depending the surgical method. No antibiotics are needed postoperatively, and the sutures are removed on the seventh postoperative day. Immediately after surgery, the width of the fold is ~ 3 to 4 mm with the eye open due to swelling, but it usually decreases and remains at 2 to 3 mm after 1 month.

21.9 Complications and Their Treatment

Upper blepharoplasty is the most popular facial aesthetic surgery in Asia, and ~ 10 percent of Asian patients who undergo blepharoplasty develop complications of the surgery. The following paragraphs discuss the main complications of upper eyelid blepharoplasty.

21.9.1 Hematoma

Hematoma is not a common complication of upper eyelid blepharoplasty. Because of the solid support of the eyeball beneath the upper eyelids, bleeding rarely becomes a hematoma. Bipolar cautery should be used to control bleeding, especially during the removal of septal fat.

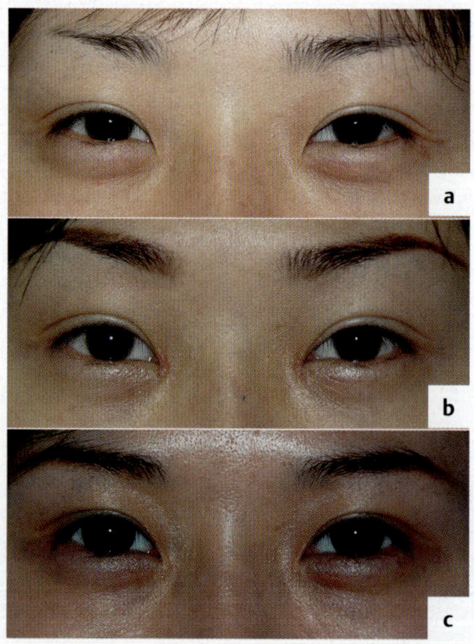

Fig. 21.20 Long-term follow up after epicanthoplasty. **(a)** A 25-year-old female with mild epicanthus underwent modified z-plasty epicanthoplasty, and was followed up at **(b)** 7 days and **(c)** 4 years. The epicanthal folds totally disappeared, the distance between the medial canthi narrowed, and the caruncles are visible. Cosmetic contact lenses are worn in **(c)**.

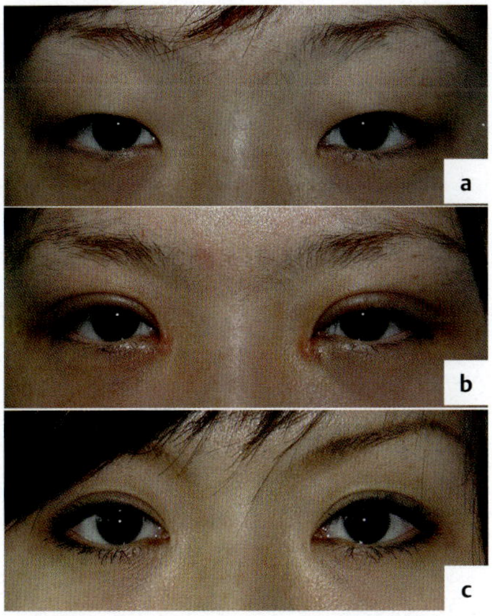

Fig. 21.21 Outcomes of full incision blepharoplasty and epicanthoplasty. **(a)** An 18-year-old female with creaseless eyelids and mild epicanthus underwent full incision blepharoplasty and epicanthoplasty, with follow-up after **(b)** 7 days and **(c)** 12 months. After blepharoplasty, her puffy upper eyelids were remarkably improved. The shape and heights of her eyelids were symmetrical and suitable for her eyes. Her caruncles were more visible and the distance between her medial canthi had narrowed after epicanthoplasty. There was no obvious scar at the medial canthus.

21.9.2 Infections

Infection seldom occurs after blepharoplasty, since the circulation surrounding the eyes is robust. Disinfection and aseptic techniques should be performed carefully.

21.9.3 Asymmetry

Asymmetry is a common complication of upper eyelid blepharoplasty, and it occurs if eyelid height or shape differs between the two eyes. To prevent asymmetry, it is necessary to perform every step carefully according to the guidelines. Attention should be paid to the following: detection of any preoperative asymmetries in the patient, especially of upper eyelids or eyebrows; adjusting the surgical plan to address the patient's original asymmetries; making identical designs on the two sides; and redoing the suturing of skin to tarsus if asymmetry has occurred. Furthermore, photography is extremely helpful for recording any tiny asymmetry in the patient.

21.9.4 Narrowing or Loss of Creases

Narrowing or loss of the crease is the most common complication of upper eyelid blepharoplasty. This complication usually occurs with the no incision method, but it can occasionally present after the full incision approach, as shown in **Fig. 21.15**. Anatomically, the mechanism of fold loss is that the adherence of the skin and tarsus is not sufficient to suspend the pretarsal skin. The possible reasons are: (1) In some puffy eyes, the soft tissue above the crease pushes the crease down and narrows it. (2) Not enough soft tissue or fat was excised from the tarsal plate and obstructs the adherence between the pretarsal skin and tarsus; this is usually caused by the imprecise technique. Even with the full incision method, it is helpful to use the anchor sutures to enhance the adherence between skin and tarsus.

21.9.5 Ptosis

Blepharoptosis is a rare complication of upper eyelid blepharoplasty. Blepharoptosis can be preoperative or postoperative. Careful examination before surgery will identify preoperative ptosis, for which the full incision method, including ptosis correction, should be used. Postoperative ptosis is usually caused by injury to the levator aponeurosis; it can be detected intraoperatively and should be corrected immediately.

21.9.6 Scarring

Scars after blepharoplasty are usually subtle, especially with the suture method and partial incision method. It is rare for a hypertrophic scar to form on the eyelid after upper eyelid blepharoplasty. Even with the full incision method, the scars are not obvious due to the lower tension on the skin and coverage by eyelid skin above the crease. The scars of epicanthoplasty are sometimes visible for 1 to 2 months, since the incisions are exposed in the medial canthus. In the patient with a tendency to scar, scars can be more obvious than normal. For hypertrophic scars, anti-scar ointments and tapes can be used.

21.10 Case Examples of Blepharoplasty and Epicanthoplasty

This chapter describes methods of upper eyelid blepharoplasty in Asians. The author prefers the full incision method combined with anchor sutures for most patients, and the epicanthoplasty for patients with epicanthus. **Fig. 21.22, Fig. 21.23,** and **Fig. 21.24** show three typical cases.

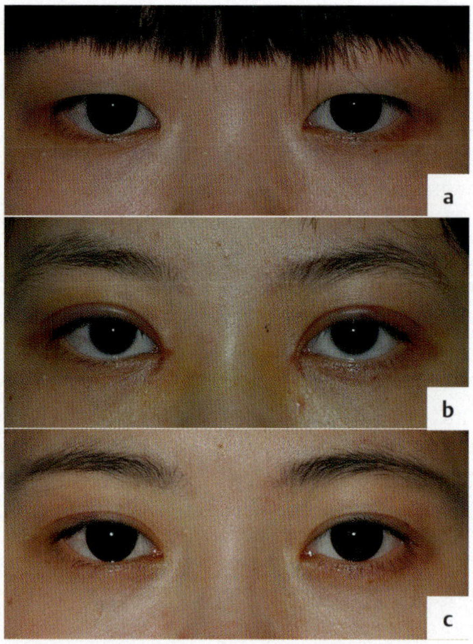

Fig. 21.22 Outcomes after full incision blepharoplasty and epicanthoplasty. **(a)** A 21-year-old female with creaseless eyelids and mild epicanthus underwent full incision blepharoplasty and epicanthoplasty, with follow-up after **(b)** 7 days and **(c)** 13 months. Her puffy upper eyelids were remarkably improved after blepharoplasty. The shape and heights of eyelids were symmetrical and suitable for her eyes. The caruncles were visible and the distance between the medial canthi was narrowed after epicanthoplasty. There was no obvious scar at the medial canthus. Cosmetic contact lenses were worn in **(a)** and **(c)**.

21.11 Conclusion

Upper eyelid blepharoplasty is the most common plastic surgery in Asia, mainly to create creases on the upper eyelids (so-called double eyelids). The mechanism of crease formation is the attachment of pretarsal skin to tarsal plate. There are three main methods: the no incision (thread embedding) method, the partial incision method, and the full incision method. Successful blepharoplasty can be achieved through an accurate preoperative design and a precise operation.

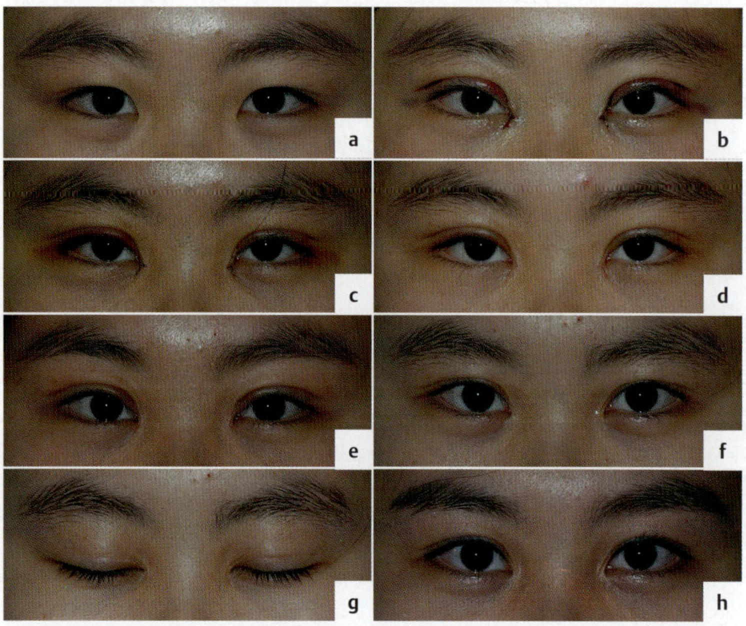

Fig. 21.23 Four-year follow-up after full incision blepharoplasty and epicanthoplasty. **(a)** A 20-year-old female with partial crease eyelids and mild epicanthus underwent full incision blepharoplasty and epicanthoplasty, with follow-up **(b)** immediately, **(c)** 3 days, **(d)** 7 days, **(e)** 20 days, **(f,g)** 7 months, and **(h)** 48 months after surgery. Swelling and bruising presented after surgery and were almost gone by postoperative day 20. Postoperatively, her puffy upper eyelids were remarkably improved. The shape and heights of her eyelids were symmetrical and suitable for her eyes. The caruncles were visible and the distance between the medial canthi had narrowed after epicanthoplasty. **(g)** There was no obvious scar on the eyelids and medial canthus.

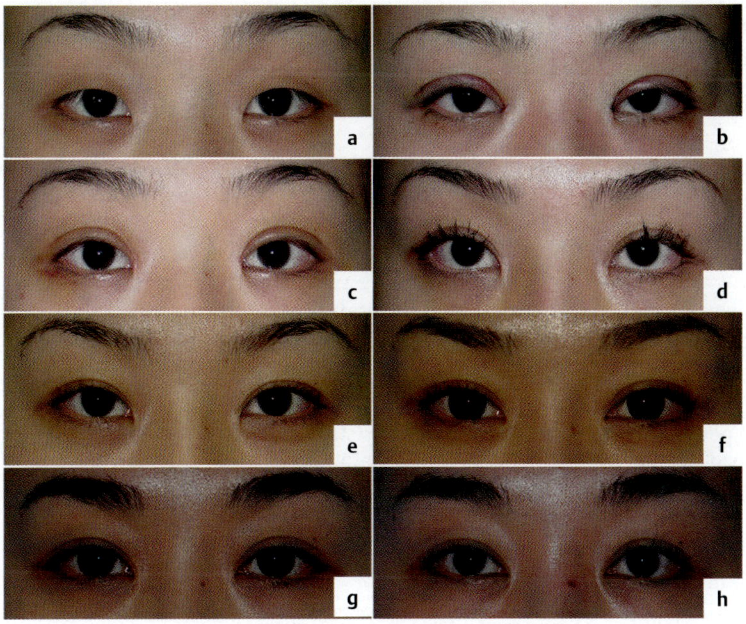

Fig. 21.24 Ten-year follow-up after full incision blepharoplasty and epicanthoplasty. **(a)** A 21-year-old female with creaseless eyelids and mild epicanthus underwent full incision blepharoplasty and epicanthoplasty, with follow-up **(b)** immediately and after **(c)** 7 days, **(d)** 6 months, **(e)** 8 months, **(f)** 54 months, **(g)** 66 months, and **(h)** 124 months. Postoperative bruising disappeared after 7 days, and no swelling could be found 6 months after surgery. Her puffy upper eyelids were remarkably improved and the distance from eyebrows to eyelids was narrowed after blepharoplasty. Both shape and heights of the eyelids were symmetrical and suitable for her eyes, and were durable and reliable for more than 10 years. The caruncles were visible and the distance between the medial canthi had narrowed after epicanthoplasty. There was no obvious scar at the medial canthus.

References

1. Sayoc BT. Plastic construction of the superior palpebral fold in slit eyes. Bull Phil Ophthal Otolaryngol Soc 1953;1:2
2. Kim DW, Bhatki AM. Upper blepharoplasty in the Asian eyelid. Facial Plast Surg Clin North Am 2007;15(3): 327–335, vi
3. Millard DR Jr. Oriental peregrinations. Plast Reconstr Surg (1946) 1955;16(5):319–336
4. Fernandez LR. Double eyelid operation in the Oriental in Hawaii. Plast Reconstr Surg Transplant Bull 1960; 25(3):257–264
5. Jeong S, Lemke BN, Dortzbach RK, Park YG, Kang HK. The Asian upper eyelid: an anatomical study with comparison to the Caucasian eyelid. Arch Ophthalmol 1999;117(7):907–912
6. Larrabee WF Jr, Makielski KH, Henderson JL. Surgical Anatomy of the Face. 2nd ed. Philadelphia: Lippincott Williams & Wilkins; 2004:128–143
7. Cheng J, Xu FZ; JianCheng. Anatomic microstructure of the upper eyelid in the Oriental double eyelid. Plast Reconstr Surg 2001;107(7):1665–1668
8. Onizuka T, Iwanami M. Blepharoplasty in Japan. Aesthetic Plast Surg 1984;8(2):97–100
9. Liu D, Hsu WM. Oriental eyelids. Anatomic difference and surgical consideration. Ophthal Plast Reconstr Surg 1986;2(2):59–64
10. Han MH, Kwon ST. A statistical study of upper eyelids of Korean young women. J Korean Soc Plast Reconstr Surg 1992;19(6):930–935
11. Liao WC, Tung TC, Tsai TR, Wang CY, Lin CH. Celebrity arcade suture blepharoplasty for double eyelid. Aesthetic Plast Surg 2005;29(6):540–545
12. Kim BG, Youn DY. Management of adhesion using a pretarsal fibromuscular flap or graft in secondary blepharoplasty. Plast Reconstr Surg 2006;117(3):782–789, discussion 790–791
13. Chen SH, Mardini S, Chen HC, et al. Strategies for a successful corrective Asian blepharoplasty after previously failed revisions. Plast Reconstr Surg 2004;114(5): 1270–1277, discussion 1278–1279
14. Perin LF, Helene A Jr, Fraga MF. Sutureless closure of the upper eyelids in blepharoplasty: use of octyl-2-cyanoacrylate. Aesthet Surg J 2009;29(2):87–92
15. Wu S, Shi H, Yan S, Sun Y, Pan L, Wu H. Combined anchor suture with external upper eyelid blepharoplasty in Asian patients. Arch Facial Plast Surg 2010;12(4):230–234
16. Flowers RS. Upper blepharoplasty by eyelid invagination. Anchor blepharoplasty. Clin Plast Surg 1993;20(2): 193–207
17. Chuangsuwanich A. Short incisional double-eyelid blepharoplasty for Asian patients. Aesthet Surg J 2006; 26(3):280–286
18. Kim JW, Lee JO. Asian blepharoplasty with a short-pulsed contact Nd-Yag laser: limited-incision resectable laser double fold with internal medial and lateral functional epicanthoplasty. Aesthetic Plast Surg 1998;22(6):433–438

22 Surgical and Nonsurgical Techniques for Treating the Square Jaw

Xiongzheng Mu and Yingzhi Wu

22.1 Introduction

A square jaw is commonly seen in East Asians and is considered aesthetically unfavorable. When a square jaw is combined with a prominent malar complex, the facial contour can appear square, with a masculine, obstinate, and unlucky image. Patients often complain about having a square-shaped face, not only those with a square jaw but also those with a normal oval face. Melon seed–shaped or oval faces are the favored facial contours because they look like the faces of movie stars.

A square jaw is mostly due to two factors: hypertrophy of the masseter muscle and a prominent mandibular angle. Based on cadaver measurements and three-dimensional computed tomography (CT), the average mandibular angle is ~ 110 degrees in East Asians. If the mandibular angle is less than 100 degrees, the patient is most likely to have a square jaw. Several techniques have been developed to help the patient get a melon seed–shaped or oval face. The technique applied depends on the patient's particular characteristics. The techniques are basically divided into two categories: surgical and nonsurgical.

22.2 Nonsurgical Technique

The nonsurgical technique is mainly used for patients who have a hypertrophied masseter muscle without a prominent mandibular angle. Asians tend to have more-developed mandibles than Westerners. Data show that the distance between the gonions is 12 to 20 mm longer in Korean women than in Caucasians.[1] In addition, benign hypertrophy of the masseter muscle is common in Asians and contributes to an undesirable quadrangular and wide lower face. There is high demand for a slim mandible in Asians, and the use of botulinum toxin type A (BTA) to improve a square-jawed appearance is common.

Injection of BTA is one of the most widely performed cosmetic procedures in the world. The first medical use of BTA was reported in 1980,[2] and the first cosmetic use of BTA—as a safe and effective treatment for glabellar lines—was described in a seminal paper published in 1992.[3] In Asian countries, the use of BTA in cosmetic procedures started when commercial preparations of BTA became available, roughly 1999.[4] Use of BTA injection for a hypertrophied masseter is in high demand in Asia, and good results can be achieved with repeated injections. There are two main techniques of injection: (1) one-point injection and (2) three-point injection. For both techniques, physicians should ask patients to clench their teeth to set the boundary of the safe zone. The safe zone is a rectangular area defined by linking the lower border of the mandible, the tragus–mouth corner line, and the anterior and posterior borders of the masseter.[1] Injection into this zone is highly effective and safe.

22.2.1 Reconstitution

The volume of reconstitution can be adapted according to the quantity of product. We recommend reconstituting a vial of BTA (100 U) in preservative-free 0.9% saline (2.0 mL).

Syringe and Needle for Injection

A 1 mL insulin syringe marked with graduations of 0.01 mL is recommended for reconstitution. A 30G-13 mm needle is standard and is recommended for the injection.

One-Point Injection Technique

Penetrate into the thickest (middle) portion of the masseter muscle 1.5 cm from the border of the mandibular angle and inject 10 U, then draw back the needle under the dermis, and while directing the needle anteriorly, posteriorly, inferiorly, and superiorly, inject 10 U, respectively. A total dose of 50 U is recommended **(Fig. 22.1)**.

Three-Point Injection Technique

The first injection is administered into the thickest (middle) portion of the masseter muscle 1.5 cm from the border of the mandibular angle. Two other points are located anterior and posterior to the center. Together, the three points form a triangle. A total dose of 50 to 60 U is recommended (8–10 U per point) **(Fig. 22.2)**.

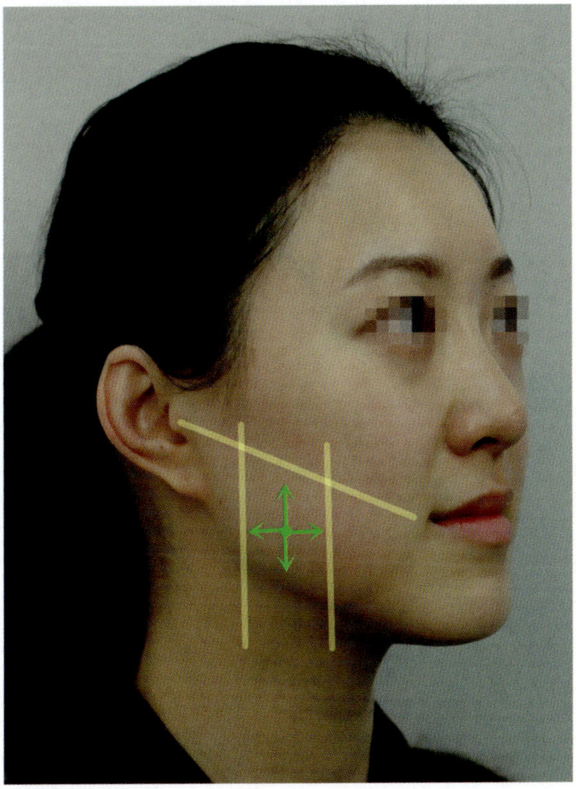

Fig. 22.1 One-point injection.

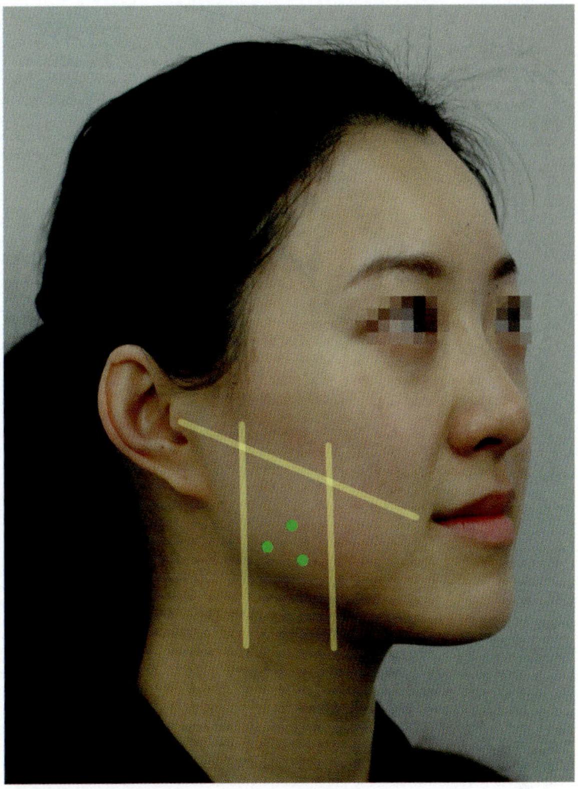

Fig. 22.2 Three-point injection technique.

22.3 Surgical Technique

22.3.1 Mandibular Reshaping Methods and Inclined-Fullness Osteotomy

General anesthesia with nasal intubation is given to all patients. An intraoral incision is made 0.5 to 1 cm away from the attached gingiva along the lower buccal mucosa, beginning at the second premolar and ending at the occlusal plane. Subperiosteal undermining is performed meticulously to expose the lateral-inferior part of the mandibular angle and the body of the mandible. Precautions are taken to protect the mental nerve until sufficient exposure has been achieved.

Bur and Shaving Method

In cases of a moderately prominent or outward type of mandibular angle, the patient usually undergoes bone shaving by burring, chiseling, and/or chipping of the outer cortex of the mandibular angle in the early period.

Mandibular Angle Reduction Osteotomy

For cases of a severely prominent or inward type of mandibular angle, angle osteotomy is used. Usually, the direction line is marked with an electric grinder before the osteotomy. The full thickness of the mandibular angle is then removed with an oscillating saw, including equal amounts of the outer and inner cortexes.

Outer Cortex-Splitting Osteotomy

In cases of a moderately prominent or inward type of mandibular angle, a sagittal osteotomy of the outer cortex is performed in the mandibular angle area (**Fig. 22.3**). The prominence of the region between the molar teeth and the external oblique line is the key factor for evaluating the possibility of split cortical osteotomy. The osteotomy line is first labeled by using an electric drill. The horizontal line on the ramus and the perpendicular line on the mandibular body are then cut superficially on the outer cortex. After that, split cortical osteotomy is performed to remove half the thickness of the outer cortex, thus reducing the lateral projection of the lower face.

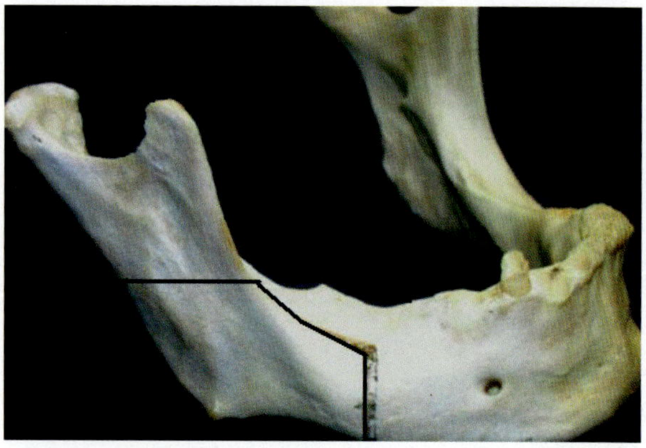

Fig. 22.3 Design of outer cortical split mandibular osteotomy.

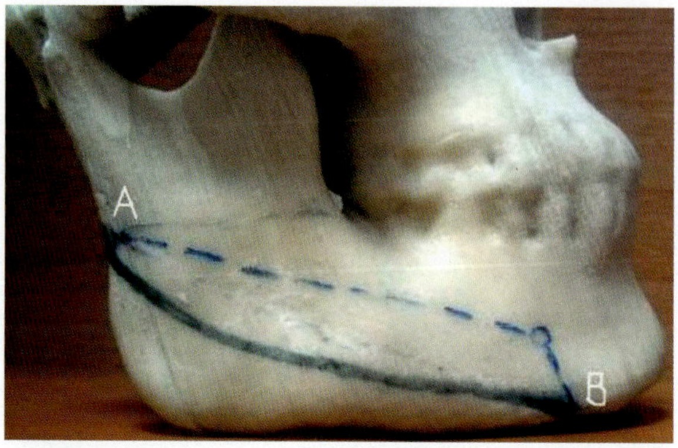

Fig. 22.4 The marking of the inclined-fullness mandibular angle and margin osteotomy.

Inclined-Fullness Osteotomy in the Mandibular Angle and Margin

In 2000, the authors modified the conventional procedure to include inclined-fullness osteotomy in the mandibular angle and margin area; this technique has been preferred in many recent cases. The design of the osteotomy is as follows **(Fig. 22.4)**: (1) The starting point of the osteotomy is the intersection where the occlusal plane meets the posterior edge of the ramus (point A). (2) The end point of the osteotomy is the intersection where the vertical line from the second premolar meets the edge of the mandible (point B). Usually, the position of the mental foramen is just beneath the second premolar. We can also set point B according to the mental foramen shown on a cephalogram. (3) For a curved osteotomy, the curvilinear osteotomy line is drawn from point A to point B. The actual osteotomy procedure has two steps. First, the upper half of the curvilinear line is cut with a reciprocating saw, with more outer plate removed than inner plate in the mandibular angle portion. Then, a second osteotomy is performed on the lower half of the curvilinear line, also with more outer plate removed than inner plate in the mandibular margin. The two surgical steps can be helpful to avoid damage to the alveolar nerve **(Fig. 22.5)**.

Mandibular angle osteotomy was first introduced by Beckers,[5] who used an external approach. This technique was considered acceptable until Converse[6] reported a method using an intraoral incision. Both methods used linear osteotomies, which did not adapt to the East Asian aesthetic concept, and usually resulted in a "second mandibular angle." Baek[7] proposed a multi-osteotomy method to overcome this disadvantage; however, it was complicated, and the patient did not present a natural mandibular outline. The authors use the term *mandibular reshaping* instead of describing reduction osteotomies in the lower mandibular region. Actually, recontouring surgery of the lower face includes not only mandibular angle reduction but also a reduction of the thickness of the mandibular body and body margin. Outer cortex-splitting osteotomy was reported for reduction mandibuloplasty.[8] Although it is a simple method, it has limited effectiveness. The author further modified this procedure to a sagittal outer cortex–splitting osteotomy. However, although it could remove half the thickness of the outer cortex and relieve the lateral projection of the lower face, it did not change the angle between the ramus plane and the mandibular plane. Female patients still complained about a postoperative masculine appearance from the lateral view. Furthermore, a splitting osteotomy could decrease the rigidity of the mandible and increase fracture risk. In contrast, the inclined-fullness osteotomy has key modifications so that it not only could achieve a natural mandibular margin outline that is well connected to the chin, but also could reduce the full thickness of the mandibular angle area without damaging the solidity of the mandible, and could alter the angle between the ramus plane and the mandibular plane in a one-stage operation **(Fig. 22.6)**. The problem was how to

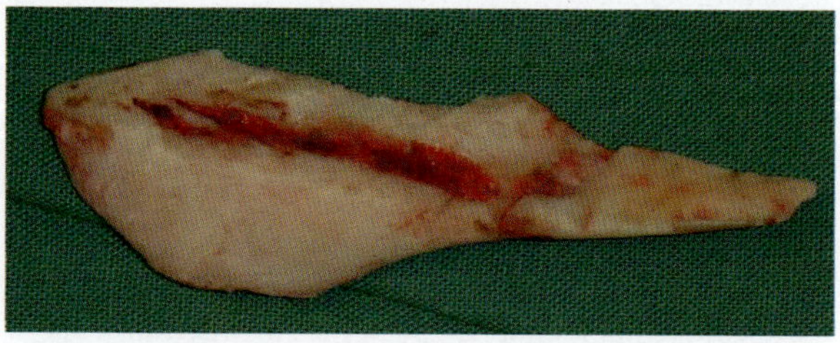

Fig. 22.5 Specimen after inclined-fullness mandibular angle and margin osteotomy.

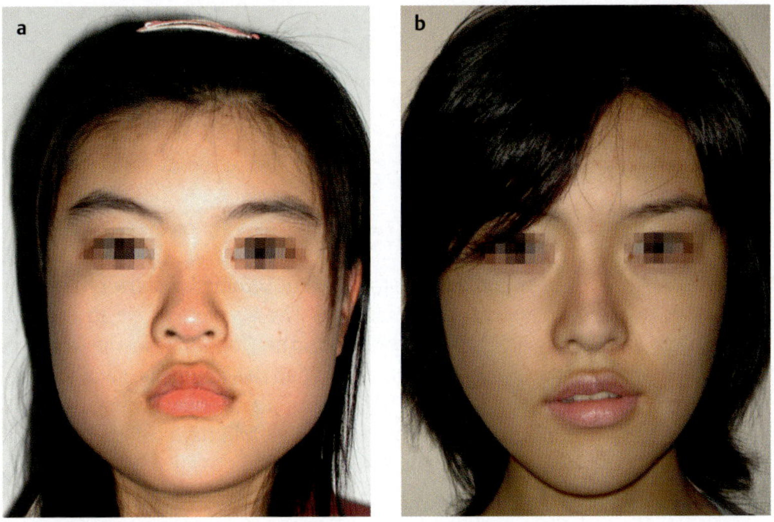

Fig. 22.6 A patient with a square-shaped face who underwent inclined-fullness mandibular reshaping. **(a)** Preoperative frontal view. **(b)** Postoperative frontal view.

determine the location of the new mandibular angle. The new mandibular angle was usually set at a point inferior to the earlobe (no more than 1 cm). Simultaneous soft tissue decrement was considered as a supplementary way to narrow the lower face. After surgery for mandibular reshaping, the masseter would have volumetric atrophy of 30%,[9] but in the aging patient (e.g., a woman older than 45 years), although mandibular angle reduction actually can smooth the prominent lower face, loss of soft tissue, such as buccal fat and parts of the masseter, will probably result in drooping of the skin of the lower face and other signs of aging in the future. In our patients, although a large number of inclined-fullness mandibulectomies and procedures for complete cortical bone removal of the lateral mandible were performed for sufficient reduction in facial width and mandibular prominence, oral function (e.g., biting strength, occlusion, and temporomandibular joint function) examined postoperatively showed a satisfactory outcome. Transient alveolar nerve injury still occurred in four cases, and it caused numbness of the mental foramen area. It is necessary to mark the anatomical structure of the alveolar nerve before surgery to avoid mistaking the location of the nerve. Careless work or mistakes caused by a less-experienced surgeon that cause mandibular fracture will probably lead to nerve injury. It should be emphasized that inclined-fullness osteotomy must be performed under the direction of an experienced and skilled surgeon.

References

1. Ahn BK, Kim YS, Kim HJ, Rho NK, Kim HS. Consensus recommendations on the aesthetic usage of botulinum toxin type A in Asians. Dermatol Surg 2013;39(12):1843–1860
2. Scott AB. Botulinum toxin injection into extraocular muscles as an alternative to strabismus surgery. J Pediatr Ophthalmol Strabismus 1980;17(1):21–25
3. Carruthers JD, Carruthers JA. Treatment of glabellar frown lines with C. botulinum-A exotoxin. J Dermatol Surg Oncol 1992;18(1):17–21
4. Rho NK, Kim HS, Kim YS, et al. Botulinum toxin type A for facial wrinkles and benign masseter hypertrophy in Korean patients. Korean J Dermatol 2010;48:823–831
5. Beckers HL. Masseteric muscle hypertrophy and its intraoral surgical correction. J Maxillofac Surg 1977;5(1): 28–35
6. Converse JM. Deformities of the jaw. In: Converse JM, ed. Reconstructive Plastic Surgery. Philadelphia, PA: WB Saunders; 1977:1406–1408
7. Baek SM, Baek RM, Shin MS. Refinement in aesthetic contouring of the prominent mandibular angle. Aesthetic Plast Surg 1994;18(3):283–289
8. Han K, Kim J. Reduction mandibuloplasty: ostectomy of the lateral cortex around the mandibular angle. J Craniofac Surg 2001;12(4):314–325
9. Gui L, Yu D, Zhang Z, Changsheng LV, Tang X, Zheng Z. Intraoral one-stage curved osteotomy for the prominent mandibular angle: a clinical study of 407 cases. Aesthetic Plast Surg 2005;29(6):552–557

23 Surgical Techniques for the Correction of Hanging Ala

Eduardo C. Yap

23.1 Introduction

East Asian noses, especially Southeast Asian noses, have some degree of hanging ala **(Fig. 23.1)** because of the thick, fibrous skin–soft tissue envelope (S-STE). The hanging ala somehow distorts the ala–columella relationship, often resulting in a lack of columellar show.

23.2 Anatomical Landmarks

Gunter[1] analyzed the ala–columella relationship by drawing an imaginary line bisecting the oblong formed by the alar rim margin and the inferior margin of the columella. The line should bisect it equally 1 to 2 mm **(Fig. 23.2)**. Gunter[1] derived a classification of ala–columella relationships **(Fig. 23.3)**. Class I has excessive columellar show. Class II has alar retraction. Class III has a combination of alar retraction and hanging columella. Class IV is hanging ala. Class V has a retracted columella, while class VI has the combination of hanging ala and retracted columella. Since most Southeast Asian noses have an underdeveloped anterior nasal spine, the columella does not show much, so the columella may appear retracted. Soft tissues are usually thick, resulting in an excessive alar rim. Hence, Southeast Asian noses are usually in classes IV to VI.

23.3 Surgical Techniques

There should be 1 to 2 mm of columellar show on the lateral view of a normal nose.[1] The ala should have an arc with its peak at midportion. On the frontal view, the alar rim should arc and end higher than the columella, giving a gull-wing appearance.[2] A hanging ala is noted when the arc is not present or is not high enough to have columellar show **(Fig. 23.4** and **Fig. 23.5)**.

A hanging ala can be lifted by elliptical excision of the alar rim skin and subcutaneous tissue via two approaches: externally, at the alar skin, or internally, at the vestibular skin.[1,3,4,5] The amount of tissue excised depends greatly on the experience and aesthetic judgment of the surgeon. There are no landmarks to follow when doing such a procedure, with the risk of a suboptimal aesthetic result.

External excision of the hanging ala usually results in visible scars and thinning of the alar rim. Sometimes, vestibular vibrissae are everted at the alar rim. The external approach is the usual approach for most surgeons. The internal approach, with elliptical excision of the vestibular skin, is discussed by several authors, but again, there are no landmarks to follow.[1,4,5]

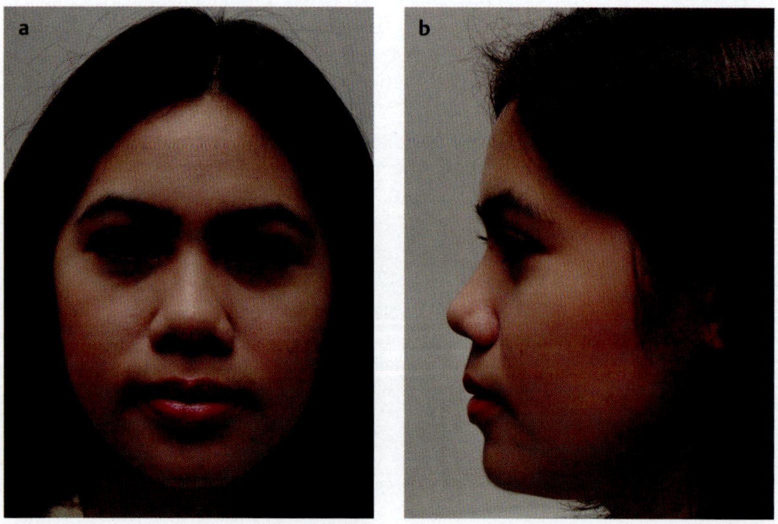

Fig. 23.1 (a,b) The typical hanging ala.

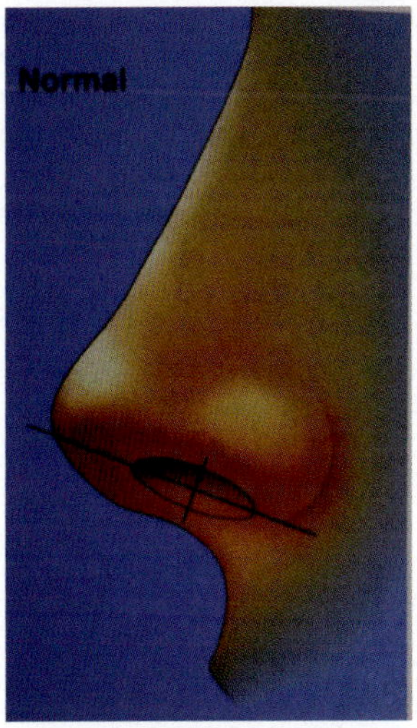

Fig. 23.2 Normal ala–columella relationship. Lateral view. A line should bisect equally the oblong formed by the alar rim and the inferior margin of the columella. (Used with permission from Gunter JP, Rochrich RJ, Adams WP Jr. Dallas Rhinoplasty, 2nd ed. QMP; 2007:403.)

23.3.1 Sail Excision Technique for the Correction of the Hanging Ala

The author has devised a method of precise correction of hanging ala via excision of a triangular piece of vestibular skin shaped like the sail of a sailboat. The technique is called sail excision of the hanging ala **(Fig. 23.6)**.[6] There are four landmarks to use for the triangle in this technique:

1. The apex. The apex of the sail can be precisely determined by pinching the nostril to elicit a fold or notch at the anterior edge of the alar rim. It also corresponds to the peak of the gull wing on the frontal view **(Fig. 23.7)**.
2. The caudal side. The alar rim corresponds to the caudal side of the sail. It is determined by the medial margin of the alar rim. On some occasions, the alar rim may be thick. The incision can be made more lateral, to include more skin and subcutaneous tissue. The reference for thickness is the anterosuperior end of the alar rim **(Fig. 23.8)**.

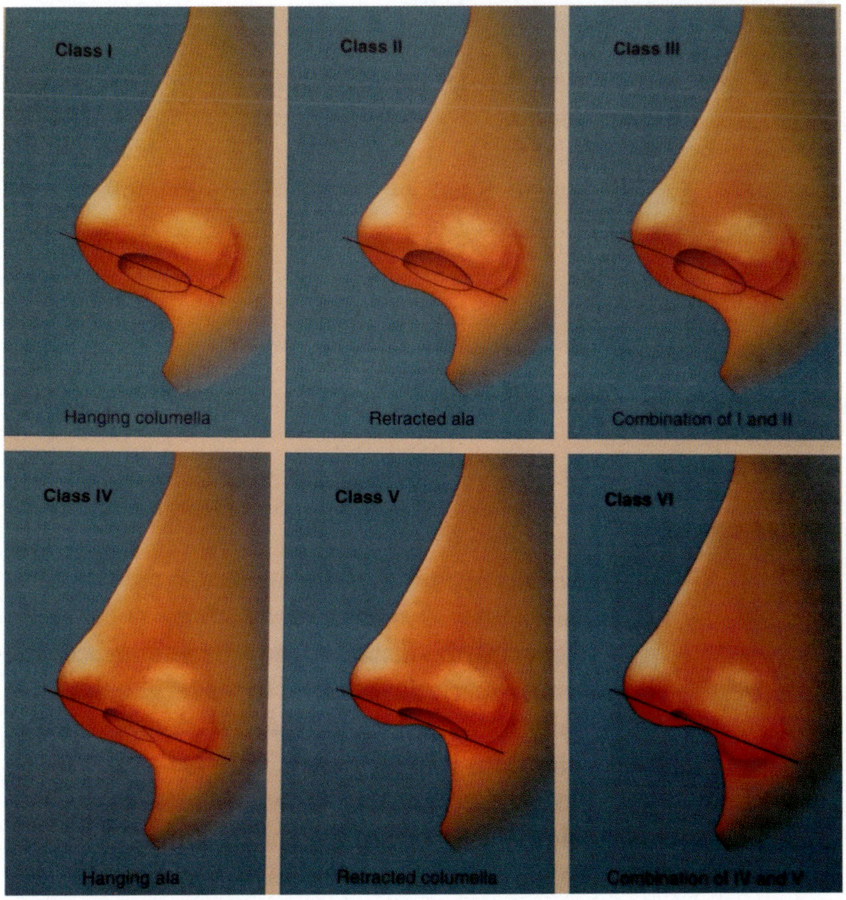

Fig. 23.3 Classification of ala–columella relationships. (Used with permission from Gunter JP, Rochrich RJ, Adams WP Jr. Dallas Rhinoplasty, 2nd ed. QMP; 2007:404.)

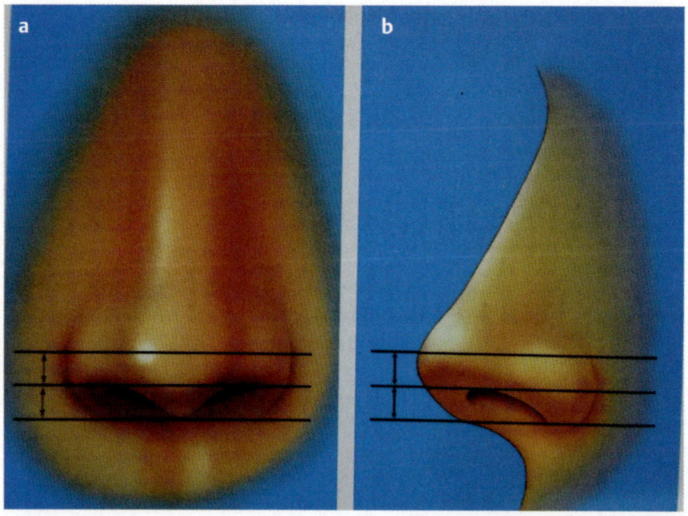

Fig. 23.4 (a,b) Normal ala–columella relationship. Frontal view. The vertical distance between the columella-lobular angle and the tip-defining points is divided in half by a horizontal line adjacent to the highest point of the alar rims. (Used with permission from Gunter JP, Rochrich RJ, Adams WP Jr. Dallas Rhinoplasty, 2nd ed. QMP; 2007:402.)

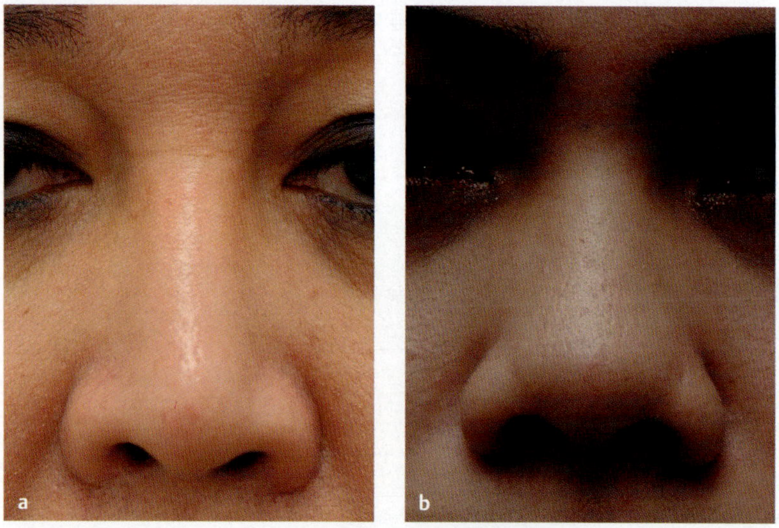

Fig. 23.5 (a) A nose with a good ala–columella relationship. **(b)** A nose with hanging ala.

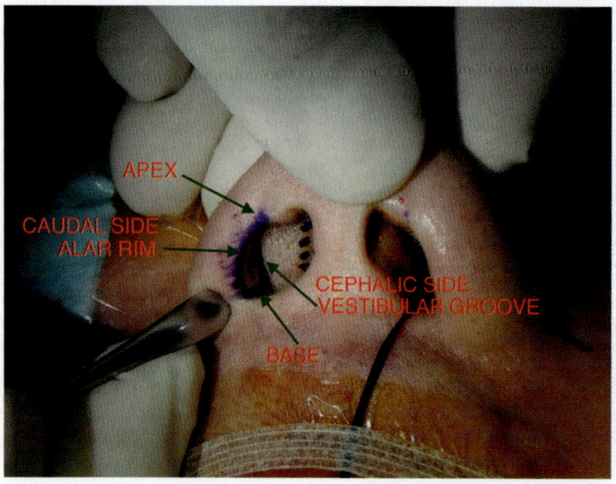

Fig. 23.6 The sail design.

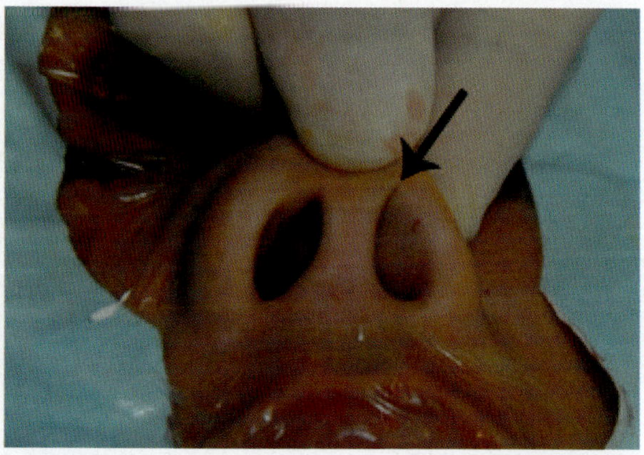

Fig. 23.7 The apex can be located by pinching the nostril.

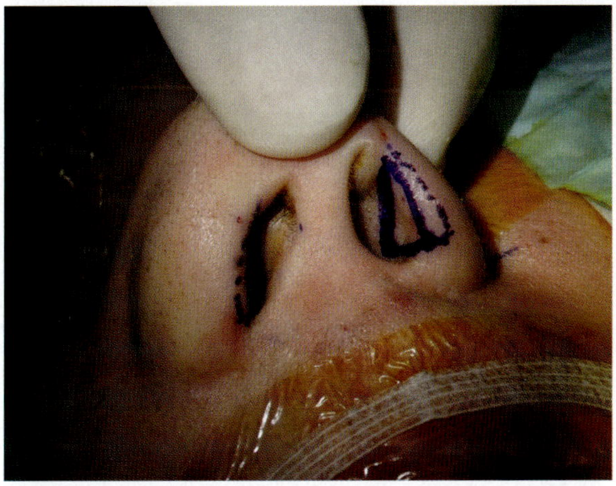

Fig. 23.8 The excision of the caudal side can be extended more laterally following the thickness at the anterior portion of the alar rim. Take note of the immediate postoperative look of the left alar rim.

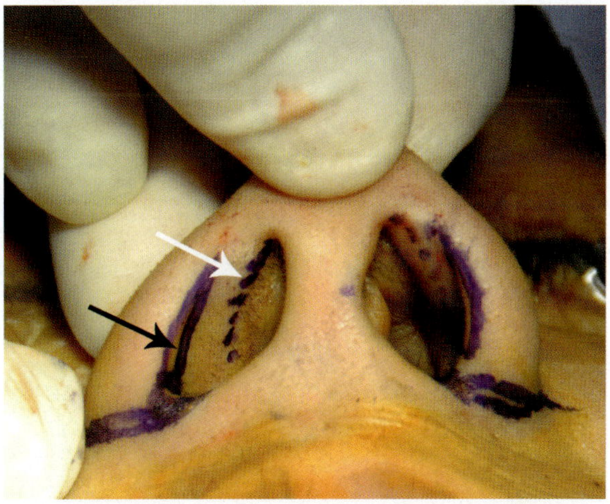

Fig. 23.9 An example with the sail pattern marked. Note that the vestibular skin groove is different from the caudal edge of the lower lateral cartilage.

3. The cephalic side. The cephalic side of the sail corresponds to a groove or skin depression in the lateral wall of the nasal vestibule. It is a few millimeters lateral to the caudal edge of the lower lateral cartilage. This landmark is termed the vestibular skin groove. The vestibular skin groove should not be mistaken for the lower lateral cartilage **(Fig. 23.9)**.
4. The base. The base is a line drawn just lateral to the nasal sill connecting the caudal side (alar rim) and the cephalic side (vestibular skin groove). The length of the base may vary from 3 mm to 10 mm. The actual lift can be estimated by dividing the length of the base in half: e.g., a 5 mm base can give an alar lift of 2.5 mm **(Fig. 23.10)**.

If alar base plasty is needed, this is marked prior to sail excision. About 1 to 1.5 mm of vestibular skin is left intact between the sail and alar base plasty to ensure symmetry of the nostrils during closure and to prevent scarring at the nasal sill **(Fig. 23.11)**.

In noses with normal alar width but with hanging alar rim and alar base, simultaneous lift can be achieved by excising the nasal floor in continuum with the lateral vestibular wall, resulting in an ellipse **(Fig. 23.12)**.

After excision of the skin and subcutaneous tissue, lifting is achieved by inward rolling of the alar rim to the vestibular skin groove, including the base, using nylon 6–0 simple interrupted sutures. Meticulous skin-to-skin contact closure should be achieved to avoid a thick scar. Because of the unequal lengths in closure, adjustments are

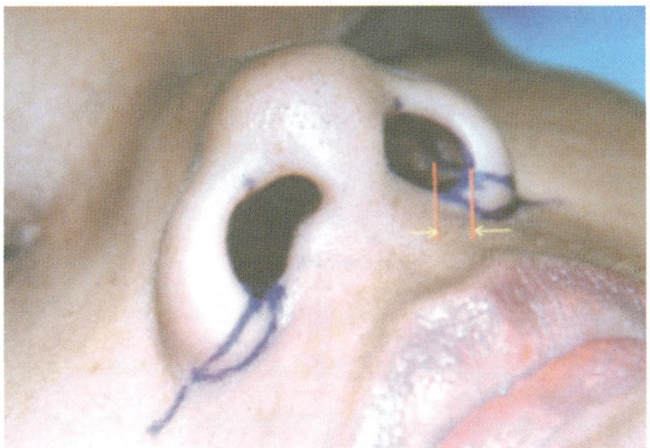

Fig. 23.10 The expected amount of lift can be predicted by calculating half of the base length.

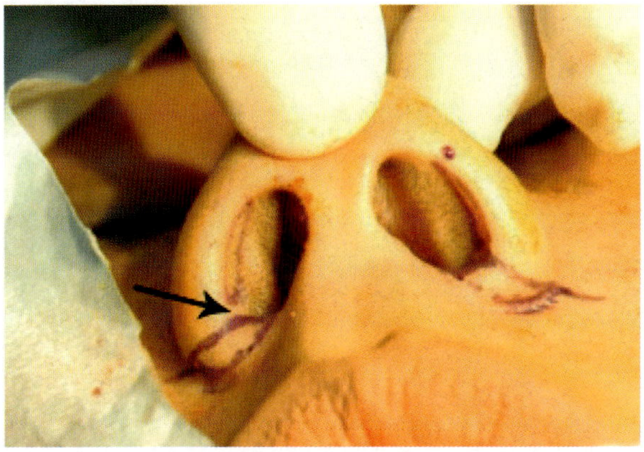

Fig. 23.11 1.0 to 1.5 mm of vestibular skin is preserved if an alar lift procedure will be done simultaneously with alar base plasty.

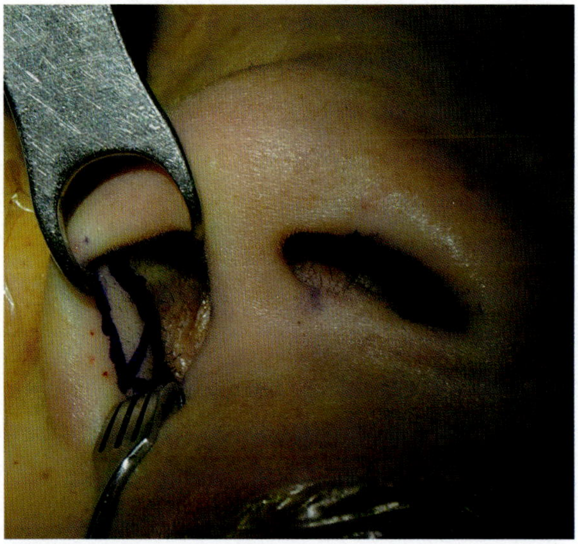

Fig. 23.12 Noses with normal nostril sill width can have a simultaneous lift of alar rim and base via an ellipse excision in the lateral vestibular wall in continuum with the nasal sill.

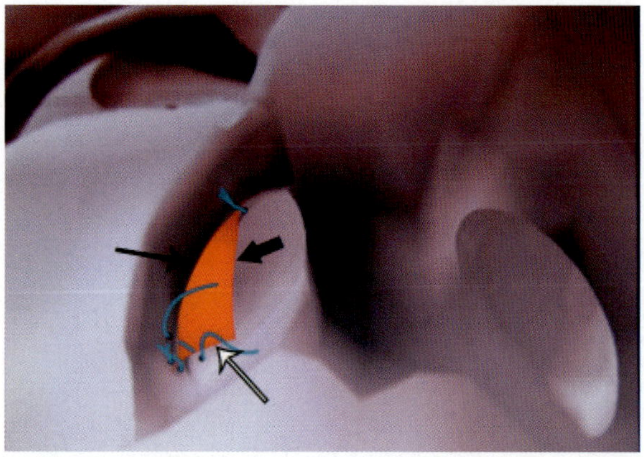

Fig. 23.13 Closure of the defect involves two unequal lengths; alar rim coapts with the vestibular groove and base.

required to achieve a smooth contour of the new alar rim (**Fig. 23.13**).

The scars are generally good looking and acceptable (**Fig. 23.14**). The initial cross-hatch marks of the sutures disappear in a few weeks.

23.4 Conclusion

In summary, sail excision of the hanging ala uses consistent landmarks and ensures a good aesthetic result. The landmarks are the apex, alar rim, and vestibular skin groove. Among these landmarks, the vestibular skin groove is fixed in its location. In noses with a good ala–columella relationship, as is seen commonly in Caucasians, the groove is noted to be near the alar rim (**Fig. 23.15**). However, in East Asian noses with hanging ala, the distance between the alar rim and the vestibular skin groove is greater (**Fig. 23.16**). Under light microscopy, the vestibular skin groove reveals a change in the orientation of nasalis muscle fibers, resulting in a linear depression in the lateral vestibular wall (**Fig. 23.17**). By following the vestibular skin groove as the inner limit of excision and by allowing the alar rim skin to roll inward, one is assured of symmetry and a better ala–columella relationship. Meticulous closure of the defect almost always heals with a nice-looking scar. The linear scar is located in the inner lateral vestibular wall, making it all the more inconspicuous. The new alar rim skin is smooth, with no scar, in contrast to the external method of correction, which usually leaves scars at the rim.

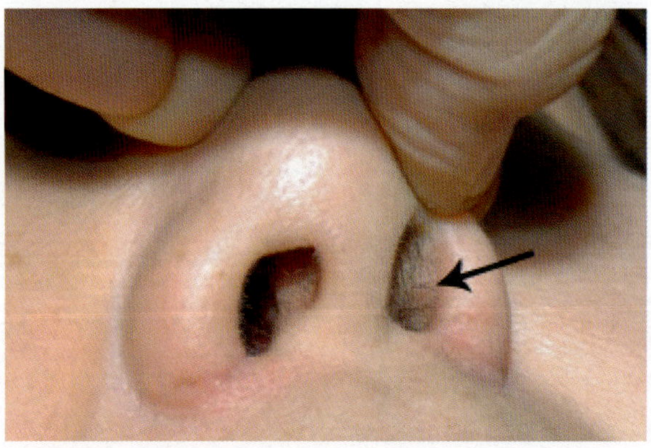

Fig. 23.14 The scar is hidden in the nasal vestibule and is generally good looking and acceptable.

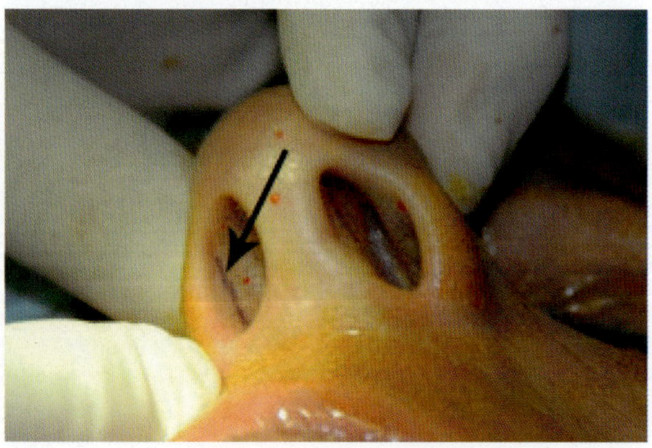

Fig. 23.15 The vestibular groove in a Caucasian nose.

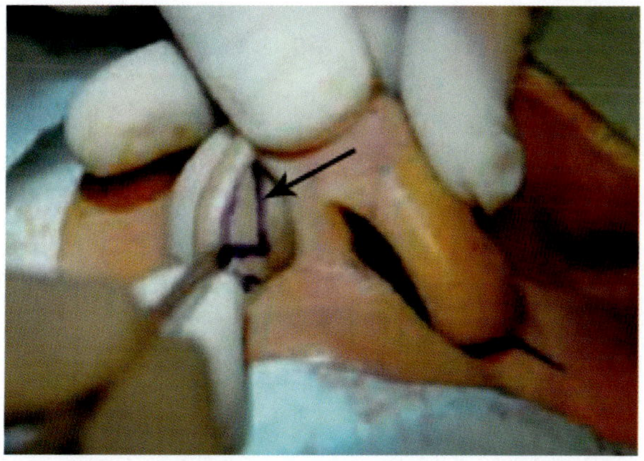

Fig. 23.16 The vestibular groove in an Asian nose.

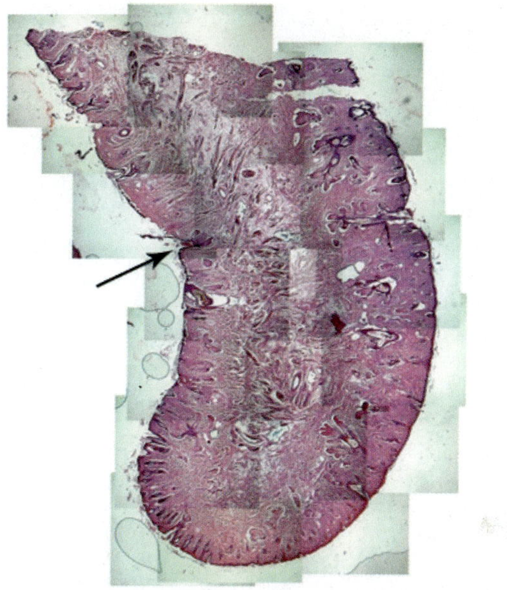

Fig. 23.17 Microscopic view of the vestibular skin groove at the lateral vestibular wall, showing the depression, which is due to the directional orientation of nasalis muscle.

Another advantage of sail excision is that it can give counter-rotation to the tip because the rim is elevated, resulting in a better columellar show. This procedure complements Asian rhinoplasty because the majority of Asian tips are slightly rotated.

A summary of the sail excision technique for hanging ala is seen in **Fig. 23.18**. Preoperative and postoperative photos are shown in **Fig. 23.19**.

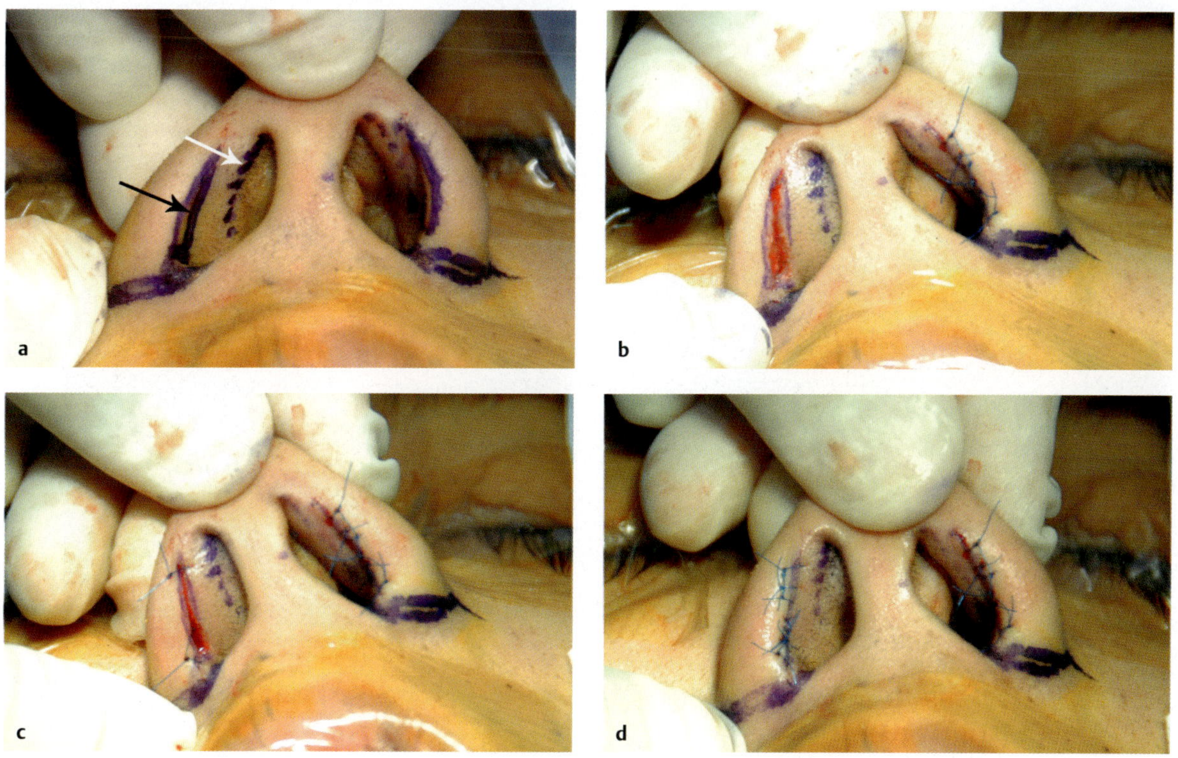

Fig. 23.18 Summary of sail excision for correction of hanging ala. **(a)** Marking of sail. **(b)** Excision of skin and subcutaneous tissue, right ala. Note the finished trimming in the left ala. **(c)** Nylon 6–0 is used for closure of the defect, which proceeds from both ends to avoid dog-ear deformity. **(d)** Immediately postoperative.

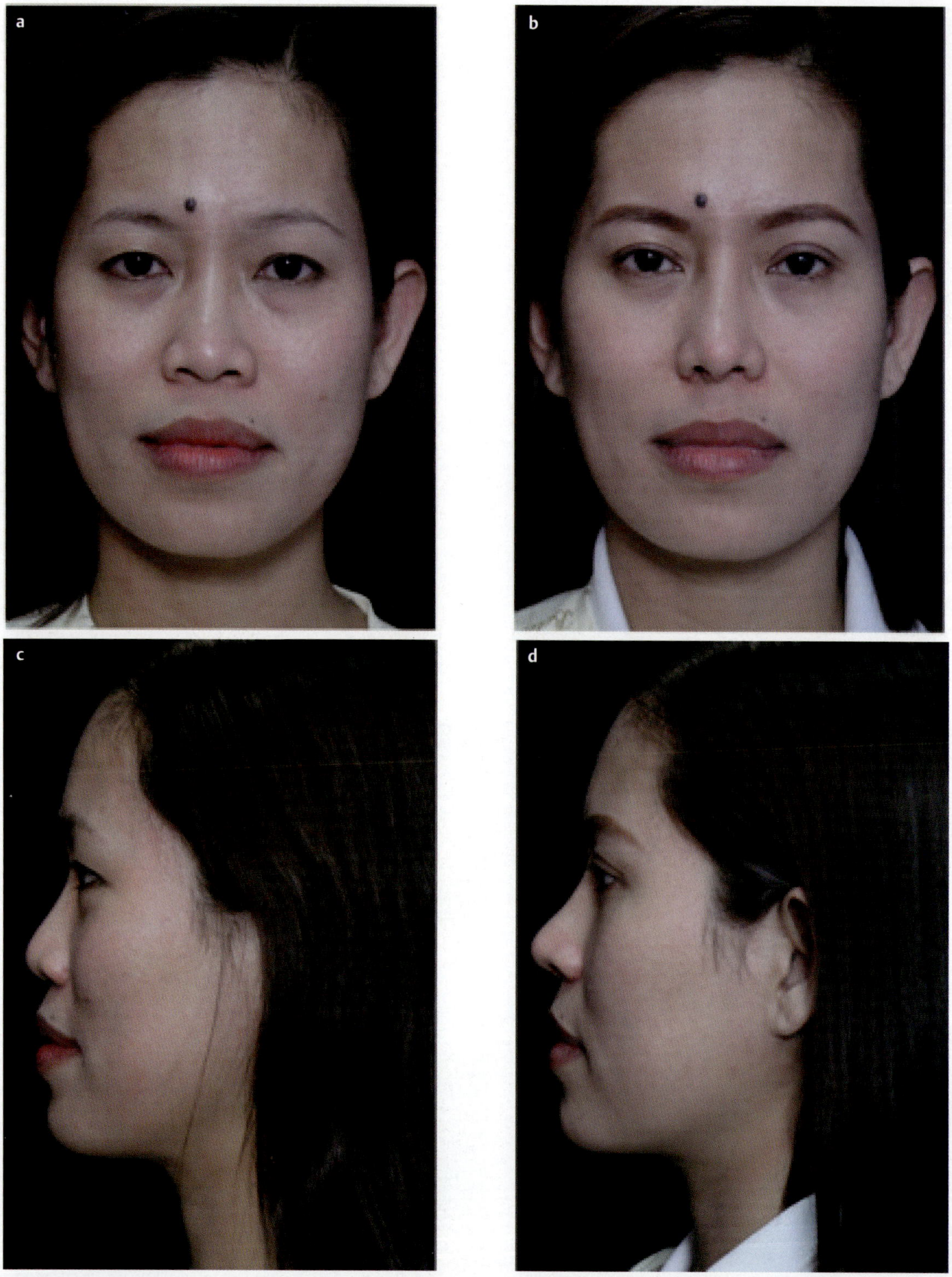

Fig. 23.19 **(a,c)** Preoperative and **(b,d)** postoperative views of alar lift surgery via sail excision. Dorsal augmentation and tip surgery were also performed.

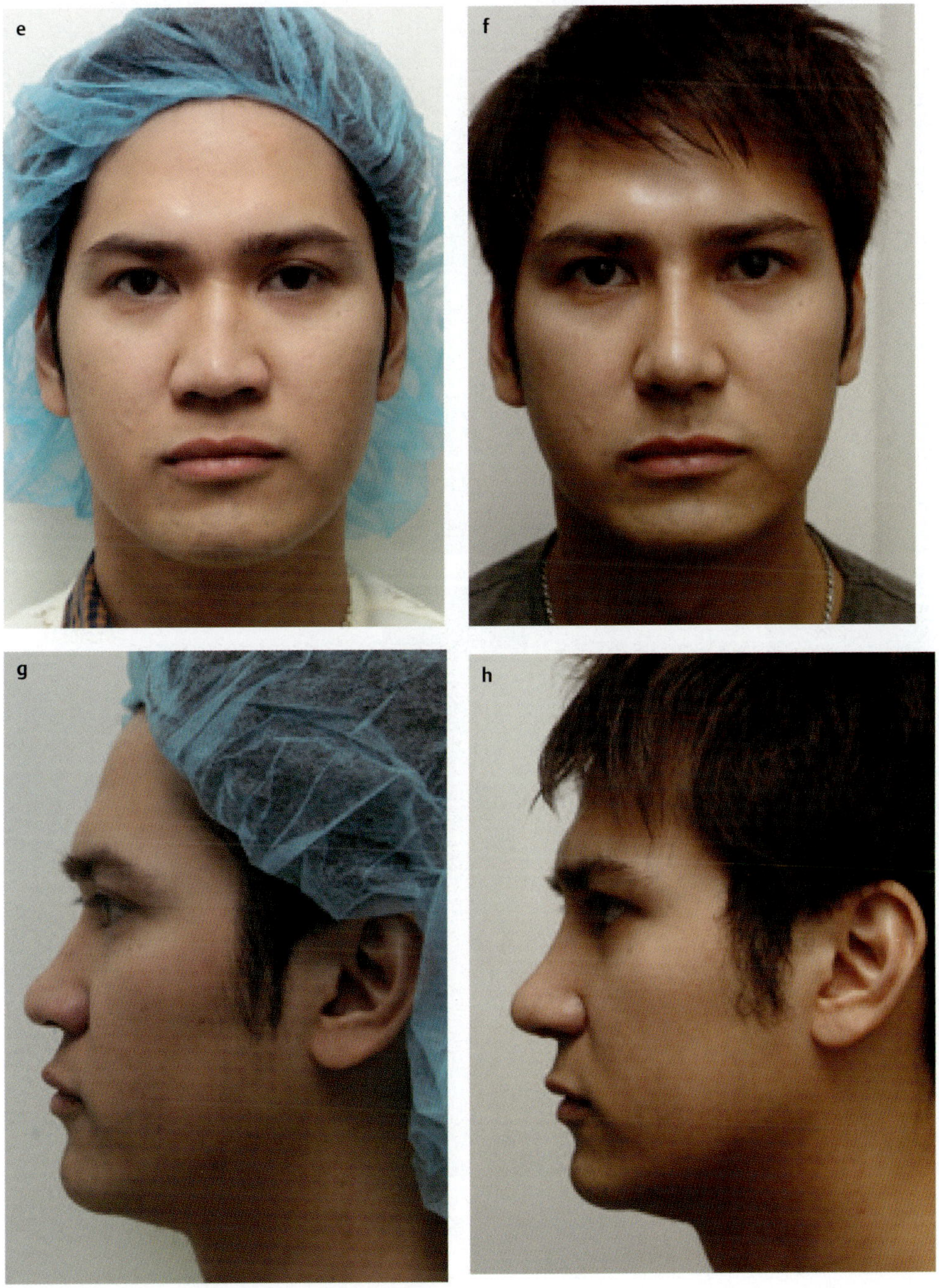

Fig. 23.19 *(Continued)* **(e,g)** Preoperative and **(f,h)** postoperative views of alar lift surgery via sail excision. Dorsal augmentation and tip surgery were also performed. *(Continued on page 278)*

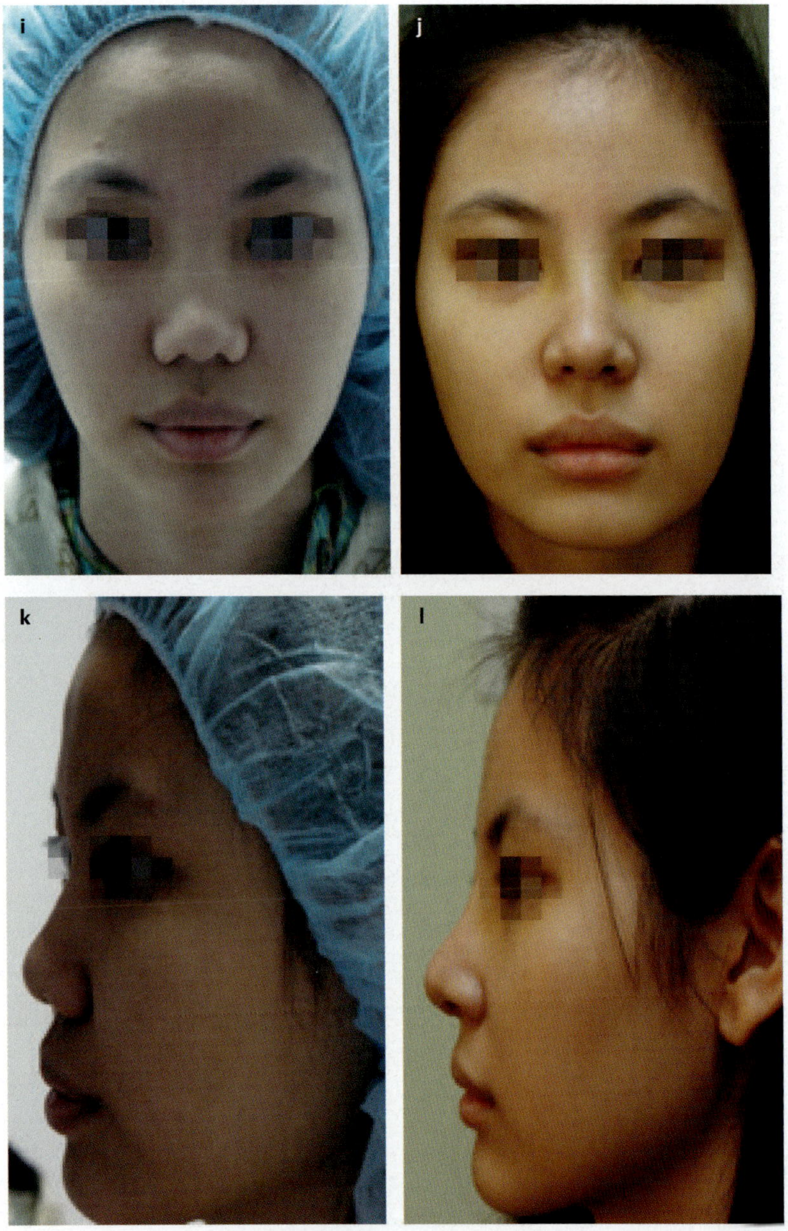

Fig. 23.19 *(Continued)* **(i,k)** Preoperative and **(j,l)** postoperative views of alar lift surgery via sail excision. Dorsal augmentation and tip surgery were also performed.

References

1. Gunter JP, Rochrich RJ, Adams WP Jr. Dallas Rhinoplasty. Vol. 1. QMP; 2007:401–409
2. Papel ID, et al. Facial Plastic and Reconstructive Surgery, 3rd ed. New York, NY: Thieme; 2009:482
3. Ellenbogen R, Blome DW. Alar rim raising. Plast Reconstr Surg 1992;90(1):28–37
4. Millard DR Jr. Alar margin sculpturing. Plast Reconstr Surg 1967;40(4):337–342
5. McKinney P, Stalnecker ML. The hanging ala. Plast Reconstr Surg 1984;73(3):427–430
6. Yap E. Improving the hanging ala. Facial Plast Surg 2012;28(2):213–217

24 Minimally Invasive Techniques in East Asian and Southeast Asian Peoples: What Do Patients Want?

Ian Loh Chi Yuan, Valerie Tay, and Hyoung Jin Moon

24.1 Introduction

Asia is the world's largest and most populous continent. It houses 60% of the world's population, ~ 4 billion people, and covers 30% of Earth's land mass. The boundaries of Asia stretch from the Ural Mountains and Mediterranean Sea in the west to the Pacific Ocean in the east. Given its size, massive population, and immense ethnic diversity, a discussion of Asian preferences as a continent for minimally invasive aesthetic procedures would be difficult. As separate sections and chapters in this book discuss ethnic preferences in South Asians and Middle Eastern patients, the authors here confine their discussion to their experiences with minimally invasive aesthetic procedures in East and Southeast Asian patients.

24.2 Key Differences Influencing Asian Preferences

24.2.1 Skin

Compared with Caucasian norms, most Asian skin is significantly more pigmented, and melanogenesis after tissue injury or solar exposure is significantly higher. Focal, localized hyperpigmentation is a hallmark of Asian photoaging, while rhytids develop significantly later than in any other ethnic group, first becoming noticeable as late as the fifth decade of life in East and Southeast Asians.

Hypertrophic scarring and keloid formation are also more common in Asians due to more florid fibrogenesis after tissue injury. Asian skin also shows an increased tendency to irritability, due to a higher proportion of apocrine glands within the skin.[1]

The combination of all these factors—increased skin irritability, increased tendency toward post-inflammatory hyperpigmentation (PIH), hypertrophic scarring and keloid formation—have influenced both patients and medical practitioners to take a more conservative approach when choosing aesthetic procedures for Asian skin. The tendency toward pigmentation and dyschromia in the Asian population is also a reason why treatment for these conditions tends to be highly popular in Asia.

Ablative procedures, such as dermabrasion and ablative laser resurfacing, are less commonly performed in Asia than nonablative procedures, such as pulsed light therapy, radiofrequency, and nonablative laser resurfacing. Priming the skin adequately before treatment, and care after the procedure, are particularly important to prevent the formation of hypertrophic scarring and post-inflammatory hyperpigmentation in the Asian patient.

The authors routinely prime patients using a combination of tretinoin and hydroquinolone for 4 weeks before performing any major resurfacing procedures for patients. This regime is stopped 3 days before, and resumed 3 days after, the procedure. Patients are prescribed silicone gels for daytime and silicone gel sheets for nighttime use if any incisions are made or ulceration occurs; incisions are closely followed up for development of any hypertrophic scarring or keloids and these are aggressively treated using intralesional steroids, sometimes in combination with 5-fluorouracil for recalcitrant cases. Sun avoidance and the use of sun blocks and screens are advised for 3 months.

24.2.2 Facial Structure

In comparison to Caucasian ideals, the Asian face is broader, with a shorter lower third due to a less-projected mentum. The midface, premaxilla, and paranasal regions are often hypoplastic. The nasofrontal angle and the nasolabial angle are more obtuse. The radix is placed more inferiorly and is less projected, and the dorsum and tip are under-projected, while the columella is often retracted. These areas are often augmented using fillers in the Asian patient.[2]

The apex of the Asian brow is placed more laterally than in Caucasians, with the peak of the eyebrow frequently placed lateral to the lateral limbus of the eye. This is an important point to consider when performing a chemical brow lift using botulinum toxin in the Asian patient.[2]

The ideal classical Asian eye has long been described as being almond shaped, wider and rounder in the lateral canthal area.[2] Larger eyes are also thought to convey a sense of youthfulness and "cuteness." Requests for botulinum toxin to achieve this desired effect are common in East Asia.

24.2.3 Cultural Preferences

"Fairness camouflages a 100 flaws" is a Chinese saying highlighting the Asian obsession with pale, white, porcelain-like skin. While fairness is perceived as an aesthetically desirable trait in many cultures, nowhere else in the world is it pursued with such fervour. From topical treatments to skin resurfacing using chemical peels, lasers, and parenteral vitamin C, minimally invasive procedures aimed at reducing pigmentation and lightening skin tones are among the most popular procedures in Asia.

Specific facial features associated with femininity in Asia also include a small chin, an inverted egg-shaped small face, and a round, nonangular forehead (**Fig. 24.1**).[2] Requests for minimally invasive procedures for masseteric reduction using botulinum toxin or radiofrequency reduction are popular in Asia, while requests for forehead rounding and augmentation are also common.

Mild hypertrophy of the pretarsal orbicularis oculi is common in young Asian females, and traditionally this has been perceived as a sign of youthfulness and attractiveness. Termed *aegyo sal*, or the "lovely eye," in Korean, this appearance is created using fillers and fat grafting and is commonly requested by Asian patients (**Fig. 24.1**).[3]

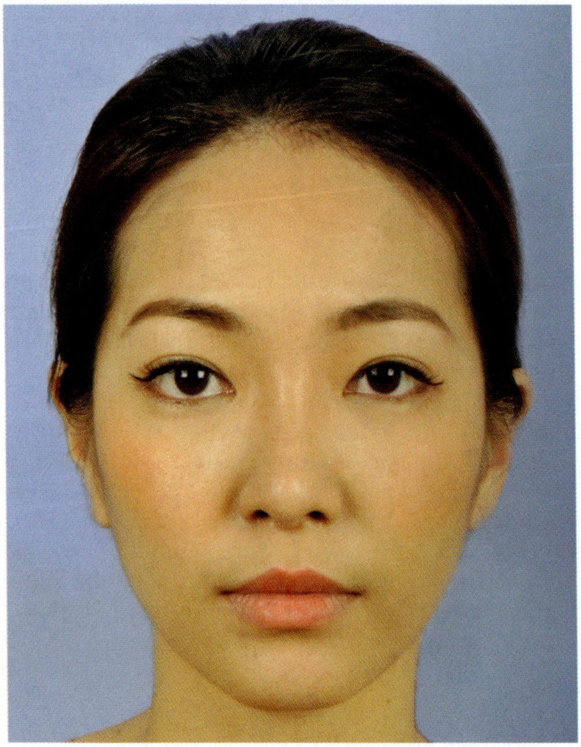

Fig. 24.1 Ideal East/Southeast Asian beauty. Picture of an aesthetically pleasing Asian woman. A fair complexion, oval face, rounded forehead, narrow mandibular width, small chin, large almond-shaped eyes, and mild hypertrophy of the pretarsal orbicularis oculi are considered attractive facial features. The Asian nose is significantly less projected and wider than in Caucasians.

24.3 Botulinum Toxin Injection

Botulinum toxin (Botox) injection is the most popular aesthetic procedure in Asia. Although the principles and techniques used are similar to those for Westerners, several important differences must be taken into account when injecting botulinum toxin in Asians.

24.3.1 Dose

Asians have significantly smaller facial mimetic muscles and being more reserved than their Western counterparts, show less facial expressivity. This means significantly reduced doses are needed when administering botulinum toxin in the Asian face (**Table 24.1**).[4]

Table 24.1 Recommended doses of botulinum toxin per site for Asian patients

Indication	Muscle	Dose (Botox units)
Glabellar frown lines	Procerus/corrugator	12
Forehead rhytids	Frontalis	12
Crow's feet	Obicularis oculi	6
Bunny lines	Nasalis	4–6
Smoker's lines	Obicularis oris	2–4
Cobbled chin	Mentalis	8
Platysma bands	Platysma	20

24.3.2 Widening of the Palpebral Fissure

A rounding of the lateral palpebral fissure can be achieved with the injection of 2 units of botulinum toxin intradermally, 3 mm below the ciliary margin, immediately lateral to the midpupillary line. Concomitant treatment of the lateral canthal region with an injection of 6 units of intradermal Botox, just lateral to the orbital margin, can further enhance this effect and result in 2 to 3 mm of palpebral fissure widening laterally.

Care must be taken to keep the injections within the dermis to avoid ocular complications. Patients who wish to retain a hypertrophic-looking pretarsal orbicularis oculi (see above: *aegyo sal*) should be advised against this procedure, as flattening of the pretarsal orbicularis oculi would result.

24.3.3 Masseteric Reduction

An excessively wide and square jaw is considered to be an unfeminine trait in Asian culture. The creation of the ideal inverted egg-shaped face can be achieved through the use of masseter muscle injection with botulinum toxin. A total of 30 units of botulinum toxin are used on each side, mainly targeting the superficial head of the masseter muscle in the inferior portion of the mandible.

Complications are rare. On occasion, an asymmetrical smile can result from diffusion of the toxin into the anterior risorius muscle. An injection placed too high under the arch can result in atrophy of the deep head, resulting in a wasted appearance. Some patients complain of a mild soreness in the jaws on mastication.[5]

24.3.4 Mesobotox

The practice of administering widely distributed, multiple intradermal injections of botulinum toxin into the face (commonly known as mesobotox, dermotoxin, or Botox lift) has been adopted in Asian aesthetic practice **(Fig. 24.2)**.[6]

Reported effects include reduction of dynamic facial lines, refinement of pore size, improvement of skin texture, and achievement of a "chemical face lift." The exact mechanism of action remains unclear, although dermal edema caused by underlying muscular paralysis and smooth muscle relaxation of the dermal vasculature are possible explanations. The lifting effects of mesobotox can be explained by the conventional mechanisms associated with botulinum toxin injection.

24.4 Filler Injections

As with trends in aesthetic procedures across the globe, minimally invasive procedures like filler injections are rapidly gaining popularity in Asia as well. In particular, filler injections are used not just for rejuvenating a volume-depleted face, but also for enhancement and augmentation in younger patients. In Asians, augmentations of the nose, chin, paranasal region, and jaw line are particularly popular, as these tend to be more deficient in Asians. While several of these applications are elaborated on in other chapters, a detailed description of filler rhinoplasty technique is included here.

24.4.1 Filler Rhinoplasty

One of the most popular procedures performed on Asians is augmentation rhinoplasty with fillers. Compared with surgical rhinoplasty, filler rhinoplasty has little down time, no donor-site morbidity, and results that are appreciated immediately.

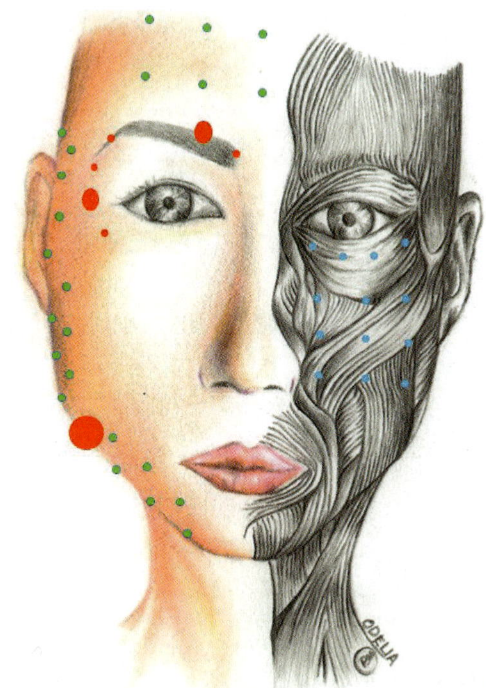

a

b

Symbol	Depth	Dose
●	IM	10
●	IM	3
•	IM	2
•	ID	0.4
•	ID	0.2

Fig. 24.2 **(a)** Sites and **(b)** doses for mesobotox injection. IM, intramuscular; ID, intradermal. All injections listed in Botox units.

The typical Asian patient has a flat and broad nasal dorsum and a poorly defined, bulbous tip with thick skin. The goals for augmentation rhinoplasty in Asians are to improve projection of the dorsum and tip, refine the tip, lengthen the nose, and modify the nasolabial angle.

24.4.2 Patient Selection

Patients who are suitable for injection rhinoplasty are those with a mild hump nose, a mildly deviated nose, a well-projected nasal tip with flat radix, or those with slight asymmetry (**Fig. 24.3**).

The patients who are less likely to achieve good results are those with a large hump, short contracted nose, bulbous tip, or severe deviation. Such patients are not expected to have good results, and one should counsel these patients that surgery may be more successful.

24.4.3 Technique

Injection rhinoplasty starts with injection of the columella, followed by the dorsum and tip.

24.4.4 Columella and Nasal Spine

Filling the area around the nasal spine has the effect of elevating the nasal tip and can alter an acute nasolabial angle to one that is more obtuse. After injecting the filler, check that it is not bulging laterally to obstruct the nasal passages, and mold it to the midline if necessary. Usually, ~ 0.5 mL of filler is used.

Injecting filler into the columellar space can correct a retracted columella. Usually, 0.2 to 0.3 mL of filler is used.

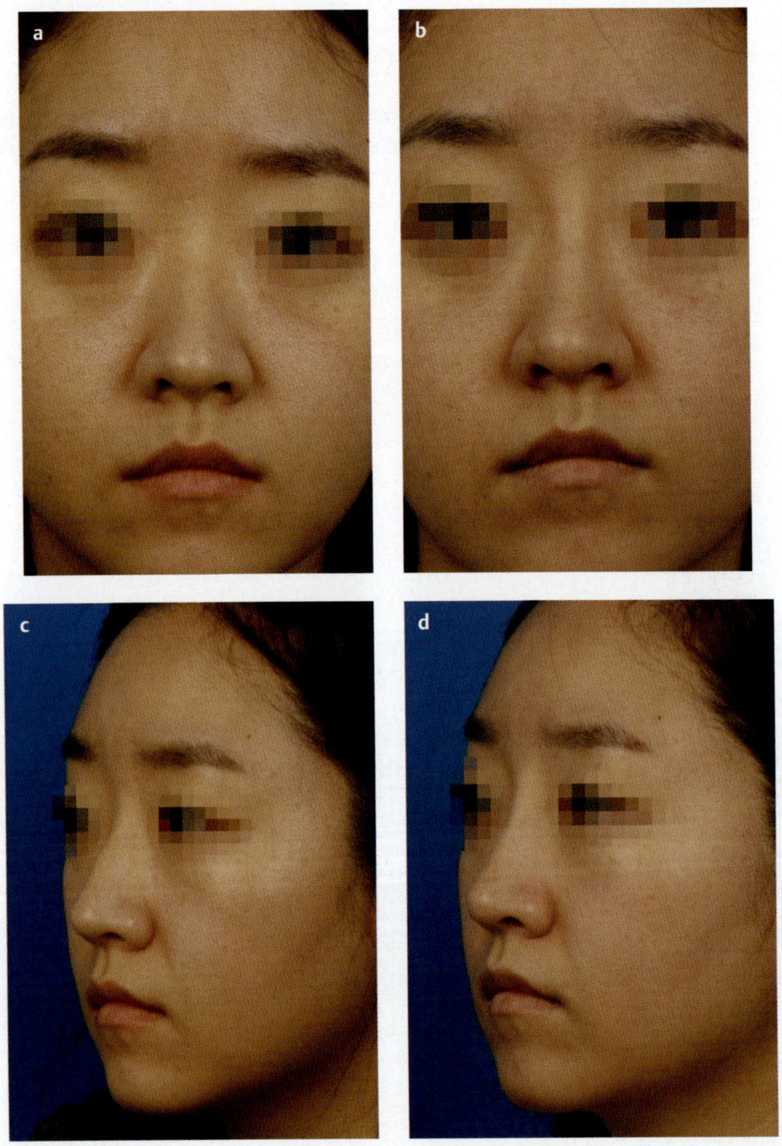

Fig. 24.3 Filler rhinoplasty results. Patient with an under-projected radix; the dorsal contour has been improved after filler injection. **(a)** Frontal view, before filler rhinoplasty. **(b)** Frontal view, after filler rhinoplasty. **(c)** Oblique view, before filler rhinoplasty. **(d)** Oblique view, after filler rhinoplasty.

24.4.5 Dorsum

The filler procedure for the nasal dorsum requires dividing the nose into four sections, i.e., the radix, rhinion, supratip, and tip. The radix and the supratip regions have thick soft tissue, and the underlying structure (bone and cartilage, respectively) is concave. Therefore, a relatively large filler volume has to be injected into these regions to avoid depressions at the nasion and the supratip due to pressure from the overlying soft tissue. The order of injection should be as follows: radix, rhinion, tip, and, finally, the supratip area. Major blood vessels and nerves of the external nose are located in the SMAS layer or the superficial fatty layer. Therefore, the ideal layer for filler injection is the deep fatty layer located between the SMAS and the perichondrium or periosteum, to minimize damage to the vessels or the nerves.

24.5 Fat Grafting

Fat grafting is a popular procedure in Asian patients who want to use autologous material and to achieve a more permanent result. It is a procedure familiar to surgeons practicing aesthetic facial surgery. The transplant of autologous fat has been reported for over a century. As with fillers, fat grafting can be done for rejuvenation or for enhancement of facial features.

The initial consultation should allow one to discern the patient's main concerns, such as reversal of aging-related changes or a desire for better proportions. History taking should include history of previous surgery, prior use of fillers, and sites of previous fat harvest or liposuction.

For Asians, the regions that are frequently grafted are the forehead, nasojugal fold, nasolabial fold, and the chin. Overall, Asians find an oval face to be aesthetically pleasing. However, Koreans prefer a larger forehead than the Japanese prefer, which may explain why forehead augmentation is more frequently performed in Koreans.[7]

24.5.1 Procedure

Fat is harvested using tumescent technique from the medial or lateral thighs with a 20 cm long cannula. There has been no evidence showing superiority of centrifuged fat or filtered fat; the senior author's preferred method is to centrifuge the harvested fat for 2 minutes at 3,000 rpm.

Structural fat grafting is then performed in the face using a 17 gauge cannula. An awl is used to create entry points that will allow even distribution of fat, and fat is injected using a combination of straight and curved cannulas to create the desired volume and contour. It is imperative that small deposits of fat are injected with each pass, as larger deposits result in a higher rate of resorption. The graft should also be deposited at multiple levels, not in a single tissue plane. The authors' usual practice is to overcorrect at the first treatment, in anticipation of fat resorption in the postoperative period.

Remaining fat that is not used at the first treatment is kept frozen at 4°C. The second treatment is usually scheduled ~ 6 weeks later. For the second treatment, the frozen fat is thawed gradually at room temperature.

24.5.2 Complications

In performing fillers and fat grafting for the face, complications like asymmetry, acne, and surface irregularities can occur. The most serious complication is arterial embolization, which can cause skin necrosis, or even blindness. The surgeon must be familiar with the anatomy and vascular supply of the face and must be knowledgeable about the danger zones, especially when injecting the glabella, nose (supratip), and nasolabial fold. The vessels that should be avoided are the supratrochlear, the dorsal and lateral nasal, and facial arteries.

24.6 Skin Resurfacing and Pigmentation

A plethora of devices are available for skin rejuvenation, and the ablative lasers are considered the gold standard. In this chapter, we discuss nonablative techniques, which are popularly used in aesthetic clinics throughout Asia, and we examine the evidence for, and effectiveness of, these different modalities. Due to Asians' greater tendency toward post-inflammatory hyperpigmentation, we advocate a graduated approach to skin rejuvenation, starting with radiofrequency and pulsed light technology before moving to more invasive methods, such as fractionated and ablative lasers.

24.6.1 Radiofrequency (RF) Devices

The use of RF for dermal tightening has been popular since the early 2000s; it is used for nonablative skin rejuvenation, atrophic scar revision, and treatment of hypertrophic scars and keloids.[8]

24.6.2 Mechanism of Action

The principle of RF in skin rejuvenation is using the tissues' natural resistance to the movement of electrons within the radiofrequency field (Ohm's law), resulting in the generation of thermal energy in the deep dermis. Repeated application of thermal energy results in the contraction and thickening of the collagen fibers. Temperatures of 57° to 75°C are ideal for collagen shrinkage.[9]

24.6.3 Evidence

In 2003, Fitzpatrick and colleagues published results of a multicenter clinical trial utilizing the first RF (monopolar) device (Thermage ThermaCool System, Thermage, Inc., Hayward, CA). In this study, 86 patients received a single treatment to the forehead and temple area. The study showed that 83.2% of the periorbital areas showed at least a 1-point improvement in Fitzpatrick wrinkle score, 14.3% showed no change, and 2.5% worsened. Photographic analysis showed improvement of eyebrow lift in 61.5% of patients.[10]

Koch and colleagues also noted that 60% of patients had significant brow elevation with one treatment, and 80% of patients showing significant elevation after four treatments.[11] Fritz and colleagues noted significant improvement in nasolabial folds, with best results being seen at 1 to 4 months.

24.6.4 Limitations and Side Effects

The selection of patients for RF facial rejuvenation is important. Best results are seen in patients with mild to moderate wrinkling and without excessive sagging skin. Main side effects were transient erythema and edema. Rarely, superficial burns, due to uneven electrode contact with the skin, and fat atrophy may occur.

24.6.5 Multimodality Treatments

In recent years, new modalities incorporating RF have been introduced. The combination of bipolar RF and optical energy is postulated to be synergistic, allowing each method to achieve the ideal skin temperature at lower energies, hence reducing discomfort and complications. An example is the Aurora SR system (Syneron, Inc., Yokneam, Israel), which is FDA-approved.

Fractional RF is a newer nonablative approach. Typically, a bipolar microneedle delivery system (ePrime system; Syneron Medical Ltd) is used, in which the skin in contact with the microneedles is heated while the adjacent areas are spared, contributing to accelerated wound healing.[12]

24.7 Platelet-Rich Plasma (PRP)

24.7.1 Mechanism of Action

The α-granules of activated concentrated platelets secrete growth factors, such as platelet-derived growth factor (PDGF), transforming growth factor (TGF), vascular endothelial growth factor (VEGF), and insulin-like growth factor (IGF).

PRP has the ability to stimulate wound healing and minimize bleeding, so it is widely used in many clinical situations, such as tendon injuries, facial skeletal defects, and chronic wounds, just to name a few.

24.7.2 Evidence

PRP use is extremely popular in Asian aesthetic practice, but high-quality studies attesting to its efficacy are scant. Kim et al conducted an in vitro study to determine the effects of PRP or platelet-poor plasma (PPP) on dermal fibroblasts.[13] Calcium chloride and thrombin were added to PRP or PPP to form activated PRP or PPP (aPRP or aPPP). The aPRP or aPPP mixture was then added to human-skin-derived dermal fibroblast cells in a Petri dish, and compared with the control. Both aPRP and aPPP stimulated an increase in fibroblast proliferation, procollagen type I carboxy-terminal peptide, and type I collagen in comparison to the control.

The use of PRP in combination with laser therapy has also been studied. Shin et al conducted a single-blinded randomized controlled trial to study the efficacy of combined PRP (topically applied) and fractional laser treatment or fractional laser treatment alone.[14] The group that received combination treatment had better self-reported satisfaction rates. They also found objective improvement in skin elasticity, a lower erythema index, and an increase in collagen density. However, the objective clinical assessment by two blinded reviewers showed no statistical difference between the two groups.

There have also been studies of the use of PRP combined with fractional ablative carbon dioxide laser for the treatment of atrophic acne scars in blinded, randomized, controlled split-face trials. Both studies found that there was significantly better clinical improvement on the side with combination treatment, with fewer side effects and faster recovery. There appeared to be no difference in terms of clinical improvement whether PRP was topically applied or administered intradermally (Gawdat).[15,16]

There has been only one study of the use of PRP as a single-modality skin treatment.[17] Most studies so far have only used it as an adjuvant therapy, after laser treatment or facial rejuvenation surgery. Nevertheless, the results have been promising, and certainly the use of PRP as single-modality treatment for facial rejuvenation should be investigated in the future (**Fig. 24.4**).

24.8 Radiofrequency for Reduction of the Masseters

When compared with botulinum toxin, radiofrequency (RF) ablation to reduce masseteric hypertrophy may be superior in terms of volume reduction and longevity.[18,19] RF ablation has been popularized among Asian surgeons

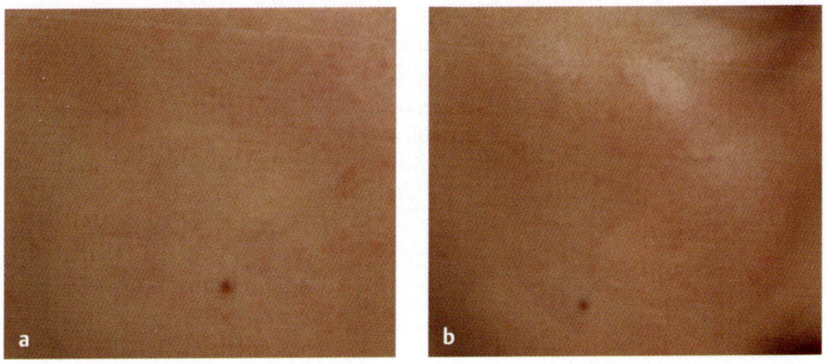

Fig. 24.4 Close-up view of skin in malar area **(a)** before and **(b)** after PRP treatment. The pore size has been reduced, the skin surface appears smoother, and skin texture has been improved.

in recent years, and limited studies suggest it has excellent safety and minimal morbidity. Rare but reported complications include transient masseteric edema and trismus, hematoma formation, injury to the facial nerve, and sialocele formation.

There is currently a lack of good scientific data on the exact anatomical sites for RF application and total energy required to achieve adequate volume reduction. The lack of RF probes specifically designed for this purpose is also of concern, with most authors using modified or custom-made probes introduced into the lower third of the masseter through an intraoral approach. However, more research into this promising new technique over the next few years will undoubtedly lead to widespread acceptance of this method as an alternative to botulinum toxin injection.

24.9 Conclusion

The choice and application of minimally invasive procedures in the Asian population are strongly influenced by cultural preferences and ethnic differences in anatomy and physiology. An appreciation of these differences is of paramount importance in achieving a satisfactory outcome when treating the Asian patient.

References

1. Rawlings AV. Ethnic skin types: are there differences in skin structure and function? Int J Cosmet Sci 2006;28(2):79–93
2. Sim RS, Smith JD, Chan AS. Comparison of the aesthetic facial proportions of southern Chinese and white women. Arch Facial Plast Surg 2000;2(2):113–120
3. Chen MC, Ma H, Liao WC. Anthropometry of pretarsal fullness and eyelids in oriental women. Aesthetic Plast Surg 2013;37(3):617–624
4. Ahn BK, Kim YS, Kim HJ, Rho NK, Kim HS. Consensus recommendations on the aesthetic usage of botulinum toxin type A in Asians. Dermatol Surg 2013;39(12):1843–1860
5. Xie Y, Zhou J, Li H, Cheng C, Herrler T, Li Q. Classification of masseter hypertrophy for tailored botulinum toxin type A treatment. Plast Reconstr Surg 2014;134(2):209e–218e
6. Seo KK. Clinical tips and recent advancements in cosmetic uses of botulinum toxin including mesobotox. J Korean Med Assoc 2000;48:1225–1232
7. Dobke M, Chung C, Takabe K. Facial aesthetic preferences among Asian women: are all Oriental Asians the same? Aesthetic Plast Surg 2006;30(3):342–347
8. Meshkinpour A, Ghasri P, Pope K, et al. Treatment of hypertrophic scars and keloids with a radiofrequency device: a study of collagen effects. Lasers Surg Med 2005;37(5):343–349
9. Sukal SA, Geronemus RG. Thermage: the nonablative radiofrequency for rejuvenation. Clin Dermatol 2008;26(6):602–607
10. Fritz M, Counters JT, Zelickson BD. Radiofrequency treatment for middle and lower face laxity. Arch Facial Plast Surg 2004;6(6):370–373
11. Koch RJ. Radiofrequency nonablative tissue tightening. Facial Plast Surg Clin North Am 2004;12(3):339–346, vi
12. Hruza G, Taub AF, Collier SL, Mulholland SR. Skin rejuvenation and wrinkle reduction using a fractional radiofrequency system. J Drugs Dermatol 2009;8(3):259–265
13. Kim DH, Je YJ, Kim CD, et al. Can platelet-rich plasma be used for skin rejuvenation? Evaluation of effects of platelet-rich plasma on human dermal fibroblast. Ann Dermatol 2011;23(4):424–431
14. Shin MK, Lee JH, Lee SJ, Kim NI. Platelet-rich plasma combined with fractional laser therapy for skin rejuvenation. Dermatol Surg 2012;38(4):623–630
15. Lee JW, Kim BJ, Kim MN, Mun SK. The efficacy of autologous platelet rich plasma combined with ablative carbon dioxide fractional resurfacing for acne scars: a simultaneous split-face trial. Dermatol Surg 2011;37(7):931–938

16. Gawdat HI, Hegazy RA, Fawzy MM, Fathy M. Autologous platelet rich plasma: topical versus intradermal after fractional ablative carbon dioxide laser treatment of atrophic acne scars. Dermatol Surg 2014;40(2):152–161
17. Nofal E, Helmy A, Nofal A, Alakad R, Nasr M. Platelet-rich plasma versus CROSS technique with 100% trichloroacetic acid versus combined skin needling and platelet rich plasma in the treatment of atrophic acne scars: a comparative study. Dermatol Surg 2014;40(8):864–873
18. Jin Park Y, Woo Jo Y, Bang SI, et al. Radiofrequency volumetric reduction for masseteric hypertrophy. Aesthetic Plast Surg 2007;31(1):42–52
19. Huang JL, Chen G, Chen XD, Zhou BR, Luo D. A comparative study of the efficacy and safety of radiofrequency ablation and botulinum toxin A in treating masseteric hypertrophy. Exp Ther Med 2014;7(5):1203–1208

Section V

The Mediterranean and Middle Eastern Perspective

25 Aesthetic, Ethnic, and Cultural Considerations and Current Cosmetic Trends in the Mediterranean and Middle East

Fazil Apaydin

25.1 Introduction

There are 32 countries bordering the Mediterranean Sea, in what is defined as the Middle East.[1,2] Throughout recorded history, there were always close trade relations among the people who lived in the area. There have also been continual migrations of populations, depending on the economic situation and living conditions; therefore, there is a great variety of ethnic groups in this part of the world. Due to globalization, the aesthetic trends in these countries are becoming similar to Western trends. However, there are still ethnic and cultural differences. The aim of this chapter is to discuss the trends within this population.

25.2 Facial Features and Aesthetic Considerations

The special difficulty among the populations in these regions is ethnical and cultural variability. Farkas et al[3] have done a very comprehensive study comparing anthropometric data from 25 countries across the world to norms established previously for North American whites (NAW).[4] They reported no significant difference between the people of European countries and NAWs. Therefore, the people living in the Euro-Mediterranean countries that were included in the study, namely Italy, Greece, Croatia, and Slovenia, showed anthropometric measurements similar to those of the NAW. These findings make sense because the ancestors of NAW were mainly from European countries. In the Farkas study, the forehead heights in Croatian males and Iranians were found to be significantly smaller. No significant differences in ear lengths were reported among the Caucasians and Middle Eastern groups (Turkey, Iran, and Egypt were included in the study). Mandibular width was extremely significantly increased in both sexes in Italians, male Turks, and Iranian females. In the Middle Eastern female groups, the three vertical measurements were identical with those in NAW in Turks only. In Iranian females, face height was found to be significantly greater, whereas both face height and lower face height were significantly smaller in Egyptian females. In Turkish males and females, bi-ocular width was significantly greater. In Iranians, the intercanthal width and eye fissure length were significantly smaller in both sexes, whereas the bi-ocular width in males was very significantly greater and in females extremely significantly smaller. Nose height was reported to be significantly greater in Greek females, in Iranians of both sexes, and in Turkish females.

The characteristics of the Middle Eastern nose have been reported as a dorsal hump, over-projected radix, thick skin, wide upper two-thirds, nasal deviation, poorly defined and under-projected tip, weak lower lateral cartilages, acute nasolabial angle, and nostril tip asymmetries.[5,6,7,8,9] In one study done in a Turkish population, the major reasons for seeking rhinoplasty were reported to be a crooked nose, obtuse nasofacial angle, and acute nasolabial angle.[10] Interestingly, the Arabic population was reported to seek rhinoplasty for similar reasons.[11,12] Palma et al went into detail about the Italian population, stating that their roots have been influenced by people from central and northern Europe, from Spain, the Middle East, and the Arab peninsula.[13] They described four achetypes of noses: drooping, strong and prominent, heavy, and the northern nose. Likewise, there is a "Black Sea nose" in Turkey, which is characterized by being very long, with a big hump and long columella.[14] People with the Black Sea nose live in the north of Turkey, and the world record of nasal length belongs to a man from this region.[15]

25.3 Current Cosmetic Trends

People living in in the Middle East and Mediterranean countries have always been very interested in beauty. The canons of beauty that are still in use today and the aesthetic concepts prevailing throughout history originated here as well. Following the trend of the development of injectables in the last two decades, the majority of Middle Eastern people seeking rejuvenation procedures are looking for less risky noninvasive modalities, and these modalities can help to establish a special bond between the doctor and the patient. Furthermore, most patients who accept surgical rejuvenation procedures are willing because of this special bond. Botulinum toxin A and hyaluronic acid fillers are currently the mainstay of rejuvenation for many people in the Middle East and Mediterranean countries (**Fig. 25.1**). The number of patients seeking surgical procedures has dropped tremendously within the last decade. Some reasons for the trend are: (1) The cost, safety, and longevity of injectable methods have become more reasonable. As the number of companies producing injectables increased,

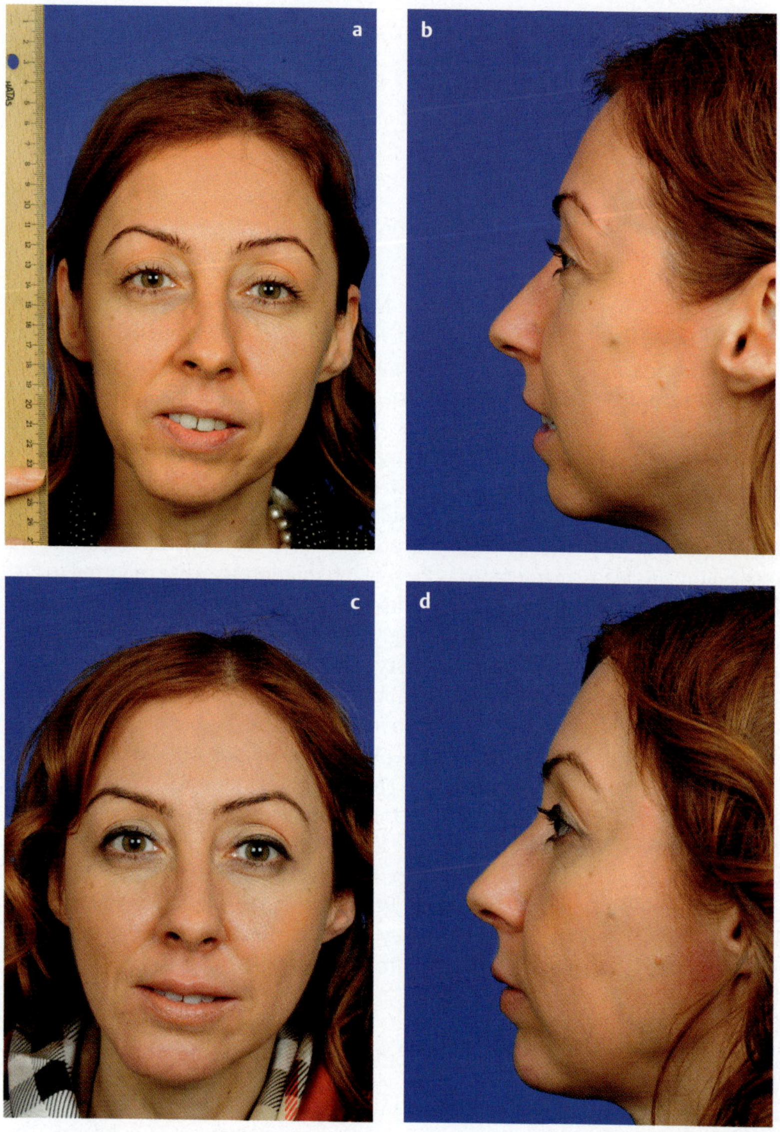

Fig. 25.1 (a,b) A 39-year-old woman with multiple asymmetries on the face and a small chin. In addition to septoplasty and nasal valve surgery, hyaluronic fillers have been injected into the corners of the mouth, chin, nasolabial sulcus, cheeks, and glabellar area. **(c,d)** Botulinum toxin A has been applied to glabella, forehead wrinkles, crow's feet, and upper lip to reduce gum-show during laughing.

competetion increased and costs decreased. (2) The specialties and the doctors applying these modalities increased in number as well. (3) There is no need for hospitalization and no need to take time off from work.

25.4 Surgical Procedures

In Turkey and in all the Middle East and Mediterranean countries, the number one operation in facial plastic surgery is still rhinoplasty, followed by blepharoplasty, and then lifting techniques, such as facelift, forehead lift, and midface lift.

25.4.1 Rhinoplasty

In all the Mediterranean and Middle Eastern countries, a dorsal hump is the main reason for rhinoplasty, and a droopy nasal tip is the second most common reason (**Fig. 25.2**). Most patients desire a smaller and upwardly rotated nose. A natural, nonoperated-looking nose is more popular in Euro-Mediterranean countries and in Turkey. However, in Iran and in many of the Arabic countries, patients want smaller, cute-looking noses. The author has been lecturing intensively in the Middle East and Mediterranean countries during the last decade and the data

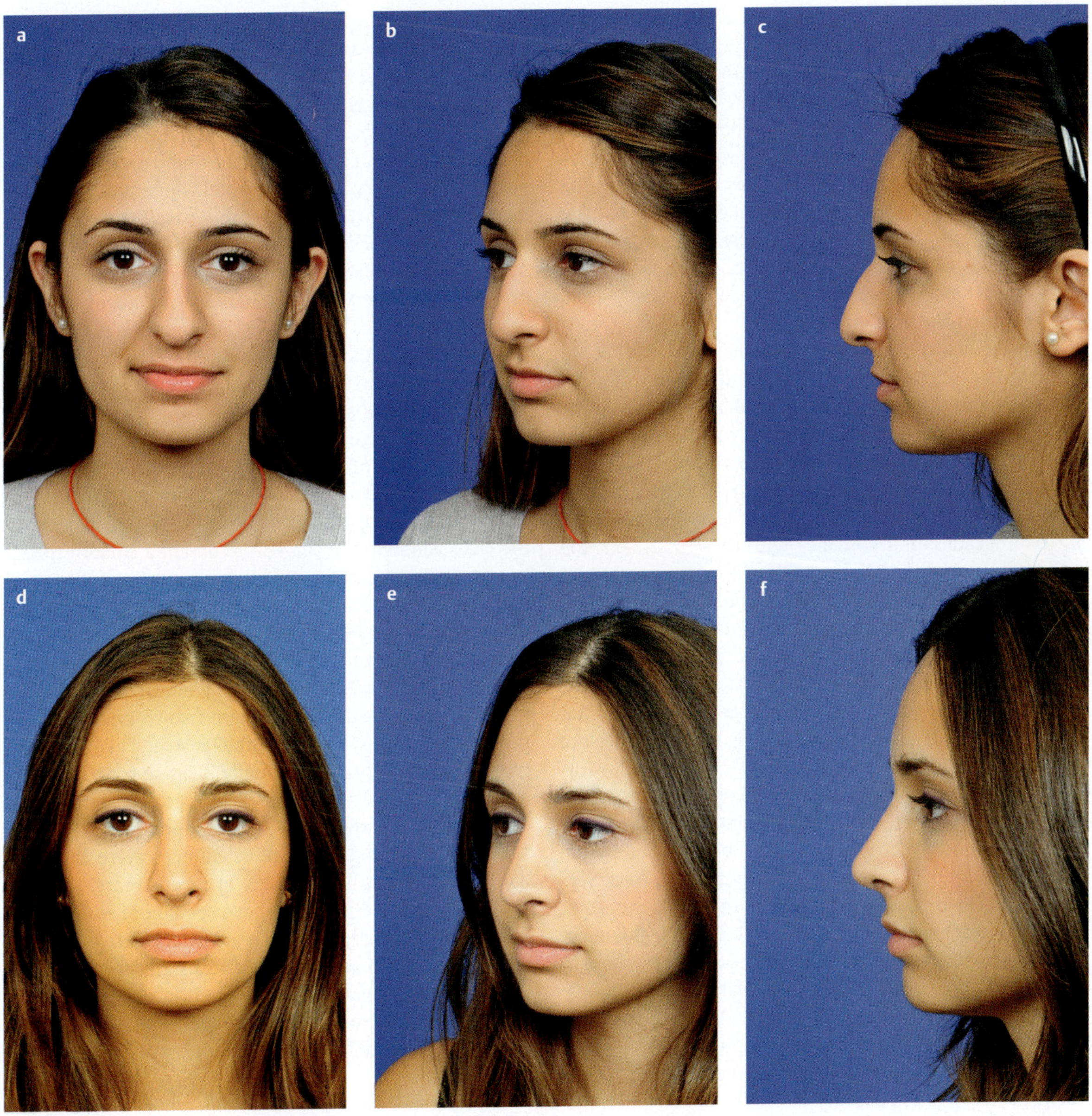

Fig. 25.2 **(a–c)** A typical Mediterranean woman at the age of 23 who underwent rhinoplasty due to dorsal hump and droopy and boxy nasal tip. Spreader flaps have been used after hump removal. Lateral crural steal, dome-equalizing sutures, transdomal sutures, and septo-columellar sutures have been utilized in addition to a columellar strut. **(d–f)** One can see the natural-looking nose with a straight dorsum and rotated tip. The skin was medium thick.

presented here are the result of extensive communication with prominent local surgeons during many meetings. In addition, in his critical analysis of 500 cases, Foda from Egypt reported the main reasons for revision rhinoplasty in the upper two-thirds of the nose as dorsal saddling, dorsal irregularities, valve collapse, open roof, and pollybeak deformities, and for the lower third as depressed tip, tip over-rotation, tip asymmetry, retracted columella, and alar notching.[16] Foda's study includes mostly patients from the Middle East, and it shows the patients' desire for smaller noses and that the complications resulted mostly from over-resection and over-rotation.

The external approach is more widely used within the last two decades in the Middle East and Mediterranean countries. The main reason is the ease of exposing all the structures without a distorted view, which helps a novice surgeon to understand rhinoplasty better. Besides, the majority of prominent practitioners of rhinoplasty from all over the world favored its use in their lectures within the last two decades. In accordance with these teachings, the external approach has been employed by the masters in Mediterranean and Middle Eastern countries extensively. Having said that, it should also be stated that there are still very reputable surgeons who always favored endonasal approaches as well. It can be said that the general opinion nowadays is that it is the result that matters, and that patients care more about a good-looking nose, regardless of the surgical approach.

In parallel with the high demand for rhinoplasty, there is a tremendous increase in the number of young rhinoplasty surgeons. According to an unpublished poll by the Turkish Society of Otorhinolaryngology, Head & Neck Surgery in 2013, the surgical procedure that residents most wanted to learn was rhinoplasty. In the author's opinion, the main reason for this trend is the successful implementation of rhinoplasty and other facial plastic surgery procedures in Turkey.

Tip sutures have become more popular than tip grafts within the last decade, although structural rhinoplasty surgeons still use grafts relatively often. The domal and transdomal sutures are the most popular suture techniques, followed by the septocolumellar suture. The columellar strut is used very often to support the tip in the external rhinoplasty approach **(Fig. 25.2)**. The use of shield grafts has gone out of favor within the last decade in comparison to the previous decade because of the likelihood for the graft to show in the long-term follow-up.[17,18,19]

It is also the author's observation that hump removal should be done differently in Middle Eastern countries. In Caucasians, it is said that a small hump should be left by taking the skin thickness variations into account.[20,21] Having followed this principle years ago in some patients, the author ended up with a residual hump in some cases. Therefore, I started dehumping the dorsum in a linear fashion both in males and females, which helped me to obtain more predictable results. The reason may be the difference in skin thickness and the different soft tissue response between the population groups.[19]

Before hump removal, the mucosa should be detached from the nasal septum and upper lateral cartilages to permit extramucosal resection. En bloc hump removal was the norm 10 years ago, whereas the detachment of the upper lateral cartilages (ULCs) from the nasal septum before hump removal has been more popular within the last decade. The middle vault reconstruction has been more seriously addressed with the widespread use of spreader grafts and spreader flaps as well.[22,23] Unless it is a crooked nose, spreader flaps are the author's first choice for a variety of reasons. First, the springiness of the ULCs is very effective in opening the internal valve angle. Second, no additional cartilage is needed to reconstruct the width needed, because turning in the ULCs supplies enough space to create brow–tip aesthetic lines and prevent an inverted-V deformity. Third, the continuation of the cephalic part of the ULCs can help the surgeon to obtain a smooth transition at the keystone area, although the surgeon might need some time to get used to the technique. In primary rhinoplasty, two types of turned-in flaps are used: spreader flaps and lateral crural turn-in flaps,[24] and the flaps help the surgeon to preserve the integrity of the internal and external valves as well. In addition to these two techniques, if the resected hump is used as a columellar strut, I like using this type of rhinoplasty as "minimally invasive functional rhinoplasty," because maximum effort is given to reconstruct the internal and external valves and support the tip.

For bony hump removal, osteotomes were the standard instrument a decade ago. In recent years, tungsten carbide rasps of various sizes have been more widely used. Rasps with coarse teeth are very efficient in removing big amounts of bone, whereas finer rasps are used to polish bony surfaces. In parallel with the advances in endoscopic sinus surgery, increasingly sophisticated powered instrumentation that can be used for rhinoplasty has been developed as well.[25,26,27]

Recurrent crooked nose is a potential complication. The main reason for this complication is failure to correct severe septal deviations. In severely deviated noses, segmental reconstruction[28] and subtotal reconstruction[29,30] techniques gained more popularity during the last decade against the extracorporeal technique.[31] In my opinion, the advances in the former techniques opened new horizons allowing surgeons to obtain more predictable results by simpler techniques. In traumatic or severe deviations, the author follows the principles of segmental nasal reconstruction during the primary surgery, where reconstruction is much easier than in revision cases. In primary cases, the bony septum is a valuable graft source. Straight pieces obtained from thin ethmoid or "thinned" vomer can be used for stenting the deviated dorsal and/or caudal segments of the cartilaginous septum.[32] In revision cases, conchal or costal cartilage may be needed for reconstruction.[28] A new and valuable technique is the oblique-split method, a technique that diminishes the risk of warping and allows the surgeon to obtain many cartilage grafts from the rib cartilage.[33]

Over-reduction of the hump is a major problem encountered in Middle Eastern patients. Unfortunately, this is mainly due to the surgeon's attempt to meet the patient's excessive demand. Therefore, a surgeon from the Middle East should learn to balance the patient's demands. In revision surgery for these patients, often the septal cartilage is not enough and additional cartilage from the ear and rib is needed. The Turkish delight technique for augmenting the nasal dorsum[34] has been repopularized by the use of temporalis fascia instead of Surgicel (Ethicon, Inc.).[35] This technique has become well accepted in Middle East in the last decade, and the author is fond of it as well. The author is content using slices obtained by the oblique-split technique for augmentation in addition to using them for reconstruction.[33]

The radix is very shallow in some patients with an osseocartilaginous hump. The radix does not have a predictable response when hump removal is undertaken; for one thing, it is covered by relatively thicker muscle, such as the procerus, and it has thicker skin. That may be why lowering the bony dorsum does not give a good soft tissue response. In a study done by Guyuron, if the intention is to lower the radix by 1 mm, 4 mm of bone should be removed, i.e., there is a 1:4 ratio.[36] That is why the surgeons should not be very obsessive with this zone and should explain the situation very carefully to patients.

In the more southern countries, such as Saudi Arabia, Iran, and Egypt, patients' thick skin is a big problem in rhinoplasty. Experienced surgeons in the region usually know not to resect more, but, on the contrary, resect less and support more. However, prominent surgeons still make aggressive resections in patients with thick skin. It is the surgeon's duty to warn all his patients with thick skin that an ideal result is not possible and to try to lower the patient's expectations. We should also inform patients that their skin will stay swollen longer than normal. Unfortunately, surgeons operating in southern countries encounter a majority of patients with thick skin. That is why they apply triamcinolone routinely in most cases.[37,38]

25.4.2 Aesthetic Surgery

Blepharoplasty

Upper blepharoplasty is a fairly straightforward procedure that is often sought by patients. Excision of skin and a small strip of muscle is the most popular method in Middle Eastern and Mediterranean countries. Fat removal is usually limited very selectively to the medial fat pocket. Trends in lower blepharoplasty have followed changes in other parts of the world. Instead of removing fat tissue from all the compartments, the tendency is now to go for fat preservation. My favorite technique nowadays is fat repositioning, which also helps to correct tear-trough deformity and lid-cheek depression in many cases (**Fig. 25.3**).[39,40,41]

Facelift

The majority of patients are usually frightened by the details of facelift because of potential complications. However, to get the best improvement, if they are well informed, they usually accept surgery. In recent years, there is a tendency for less invasive SMAS techniques[42] and short-scar facelifts,[43] rather than deep-plane procedures, because some long-term studies done by very experienced surgeons showed similar results in the long-term follow-up (**Fig. 25.3**).[44] In Turkey and surrounding countries, the tendency among surgeons is to use less-invasive procedures when doing facelifts, not only because of the recent scientific publications, but also because there is less risk of complications. Moreover, as happens in rhinoplasty, the patients do not care much about the technique used; they care about the result and less downtime from work.

Midface Lift

Midface lift is technically a challenging operation, and it has its potential risks of complications as well. Although it can be incuded in a traditional facelift by extending the incision to the temporal region and lifting the sagging tissues of the midface, endoscopic midface lift combined with endoscopic forehead lift[45] is more popular in Turkey and the Middle East and Mediterranean region. Having said that, midface rejuvenation has come to our attention more and more within the last decade due to advances in injectables and lipofilling.[46,47] The author has heard some prominent surgeons say during lectures that they favored injectables in this region, because surgery has its risks and difficulties.

Submentoplasty

The aging neck can be addressed alone or in combination with facelift techniques. More often, the latter is preferred. In mild cases, a simple liposuction[42] can be enough, whereas in severe sagging and fat accumulation, open removal of fat deposits and corset platysmaplasty give better results.[48,49] In Turkey, a heavy neck is not rare, and in these cases an aggressive approach to the neck together with facelift is offered to the patient. The author prefers the extended SMAS approach in these cases and usually combines it with direct fat removal and platysmaplasty.[50]

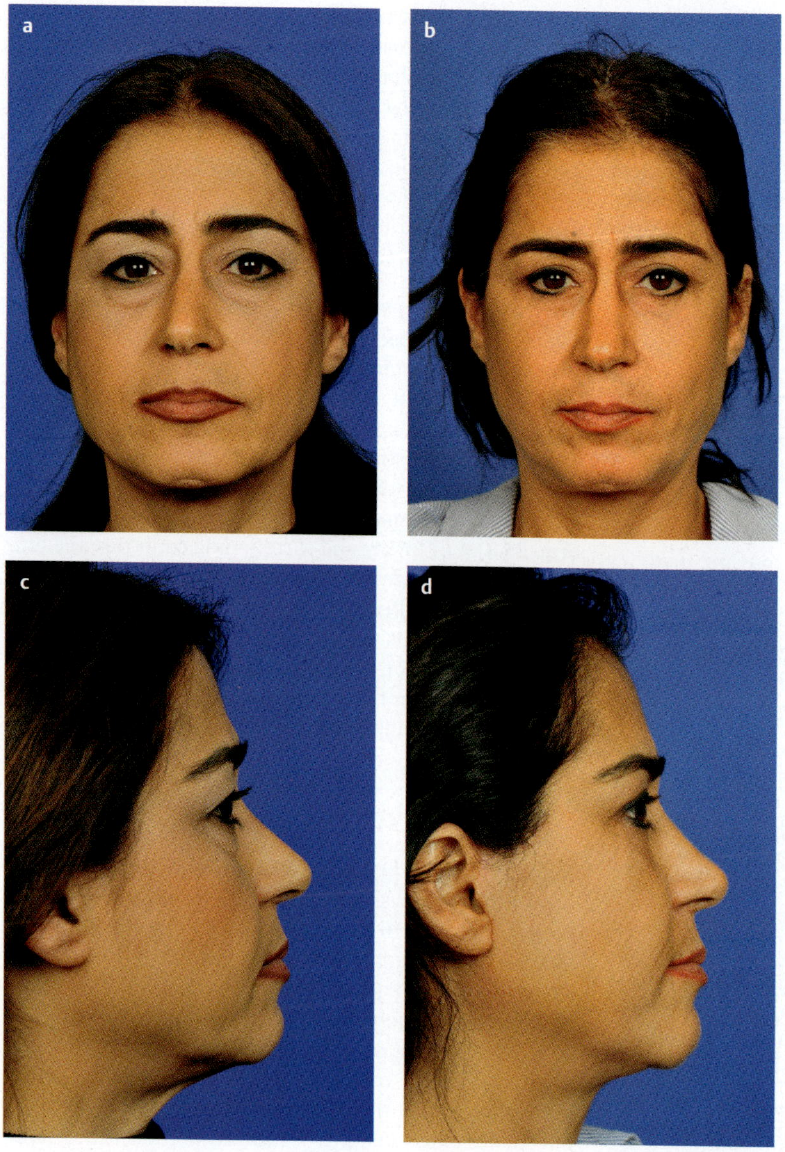

Fig. 25.3 **(a,c)** A 45-year-old woman who has a tired face and double contour due to herniation of the lower fat pads. She was also unhappy with her jowls and mild sagging of the neck. **(b,d)** She underwent blepharoplasty with fat repositioning on both sides. A short-scar facelift (MACS lift) was performed as well.

Forehead Lift

Forehead lift has been requested less often by patients within the last decade.[51,52] The main reason is the widespread use of botulinum toxin injections, which help to get rid of forehead wrinkles and to obtain browlift as well.[53] This is the trend in almost all of the Mediterranean and Middle Eastern countries. The author undertakes forehead lift usually together with endoscopic midface lift or upper blepharoplasty, and very rarely as a single procedure.

25.5 Final Recommendations and Conclusion

It should be remembered that there are 32 countries around the Mediterranean and in the Middle East. These countries have a variety of different ethnic groups with different cultural traditions as well. The facial plastic surgeon should try to learn the relevant facial characteristics and try to understand the traditions as well by visiting the countries and exchanging information with surgeons practicing there.

Facial aesthetic trends in Mediterranean and Middle Eastern countries are driven by the Western media, and patients often desire to look like the Western media icons. It should always be remembered that differences in facial proportions, variations in facial anatomy, and skin texture and thickness are the limiting factors in meeting patients' demands. The facts should be clearly expalined to patients before the application of any procedure.

25.6 Clinical Pearls

- Learn the geography, demographics, and history of the Mediterranean and Middle Eastern countries.
- Attend professional meetings organized in these countries.
- Learn the differences in facial features of people in this area.
- Do not perform aggressive resections in patients with thick skin.
- Patients in the Middle East tend to ask for smaller noses. The surgeon should educate patients about the facts and the limitations of surgery and should not attempt aggressive resections that can impair the airway and yield an unnatural result.
- During hump resection, the surgeon should end up with a straight osseocartilaginous dorsum in patients from Turkey and the Middle East.
- The principles of aesthetic nonsurgical and surgical procedures in patients from the Middle East are very similar to those for Western patients, whereas skin care can differ.

References

1. http://en.wikipedia.org/wiki/List_of_Middle_East_countries_by_population. Accessed August 20, 2014
2. http://geography.about.com/od/lists/a/Mediterranean-Countries.htm. Accessed August 20, 2014
3. Farkas LG, Katic MJ, Forrest CR, et al. International anthropometric study of facial morphology in various ethnic groups/races. J Craniofac Surg 2005;16(4):615–646
4. Farkas LG, ed. Anthropometry of the Head and Face. 2nd ed. New York, NY: Raven Press; 1994
5. Bizrah MB. Rhinoplasty for Middle Eastern patients. Facial Plast Surg Clin North Am 2002;10(4):381–396
6. Rohrich RJ. GhavamiA. The Middle Eastern nose. In: Gunter JP, Rohrich RJ, Adams WP, eds. Dallas Rhinoplasty: Nasal Surgery by the Masters. 2nd ed. St. Louis, MO: Quality Medical Publishing; 2007
7. Rohrich RJ, Ghavami A. Rhinoplasty for Middle Eastern noses. Plast Reconstr Surg 2009;123(4):1343–1354
8. Daniel RK. Middle Eastern rhinoplasty in the United States: Part I. Primary rhinoplasty. Plast Reconstr Surg 2009;124(5):1630–1639
9. Azizzadeh B, Mashkevich G. Middle Eastern rhinoplasty. Facial Plast Surg Clin North Am 2010;18(1):201–206
10. Gode S, Tiris FS, Akyildiz S, Apaydin F. Photogrammetric analysis of soft tissue facial profile in Turkish rhinoplasty population. Aesthetic Plast Surg 2011;35(6):1016–1021
11. Al-Qattan MM, Alsaeed AA, Al-Madani OK, Al-Amri NA, Al-Dahian NA. Anthropometry of the Saudi Arabian nose. J Craniofac Surg 2012;23(3):821–824
12. Boccieri A. The surgical approach to the Mediterranean nose. Facial Plast Surg 2010;26(2):119–130
13. Palma P, Bignami M, Delù G, De Bernardi F, Castelnuovo P. Rhinoplasty for the Mediterranean nose. Facial Plast Surg 2003;19(3):279–294
14. Tuncel U, Turan A, Kostakoğlu N. Digital anthropometric shape analysis of 110 rhinoplasty patients in the Black Sea Region in Turkey. J Craniomaxillofac Surg 2013;41(2): 98–102
15. http://www.guinnessworldrecords.com/longest-nose-on-a-living-person/. Accessed August 23, 2014
16. Foda HM. External rhinoplasty: a critical analysis of 500 cases. J Laryngol Otol 2003;117(6):473–477
17. Tardy ME Jr, Patt BS, Walter MA. Transdomal suture refinement of the nasal tip: long-term outcomes. Facial Plast Surg 1993;9(4):275–284
18. Toriumi DM. New concepts in nasal tip contouring. Arch Facial Plast Surg 2006;8(3):156–185
19. Apaydin F. Rhinoplasty in the Middle Eastern nose. Facial Plast Surg Clin North Am 2014;22(3):349–355
20. Toriumi DM, Becker DO. Rhinoplasty Dissection Manual. Philadelphia, PA: Lippincott; 1999
21. Rohrich RJ, Muzaffar AR, Janis JE. Component dorsal hump reduction: the importance of maintaining dorsal aesthetic lines in rhinoplasty. Plast Reconstr Surg 2004;114(5):1298–1308, discussion 1309–1312
22. Sheen JH. Spreader graft: a method of reconstructing the roof of the middle nasal vault following rhinoplasty. Plast Reconstr Surg 1984;73(2):230–239
23. Byrd HS, Meade RA, Gonyon DL Jr. Using the auto-spreader flap in primary rhinoplasty. Plast Reconstr Surg 2007;119(6):1897–1902
24. Apaydin F. Lateral crural turn-in flap in functional rhinoplasty. Arch Facial Plast Surg 2012;14(2):93–96
25. Davis RE, Raval J. Powered instrumentation for nasal bone reduction: advantages and indications. Arch Facial Plast Surg 2003;5(5):384–391
26. Avşar Y. Nasal hump reduction with powered micro saw osteotomy. Aesthet Surg J 2009;29(1):6–11
27. Avsar Y. The oscillating micro-saw: a safe and pliable instrument for transverse osteotomy in rhinoplasty. Aesthet Surg J 2012;32(6):700–708
28. Apaydin F. Segmental reconstruction for nasal septal deviation. Facial Plast Surg 2013;29(6):455–463
29. Toriumi DM. Subtotal reconstruction of the nasal septum: a preliminary report. Laryngoscope 1994;104(7): 906–913
30. Toriumi DM. Subtotal septal reconstruction: an update. Facial Plast Surg 2013;29(6):492–501

31. Gubisch W. The extracorporeal septum plasty: a technique to correct difficult nasal deformities. Plast Reconstr Surg 1995;95(4):672–682
32. Apaydin F. Bone recycling in nasal septal reconstruction. Facial Plast Surg 2013;29(6):473–478
33. Taştan E, Yücel ÖT, Aydin E, Aydoğan F, Beriat K, Ulusoy MG. The oblique split method: a novel technique for carving costal cartilage grafts. JAMA Facial Plast Surg 2013;15(3):198–203
34. Erol OO. The Turkish delight: a pliable graft for rhinoplasty. Plast Reconstr Surg 2000;105(6):2229–2241, discussion 2242–2243
35. Daniel RK, Calvert JW. Diced cartilage grafts in rhinoplasty surgery. Plast Reconstr Surg 2004;113(7):2156–2171
36. Guyuron B. Precision rhinoplasty. Part II: Prediction. Plast Reconstr Surg 1988;81(4):500–505
37. Hanasono MM, Kridel RW, Pastorek NJ, Glasgold MJ, Koch RJ. Correction of the soft tissue pollybeak using triamcinolone injection. Arch Facial Plast Surg 2002;4(1):26–30, discussion 31
38. Guyuron B, DeLuca L, Lash R. Supratip deformity: a closer look. Plast Reconstr Surg 2000;105(3):1140–1151, discussion 1152–1153
39. Hamra ST. The role of orbital fat preservation in facial aesthetic surgery. A new concept. Clin Plast Surg 1996;23(1):17–28
40. Goldberg RA, Edelstein C, Shorr N. Fat repositioning in lower blepharoplasty to maintain infraorbital rim contour. Facial Plast Surg 1999;15(3):225–229
41. Baker SR. Orbital fat preservation in lower-lid blepharoplasty. Arch Facial Plast Surg 1999;1(1):33–37
42. Tardy ME, Thomas JR, Brown RJ. Facial Aesthetic Surgery. St. Louis, MO: Mosby; 1995
43. Tonnard P, Verpaele A, Monstrey S, et al. Minimal access cranial suspension lift: a modified S-lift. Plast Reconstr Surg 2002;109(6):2074–2086
44. Alpert BS, Baker DC, Hamra ST, Owsley JQ, Ramirez O. Identical twin face lifts with differing techniques: a 10-year follow-up. Plast Reconstr Surg 2009;123(3): 1025–1033, discussion 1034–1036
45. Quatela VC, Jacono AA. The extended centrolateral endoscopic midface lift. Facial Plast Surg 2003;19(2): 199–208
46. Verpaele A, Strand A. Restylane SubQ, a non-animal stabilized hyaluronic acid gel for soft tissue augmentation of the mid- and lower face. Aesthet Surg J 2006;26(1S): S10–S17
47. Meier JD, Glasgold RA, Glasgold MJ. Autologous fat grafting: long-term evidence of its efficacy in midfacial rejuvenation. Arch Facial Plast Surg 2009;11(1):24–28
48. Feldman JJ. Neck Lift. St Louis, MO: Quality Medical Publishing; 2006
49. Feldman JJ. Corset platysmaplasty. Plast Reconstr Surg 1990;85(3):333–343
50. Perkins SW, Waters HH. The extended SMAS approach to neck rejuvenation. Facial Plast Surg Clin North Am 2014;22(2):253–268
51. Ramirez OM. Endoscopic subperiosteal browlift and facelift. Clin Plast Surg 1995;22(4):639–660
52. Villano ME, Leake DS, Jacono AD, Quatela VC. Effects of endoscopic forehead/midface-lift on lower eyelid tension. Arch Facial Plast Surg 2005;7(4):227–230
53. Maas CS, Kim EJ. Temporal brow lift using botulinum toxin A: an update. Plast Reconstr Surg 2003;112(5, Suppl):109S–112S, discussion 113S–114S

26 Rhinoplasty in Mediterranean Patients

Pietro Palma and Iman Khodaei

26.1 Introduction

In recent years, "ethnic beauty" has become a hot topic in facial plastic surgery,[1,2,3,4,5,6,7,8,9] but most of the information about ethnic facial plastic surgery in books, articles, and conference presentations should be assessed carefully by rhinoplasty surgeons, because maintenance of ethnic facial features is a highly complex problem.

In the authors' view, ethnic rhinoplasty is more an issue for article writers than a real concern of patients requesting rhinoplasty. Concepts of beauty are shared across the globe,[10] and facial aesthetic values are becoming global and more uniform with time.[11] This is probably related to the dissemination of the "ideal look" by trend-setters in the fashion and entertainment industries. The authors' practice proves that patients, especially younger patients, ask for changes that will make them look like images they see in glossy magazines and on the Internet. Their desires are less linked to maintaining ethnic features than to looking like their idols in fashion, sports, music, and the movies.

Aesthetic trends are also influenced by marketing changes worldwide. For instance, it is now rare to see the diamond-shaped nasal tip[12] on models depicted in advertisements for perfumes, jewels, or glasses. On the contrary, it has become more and more common to see models with softer tip contours (the smooth single tip[13]), probably because of the changing demography of consumers. The most quickly growing market is in Asian countries, and the diamond-shaped tip is not a common feature of Asian noses.

However, in certain parts of the world, a desire to maintain local characteristics has taken root. Much of the reaction against creating Western noses in the East is a political issue. Examples of this can be seen in India and the Middle East, where patients simply request a better profile and less exuberant ethnic characteristics. In contrast, in Japan, the demand for augmentation rhinoplasty and blepharoplasty to look more American arose after the World War II. This may be interpreted as an attempt to blend in with the dominant Western culture.

In other places, strong ethnic features are the rule, as among the Aborigines of Australia, the people of West Africa, and the Indians of South America, for example. Here, the ethnic nose really comes into its own light. In these cases, the surgeon must ensure that ethnic features are maintained. A small nose on a face of Aztec origin would look out of place.

So, there are good reasons for believing that rhinoplasty surgeons are facing a dramatic change in the demography of their patients, and that change requires a serious rethinking of patient selection and the choice of the techniques to be used in an individual rhinoplasty patient.

26.2 Overview of the Mediterranean Nose

The definition of what an "average" Mediterranean nose should look like is not easy.[14,15] Since ancient times, large numbers of people have moved from Europe to Asia, and in the opposite direction as well, so that in any southern Mediterranean country, it is common to see examples of Semitic noses, Oriental noses, Roman noses, and noses with Slavic features.

Therefore, the idea of an ethnic nose may not be applicable in Mediterranean countries, the Near East, and the Middle East. It is now completely ordinary to find people in Mediterranean countries who have features from many different races. Furthermore, current migration flows will inevitably result in more complex mixed-race presentations in the future.

With the rise of facial aesthetic surgery, and rhinoplasty in particular, it has become apparent that a single formula for beauty cannot be applied in all regions of the world. Each area has its own particular characteristics that must be defined and described with anthropometric measurements or photographic analysis. The wishes of the individual patient and the ramifications of aesthetic principles from one side of the globe to the other must also be considered.[16,17] In this regard, the Mediterranean nose poses unique challenges for the surgeon. From ancient times, Mediterranean countries have experienced mass migrations, and exchange of people between Europe, North Africa, and the Near East. This has led to certain unique nasal characteristics, such as a prominent profile, ptotic or broad tip, and thick skin in the lower nasal third.[18,19] Specifically, in Mediterranean noses, the thicker than ideal skin on the tip, absolute or relative dorsal hyperprojection, tip malposition, and presence of weak lower lateral cartilages (LLCs) have posed a significant challenge to rhinoplasty surgeons over the past 30 years.

26.3 Peculiarities–Nature of the Problem

Three clinical situations frequently encountered in the senior author's (PP) rhinoplasty practice have been chosen as the most paradigmatic challenges of the Mediterranean nose. The three situations have in common forward over-projection of the cartilaginous septum, so they can be grouped under the definition of tension nose. In essence, a tension nose is the result of an over-projection of the middle third of the nose so that it looks too massive for that particular individual's nasal and facial proportions. While this is somewhat true, as surgeons we need to define the clinical presentation, the factors that contribute to nasal size, and specific surgical options.

The common denominator is an over-projection of the cartilaginous pyramid, i.e., from the anterior septal angle to the point of maximal dorsal projection. This condition leads to some secondary changes that have different expressions from patient to patient, such as stretching of the soft tissue envelope, narrowing of the internal valve, apparently malpositioned LLCs, thin and weak alar walls, and slit-like openings of the external nostrils. These findings are often accompanied by an over-projection of the anteroinferior nasal spine and hyperactivity of the depressor septi nasi muscle.

There may also be an associated nasal valvular dysfunction due to narrowing of the the internal valve angle and the distortion of the upper lateral cartilages (ULCs) and LLCs.[20,21]

In a nose where the LLCs are disproportionately large and/or malpositioned, but the septum is moderately sized, the term *tension nose* is inappropriate.

The authors classify tension nose into various types, depending on the surface landmarks: nasion, anterior septal angle, pronasale in static and dynamic conditions, alar rim configuration, and subnasale. However, it is important to realize that these three categories may be found in various combinations with each other.

Of course, individual special features are to be taken into account and should be specifically addressed both in formulating the surgical plan and in performing surgery.

26.3.1 Type A

The type A tension nose is characterized by a prominent, often cephalically positioned nasion; over-projection of the three arches of the nasal pyramid (bony vault, cartilaginous vault, tip); a prominent nasal spine; a crowded columella-lip junction; an obtuse columellar-labial angle; and tip animation **(Fig. 26.1)**.

26.3.2 Type B

In the type B tension nose, the relevant anomalies are over-projection of the cartilaginous framework that may or may not be associated with over-projection of the bony vault; relative/absolute under-projection of the nasal tip and/or under-rotation of the nasal tip; straight or acute columellar-labial angle; and tip animation **(Fig. 26.2)**.

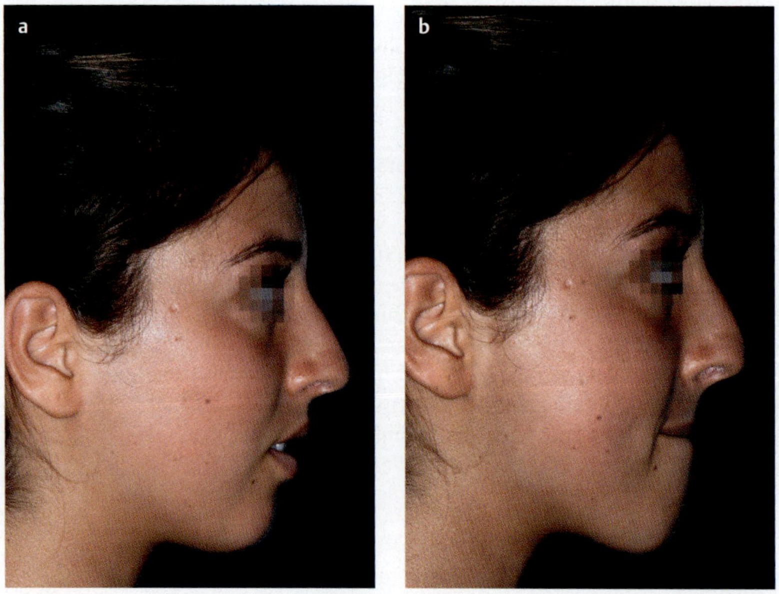

Fig. 26.1 (a,b) Type A tension nose. Type A is characterized by a prominent, often cephalically positioned nasion; over-projection of the three arches of the nasal pyramid (bony vault, cartilaginous vault, tip); prominent nasal spine; crowded columella-lip junction; obtuse columellar-labial angle; and tip animation.

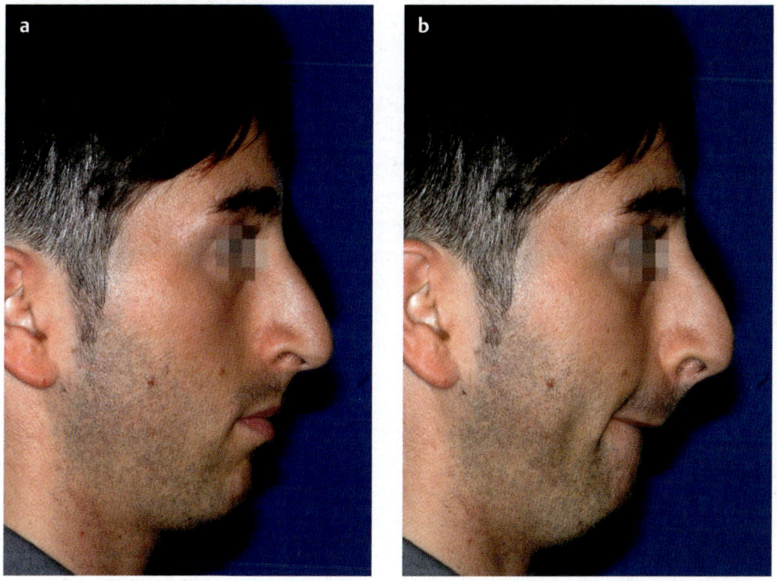

Fig. 26.2 **(a,b)** Type B tension nose. The relevant anomalies are over-projection of the cartilaginous framework that may or may not be associated with over-projection of the bony vault, relative/absolute under-projection of the nasal tip and/or under-rotation of the nasal tip, straight or acute columellar-labial angle, and tip animation.

26.3.3 Type C

The type C tension nose presents with a deep and caudal nasion, causing a low radix appearance; under-projection of the upper part of the bony vault; over-projection of the cartilaginous vault; under-projection and/or under-rotation of the nasal tip; straight/acute columellar-labial angle; and tip animation. It is the paradigmatic "pseudo-hump" trap **(Fig. 26.3)**.

The three different clinical types require distinct surgical options.

26.4 Preoperative Analysis

26.4.1 Clinical Assessment

The main presenting feature is a nose that is too large for the patient's face. This is immediately obvious as the patient walks into the consultation room.

Patients with this condition often reveal a state of profound psychological distress, because they have been the object of negative remarks from their peers. Their distress is a strong motivating factor in their quest for rhinoplasty.

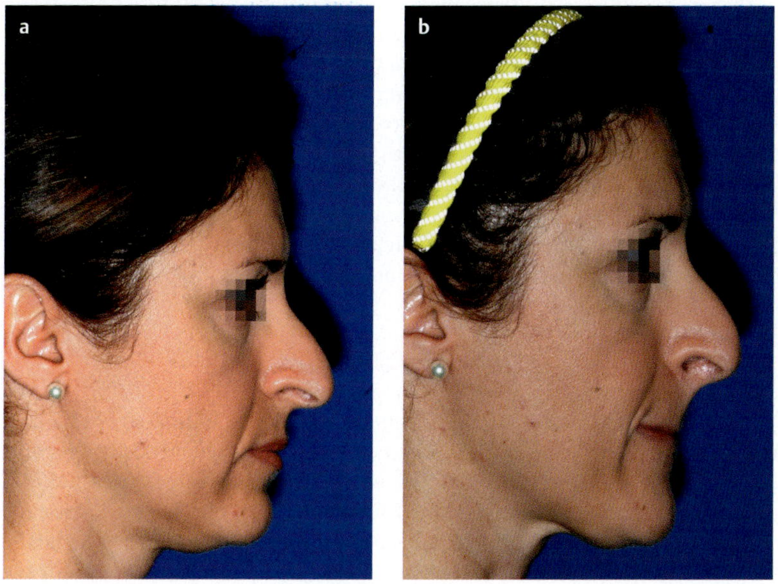

Fig. 26.3 **(a,b)** Type C tension nose. Type C presents a deep and caudal nasion, causing a low radix appearance, under-projection of the upper part of the bony vault, over-projection of the cartilaginous vault, under-projection and/or under-rotation of the nasal tip, straight/acute columellar-labial angle, and tip animation. Type C tension nose is the paradigmatic pseudo-hump.

Improvement of the physical appearance of the nose is more important to these patients than improvement of function when the two challenges coexist in the same individual.[22,23,24] It is of paramount importance to establish exactly what the patient wants in terms of cosmetic and functional improvement and to address the issue of the balance between functional improvement and aesthetic appearance. In the authors' experience, this is a critical aspect for clarification as early as possible in the surgeon–patient interaction. In a significant number of cases, grafting procedures are indicated for functional purposes that may ultimately result in widening of the midnose and/or alar sidewalls. In the authors' patient population, a significantly large number of individuals, especially women, dislike the "swollen" appearance of the inferior nasal two-thirds, and often reject the option of structural, supporting grafts in these critical areas despite the beneficial functional result. These considerations should be clearly reviewed during the second meeting with the patient, and they must reported in detail on the consent form.

26.4.2 Inspection

Systematic examination of the nose is designed to glean as much information as possible in a relatively short period. The authors begin by sitting in front of the patient and assessing the brow–dome lines (BDLs),[25,26] and then analyze the light/shade interplay on both the midline of the patient's nose and at the nose-cheek junction. Ideally, a central area of light reflection, with a light–shadow border on each side, is visible. The two borders are the actual BDLs. Lateral to each BDL, there will be an area of shadow on the nasal sidewall up to the transition to the periorbital/cheek area.

The alar–columellar relationship (ACR), which is sometimes described as a gull in flight, depends on the size and orientation of the LLCs, caudal septum position and length, conformation of the middle crura, and position/size of the nasal spine. In a tension nose, the LLCs are often distorted due to the large septum pushing them through a posterolateral vector. This may create the illusion that the altered LLC configuration represents a major deformity of the tip, rather than being a consequence of the protruding septum. It is the authors' policy to execute a significant primary septoplasty that will alleviate LLC distortion, and then to plan specific surgery on the tip cartilages. After proper septal surgery, the "real" over-projection of the dorsum will become immediately obvious from the lateral viewpoint. Often, the lateral view of the face will also reveal the effects of an overly active depressor nasi septi muscle when the patient smiles: the upper lip will shorten and the tip may de-rotate. The nose should always be carefully inspected for signs of previous surgery, such as a columellar or alar base scar, as some tension nose patients have already had surgery but are not fully satisfied with the results.

The second step is to observe the patient during quiet respiration with the mouth closed, and to watch for evidence of collapse of the lateral walls of the cartilaginous pyramid. The next step is the forced inspiration test, in which the patient is asked to obstruct each nostril gently and to breathe only through the unobstructed side. This forces a larger amount of air displacement through the region of the external valve and makes its dysfunction more obvious. Lifting the cheek laterally can improve the airflow, which is known as a positive Cottle sign. The surgical implications of a positive Cottle sign are generally overestimated, because the sign does not provide a clear indication of the anatomical site of dynamic obstruction. On the contrary, the curette wax test is much more specific in defining the location of collapsible areas: a curette wax is introduced inside the mid-lower nose and gently pushed outward when the patient inspires. The patient will precisely indicate the epicenter(s) of collapsibility located where the outward pulls ameliorate significantly breathing performance.[27] This test is routinely repeated immediately before surgery, and the areas of major collapsibility are carefully traced on the external skin with a marking pen. These areas will need structural support.

26.4.3 Palpation

Palpation of the nose is extremely important, because rhinoplasty is mainly a tactile form of surgery. The surgeon must manually assess the quality and thickness of the skin–soft tissue envelope (S-STE); the size, firmness, and orientation of both ULCs and LLCs; position, configuration, and tensile strength of the caudal septum as well its relation to the membranous septum and nasal spine. Then the surgeon should gently press on the nasal tip and release the pressure while looking at, and feeling the response of, the tissues under his/her finger. This tip recoil test differs greatly depending on the type of tension nose: type A will not show a weakness or delay in response, whereas type C will have a weak and delayed reaction.

In these patients, the nasal spine has to be systematically evaluated. Usually, the spine can be palpated with the ventral aspect of the examiner's thumb as it makes its way to the base of the columella. When the spine is large, it may even reach halfway up the columella. This fact needs to be noted for surgical planning.

26.4.4 Nasendoscopy

All rhinoplasty patients need to be examined with a nasendoscope prior to surgery. There are several good reasons for this policy: rhinosinusitis is a prevalent disease that is regularly seen in ENT clinics; signs of coincidental disease, such as early nasal polyposis or past surgery, should not be missed; and the angle of the internal valve may have already been altered by trauma or distorted by an overly large septum. Specific attention should be paid to the cicatricial sequelae of past surgery: webbing, circumferential stenosis along the contour of the internal nasal valve, and quality of scarring at the level of previous vestibular incisions must be systematically sought and reported on the preoperative worksheet. Finally, endoscopy provides the surgeon with vital photodocumentation that helps in assessment of the effects of surgery postoperatively. Photodocumentation is now readily available through adaptors for smartphones and it should be made part of the patient's notes.

26.4.5 Facial Photography

There are many fine texts on the subject of taking photographs; however, obtaining consistently excellent photographs requires skill, patience, practice, and a systematic approach. The authors take photographs in the following sequence because the analysis leads to surgically relevant conclusions: frontal static, frontal dynamic (patient smiles), base-radix, base, lateral static, lateral dynamic (patient smiles), second lateral dynamic to show the prominence of the anterior angle (patient pulls the upper lip downward), three-quarter views from each side, and helicopter views.

26.5 Surgical Solutions

The wealth of information provided by the first consultation, examination, and photography is used to analyze the situation and to create a plan for surgery. Photographic analysis concentrates on surgically relevant and useful landmarks (measuring every single possible angle and line is neither productive nor helpful). Each patient has cultural considerations that need to be recognized when undertaking the facial analysis. Therefore, facial analysis needs to be patient specific and culturally relevant. Computer-assisted simulations are created that combine the result of facial analysis with the patient's desires. The patient is duly informed that simulations are not exactly predictive of the result, but instead suggest the possibilities. The main goal of the simulations is to create an individualized operative plan.

The findings of the photo-analysis and the simulations are discussed with the patient in a compulsory second consultation. Performing rhinoplasty based on a single preoperative meeting is a recipe for disaster. Once the surgical goals have been agreed upon, the operation can go ahead.

The patient's photographs, facial analysis results, and surgical plan are taken into the operating room. While the main aims of surgery, de-projection, reestablishing surface aesthetics, and possible increased rotation, may also be achieved by an external approach,[28] the authors manage the tension nose endonasally.[29]

Treatment of a tension nose depends on adequate preoperative diagnosis of the factors that create the impression of a large nose. Clinical and photographic assessment will clearly identify the culprit and will direct the specific surgical plan toward the main causes of the problem. Septoplasty is the key to a successful outcome, but it needs to be done in a stepwise manner. The refashioned septum needs to support the tip, to project onto the midline of the two parallel brow–dome lines, and to recreate a proportionate alar-columellar relationship.

Whenever possible, the unity of the septolateral cartilage is maintained, and the extramucosal approach[30] represents the workhorse for managing the cartilaginous vault. Hump removal is executed sequentially, first cartilage and then bone, but in one piece as it guarantees a smooth transition at the rhinion area. Because the majority of noses undergoing rhinoplasty are asymmetric, osteotomies should reflect this fact.

The approach to the tip needs to be flexible, to accommodate the specific anatomy and the patient's desires. For the majority of patients, the endonasal "extended" transcartilagenous approach is used. When complete visualization of the cartilaginous skeleton of the tip is needed, the authors resort to infracartilaginous, transvestibular, or delivery approaches, depending on the techniques to be used. A variety of sutures can be used in the different approaches.

Grafts are utilized judiciously. In most cases, their use is aimed at creating surface aesthetic lines and softening contours. Sometimes they are employed to regain structural firmness.

The tension nose is an opportunity for the use of endonasal hybrid rhinoplasty (EHR).[31] EHR refers to the combination of the best of both worlds: the lessons learnt from the external approach, mainly grafting procedures and suturing techniques, are combined with the philosophy of minimal tissue damage of endonasal surgery to create an alternative third path for rhinoplasty.

After administration of general anesthesia, the patient is draped, and the head of the bed is elevated by 30 degrees to decrease venous pressure in the face. Use of local anesthesia with epinephrine is limited to the infraorbital nerve, osteotomy lines, caudal septum, and premaxillary region. Distortion of the tip and dorsum by injection is undesirable. Use of bipolar diathermy is limited to the deviated nasal septum (DNS) muscle in order to minimize postoperative upper lip contusion and hematoma.

Septal surgery is the most important part of the rhinoplasty in these patients and needs detailed attention. First, expose the caudal septum and raise submucoperichondrial flaps to expose the bony-cartilaginous junction between the septum and adjacent bony structures. In revision cases, when finding the correct plane proves to be difficult, use magnification with loupes, and approach the problem inferocaudally, creating a pocket in front of the nasal spine, severing scar tissue, and exposing the nasal spine and medial aspect of the pyriform aperture. The size of the spine should already be known from the clinical examination of the patient. A spine and its wings need to have appropriate size and orientation. Both of these factors can be corrected surgically by gently rasping when appropriate, or at times by more rigorous excision if necessary. In the authors' experience, the reduction of the spine is an important first step in de-projecting a tension nose, together with well-planned and precisely executed inferior and posterior chondrotomies of the quadrangular cartilage. The combination of these maneuvers will allow the posterior septal angle to be repositioned onto the nasal spine so that the septum may be returned to its new, more anatomically appropriate position. Reevaluate the lateral profile at this point: the reduction in projection will be immediately apparent. Also, the frontal view should be reevaluated at this point: most of the time, resizing of the quadrangular cartilage (through ad hoc horizontal and longitudinal wedge resections) will correct most of the malposition of the cartilaginous pyramid. The explanation for such a dramatic change lies in the native imbalance between the oversized cartilaginous septum and its mucoperichondrial envelope. The septal cartilage is stretched inside a relatively smaller envelope, thus producing a distortion of the quadrangular cartilage on the sagittal plane. This results in a C-shaped or inverted C-shaped configuration of the septal cartilage and the cartilaginous dorsum.

The next task is reshaping the intermediate and anterior septal angles. This can be achieved by excising a U-shaped piece of caudal septum that starts at the newly created posterior septal angle and continues anteriorly to include the intermediate septal angle, and then climbs superiorly to reduce the height of the anterior septal angle. The level of the newly created anterior septal angle shows significant gender differences: a light supratip dip is specially desired by most of the authors' female patients.

The intermediate septal angle is often overlooked, although it plays a significant role in the aesthetic contour of the columella–upper lip junction. Standard use of columellar strut tends to flatten and straighten the contour of the caudal septum. Endonasal surgery provides a more flexible way to deal with such a relevant aesthetic landmark. A more aesthetic intermediate angle can be recreated in both male and female patients with gently crushed cartilage at the end of the operation; otherwise the columella will look unnaturally straight.

Next it is time to reassess the size and projection of the nose. This step will reduce the undesirable aesthetics parameters.

Finally, if the above two steps have not been enough, a posterior chondrotomy can further de-project the nose, and it should be performed with great care. The junction of the cartilaginous and bony septum is confirmed by sight and palpation. Using a Freer elevator, the separation of cartilage from bone is started inferiorly, and then the instrument ascends toward the junction between the ULCs and nasal bones, without ever reaching it (**Fig. 26.4**). The amount of de-projection gained is proportional to the amount of vertical ascent along the bony-cartilaginous junction: the higher the dissociation, the larger the amount of de-projection gained. The endonasal aspect of the keystone area must never be violated, so posterior chondrotomy should always keep 1 cm of untouched connection between quadrangular cartilage and perpendicular plate.

From the previous discussion, it is apparent that there are two pivot points that are vital for septal stability: the posterior septal angle–spine junction, and the keystone area. The spine may be carefully altered while maintaining a close relation with the posterior septal angle, which should ideally rest on the nasal spine without surpassing it. The keystone area is definitely the core in the management of the tension nose. Many tension nose patients require dorsal humpectomy, which can result in dissociation of the ULCs from both the septum and the central portion of the overlying nasal bones. Before routinely splitting at full thickness the septum–ULC junction and routinely placing a spreader graft, the implications of these steps

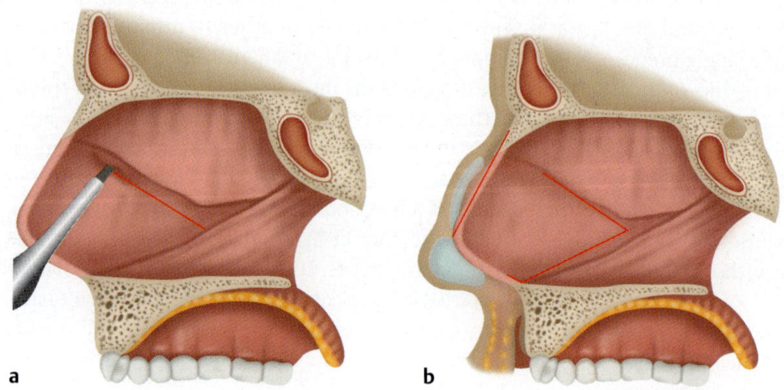

Fig. 26.4 **(a)** Posterior chondrotomy is started inferiorly, and then the instrument ascends toward the junction between the upper lateral cartilages and the nasal bones, without ever reaching it. **(b)** The posterior chondrotomy should always keep 1 cm of untouched connection between quadrangular cartilage and perpendicular plate.

should be carefully considered. In many cases, the amount of cartilaginous hump to be removed is not large enough to result in a complete separation of the natural "spreading relation" of the septolateral cartilaginous unit. Second, positioning spreader grafts will broaden the dorsum of the nose, which many patients do not desire, and may distort the BDLs. Moreover, the spreader grafts—when aimed at opening the internal valve—must be harvested with significant thickness and, therefore, intrude into the valve area, contributing to reduction of its cross-sectional area, which is the main resistive area of the whole airway. In the authors' hands, the autospreader technique[32] proved to be cumbersome to perform and did not provide reproducible effects. Instead, a fold of mucosa released from the ULC-septal junction ("extramucosal" technique of Robin) may be interposed between the two structures. This mucoperichondrial tunneling can be executed either via intercartilaginous **(Fig. 26.5)** or hemitransfixion **(Fig. 26.6)** incisions. The extramucosal technique produces a softer spreading effect that helps to prevent a decrease in the crucial angle of the internal valve (middle vault protection) **(Fig. 26.7)** without causing problems due to spreader graft positioning. A relevant variation used by the authors in preventing the inverted-V deformity, especially in the type A variant of the tension nose, is to minimize the extent of the dissection plane over the bony-cartilaginous vault junction and bony vault. In these cases, the dissection is just above the periosteum and is strictly limited to the area of the hump to be removed **(Fig. 26.8)**. Preservation of the junction between the ULCs and the nasal bones lateral to the hump is critical in preventing an inverted-V deformity. For such a purpose, an accurately sharpened osteotome for humpectomy is by far preferable to rasps, whose up-and-down movements can easily jeopardize the integrity of the bony-cartilaginous vault junction lateral to the hump. Hump removal is executed sequentially, first cartilage and then bone, but in one piece, as it guarantees a smooth transition at the rhinion area.

The pattern of osteotomies is dictated by the facial photographic analysis. Because most noses are asymmetrical, osteotomies should reflect this fact. Internal basal osteotomies start just above the head of the inferior turbinate, and follow a high-low-high pattern up to the junction with the frontal bone. The thick, solid frontal bone will represent the pivot point, where a medial-downward rotation of the hand creates a back-fracture and mobilizes the bony wall to close the open roof. This osteotomy sequence makes paramedian osteotomies unnecessary in most cases. Should osteotomy result in inadequate infracture, a superiorly placed percutaneous transverse osteotomy will also be required. In performing infracture maneuvers, the use of fingers should be extremely gentle in order not to detach the ULCs from the overlying bones lateral to the dehumped area.

After dorsal work, the tip is addressed. Do the LLCs still appear disproportionate or malrotated and is the alar rim malpositioned? Often, reduction of a very large septum gets rid of this illusion and may obviate the need for surgery to modify it. For the majority of patients, the first author utilizes the endonasal "extended" transcartilaginous approach,[33] executed through intracartilaginous

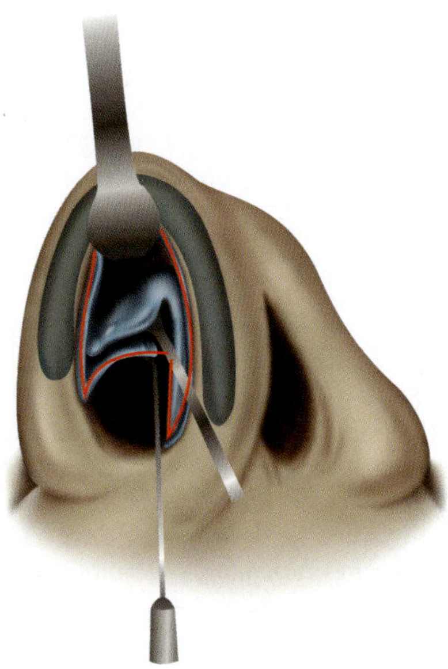

Fig. 26.5 Mucoperichondrial tunneling ("extramucosal" technique) under the cartilaginous vault executed via intercartilaginous incision.

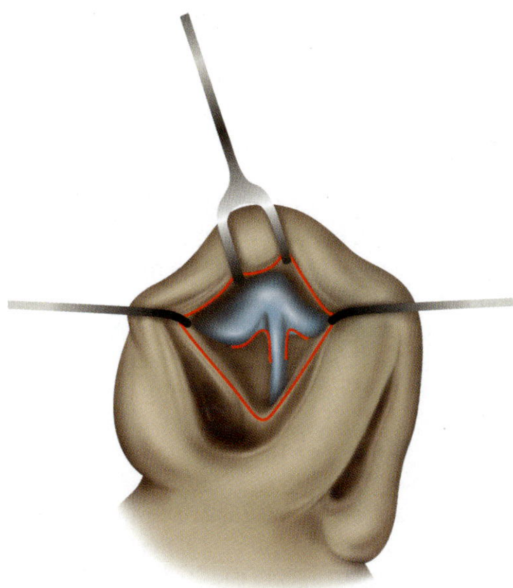

Fig. 26.6 Extramucosal dissection performed through hemitransfixion incision.

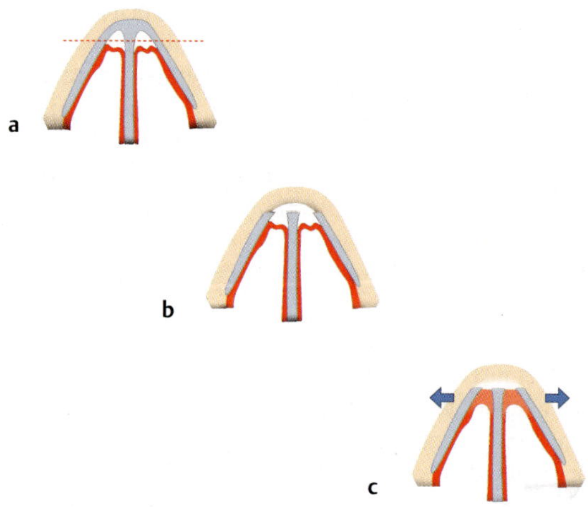

Fig. 26.7 (a–c) Middle vault protection. The tissue surplus produced by the "extramucosal" dissection determines a soft spreading effect, preventing both inward collapse of the upper lateral cartilages and a decrease in the crucial angle of the internal valve.

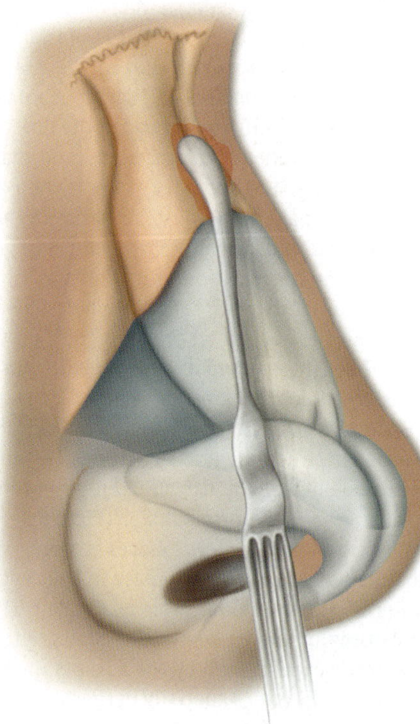

Fig. 26.8 In the high, narrow nose with short nasal bones, dissection over the bony dorsum is performed just above the periosteum and is strictly limited to the area of the hump to be removed, in order not to jeopardize the junction between the upper lateral cartilages and the nasal bones lateral to the hump.

incisions. This approach not only provides direct access to the areas of the lateral crura that need resculpting, but also for refining the scrolls as required. Many sutures and grafts can be used through the transcartilagenous approach and concurrent endonasal incisions: hemitransfixion, partial infracartilaginous, or slot "custom-made" incisions. The extended transcartilagenous approach allows for greater flexibility in dealing with complex tip problems and in the creation of surface aesthetics. When a complete visualization of the cartilaginous skeleton of the tip is needed, the authors resort to infracartilaginous or delivery approaches.

The type C tension nose poses special problems that require a change in strategy. After the septal work, the tip is approached before the dorsum, as the repositioning and stabilization of the pronasale will dictate the degree of dorsal reduction. In this case, the main tool is the intracolumellar strut, which is positioned through the hemitransfixion incision. At the end of the operation, further stabilization is achieved by the tongue-in-groove suture. Special attention is paid to the alar rim, which may present an unsightly "Chinese hat" configuration. This can be part of the so-called cephalic malposition of the lateral crura. In these cases, the authors refrain from aggressive surgery. Caudal rim displacement is managed through a partial infracartilaginous approach and utilization of a custom-shaped graft sutured caudally to the arched part of the lateral crura. This lateral crura is kept in a more caudal position after dissection from the underlying SMAS, and placement of a SMAS-anchoring infracartilaginous suture.

The final check of the nose includes inspection of the major lines of importance, such as the BDLs, and symmetries from frontal, lateral, and helicopter views. Using crushed cartilage in precise slots restores surface aesthetics.

26.6 Outcomes

Fig. 26.9 shows preoperative views and **Fig. 26.10** shows postoperative results for a young adult female.

26.7 Conclusion

Each population has certain cultural requirements that need to be taken into consideration when undertaking facial analysis. Globalization has produced dramatic changes in patients' requests, especially among younger patients. Patients' desires are less linked to maintaining ethnic features and more linked to looking like their idols in fashion, sports, music, and the movies. Such a unified aesthetic ideal requires rethinking of traditional rhinoplasty and adjustment of the canons of nasal aesthetic analysis.

In modern rhinoplasty practice, nasal and facial analysis need to be patient-specific and culturally relevant. Similarly, the imposition of a cloned treatment plan in each case should be abandoned in favor of patient-centered rhinoplasty.

These complex considerations have a major effect on patient selection, surgical planning, and performance of surgery.

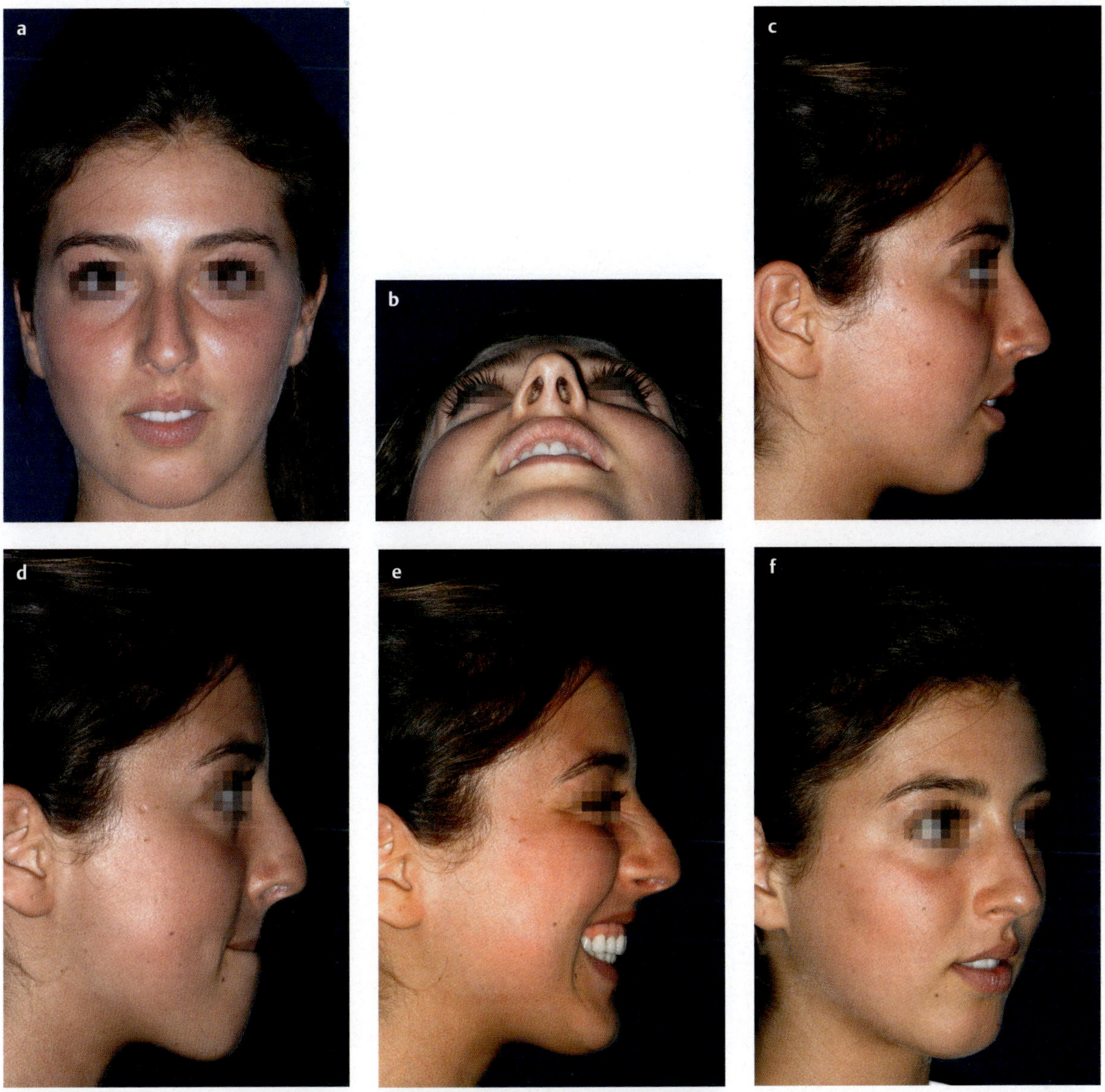

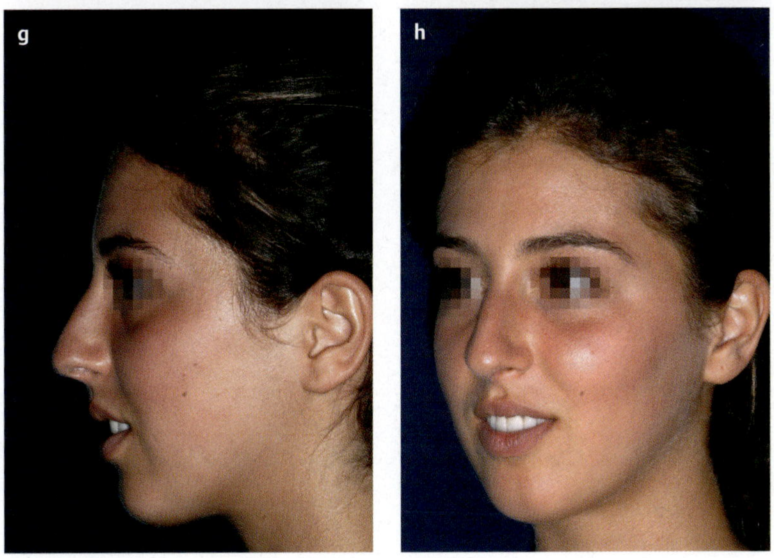

Fig. 26.9 **(a–h)** Preoperative views of a young adult female. Operation highlights are: septoplasty, depressor septi nasi release, spine reduction, and debulking of the soft tissues between the feet of the medial crura via hemitransfixion incision; transcartiliginous approach for tip and scroll sculpting; creation of submucosal tunnels under the cartilaginous vault extended to the bony vault to create a "spreader effect"; hump removal; basal osteotomies and infracture without paramedian osteotomies; subdomal sutures to improve tip definition/width angles; alar rim contour grafts through "slot" infracartilaginous incisions; caudal composite infratip shortening of the septum; tongue-in-groove suture.

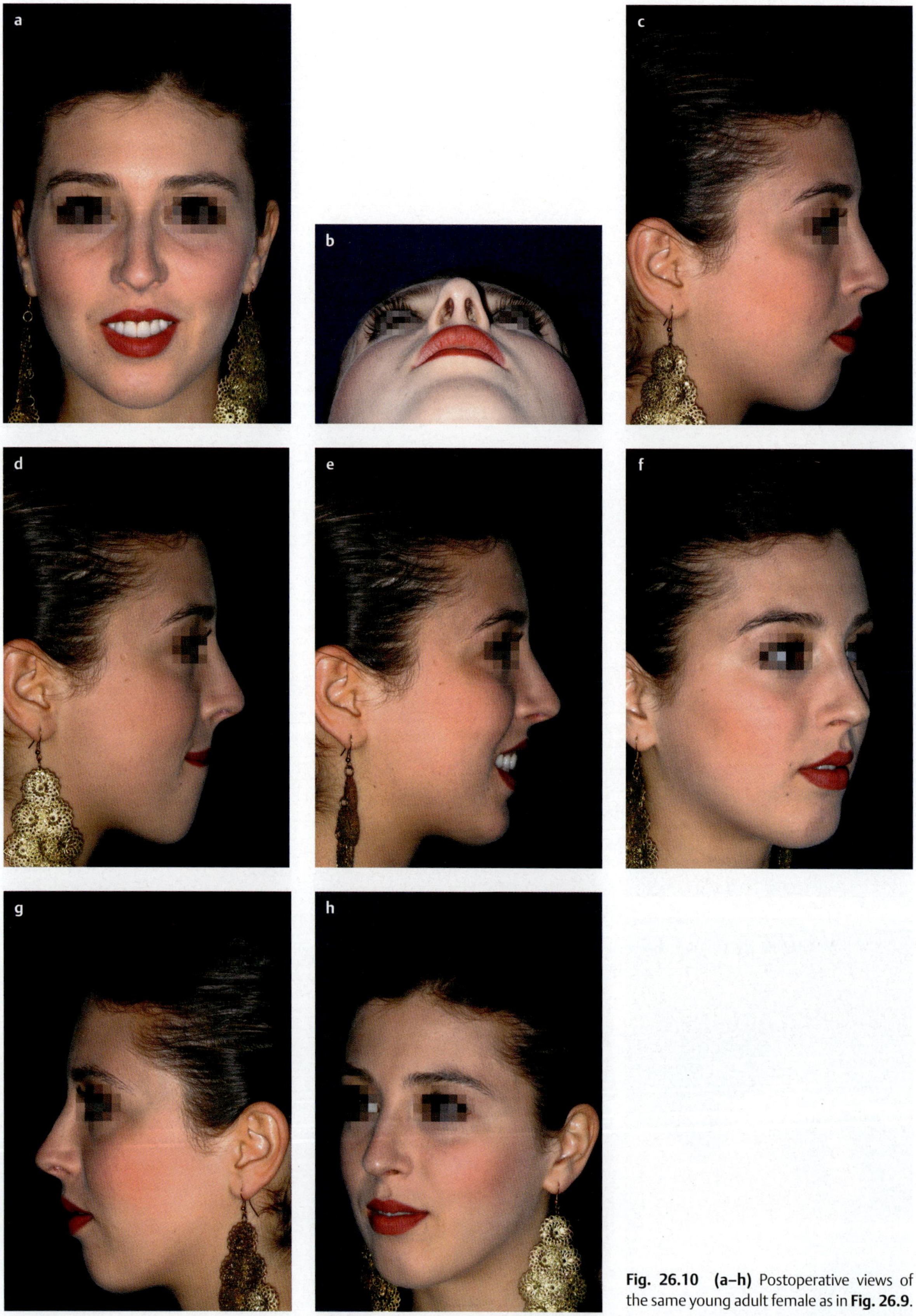

Fig. 26.10 (a–h) Postoperative views of the same young adult female as in **Fig. 26.9**.

Collective experience has clearly demonstrated that there is no single best approach that answers all the demands of our patients. While some patients require major structural changes, others need only subtle changes in surface aesthetics. Applying the same techniques in all cases can result in inadequate surgery, rather than tailor-made, patient-centered surgery. Endonasal hybrid rhinoplasty, which combines the best techniques from endonasal and external approaches, can adequately deal with the problems encountered in the management of the Mediterranean nose.

References

1. Sturm-O'Brien AK, Brissett AEA, Brissett AE. Ethnic trends in facial plastic surgery. Facial Plast Surg 2010;26(2): 69–74 10.1055/s-0030-1253496
2. Leong SC, Eccles R. Race and ethnicity in nasal plastic surgery: a need for science. Facial Plast Surg 2010;26(2): 63–68 10.1055/s-0030-1253505
3. Cobo R. Hispanic/Mestizo rhinoplasty. Facial Plast Surg Clin North Am 2010;18(1):173–188
4. Cobo R. Facial aesthetic surgery with emphasis on rhinoplasty in the Hispanic patient. Curr Opin Otolaryngol Head Neck Surg 2008;16(4):369–375 10.1097/MOO.0b013e3283071426
5. Milgrim LM, Lawson W, Cohen AF. Anthropometric analysis of the female Latino nose. Revised aesthetic concepts and their surgical implications. Arch Otolaryngol Head Neck Surg 1996;122(10):1079–1086
6. Choi JY, Park JH, Javidnia H, Sykes JM. Effect of various facial angles and measurements on the ideal position of the nasal tip in the Asian patient population. JAMA Facial Plast Surg 2013;15(6):417–421
7. Jang YJ, Yu MS. Rhinoplasty for the Asian nose. Facial Plast Surg 2010;26(2):93–101 10.1055/s-0030-1253507
8. Patel AD, Kridel RWH. African-American rhinoplasty. Facial Plast Surg 2010;26(2):131–141 10.1055/s-0030-1253499
9. Apaydin F. Rhinoplasty in the Middle Eastern nose. Facial Plast Surg Clin North Am 2014;22(3):349–355 10.1016/j.fsc.2014.04.009
10. Sands NB, Adamson PA. Global facial beauty: approaching a unified aesthetic ideal. Facial Plast Surg 2014;30(2): 93–100 10.1055/s-0034-1371905
11. Perrett DIMK, May KA, Yoshikawa S. Facial shape and judgments of female attractiveness. Nature 1994; 368(6468):239–242
12. Gunter JP. Facial analysis for the rhinoplasty patient. In: 1995 Dallas Rhinoplasty Symposium 12th Annual. Dallas, TX: UT Southwestern Medical Center at Dallas; 1995:17–27
13. Palma P, Khodaei I. Dichotomy of rhinoplasty practice: from the conference floor to the operating room. Facial Plast Surg 2014;30(2):103–112
14. Palma P, Bignami M, Delù G, De Bernardi F, Castelnuovo P. Rhinoplasty for the Mediterranean nose. Facial Plast Surg 2003;19(3):279–294
15. Erol OO. Tip rhinoplasty in broad noses in a Turkish population: Eurasian noses. Plast Reconstr Surg 2012;130(1): 185–197 10.1097/PRS.0b013e318254ca1d
16. Moss JP, Linney AD, Grindrod SR, Arridge SR, Clifton JS. Three-dimensional visualization of the face and skull using computerized tomography and laser scanning techniques. Eur J Orthod 1987;9(4):247–253
17. Tuncel U, Turan A, Kostakoğlu N. Digital anthropometric shape analysis of 110 rhinoplasty patients in the Black Sea Region in Turkey. J Craniomaxillofac Surg 2013;41(2): 98–102 10.1016/j.jcms.2012.05.014
18. Boccieri A. The surgical approach to the Mediterranean nose. Facial Plast Surg 2010;26(2):119–130
19. Higuera S, Hatef DA, Stal S. Rhinoplasty in the Hispanic patient. Semin Plast Surg 2009;23(3):207–214 10.1055/s-0029-1224800
20. Sputh CB. The tension nose. Rhinology 1985;23(1): 79–80
21. Barelli PA. The tension nose. In: Barelli PA, ed. The Collective Writings and Reprints of Maurice H. Cottle, M.D. Kansas City, MO: University of Missouri Kansas City School of Dentistry; 1982:209–220
22. Dinis PB, Dinis M, Gomes A. Psychosocial consequences of nasal aesthetic and functional surgery: a controlled prospective study in an ENT setting. Rhinology 1998;36(1):32–36
23. McKiernan DC, Banfield G, Kumar R, Hinton AE. Patient benefit from functional and cosmetic rhinoplasty. Clin Otolaryngol Allied Sci 2001;26(1):50–52
24. Hay GG, Heather BB. Changes in psychometric test results following cosmetic nasal operations. Br J Psychiatry 1973;122(566):89–90
25. Palma P, Khodaei I, Tasman A-J. A guide to the assessment and analysis of the rhinoplasty patient. Facial Plast Surg 2011;27(2):146–159
26. Palma P, Khodaei I. Functional and aesthetic analysis of the nose. In: Ahmad Z, Morton R, Giles M, eds. Practical Otolaryngology—Head & Neck Surgery: A Symptom-Oriented Approach. Philadelphia, PA: Jaypee Medical Publishers; in press
27. Smith TL. Evidence-based clinical practice in otolaryngology. Otolaryngological Clinics of North America 2012;45(5)
28. Johnson CM Jr, Godin MS. The tension nose: open structure rhinoplasty approach. Plast Reconstr Surg 1995;95(1): 43–51
29. Tasman AJ, Palma P. The infracartilaginous approach revisited. Arch Facial Plast Surg 2008;10(6):370–375
30. Robin JL. Extramucosal method in rhinoplasty. Aesthetic Plast Surg 1979;3(1):171–178
31. Palma P, Khodaei I. Hybrid rhinoplasty: the 21st century approach to remodeling the nose. Arch Facial Plast Surg 2010;12(6):412–414
32. Yoo S, Most SP. Nasal airway preservation using the autospreader technique: analysis of outcomes using a disease-specific quality-of-life instrument. Arch Facial Plast Surg 2011;13(4):231–233
33. Palma P. Rhinoplasty: Endonasal strategies. In: Myers EN, ed. Master Techniques in Otolaryngology—Head and Neck Surgery. Philadelphia, PA: Lippincott Williams & Wilkins; in press

27 Managing the Long, Droopy Nasal Tip

Hossam M. T. Foda

27.1 Introduction

The droopy nasal tip is a deformity in which the nasal tip is inferiorly rotated, leading to an increase in the length of the nose and contraction of the nasolabial angle.[1] The droopy tip deformity, besides being cosmetically unattractive, may interfere with normal nasal functions by restricting the airflow through the nares. This can be demonstrated by the subjective improvement in breathing that occurs with manually lifting the droopy tip.

The causes of the droopy tip may be broadly divided into two groups, the first group includes an "abnormal" alar cartilage with excessively long lateral crura, vertically oriented lateral crura with high abutment to the pyriform aperture, or short, weak medial crura. The second group comprises a "normal" alar cartilage complex that is inferiorly displaced by the effect of extrinsic forces. The forces may be pushing from above, as in the case of long upper lateral cartilages, a high anterior septal angle, and overdeveloped caudal septum; or the forces may be pulling from below, as with thick, heavy nasal skin, overactive depressor septi nasi muscle, or the effect of gravity in cases with poor nasal tip support as a result of aging or previous surgeries.[2]

The ultimate goal, in correcting the droopy tip, is to relocate the alar cartilages in a more cephalically oriented position. This can be achieved through directly modifying the alar cartilages or by using complementary procedures on structures closely related to the alar cartilages. These procedures may include excision of the overdeveloped scrolls of upper lateral cartilages, lowering the anterior septal angle, shortening the caudal septum, and weakening of depressor septi nasi muscle.[2] The aim of such procedures is to eliminate the forces that inferiorly displace the tip cartilages, thus making their cephalic repositioning easier during alar cartilage modification.

Our preferred alar cartilage modifying techniques to correct the droopy nasal tip are the lateral crural steal (LCS),[3] lateral crural overlay (LCO),[4] and the tongue-in-groove technique (TIG).[5] Although these three techniques can result in predictable degrees of cephalic rotation of the nasal tip, it's important to understand that the achieved degree of rotation can be maintained only in the presence of an adequate amount of tip support.[6,7]

In summary, our strategy in correcting the droopy nasal tip is to eliminate the forces that inferiorly displace the alar cartilages before adopting any alar cartilage modifying technique, then to increase the tip support to maintain the effect of the alar cartilage modifying technique adopted.

27.2 Tip Dynamics

Both the tripod concept described by Anderson[8] in 1969 and its recent modernization into the M-arch model by Adamson[9] are very helpful for understanding the effects that alar cartilage modifying techniques have on the degree of tip projection and rotation. In the tripod theory, the cartilaginous framework of the nasal tip is likened to a tripod, with two upper legs formed by the lateral crura on each side and one lower leg formed by the conjoined medial crura. According to the tripod analogy, LCS, which shortens the lateral crura and lengthens the medial crura, should move the tip upward and forward, resulting in an increase in both tip rotation and projection. On the other hand, LCO, which shortens the lateral crura, should pull the tip upward and backward, leading to an increase in rotation and a decrease in projection. Finally, the TIG, which moves the alar cartilages (the whole tripod) upward and fixes them to the caudal septum, will move the tip upward, thus increasing the amount of tip rotation but with no significant change in projection. The effects of the three techniques on the degree of projection and rotation were objectively assessed and were proved to conform very well with the tripod concept.[2,10,11]

27.3 Physical Examination

It is necessary to fully examine the nose both externally and internally. The first thing to evaluate is the thickness of the nasal skin and then the degree of tip support available, by examining alar cartilage size, strength, and orientation as well as the condition of caudal septum and the anterior nasal spine. This is followed by careful assessment of the tip and alae. The tip is evaluated for its degree of projection and rotation and any broadness, bifidity, or deflection, while the alae are examined for their thickness and any degree of retraction, collapse, or excessive flare.

27.4 Surgical Technique

Surgery is performed through an external rhinoplasty approach because the exposure provided allows an accurate, direct appraisal of the tip cartilages in their natural, undistorted position. The approach also permits alar cartilage modifications to be performed precisely and under direct vision. Bilateral marginal incisions are connected via an inverted-V columellar incision.[12,13] The columellar skin flap is carefully elevated off the medial crura and dissection is continued in the supraperichondrial plane to fully expose the alar cartilages. The dorsal skin flap elevation proceeds upward over the bony-cartilaginous framework while the surgeon makes sure to stay in the avascular sub-SMAS plane until reaching the nasofrontal angle. Any required dorsal modifications are made before modifying the tip cartilages to avoid inadvertent disruption of the delicate reconstructed alar cartilages. Any subcutaneous fatty tissue found between the domes or between the medial crura is carefully removed. If the medial crura are found to be weak and buckled, they are strengthened by splinting them to a strong columellar strut, making sure that the strut goes down to the premaxilla but stops short of the anterior nasal spine. This increases the support and stability of the nasal tip complex. In cases with wide lateral crura, a conservative lateral crural cephalic trim is performed, leaving a strong intact caudal strip of at least 6 mm to maintain adequate tip support; the width may be increased up to 8 mm in cases with thick, heavy nasal skin. At this stage, any projecting caudal ends (scrolls) of upper lateral cartilages are trimmed, to facilitate the upward movement of the tip cartilages by the alar cartilage modification.

27.4.1 Lateral Crural Steal

In cases with a droopy, under-projected nasal tip, the vestibular skin is undermined from the undersurface of the lateral crus, starting at the junction of the medial and lateral crura (native domes) and proceeding laterally for ~ 8 to 10 mm (**Fig. 27.1a**). This allows the lateral crura to be mobilized freely without being tethered by their skin attachments. The lateral crus on each side is then advanced medially in a curvilinear fashion onto the medial crus and fixed in its new position using a 5–0 Prolene mattress-type suture.[3,10] The entry point of the LCS suture is at the native dome, and the exit point is in the lateral crus (**Fig. 27.1b** and **Fig. 27.2a**). The location of the exit point depends on the amount of steal that needs to be achieved; in cases where 2 mm of steal is needed, the exit point has to be 4 mm lateral to the entry point, and if 4 mm of steal is needed, then the exit point has to be 8 mm lateral to the entry point. Additional narrowing and refinement are accomplished by mattressing the newly created domes together using a 6–0 Prolene transdomal suture.

The LCS suture will create a new dome that is more projected and more cephalically rotated (**Fig. 27.1c** and **Fig. 27.2c**); thus it is an ideal technique to adopt in cases with an under-projected and droopy nasal tip (**Fig. 27.3**).

27.4.2 Lateral Crural Overlay

In cases where the lateral crura are overly long, leading to an over-projected and droopy tip, an incision is planned in the lateral crus at the junction of its lateral third with the medial two-thirds (**Fig. 27.4a** and **Fig. 27.5a**), because the alar skin is relatively thicker at this area and thus can easily camouflage the cut and overlapped edges of the lateral crus. Before the cartilage cut is made, the vestibular skin is elevated off the undersurface of the lateral crus for ~ 5 mm on each side of the planned cartilaginous incision (**Fig. 27.4b**) to release the tethering forces that may prevent the free overlap of the cut edges. The cartilaginous cut is made by a no. 15 blade and extends in a straight line from the cephalic to the caudal margin of the lateral crus. The free medial segment of the lateral crus is advanced and rotated over the lateral segment to shorten the lateral crus until the desired degree of de-projection and rotation is reached.[4,10] The integrity of the lateral crus is then reestablished by fixing the overlapped segments with a 6–0 Prolene suture in a horizontal mattress fashion (**Fig. 27.4c** and **Fig. 27.5b,c**). This maneuver will move the domes upward. and backward, resulting in an increase in tip rotation and a decrease in tip projection (**Fig. 27.5b,c**); thus, LCO is an ideal technique to adopt in cases with a droopy and over-projected nasal tip (**Fig. 27.6**).

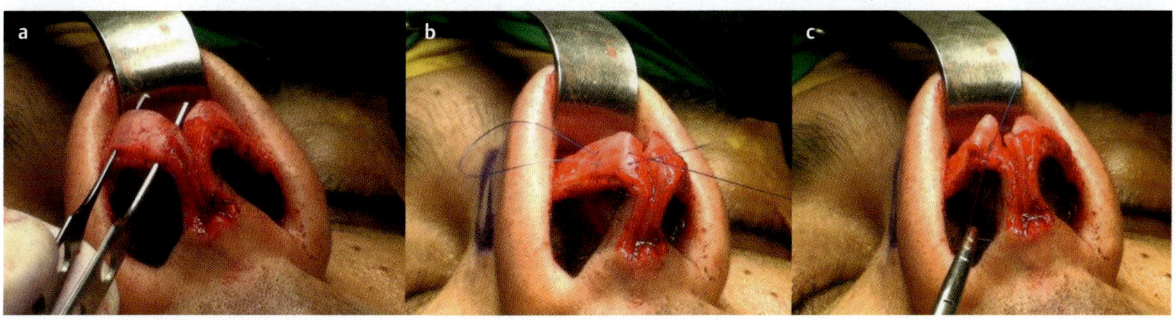

Fig. 27.1 Intraoperative steps of lateral crural steal (LCS) technique. **(a)** Undermining of vestibular skin lateral to the native dome. **(b)** LCS suture entry at native dome and exit point in the lateral crus. **(c)** Tying the LCS suture, resulting in creation of a new dome that is more projected and rotated.

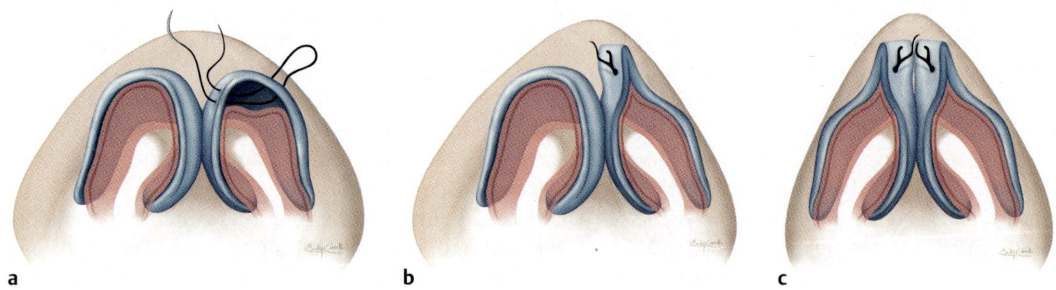

Fig. 27.2 Schematic diagram of lateral crural steal (LCS) technique. **(a)** Vestibular skin undermining and LCS suture placement. **(b)** Tying the LCS suture, resulting in a new dome that is more projected and cephalically rotated. **(c)** Completing the LCS on both sides.

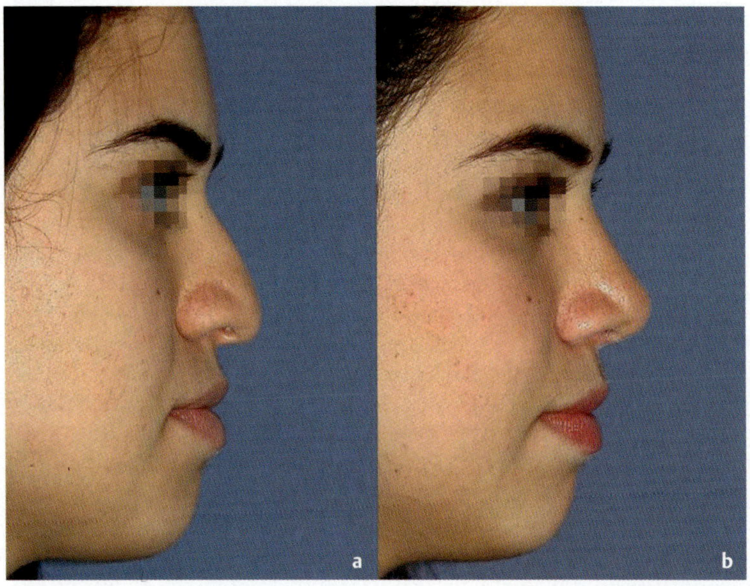

Fig. 27.3 **(a)** Preoperative view of a patient with a droopy and under-projected nasal tip. **(b)** Two-year postoperative view of the same patient after the LCS technique was used to increase the tip projection and rotation.

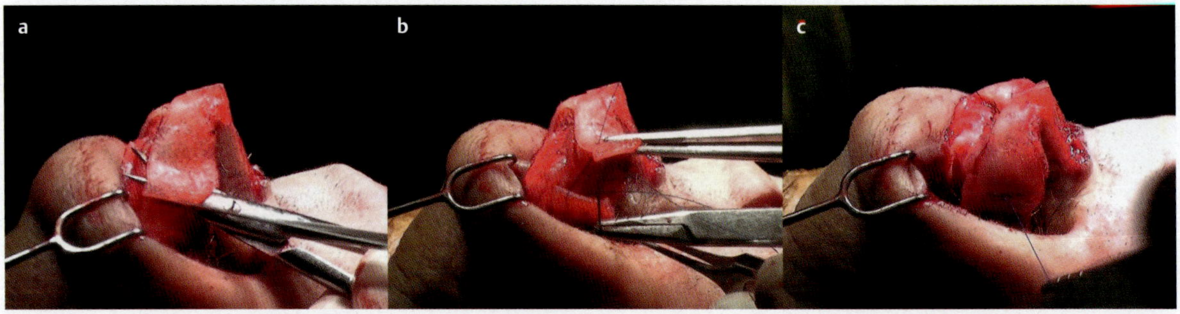

Fig. 27.4 Intraoperative steps of lateral crural overlay (LCO) technique. **(a)** Lateral crural transection. **(b)** Overlap of cut segments. **(c)** Suture fixation of the overlapped cartilages.

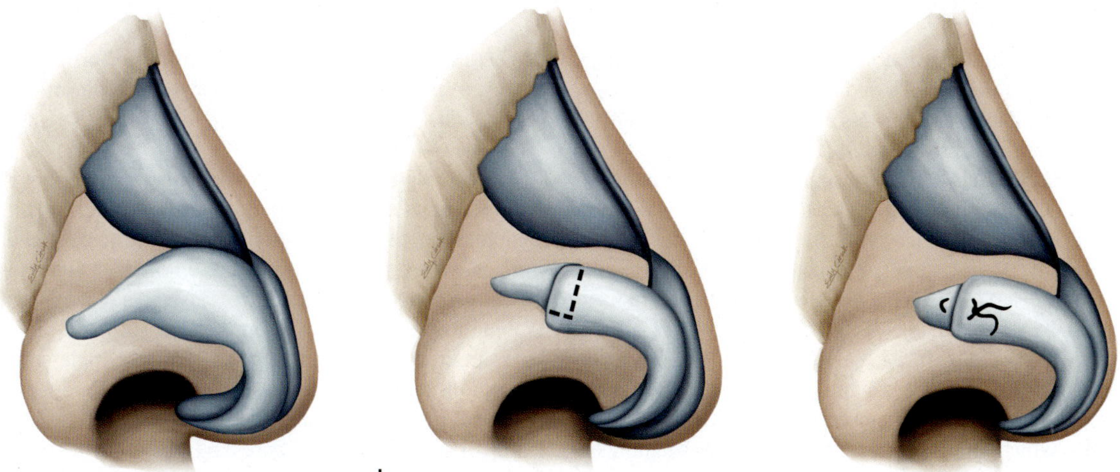

a b c

Fig. 27.5 Schematic diagram of lateral crural overlay (LCO) technique. **(a)** Long lateral crura leading to an over-projected and droopy tip. **(b)** Transection of lateral crus and overlap of cut edges will move the dome upward and backward. **(c)** Suture fixation of the overlapped segments.

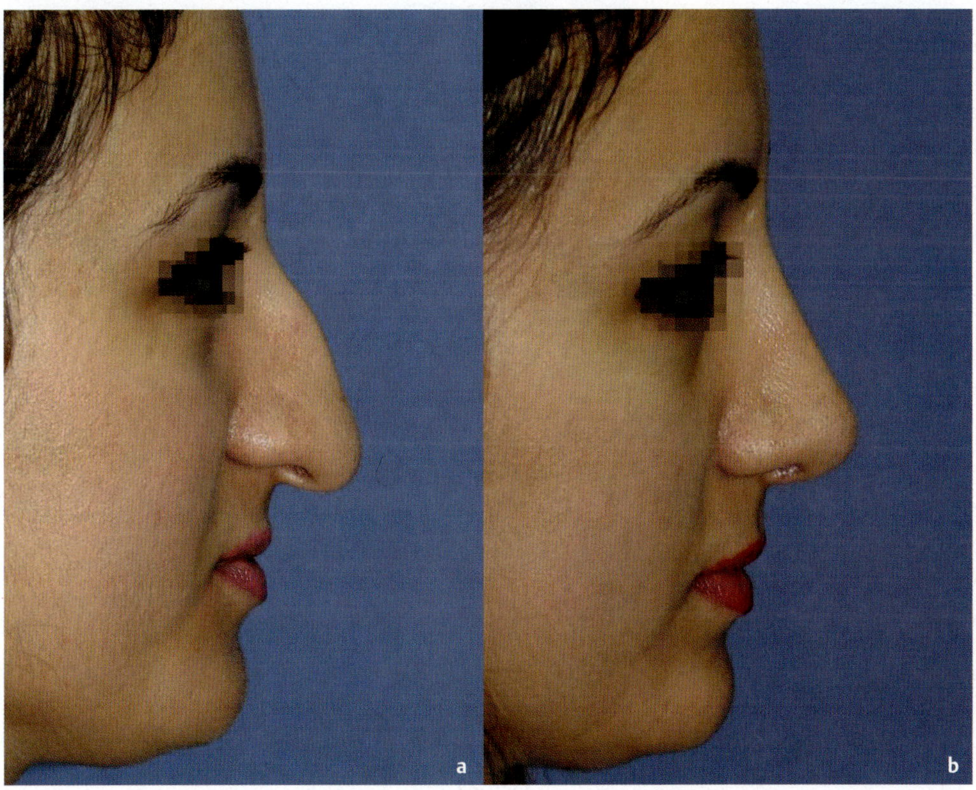

Fig. 27.6 **(a)** Preoperative view of a patient with a droopy, over-projected nasal tip. **(b)** The 3-year postoperative view of the same patient after the lateral crural overlay (LCO) technique was used to de-project and superiorly rotate the nasal tip.

27.4.3 Tongue-in-Groove

For the TIG, a full transfixion incision in the membranous septum is performed, followed by elevation of the mucoperichondrial flaps on both sides of the caudal septum. After making sure the caudal septum is lying strictly in the midline, a pocket is fashioned by retrograde dissection between the medial crura, followed by advancing the medial crura upward onto the caudal septum, which fits in the created pocket.[5] Once the desired relationship of the medial crura to the septum is achieved, these structures are fixed together by three 5–0 PDS (Ethicon, Inc.) mattress sutures (**Fig. 27.7a,b** and **Fig. 27.8a,b**). Further stabilization can be achieved by using septo-columellar sutures of 5–0 Vicryl Rapide (Ethicon, Inc.) on a short straight needle (**Fig. 27.7c**). The TIG, which moves the alar cartilages upward and fixes them to the caudal septum, will move the tip upward, thus increasing the amount of tip rotation with no significant change in projection, so it is an ideal technique to use in cases in which a droopy tip is associated with normal tip projection (**Fig. 27.9**). It is to be noted that performing a TIG in the presence of any degree of caudal septal deviation can result in distortion of the nasal tip, the columella, and the whole nasal base.

At completion of the tip remodeling, the nasal skin is redraped to its normal anatomical position and the external rhinoplasty incisions are closed, starting with the columellar incision, which is closed using a 6–0 PDS deep subcutaneous suture in a horizontal mattress fashion, followed by 6–0 Prolene interrupted sutures on the skin surface. The marginal incisions are closed using 5–0 Vicryl Rapide sutures. Meticulous taping is necessary to maintain the proper positioning of the reconstructed tip cartilages; this is performed using 0.5 inch brown Micropore tape after applying Mastisol to the skin surface, then a metal splint is positioned over the dorsum and is secured by a second layer of tape.

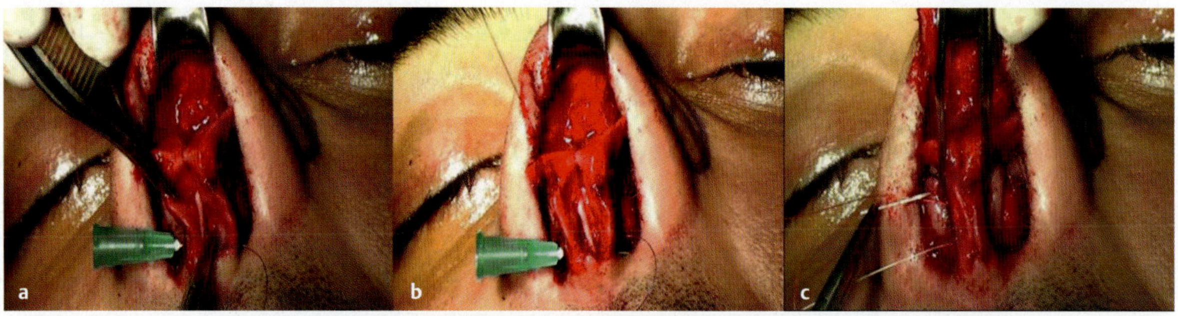

Fig. 27.7 Intraoperative steps of tongue-in-groove (TIG) technique. **(a,b)** Advancing and suturing of medial crura to the caudal septum using 5–0 PDS sutures. **(c)** Septo-columellar sutures using 5–0 Vicryl Rapide.

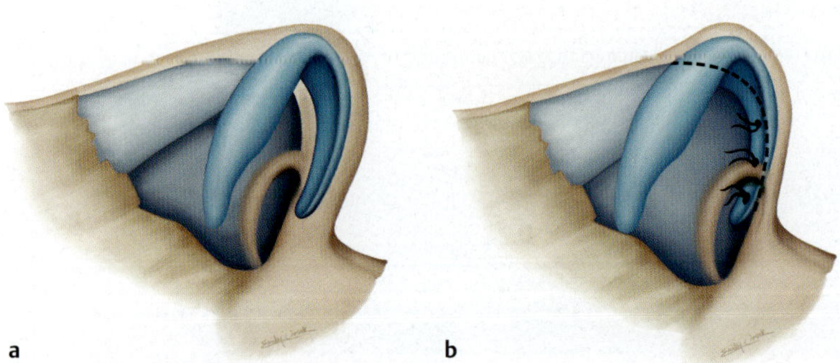

Fig. 27.8 Schematic diagram of tongue-in-groove (TIG) technique. **(a)** Preoperative relationship of medial crura to the caudal septum. **(b)** Postoperative condition after advancing and suturing of medial crura to the caudal septum.

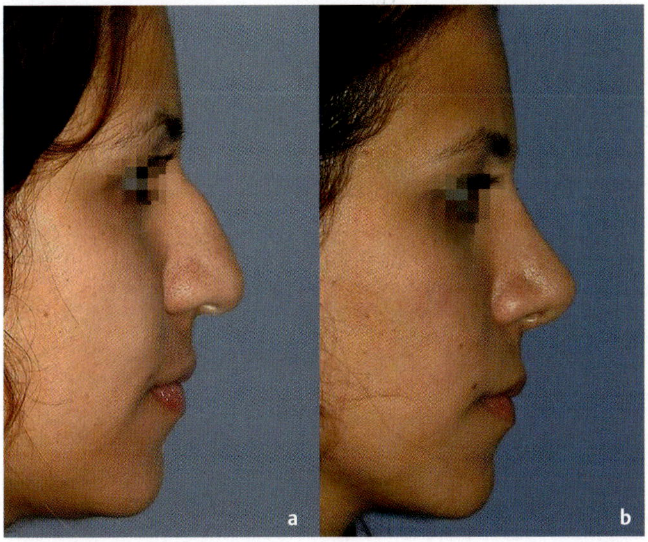

Fig. 27.9 **(a)** Preoperative view of a patient with a droopy nasal tip and normal degree of projection. **(b)** The 4-year postoperative view of the same patient after the tongue-in-groove (TIG) technique was used to increase tip rotation without changing tip projection.

27.5 Postoperative Care

To minimize postoperative facial edema, the patient is advised to sleep in the supine position with the back of the bed raised for 3 days. Oral antibiotics are given for 5 days, and the patient is instructed to use antibiotic ointment intranasally until all the sutures in the nasal cavity fall off, which may take 4 to 6 weeks. Saline nasal irrigations can be used before ointment application to decrease the stuffy nose sensation.

The splint and the columellar sutures are removed after 1 week, and the nose is taped for another week to help support the tip during the early healing phase, when new fibrous attachments are being developed between the bony-cartilaginous nasal framework and the overlying skin. Sunscreen is used on the columellar incision as well as any external alar incisions for the first 2 months.

27.6 Droopy Tip with Poor Tip Support

In cases of droopy nasal tip with poor tip support, the alar cartilage modifying techniques, alone, cannot correct the droopy tip. Poor tip support is a common finding in revision cases as well as in cases with thick, heavy nasal skin, and it can be detected by preoperative examination and confirmed by the intraoperative findings.

1. Preoperative nasal analysis for signs of loss of tip support (**Fig. 27.10**):
   - Depressed, under-projected nasal tip
   - Droopy, inferiorly rotated nasal tip
   - Acute nasolabial angle
   - Retrodisplaced nasolabial junction
   - Posteriorly inclined upper lip
   - Retracted columellar base
2. Preoperative digital palpation to evaluate the degree of tip support:
   - Press on nasal tip to detect amount of cartilage support and degree of recoil
   - Press upward on the columella to detect any caudal septal deficiency
   - Press inward on the nasolabial junction to evaluate the premaxilla and anterior nasal spine
3. Intraoperative findings in revision cases with lost tip support (**Fig. 27.11**):
   - Premaxillary bony deficiency due to previously resected, or partial resorption of, anterior nasal spine
   - Caudal septal cartilage deficiency from previous excisions or resorption
   - Medial crura may be weak, fractured, twisted, buckled, or partially missing

27.7 Restructuring the Tip Support

An external rhinoplasty approach is used to reconstruct the lost tip support using a cartilaginous caudal septum replacement (CSR) graft[14] combined with premaxillary augmentation.

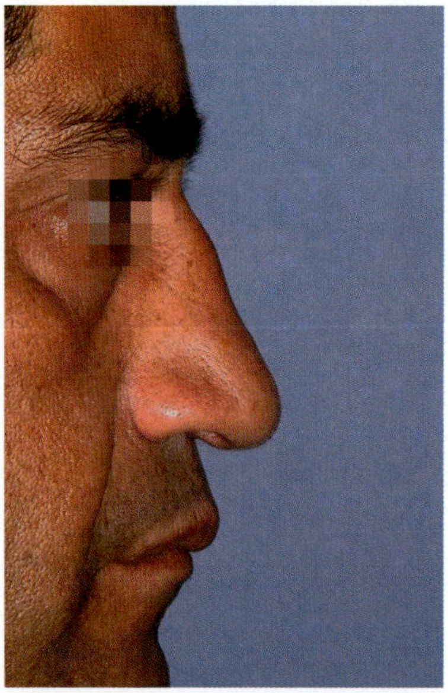

Fig. 27.10 A revision patient with premaxillary and caudal septum deficiency resulting in a depressed, droopy tip, acute nasolabial angle, retrodisplaced nasolabial junction, and posteriorly inclined upper lip.

27.7.1 Premaxillary Augmentation

A pocket is dissected between the footplates of the medial crura until the premaxilla and the anterior nasal spine are reached, although, in cases of premaxillary deficiency, they can be congenitally deficient, previously resected, or partially resorbed. In such cases, dissection is continued on both sides of the spine to create a pocket for premaxillary augmentation. In mild and moderate degrees of premaxillary deficiency, autogenous cartilage can be used after chopping it into small (1–2 mm) pieces; more finely diced cartilage doesn't give the same plumping effect in the premaxilla. In severe degrees of premaxillary deficiency, many types of implants have been used to provide premaxillary augmentation. Silastic (Dow Corning) was one of the first implants to be used in the premaxilla[15,16]; however, due to its smooth surface, it does not adhere to the surrounding tissues and is associated with a high incidence of migration and extrusion.[14,15,16] Unlike Silastic, Proplast[17,18] (Vitek, Houston, Texas) and Gore-Tex[19] (W.L. Gore & Co., Flagstaff, Arizona) are highly porous, thus inviting early tissue ingrowth and stabilization; however, they are more difficult to carve and insert and leave the patient with the rigid, unnatural feeling of a solid implant. Mersilene mesh[20] (Ethicon, Inc., Somerville, New Jersey) is our preferred implant in cases with severe premaxillary deficiency, as its lattice-like composition makes it soft and easily infiltrated by host tissue, thus leading to early fixation, and ensures a natural-feeling implant in the lower, mobile part of the nose.[20,21,22]

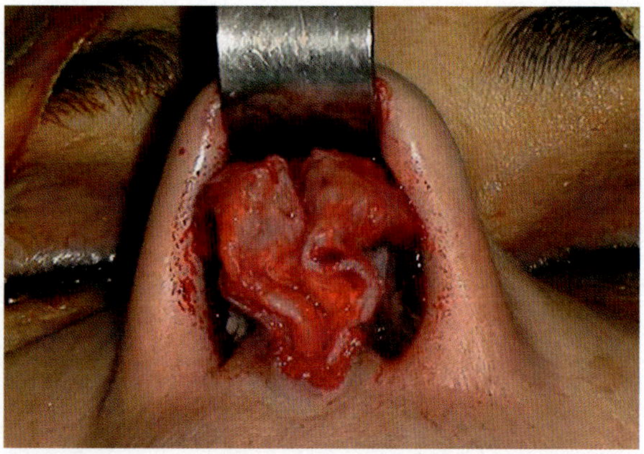

Fig. 27.11 Intraoperative view of a revision case with total loss of tip support showing weak, buckled medial crura and deficient caudal septum due to partial resection and resorption.

Another major advantage of Mersilene mesh over all other grafts and implants is its pliability, which allows the ribbon of mesh to be introduced through a small opening (**Fig. 27.12**) and to conform with and to fill out the underlying asymmetric areas of bony deficiencies. After adequate premaxillary augmentation with cartilage or mesh has been achieved, a columellar strut or CSR graft is introduced, with the surgeon making sure to mattress the medial crural footplates to the columellar graft to seal off the premaxillary pocket. This sealing of the premaxillary pocket will prevent upward migration of the cartilage pieces with cartilage augmentation and will prevent any contamination or extrusion with Mersilene mesh augmentation.

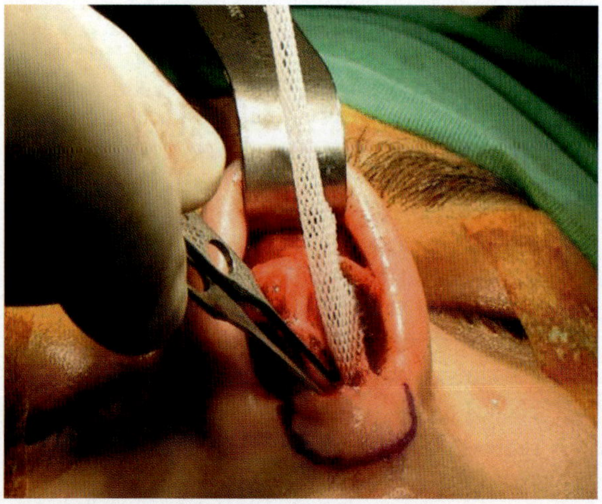

Fig. 27.12 Intraoperative view of premaxillary augmentation with Mersilene mesh.

27.7.2 Caudal Septum Replacement (CSR) Graft

Donor cartilage for the CSR graft can be obtained from multiple sources. Our first choice is autogenous septal cartilage, followed by autogenous conchal cartilage, and finally autogenous costal cartilage or irradiated costal cartilage homograft.

Graft Placement and Fixation

The extent of missing caudal septum is evaluated by instrument palpation. Occasionally, the membranous septum may be stiff on palpation, giving the impression that some cartilage is present, but on exploration only thick scar tissue from the previous surgeries is found. The medial crura are pulled apart and the thick scar tissue is excised using sharp dissection with a no. 15 blade; then fine tenotomy scissors are used to continue the dissection cephalically, making sure to stop a few millimeters before reaching the edge of the remaining septal cartilage, thus keeping the created membranous septal pocket isolated from the septum proper. The dissected pocket is then extended posteriorly between the footplates of the medial crura until reaching the premaxillary mesh. The graft is then introduced into the membranous septal pocket and is pushed downward until it is tightly pressed against the premaxillary mesh (**Fig. 27.13**). The graft is fixed in that position to the medial crura using 5–0 PDS sutures in a horizontal mattress fashion. Finally, the degree of tip projection is assessed and any excess length of the graft is trimmed to allow approximation of domes to be done above the level of the anterior end of the graft.

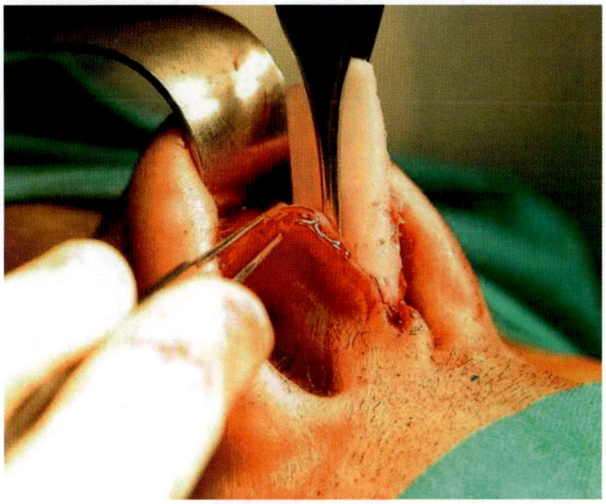

Fig. 27.13 Intraoperative view of a large caudal septum replacement (CSR) graft.

Many types and shapes of septal extension grafts have been used successfully to replace missing or weak caudal septal cartilage. The major problem with septal extension grafts is the unnatural rigidity and stiffness of the nasal lobule, which results from fixing the graft to the nasal septum either directly by suturing or via cartilage grafts.[23,24,25,226,27,28,29] On the other hand, the pocket for the CSR graft is kept separate from the septum by leaving an intact part of the membranous septum to intervene between the septum and the graft, which allows one to increase the tip support and projection while preserving some of the natural mobility of the nasal lobule (**Fig. 27.14**).

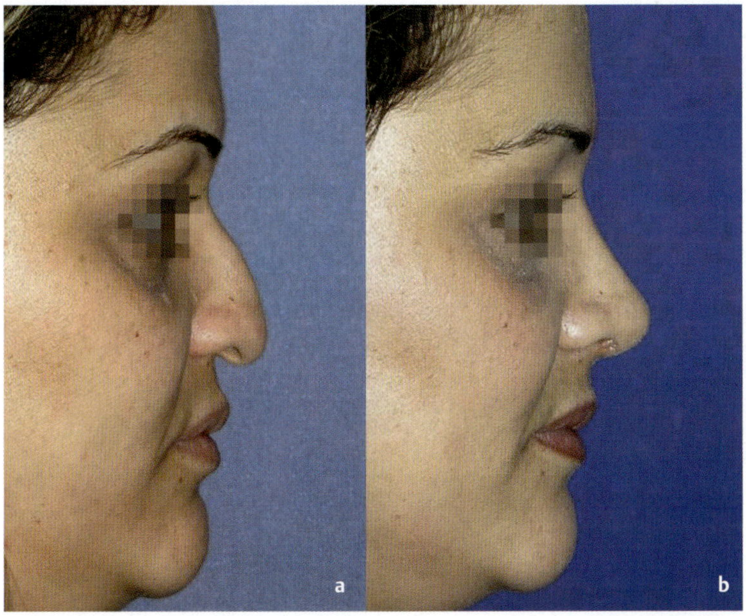

Fig. 27.14 **(a)** Preoperative view of a revision patient who had previous septal surgery with resection of the caudal septum and anterior nasal spine. **(b)** The 2-year postoperative view of the same patient after reconstruction of the tip support with a CSR graft and premaxillary augmentation with Mersilene mesh.

References

1. Simons R. Nasal tip projection, ptosis, and supratip thickening. Ear Nose Throat 1982;61:452–455
2. Foda HMT. Management of the droopy tip: a comparison of three alar cartilage-modifying techniques. Plast Reconstr Surg 2003;112(5):1408–1417, discussion 1418–1421
3. Kridel RWH, Konior RJ, Shumrick KA, Wright WK. Advances in nasal tip surgery. The lateral crural steal. Arch Otolaryngol Head Neck Surg 1989;115(10):1206–1212
4. Konior RJ, Kridel RWH. Lateral crural techniques for repositioning of the nasal tip. Oper Tech Otolaryngol--Head Neck Surg 1990;1(3):158–165
5. Kridel RWH, Scott BA, Foda HMT. The tongue-in-groove technique in septorhinoplasty. A 10-year experience. Arch Facial Plast Surg 1999;1(4):246–256, discussion 257–258
6. Janeke JB, Wright WK. Studies on the support of the nasal tip. Arch Otolaryngol 1971;93(5):458–464
7. Foda HMT. Alar setback technique: a controlled method of nasal tip deprojection. Arch Otolaryngol Head Neck Surg 2001;127(11):1341–1346
8. Anderson JR. The dynamics of rhinoplasty. In: Bustamant GA, ed. Proceedings of the Ninth International Congress of Otolaryngology, Mexico City, August 10–14, 1969. Amsterdam, the Netherlands: Excerpta Medica; 1970
9. Adamson PA, Litner JA, Dahiya R. The M-arch model: a new concept of nasal tip dynamics. Arch Facial Plast Surg 2006;8(1):16–25
10. Foda HMT, Kridel RWH. Lateral crural steal and lateral crural overlay: an objective evaluation. Arch Otolaryngol Head Neck Surg 1999;125(12):1365–1370
11. Ghazipour A, Ghadakzadeh S, Karimian N. The comparison between two different combinations of alar cartilage-modifying techniques: is lateral crural steal the choice? Eur Arch Otorhinolaryngol 2009;266(3):391–395
12. Foda HMT. External rhinoplasty for the Arabian nose: a columellar scar analysis. Aesthetic Plast Surg 2004;28(5):312–316
13. Foda HMT. External rhinoplasty: a critical analysis of 500 cases. J Laryngol Otol 2003;117(6):473–477
14. Foda HMT. The caudal septum replacement graft. Arch Facial Plast Surg 2008;10(3):152–157
15. Caronni EP. A new method to correct the nasolabial angle in rhinoplasty. Plast Reconstr Surg 1972;50(4): 338–340
16. Fanous N, Yoskovitch A. Premaxillary augmentation: adjunct to rhinoplasty. Plast Reconstr Surg 2000;106(3): 707–712
17. Kridel RWH, Kraus WM. Grafts and implants in revision rhinoplasty. Facial Plast Surg Clin North Am 1995;3:473–486
18. Cook TA, Wang TD, Brownrigg PJ, Quatela VC. Significant premaxillary augmentation. Arch Otolaryngol Head Neck Surg 1990;116(10):1197–1201
19. Schoenrock LD, Reppucci AD. Correction of subcutaneous facial defects using Gore-Tex. Facial Plast Surg Clin North Am 1994;2:373–388
20. Foda HMT. Mersilene mesh in premaxillary augmentation. Aesthetic Plast Surg 2005;29(3):169–173
21. Beekhuis GJ. Mersilene mesh to augment the nasal bridge. Am J Cosmet Surg 1986;3(2):49–53
22. McCollough EG, Weil C. Augmentation of facial defects using Mersilene mesh implants. Otolaryngol Head Neck Surg (1979) 1979;87(4):515–521
23. Slavit DH, Bansberg SF, Facer GW, Kern EB. Reconstruction of caudal end of septum. A case for transplantation. Arch Otolaryngol Head Neck Surg 1995;121(10):1091–1098
24. Pirsig W, Kern EB, Verse T. Reconstruction of anterior nasal septum: back-to-back autogenous ear cartilage graft. Laryngoscope 2004;114(4):627–638
25. Naficy S, Baker SR. Lengthening the short nose. Arch Otolaryngol Head Neck Surg 1998;124(7):809–813
26. Gruber RP. Surgical correction of the short nose. Aesthetic Plast Surg 2002;26(Suppl 1):S6
27. Guyuron B, Varghai A. Lengthening the nose with a tongue-and-groove technique. Plast Reconstr Surg 2003;111(4):1533–1539, discussion 1540–1541
28. Toriumi DM. New concepts in nasal tip contouring. Arch Facial Plast Surg 2006;8(3):156–185
29. Toriumi DM, Pero CD. Asian rhinoplasty. Clin Plast Surg 2010;37(2):335–352

28 Approaches to the Middle Eastern Nose

Sameer Ali Bafaqeeh and Tareq Alotaibi

28.1 Introduction

Rhinoplasty is one of the most challenging facial plastic operations for the Middle Eastern patient. Middle Eastern patients are defined as people of Arabic, Turkish, North African, or Persian descent. Of this population, the Arab countries have the widest geographical distribution. The Arab countries are divided into the Gulf nations (Saudi Arabia, Kuwait, Bahrain, Qatar, Oman, United Arab Emirates, and Iraq) and the non-Gulf nations on the Mediterranean Sea (Morocco, Algeria, Tunisia, Libya, Egypt, Syria, and Lebanon). Patients from non-Gulf nations usually desire more tip projection and less dorsal height than patients from Gulf countries.[1]

In Saudi Arabia, the surgeon encounters all types of Middle Eastern noses. Normal nasal anthropometric measurements are listed in **Table 28.1**. In the general Saudi population, the male nasolabial angle averages 100.4 degrees, and the female, 102.3 degrees.[2] Saudi noses have unique features (**Table 28.2** and **Table 28.3**)[2] and it is important to recognize them to avoid an operated look.

Surgery on Middle Eastern noses using techniques described for persons of European descent can be problematic. Nevertheless, there are characteristics of beauty that are agreed upon independent of race or gender. Beautiful faces and noses are those with symmetrical and harmonious features.

In this chapter, we discuss preoperative counseling, facial analysis, surgical techniques, postoperative management, and frequent complications of rhinoplasty in Middle Eastern noses.

Table 28.1 Nasal anthropometric findings (expressed as mean [SD]) in Saudi Arabian men and women

Anthropometric measure	Men (n = 104)	Women (n = 105)
Intercanthal width	31.6 (2.7)	32.6 (2.8)
Nasal root width	20.8 (2.9)	23.1 (2.4)
Nasal root slope length	19.5 (1.9)	15.2 (2.3)
Nasal width	38.5 (3.1)	35.6 (3.3)
Cutaneous upper lip	14.9 (2.4)	13.6 (2.2)
Nose height	53.5 (3.7)	49.4 (3.9)
Nasal bridge length	50.6 (4.2)	43.3 (4.1)
Nasofrontal angle	135.9 (9.6)	145.9 (6.1)
Nasolabial angle	100.4 (16.4)	102.3 (10.0)
Nasofacial angle	41.4 (6.8)	33.3 (4.1)
Nasomental angle	130.8 (4.9)	128.9 (6.5)
Glabellonasal angle	155.9 (8.4)	173.8 (5.7)
Nasal tip angle	90.5 (6.0)	97.3 (5.1)
Nasal base width	25.6 (4.9)	29.9 (3.0)
Alar length	25.8 (2.0)	24.2 (2.6)
Alar width	5.6 (0.9)	5.1 (0.9)
Columella width	9.6 (2.3)	11.4 (1.6)
Columella length	9.3 (1.9)	11.2 (1.6)
Nasal tip protrusion	20.7 (2.3)	22.1 (2.2)
Ala slope angle	92.3 (9.9)	89.3 (9.0)

28.2 Preoperative Counseling

Most of our patients who come for rhinoplasty are seen two or three times before surgery is actually scheduled. Many patients bring family members during the first consultation. It is important to define what the patient wants and if he/she wants to preserve his/her ethnic identity. It is not uncommon to deal with patients with high expectations and frequently with patients who ask the surgeon to decide on their behalf what changes should be made. Digital photography is performed during the first visit. After physical examination of the nose, digital imaging is used to show patients possible surgical options.

During preoperative counseling, it is important to assess the personality of the patient and family members through open-ended questions. We urge the patients to point out what they don't like about their nose and what changes they think should be made. To obtain satisfactory results, this discussion should involve the head of the family. Some patients cannot decide what their needs are and ask a family member to decide on their behalf. The surgeon should be careful with this type of personality and should ask the patient and the family member for a second or third visit, allowing time to decide whether a patient with this personality is a candidate for surgery.

Table 28.2 Comparison of nasal anthropometric findings (expressed as mean [SD]) in men

Anthropometric measure	Saudi Arabian (n = 104)	Chinese (n = 28)	Caucasian (n = 24)	Iranian (n = 24)	Turkish (n = 108)	African American (n = 28)	Caucasian (Canadian) (n = 60)
Intercanthal width	31.6 (2.7)	35 (0.3)*	31 (0.3)	32 (3)	N/A	N/A	N/A
Nasal root width	20.8 (2.9)	19 (0.2)*	18 (0.2)*	N/A	29.74 (0.46)*	26.8 (0.52)*	N/A
Nasal width	38.5 (3.1)	41 (0.3)*	37 (0.4)*	N/A	33.63 (0.27)*	43.5 (0.39)*	36.9 (2.8)*
Nasal bridge length	50.6 (4.2)	N/A	N/A	50 (3)	56.92 (0.44)*	52.4 (0.44)*	N/A
Nasofrontal angle	135.9 (9.6)	129.3 (6.5)*	129 (10.4)*	126 (6)*	N/A	N/A	N/A
Nasolabial angle	110.4 (16.4)	86.2 (12.5)*	96.8 (7.8)	97 (11)	N/A	N/A	N/A
Nasofacial angle	41.4 (6.8)	34.7 (6.8)*	36.7 (7)*	36 (4)*	N/A	N/A	N/A
Nasomental angle	130.8 (4.9)	N/A	N/A	125 (6)*	N/A	N/A	N/A
Nasal tip angle	90.5 (6.0)	102.6 (10.3)*	103 (9)*	N/A	N/A	N/A	N/A
Nasal base width	25.6 (4.9)	N/A	N/A	N/A	23.14 (0.28)*	N/A	35 (3)*
Alar width	5.6 (0.9)	N/A	N/A	N/A	N/A	N/A	N/A
Columella length	9.3 (1.9)	N/A	N/A	N/A	9.34 (0.15)	10.0 (0.33)	N/A
Nasal tip protrusion	20.7 (2.3)	25 (0.3)*	32 (0.2)*	N/A	N/A	N/A	N/A

*Significantly different. N/A indicates the value is not available in the study.

Used with permission from Al-Qattan MM, Alsaeed AA, Al-Madani OK, et al. Anthropometry of the Saudi Arabian nose. J Craniofac Surg 2012;23(3):821–824.

The digital photographs that were taken on the first visit are reviewed during the second visit. Possible surgical solutions are discussed and images are morphed to suggest surgical outcomes. Nevertheless, it is important that the patient understand that digital morphing is a simulation and that final results can vary from what was seen on the computer screen. This understanding helps prevent patient dissatisfaction with surgical results. Consent forms are explained, are discussed, and are signed by the patient and the family member. Sometimes, a third office visit is needed before a final decision on surgery is reached.

28.3 Facial Analysis

Older Middle Eastern patients often express the feeling that their noses are large, with boxy, droopy tips, and a deviated profile. (See box **Features of the Middle Eastern Nose on Frontal View,** box **Features of the Middle Eastern Nose on Lateral View,** and box **Features of the Middle Eastern Nose on Base View.**) They ask for conservative surgeries that can produce enough changes to make the surgery worth the money invested. Younger patients want good tip projection and rotation with a straight dorsum. Most of them have a particular "ideal" nose in mind before contacting the surgeon.

Middle Eastern patients present with variable skin thickness. The majority have normal to slightly thick skin (Fitzpatrick skin type III–IV) while a third of patients have thick, oily skin, a high density of pilosebaceous units, an amorphous tip appearance, and supratip fullness.[3,4]

Almost all patients have some degree of dorsal deviation with variable skin thickness. On the frontal view (**Fig. 28.1**), the nasal bones are commonly long and the middle vault is narrow, with long upper lateral cartilages that are wide at the scroll area.[5] The tip is dependent, with poor support, while the base is often asymmetrical and apparently wide. Asymmetry of the face in general is also very common; rarely do we come across cases where surgery can be done without osteotomies.

On the lateral view (**Fig. 28.2**), the radix can be deep and low. Many patients have a dorsal bony and cartilaginous hump, which makes spreader grafts essential to avoid middle vault deformities and functional problems. Tip projection is often inadequate and under-rotated. A droopy tip

Table 28.3 Comparison of nasal anthropometric findings (expressed as mean [SD]) in women

Anthropometric measure	Saudi Arabian (n = 105)	Chinese (n = 26)	White (n = 26)	Iranian (n = 50)	White (Canadian) (n = 60)	Indian American (n = 102)	Korean American (n = 72)	African American mean (SEM) (n = 108)
Intercanthal width	32.6 (2.8)	34 (0.3)*	29 (0.4)*	30 (3)*	N/A	31.2 (3.7)*	N/A	N/A
Nasal root width	23.1 (2.4)	19 (0.2)*	16 (0.2)*	N/A	N/A	N/A	21.1 (4.1)*	N/A
Nasal width	35.6 (3.3)	38 (0.3)*	34 (0.3)*	N/A	32.9 (2.7)*	35.6 (3.3)	35.5 (3.4)	38.0 (0.28)*
Nose height	49.9 (3.9)	N/A	N/A	N/A	N/A	45.6 (3.5)*	51.8 (4.3)*	48.0 (0.4)
Nasal bridge length	43.3 (4.1)	N/A	N/A	45 (3)*	N/A	39.2 (3.9)*	43.5 (3.9)	N/A
Nasofrontal angle	145.9 (6.1)	136.6 (6.5)*	135.3 (3.7)*	134 (8)	N/A	138.2 (8.1)*	136.8 (6.4)*	N/A
Nasolabial angle	102.3 (10.0)	87.6 (13.7)*	101.8 (8.8)	98 (10)*	N/A	97.2 (10.6)*	92.1 (9.2)*	N/A
Nasofacial angle	33.3 (4.1)	33.7 (5.5)	36.6 (5.2)*	36 (3)*	N/A	31.8 (4.5)*	32.3 (5.1)	N/A
Nasomental angle	128.9 (6.5)	N/A	N/A	124 (4)*	N/A	N/A	128 (4.1)	N/A
Nasal tip angle	97.3 (5.1)	112.3 (6.6)*	104.6 (9.3)*	N/A	N/A	N/A	N/A	N/A
Nasal base width	29.9 (3.0)	N/A	N/A	N/A	31.6 (2.8)*	31.9 (5.1)*	N/A	N/A
Alar length	24.2 (2.6)	N/A	N/A	N/A	N/A	29.2 (3.0)*	29.9 (3.1)*	N/A
Alar width	5.1 (0.9)	N/A	N/A	N/A	N/A	5.0 (0.9)	4.5 (0.8)*	N/A
Columella length	11.2 (1.6)	N/A	N/A	N/A	N/A	9.1 (1.9)*	7.5 (1.1)*	N/A
Nasal tip protrusion	22.1 (2.2)	24 (0.4)*	28 (0.3)*	N/A	N/A	19.1 (2.0)*	19.6 (1.4)*	N/A

*Significantly different. N/A indicates the value is not available in the study.

Used with permission from Al-Qattan MM, Alsaeed AA, Al-Madani OK, et al. Anthropometry of the Saudi Arabian nose. J Craniofac Surg 2012;23(3):821–824.

Features of the Middle Eastern Nose on Frontal View

- Variable nasal skin
- Deviated nasal dorsum
- Facial asymmetry, including base asymmetry
- Long nasal bones
- Narrow middle vault
- Large and long lateral crura
- Long upper lateral cartilage
- Inferior rotated tip

is one of the most frequent complaints among our patients. The ptosis can be mild, moderate, or severe according to the degree of tip rotation and projection. Depending on the severity of the tip ptosis, surgical techniques will vary.

Features of the Middle Eastern Nose on Lateral View

- Low radix
- Prominent hump
- Poor tip projection
- Hanging columella
- Acute nasolabial angle

The tip often plunges significantly upon smiling, while the columella is commonly hanging, with relatively deficient anterior nasal spine.

On the base view (**Fig. 28.3**), it is not uncommon to find the tip deviated to one side, with asymmetrical nostrils due to a dislocated caudal septum. The columella is commonly short and deviated.

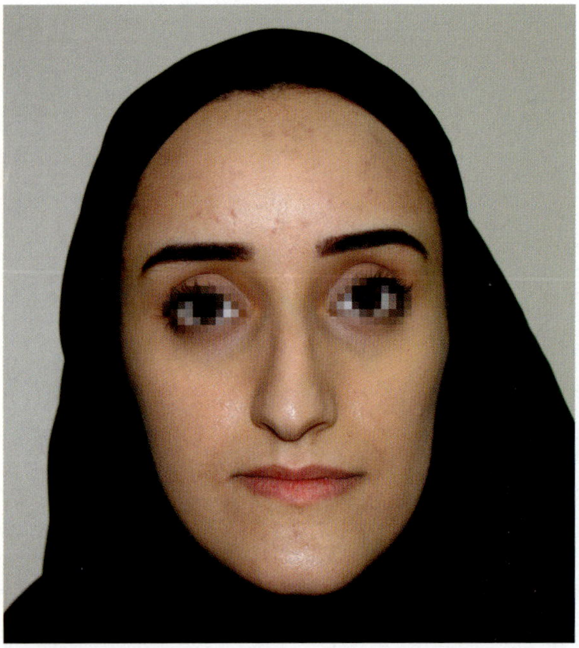

Fig. 28.1 Frontal view of a patient with typical features of a Middle Eastern nose.

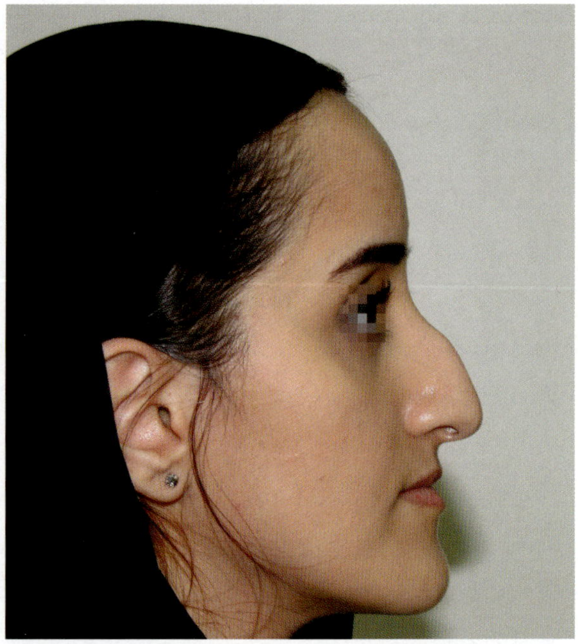

Fig. 28.2 Lateral view of a typical Middle Eastern nose.

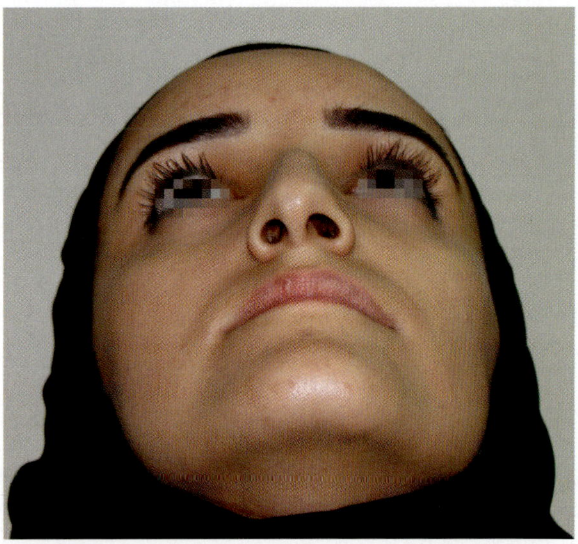

Fig. 28.3 Basilar view of a typical Middle Eastern nose.

Features of the Middle Eastern Nose on Base View

- Broad and deviated tip
- Asymmetric nostrils
- Flaring footplates
- Relatively short columella
- Dislocated caudal septum

28.4 Surgical Techniques

The fundamental concept is to set the ideal profile line first and then to create the desired tip. The problems most frequently encountered are: prominent dorsum and hump; wide bony and cartilaginous nasal vaults; a droopy nasal tip; acute nasolabial angle; thick, sebaceous, and hairy skin; asymmetrical, amorphous bulbous broad tip; and trauma-related crooked nose. A summary of possible surgical procedures is listed below.[6,7,8,9,10,11,12] The sequence of surgical steps and techniques can be modified according to the surgeon's preference.

- Open approach +/– skin defatting
- Tip analysis
- Dorsal reduction
- Septal surgery + harvesting of septal cartilage
- Osteotomies
- Spreader grafts, or auto spreader grafts
- Tip work
  - Conservative cephalic trim of alar cartilages
  - Columellar strut
  - Double-dome unit suturing technique/lateral crural steal
  - Lateral crural spanning sutures
  - Onlay tip graft +/– shield graft
  - Lateral crural overlay technique
  - Tongue-in-groove technique
- Dorsal-only graft

- Plumping graft
- Alar rim graft
- Alar base modifications

Most rhinoplasties performed by the senior author are cartilage-preserving techniques where grafts are used instead of cartilage resection.[7] This is due to the nature of skin and underlying septal and lateral cartilage. The procedure usually follows the sequence:

- Open approach with optional skin defatting
- Tip analysis
- Dorsal reduction and modification of caudal septum and the anterior septal angle as indicated
- Septal surgery, including harvesting of septal cartilage
- Osteotomies
- Insertion of spreader grafts or auto spreader grafts if possible
- Columellar strut, or extended columellar strut
- Suturing techniques in the nasal tip: transdomal sutures, lateral crural steal, alar spanning sutures
- Conservative cephalic trim of lateral crura/lateral crural turn-in flap
- Grafts in the nasal tip and dorsum: single or multiple onlay tip grafts, shield graft, and radix grafts as needed
- Lateral crural overlay technique in marked tip ptosis, especially when ptosis is combined with over-projection[10]
- Tongue-in-groove technique
- Dorsal-only graft of intact, crushed, or diced cartilage wrapped in temporalis fascia or fascia lata graft
- Premaxilla grafts (in front of nasal spine): cartilage pieces; morcelized, diced, or crushed cartilage

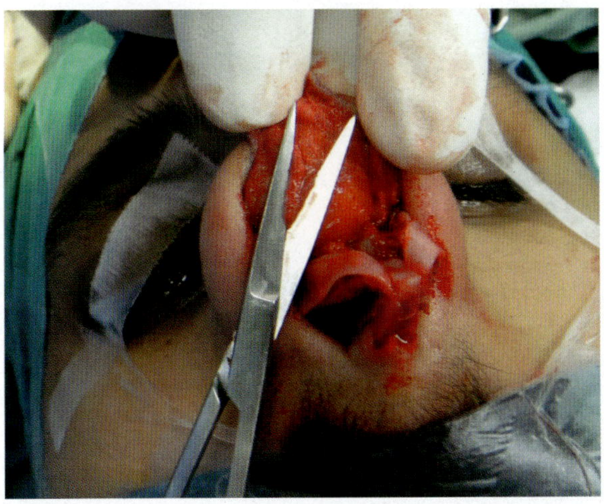

Fig. 28.4 Defatting of the skin envelope by dissection in the subdermal plane.

- Alar rim grafts
- Alar base modification as indicated

28.4.1 Skin Envelope

Surprisingly, the majority of Middle Eastern patients have normal to slightly thick skin. Saudi patients frequently have Fitzpatrick skin types III through IV. About a third of patients have thick, heavy, sebaceous skin. In these cases, defatting of the subdermal plane of the nasal tip lobule is necessary. Defatting is done using a small scissor that is positioned parallel to the dermis during debulking, to prevent injury to the subdermal plexus (**Fig. 28.4**). An Adson forceps may be used instead of scissors.

Care should be taken to avoid being too close to the dermis, which can produce irregularities and vascular compromise.[13] Thick and heavy sebaceous skin usually hides underlying irregularities. It can also produce persistent postoperative swelling and the pollybeak deformity, which can be prevented in the early postoperative period by placing nasal splints that extend inferiorly just to the area of the supratip break (**Fig. 28.5**).

28.4.2 The Dorsum

Surgical planning for the dorsum involves the height of the radix and the width of the osteocartilaginous vault. Dorsal reduction is done in an incremental fashion using a no. 11 blade for the cartilaginous vault and sharp osteotomes and rasps for the bony vault (**Fig. 28.6**). In most cases, we are dealing with an underprojecting nasal tip, so we recommend to start tip work adjustment before hump removal in order to avoid overresection. The surgeon art the end of the surgery has to keep almost 6-mm tip-to-dorsum height to prevent postoperative pollybeak or tip-to-dorsum imbalance deformity.

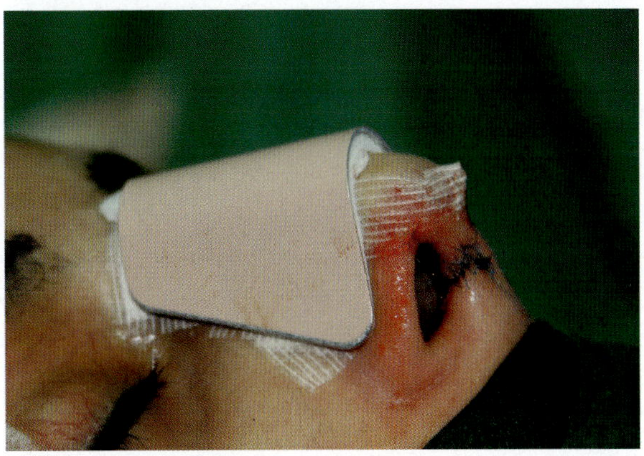

Fig. 28.5 The nasal splints are extended inferiorly just to the area of the supratip break.

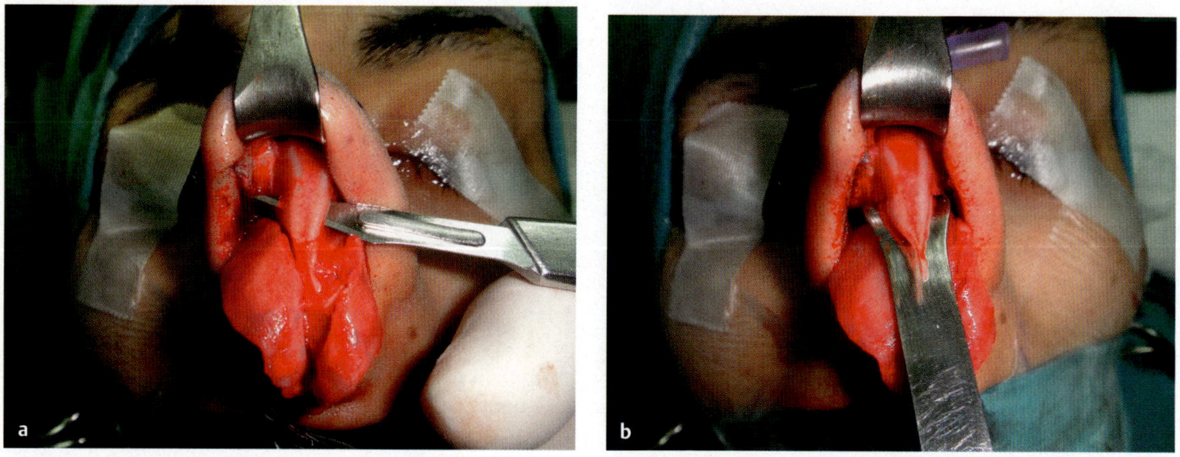

Fig. 28.6 **(a)** Starting excision of the cartilaginous hump with a no. 11 blade directed toward the anterior septal angle. **(b)** Removal of the bony hump with sharp osteotome.

Dorsal humps among our patients vary widely, but the greatest reductions are usually done on the cartilaginous hump (**Fig. 28.7**), which makes spreader grafts (**Fig. 28.8**) essential to avoid any middle nasal vault deformities (inverted-V deformity) or functional compromise of the internal nasal valve.

When necessary, double spreader grafts can be placed unilaterally to correct dorsal deviations. The first choice in spreader grafts is to use septal cartilage, but in revision cases, where there is not enough septal cartilage, several alternatives are available, including irradiated rib cartilage, autologous rib cartilage, or auricular cartilage (**Fig. 28.9**). Osteotomies, when performed, are made using a low-to-low technique, because bony width usually starts at the ascending process of the maxilla.

28.4.3 The Scroll Junction

A unique anatomical finding in Middle Eastern patients is the extreme width of the upper lateral cartilages at their junction with the lateral crus of the alar cartilage (**Fig. 28.10**). This scroll area is divided sharply. Instead of performing a cephalic trim of the lateral crus of the alar cartilage, a turn-in flap technique is used, in which the cephalic edge of the alar cartilage is folded inward and sutured in place (**Fig. 28.11**). This technique will strengthen the lateral crura, correct any convexity of the alar cartilage, and prevent postoperative alar rim notching.

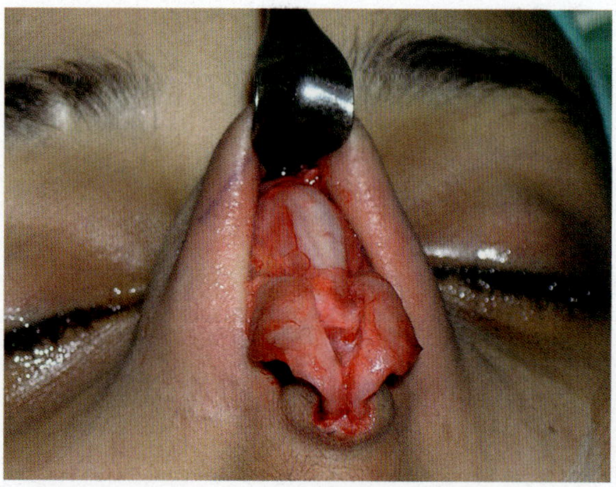

Fig. 28.7 Dorsal hump composed mainly of cartilage.

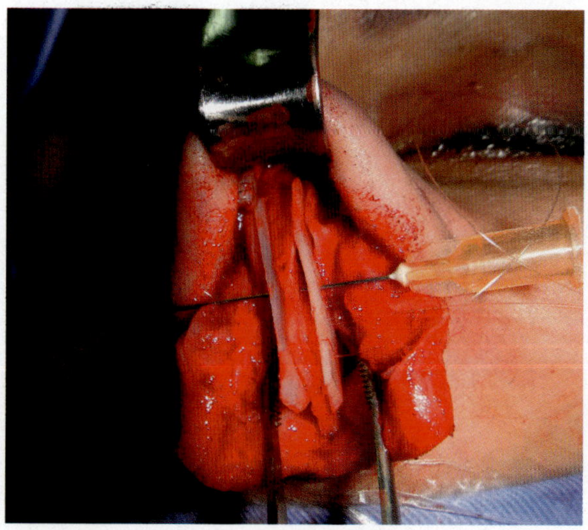

Fig. 28.8 Fixation of spreader grafts.

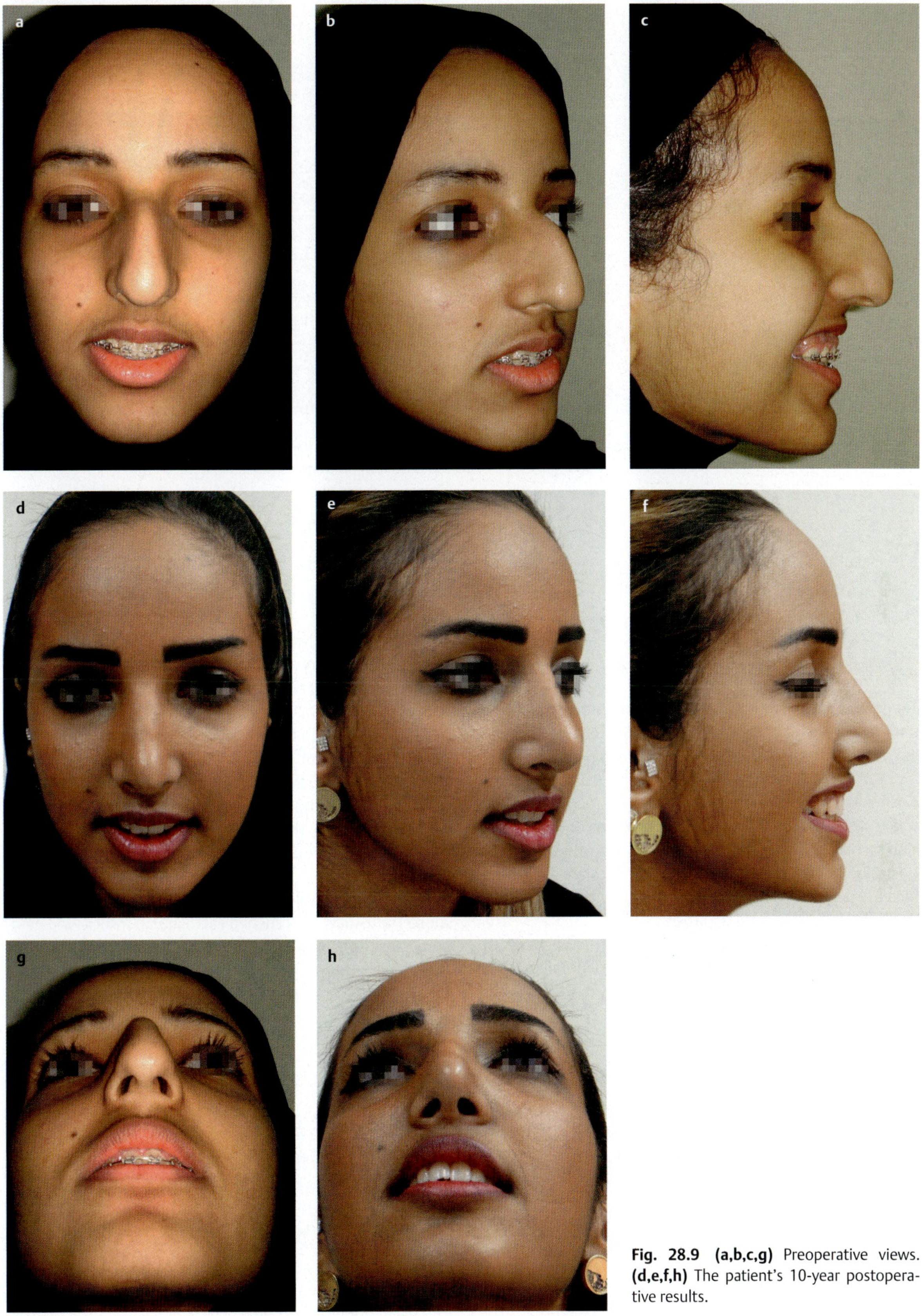

Fig. 28.9 (a,b,c,g) Preoperative views. **(d,e,f,h)** The patient's 10-year postoperative results.

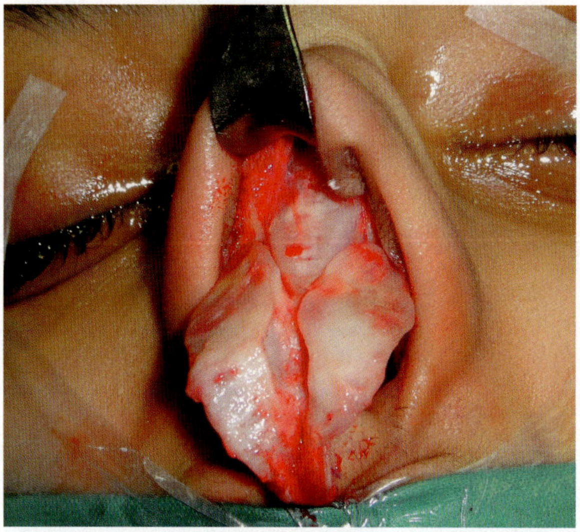

Fig. 28.10 Large scroll junction; note the size of the lower lateral cartilage.

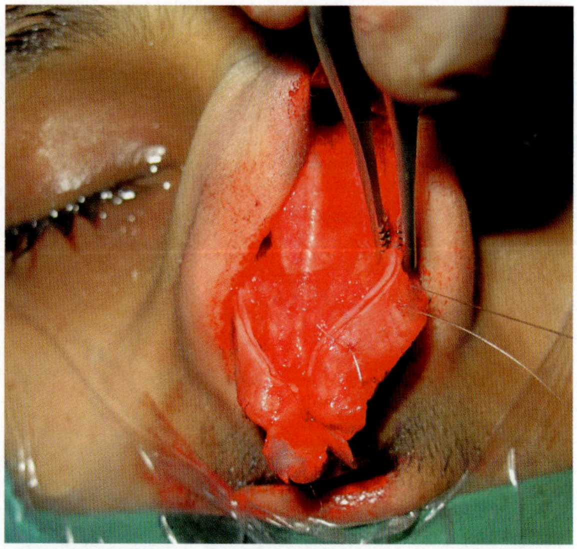

Fig. 28.11 Turn-in flap technique: cephalic trimming, with stitching of incised part under the main lateral crura.

28.4.4 Alar Cartilage

The skin envelope of Middle Eastern patients may hide the underlying details of the alar cartilage, which often requires aggressive tip-modification techniques (**Fig. 28.12**).

Middle Eastern patients' lateral crura usually are wide, nasal domes are undefined and flat, and medial crura are short, weak, and buckle easily. This anatomical shape of the alar cartilages usually results in ptotic and under-projected tips (**Fig. 28.12**). Several surgical techniques are available to increase projection and rotation of the tip; the technique used depends on the degree of tip ptosis.

In all rhinoplasties, when dealing with the nasal tip, a double-dome unit is created using horizontal mattress sutures for each dome and a transdomal mattress suture to bring both domes together. Lateral crural steal, an alar crural spanning suture, and a columellar strut are also used routinely in all patients.

In cases of mild tip ptosis, a conservative cephalic trim of the lateral crura will result in contraction of tissue in the scroll area, with a resulting upward rotation of the tip (**Fig. 28.13**). For moderate tip ptosis, an inverted triangle is removed from the caudal septum while taking care not to damage the septocolumellar ligaments (**Fig. 28.14** and **Fig. 28.15**).

Another technique is to insert plumping grafts (intact, morcelized, diced, or crushed cartilage) in front of the nasal spine, resulting in rotation of the nasal tip. This can be done through an internal or external incision (**Fig. 28.16** and **Fig. 28.17**).

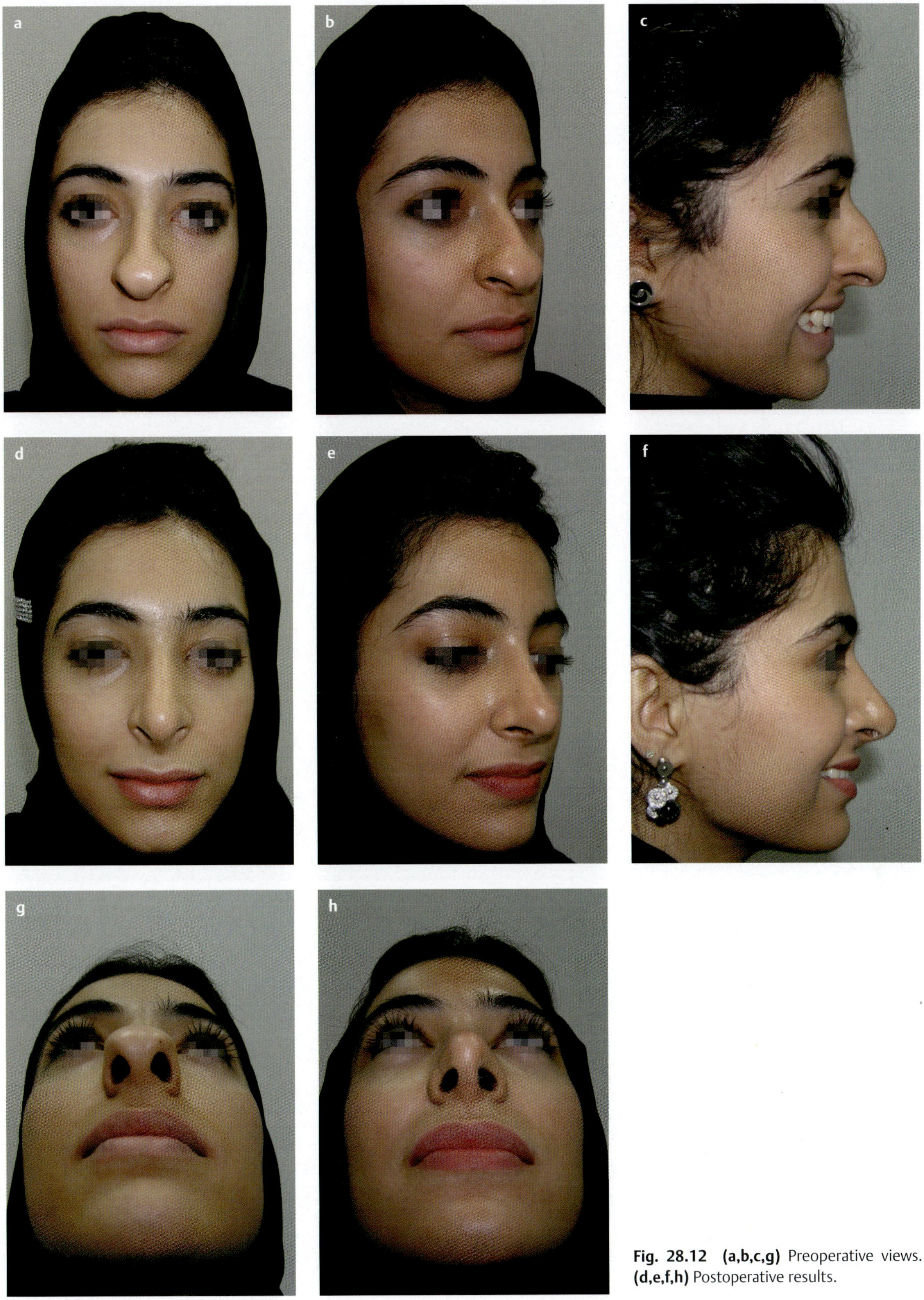

Fig. 28.12 (a,b,c,g) Preoperative views. **(d,e,f,h)** Postoperative results.

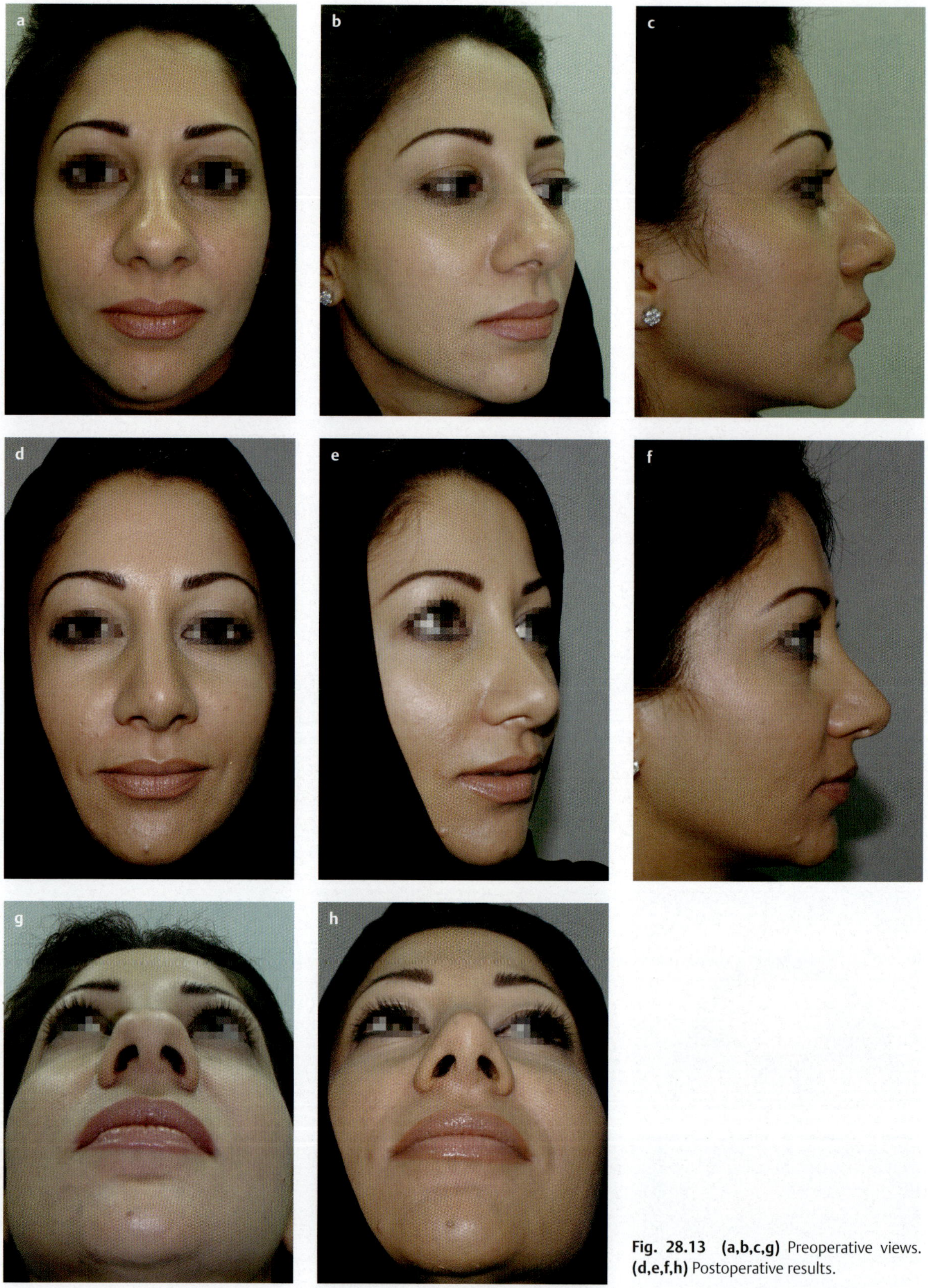

Fig. 28.13 **(a,b,c,g)** Preoperative views. **(d,e,f,h)** Postoperative results.

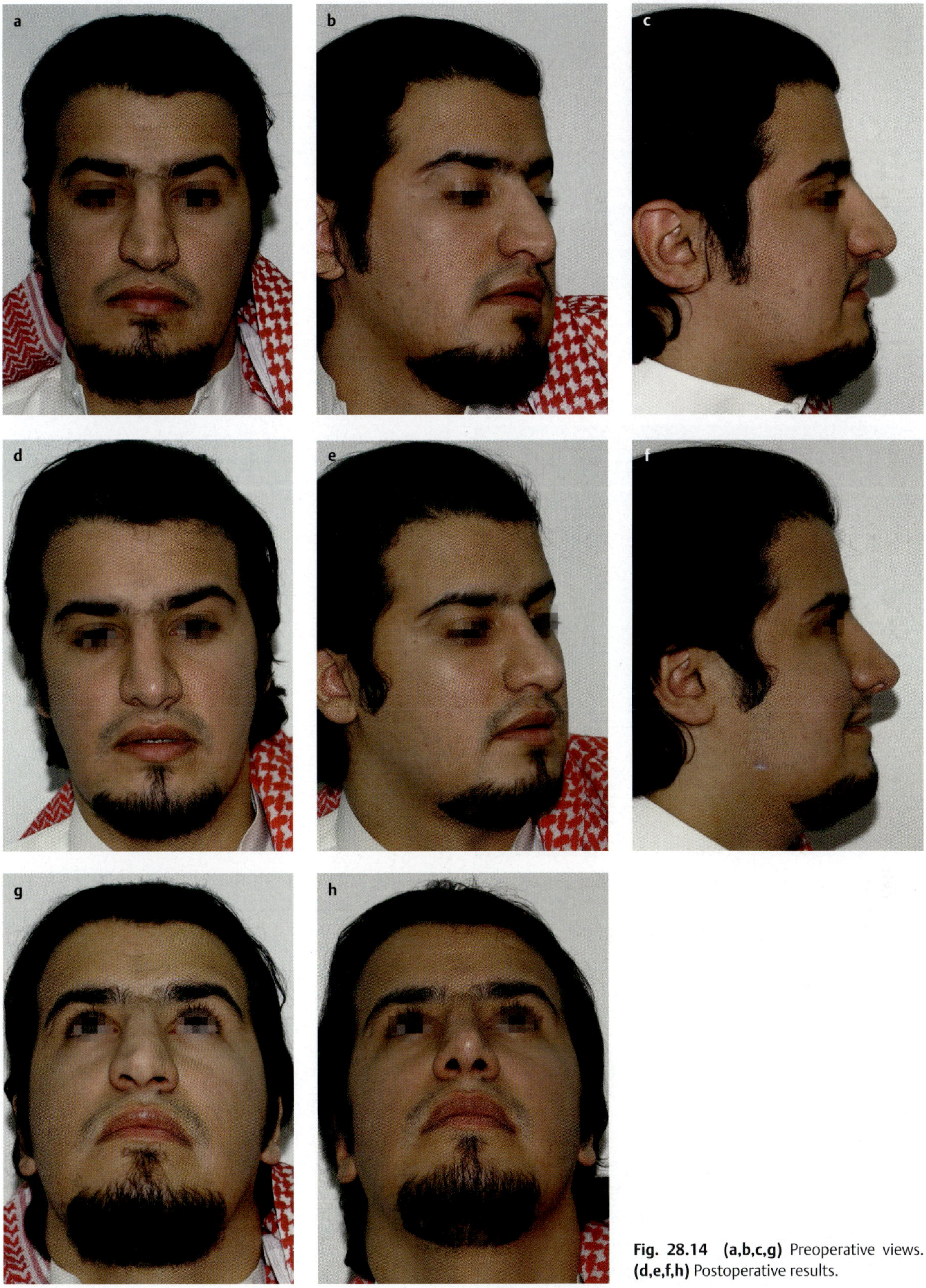

Fig. 28.14 **(a,b,c,g)** Preoperative views. **(d,e,f,h)** Postoperative results.

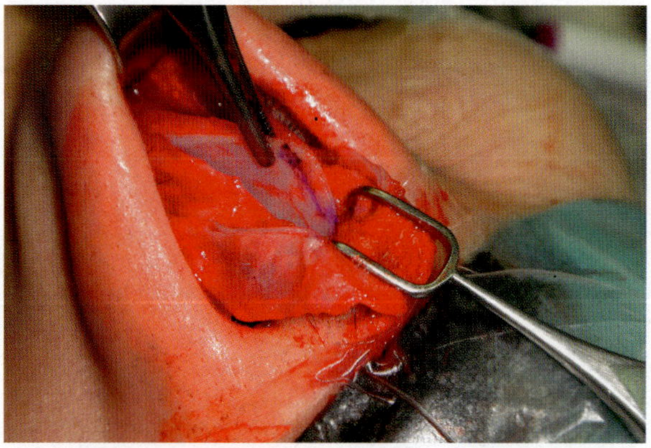

Fig. 28.15 Marking the incision site of the inverted triangle in the caudal septum.

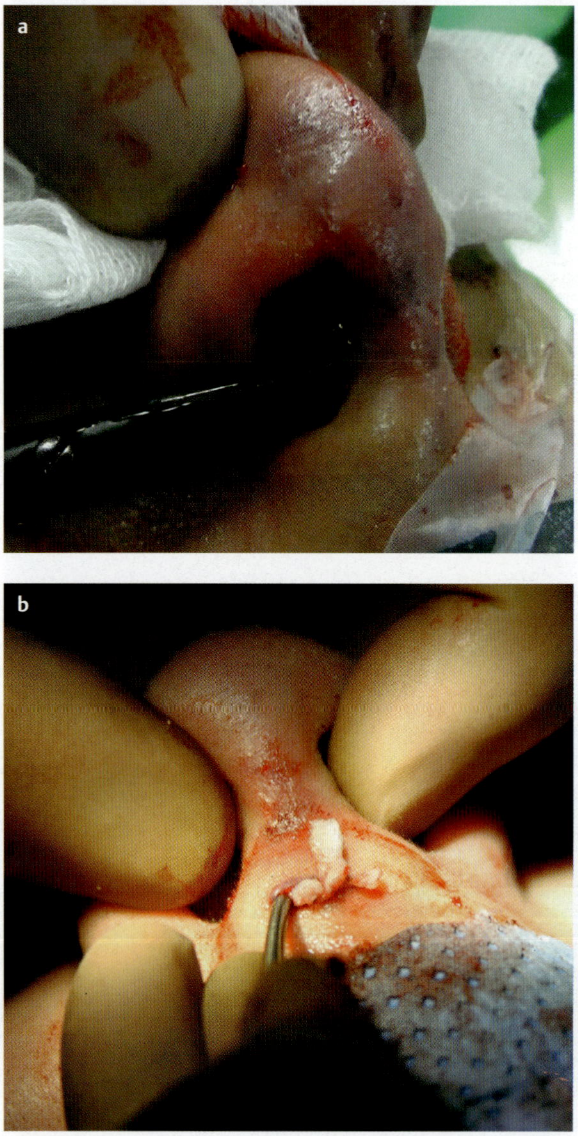

Fig. 28.16 **(a)** Insertion of plumping grafts through internal incision. **(b)** Insertion of plumping grafts through external incision.

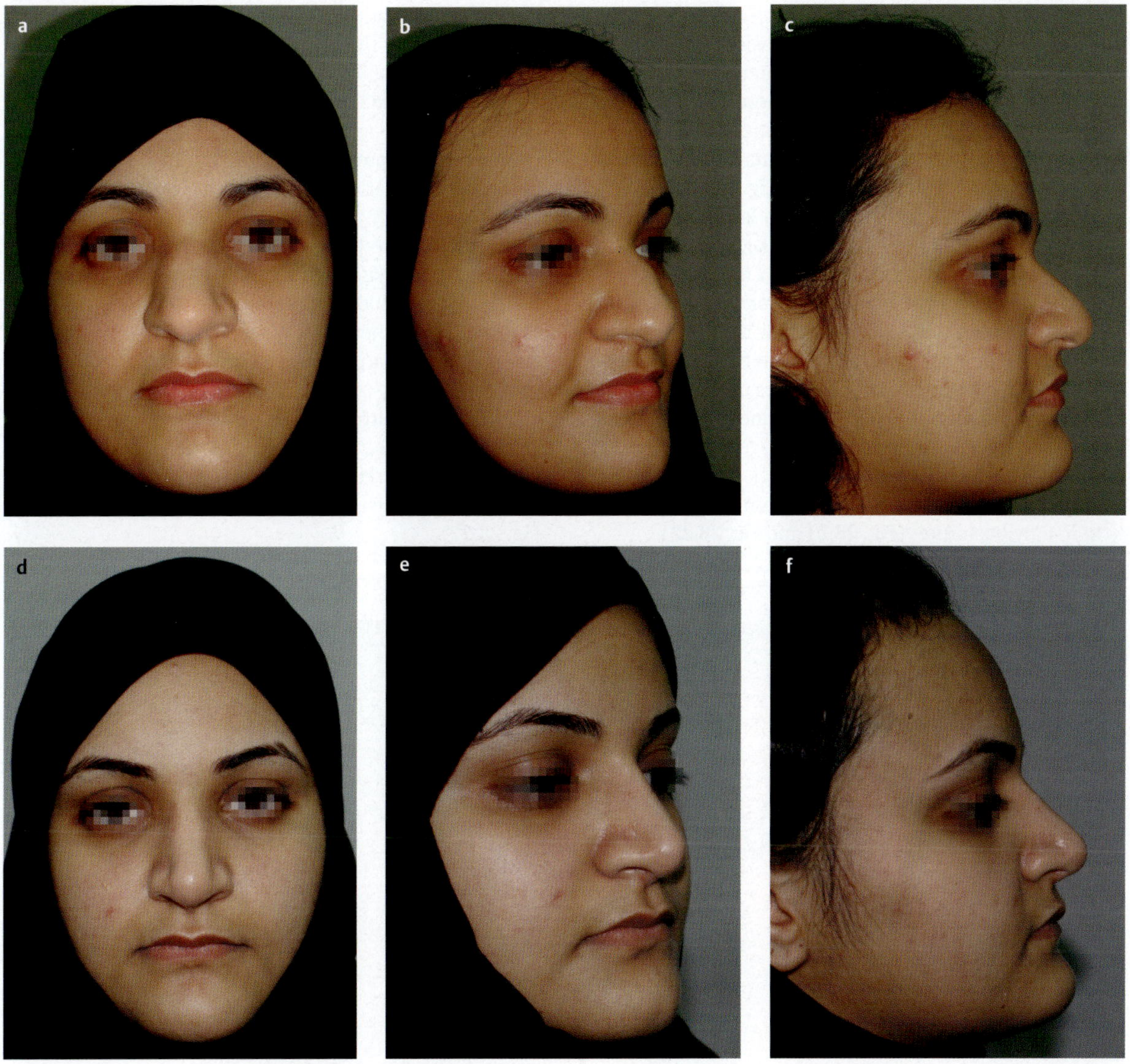

Fig. 28.17 **(a–c)** Preoperative views. **(d–f)** Postoperative results.

To increase the degree of tip projection, lateral crural steal is used. This technique involves lengthening the medial crura at the expense of the lateral crura and creating a new dome complex in a more lateral position (**Fig. 28.18** and **Fig. 28.19**). For further tip projection, onlay grafts of single or multiple pieces of intact septal cartilage can be fixed over the dome complex (**Fig. 28.20**).

In severely plunging, ptotic tips, a lateral crural overlay technique is used.[11,12] The alar cartilage is dissected free from the underlying vestibular skin in the dome and lateral crus area, and a conservative trim of the lateral crura is performed. When the skin is normal or thick, the cartilage is incised at the beginning of the posterior two-thirds. In thin-skinned patients, where the edges of the incised cartilage can be visible, the incision is done at the beginning of the posterior one-third of the cartilage. The incised segments are overlapped, with the anterior segment laid over the posterior segment and sutured in place with permanent 5–0 nylon sutures (**Fig. 28.21** and **Fig. 28.22**).

To avoid supratip fullness and to improve definition of the nasal tip after the lateral overlay technique, it is necessary to use the double-dome unit suturing technique with placement of a columellar strut (**Fig. 28.23**). Columellar struts help to strengthen the medial crura, give additional tip support, and preserve the stability of tip rotation and projection. They also correct asymmetries of the medial crura (**Fig. 28.24**).

Grafts like the lateral crura batten graft are used to camouflage any visible irregularities and to strengthen the lateral crura and, if necessary, the external nasal valve (**Fig. 28.25**). Furthermore, placing an alar rim graft will prevent postoperative alar notching and alar rim retraction (**Fig. 28.26**).

The senior author prefers to use a tongue-in-groove technique when the aim is to reduce the length of the nose in addition to correcting the ptosis. The caudal portion of the nasal septum is sutured between the two medial crura (**Fig. 28.27**).

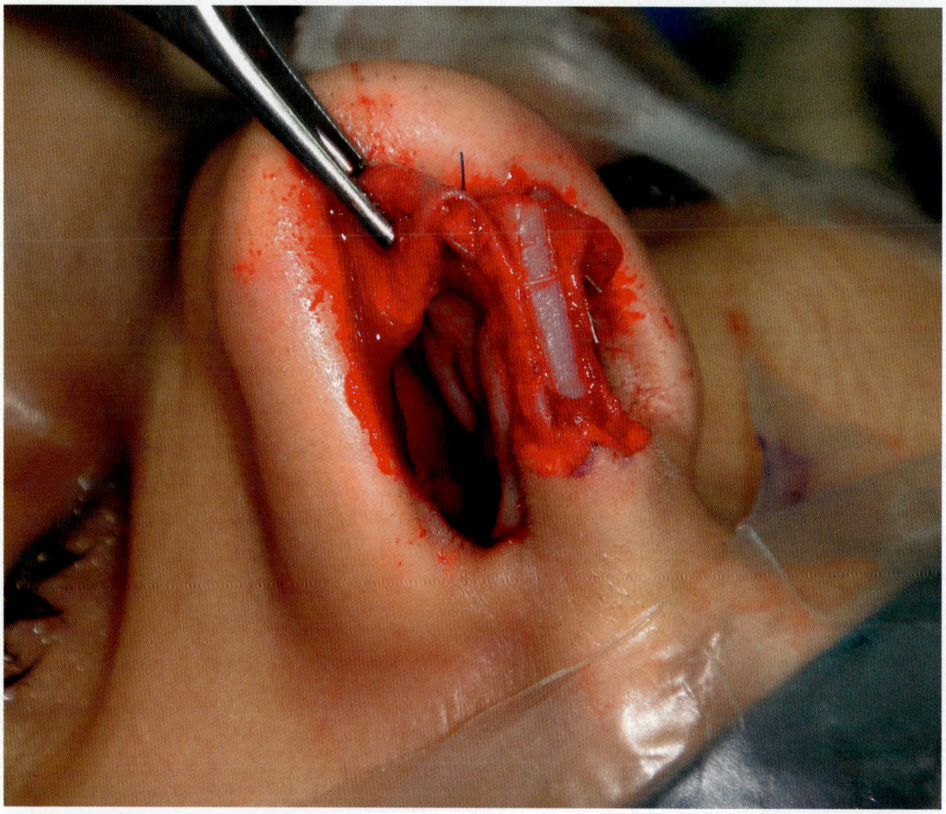

Fig. 28.18 Lateral crural steal with increasing tip projection at the right side.

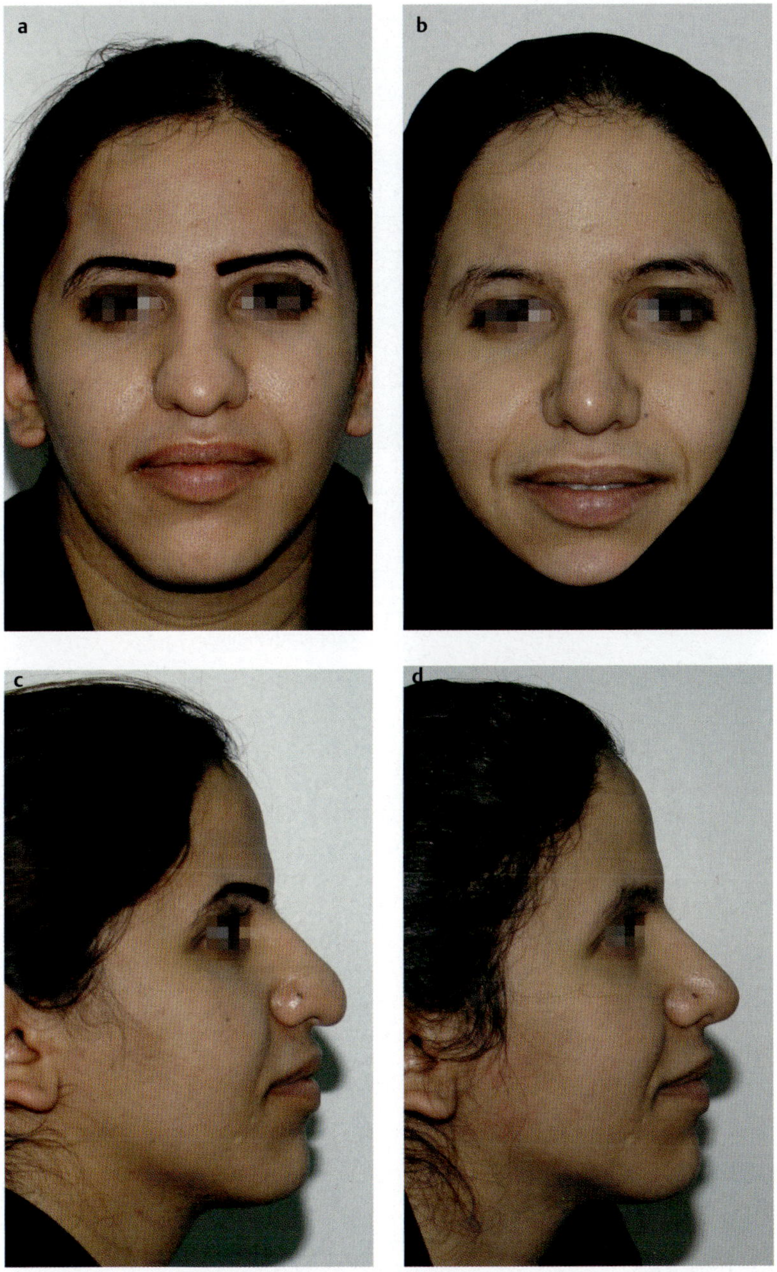

Fig. 28.19 **(a,c)** Preoperative views. **(b,d)** Postoperative results.

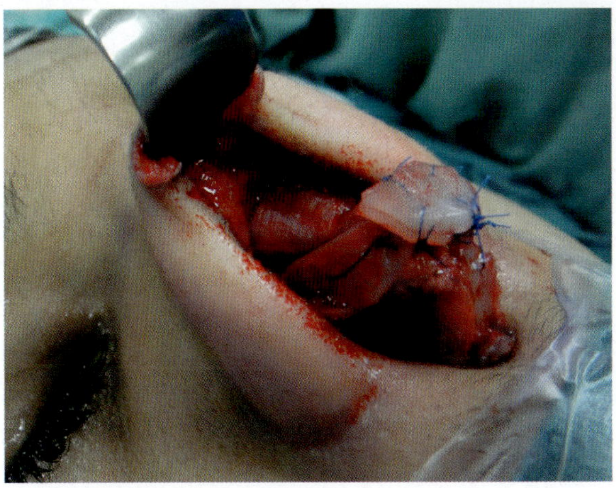

Fig. 28.20 Double-layer tip graft.

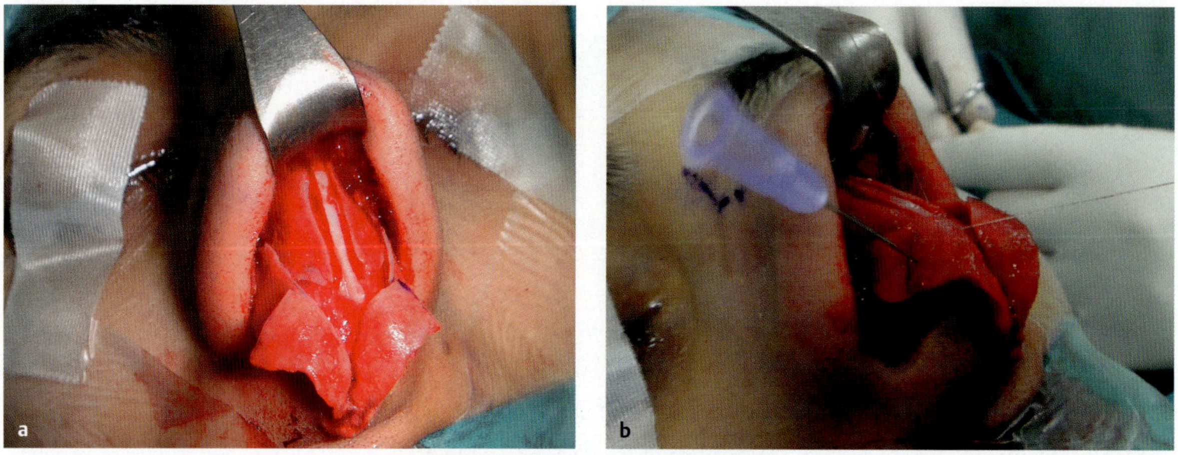

Fig. 28.21 **(a)** Cutting the lateral crura at the beginning of the posterior two-thirds (lateral crural overlay technique). **(b)** Suturing the anterior segment over the posterior segment of the lateral crura in the lateral crural overlay technique.

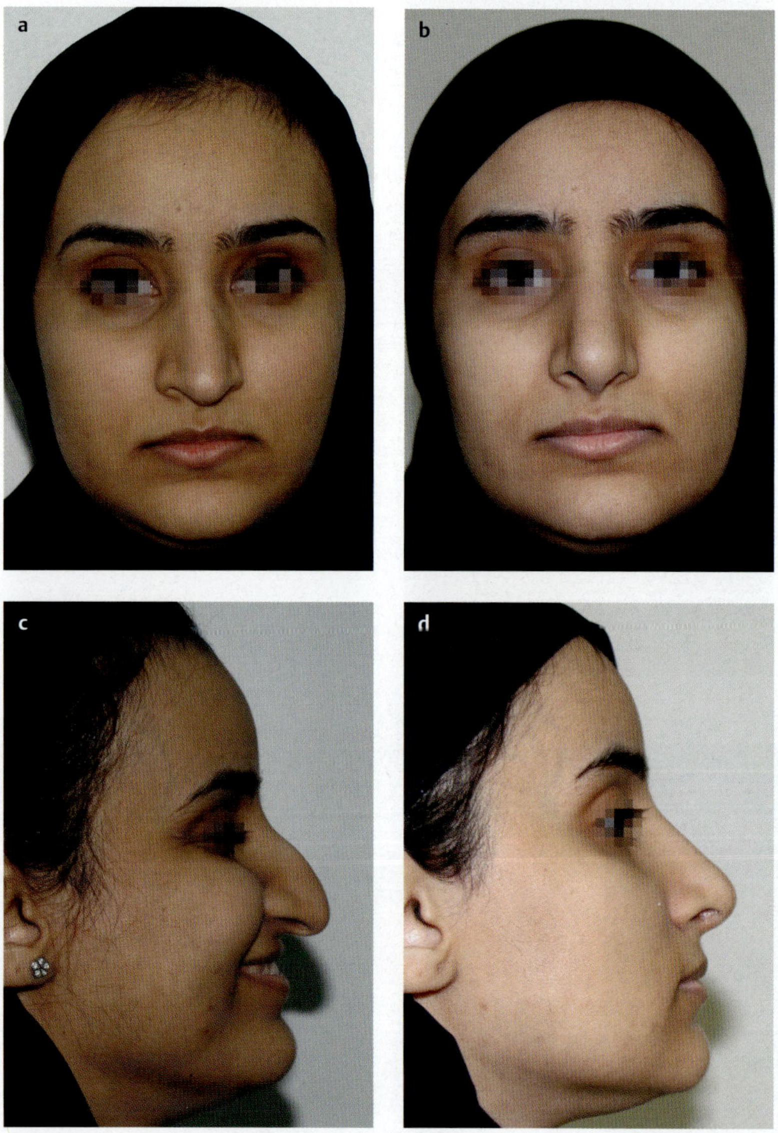

Fig. 28.22 **(a,c)** Preoperative views. **(b,d)** Postoperative views.

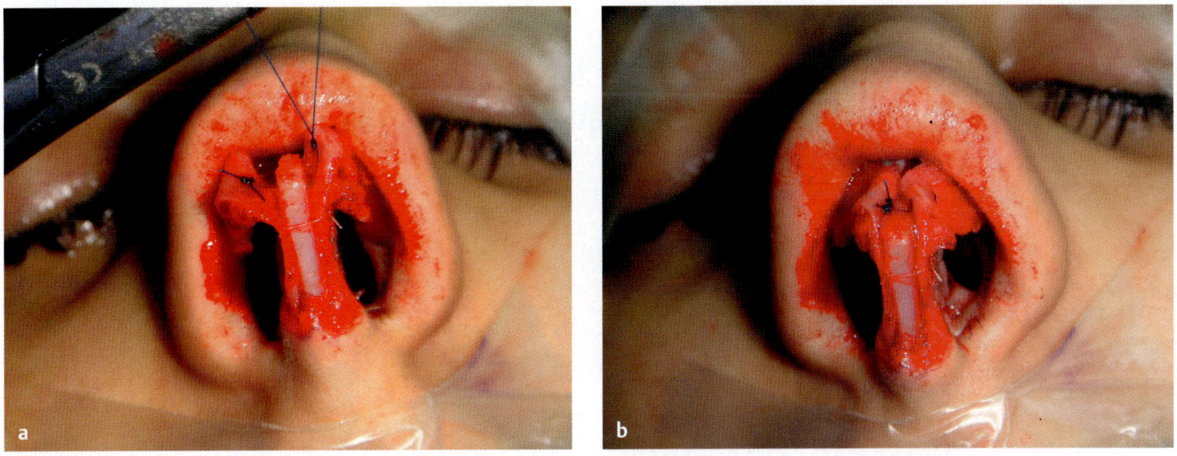

Fig. 28.23 **(a)** Showing columellar strut with horizontal mattress suture of each dome. **(b)** Double-dome technique showing the transdomal mattress suture of both new domes.

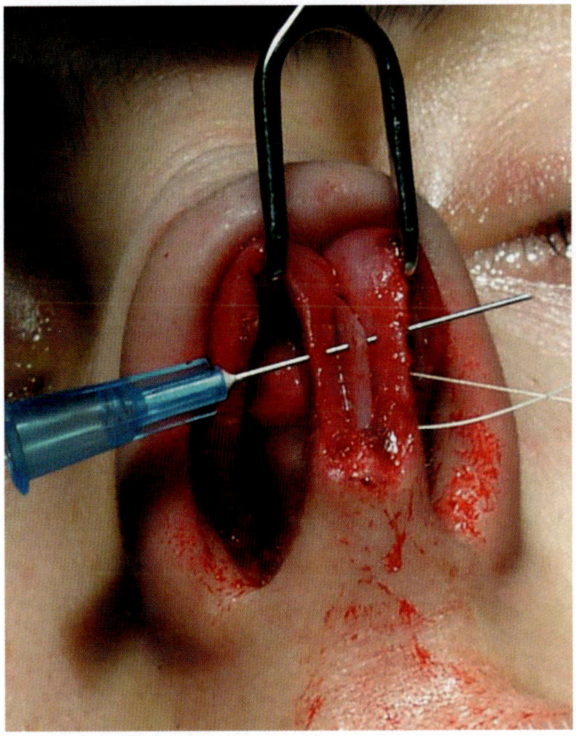

Fig. 28.24 Fixing the columellar strut.

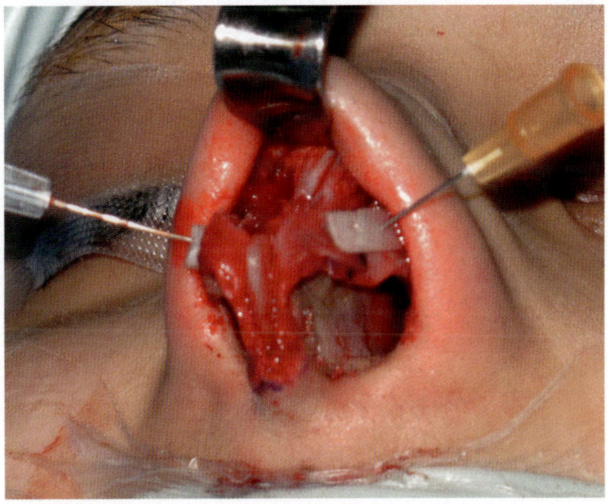

Fig. 28.25 Fixing the lateral crura batten graft.

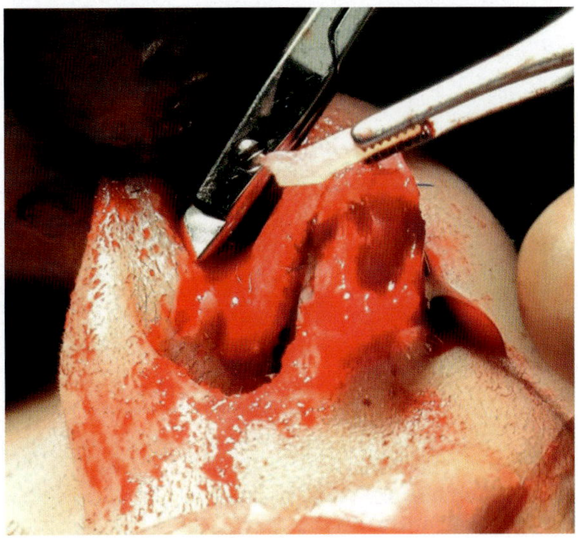

Fig. 28.26 Insertion of alar rim graft.

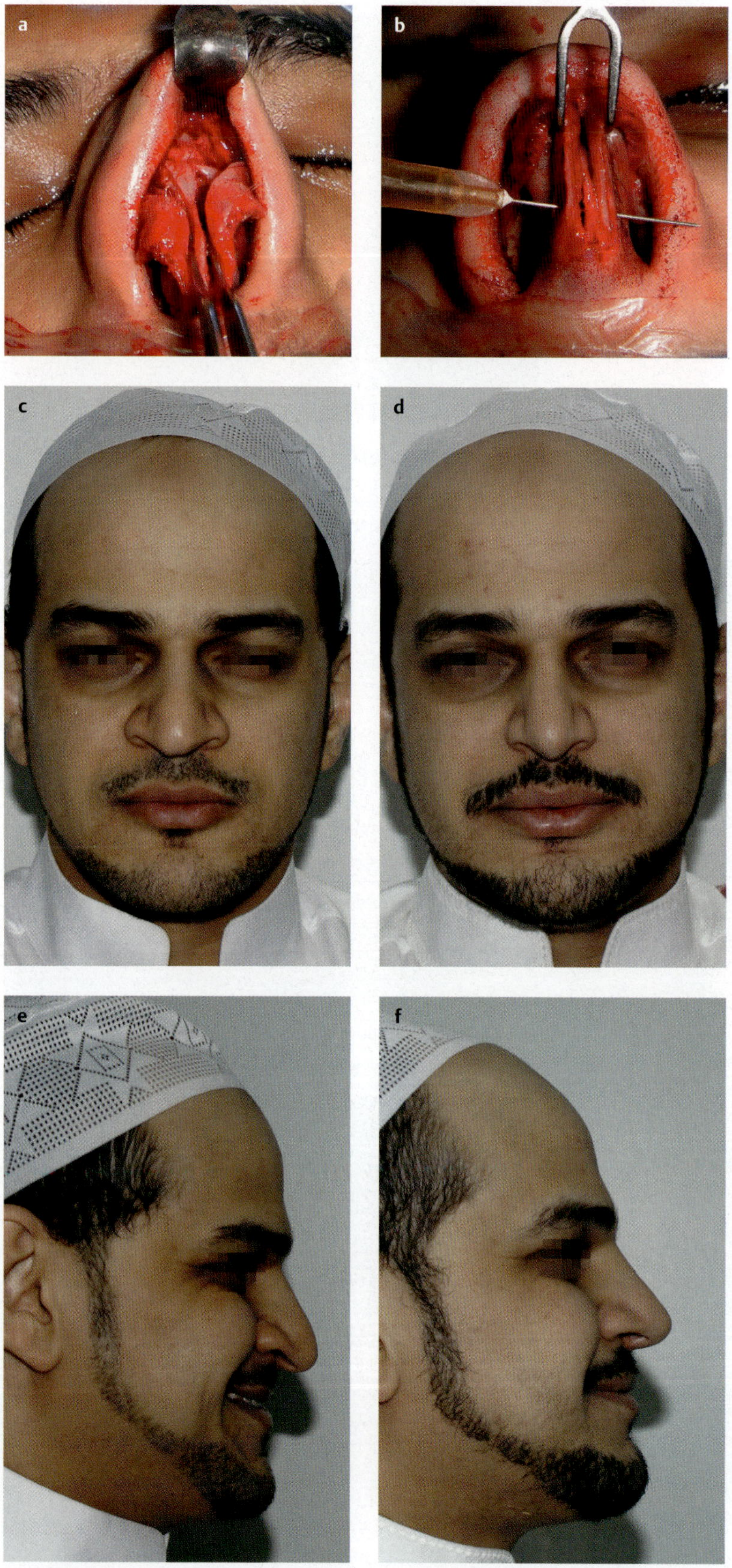

Fig. 28.27 **(a)** Bringing the caudal septum between the two medial crura. **(b)** Fixing the caudal septum between the two medial crura. **(c,e)** Patient's preoperative pictures. **(d,f)** The patient's postoperative results.

28.4.5 Alar Base

Some patients have a wide alar base that requires alar basal resection, but not as much as that required by Black, Asian, or Hispanic patients. Usually, increasing nasal tip projection and rotation will affect the shape of the alar base, so it is important to close all incisions, including marginal and transcolumellar incisions, before performing alar base modifications. It is also important to distinguish between alar flare and width of the nasal sills. We prefer to insert alar rim grafts in all cases to avoid any postoperative excessive straightening of the alar rim or alar notching.

28.5 Postoperative Period

Nasal dressing and splints are placed all the way down to the area of the supratip break, to avoid persistent postoperative swelling and supratip deformities. The external dressing is used only for 3 to 5 days to prevent any possibility of skin sloughing or skin necrosis, especially in dry and hot weather. Skin edema may last for up to 6 months. Patients are advised to perform massages over nasal skin for at least 6 weeks. Some patients note nasal dorsum deviation or tip deviation when they wake up from sleep. This may be due to the effect of gravity on the edema. Taping the supratip area at night and performing a nasal massage when waking up will help keep the nasal dorsum in an adequate position. In our patients, the columellar incision has excellent healing without noticeable scar.

28.6 Complications and Pitfalls

Complications may be the result of inadequate procedures, over-correction, or presence of nasal deformities that were not diagnosed preoperatively or during surgery. The most frequently seen are:

- Over-correction of the radix deficiency
- Pollybeak deformity
- Inverted-V deformity
- Alar retraction
- Not addressing the thick ala

A low radix will result in a flattened, washed-out appearance, which in most cases is undesirable, especially when associated with a short nose and low nasal dorsum. Over-correction of the radix deficiency can make the eyes appear too close to each other **(Fig. 28.28)**.

Pollybeak is most often the result of inadequate resection of the supratip structure, loss of tip support, or, paradoxically, excessive cartilage resection in the supratip region. This may cause a dead space filled with blood and the formation of fibro-fatty tissue that results in subcutaneous scar tissue formation, often in conjunction with thick nasal tip skin **(Fig. 28.29)**.

Thick and heavy sebaceous skin usually hides any underlying irregularities, but it may lead to persistent postoperative swelling and soft tissue supratip pollybeak deformity, which can be prevented in the early postoperative period by placing the nasal splints extended inferiorly just to the area of the supratip break.

Inverted-V deformity **(Fig. 28.30)** is a consequence of aggressive resection of the dorsal edge of upper lateral cartilage after removal of a dorsal cartilaginous hump without inserting any spreader grafts. The deformity is usually associated with internal nasal valve collapse, causing nasal obstruction.

Alar retraction can occur due to placement of overly tight transdomal and/or lateral crural spanning sutures in addition to excessive removal of the lateral crura of the lower lateral cartilages. This deformity can be corrected with placement of alar rim grafts **(Fig. 28.31)**.

28.7 Case Study

The thick ala can be corrected by performing an elliptical incision on the caudal border of the rim close to the intranasal lining. Soft tissue is excised and the incision is closed.

A 17-year-old patient presents with complaints of right nasal obstruction and nasal deviation and deformity, as shown in **Fig. 28.32**. Her 12-year postoperative results are seen in **Fig. 28.33**.

Nasal analysis includes the following:

- Moderately thick skin envelope
- Twisted narrow midvault and dorsal hump (5–6 mm)
- Underprojected and bulbous nasal tip with symmetric alar cartilages
- Alar-columellar imbalance with retracted columella
- Septal deviation
- Nostril asymmetry

Fig. 28.33 shows 12 years of postoperative photographs. An open rhinoplasty approach was performed using the following procedures:

- 7 mm dorsal hump reduction
- Bilateral spreader grafts
- Cephalic trim of alar cartilages
- Medial crural, interdomal, and transdomal sutures
- Strong columellar strut graft
- Bilaeral alar rim grafts
- Infralobular and onlay tip grafts
- Low-to-low osteotomies

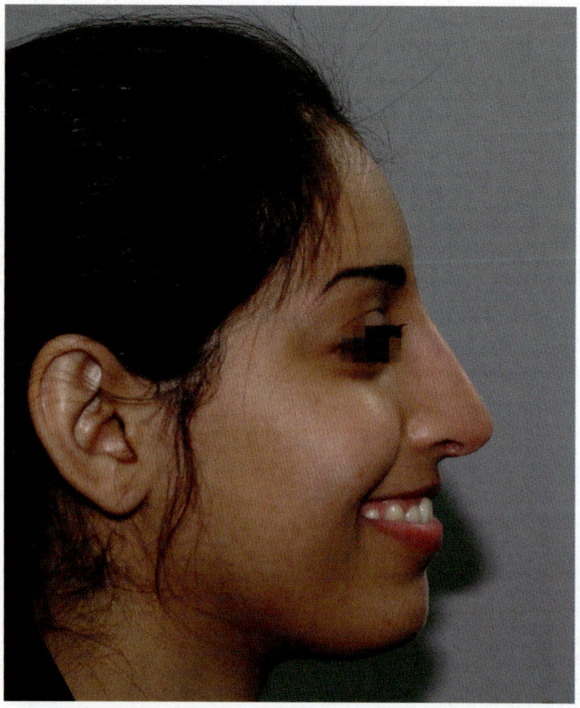

Fig. 28.28 Over-correction of the radix.

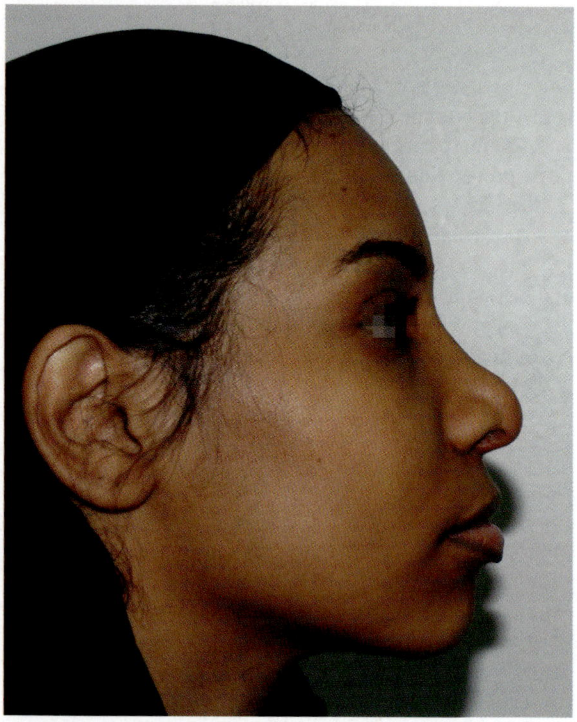

Fig. 28.29 Postoperative soft tissue pollybeak deformity.

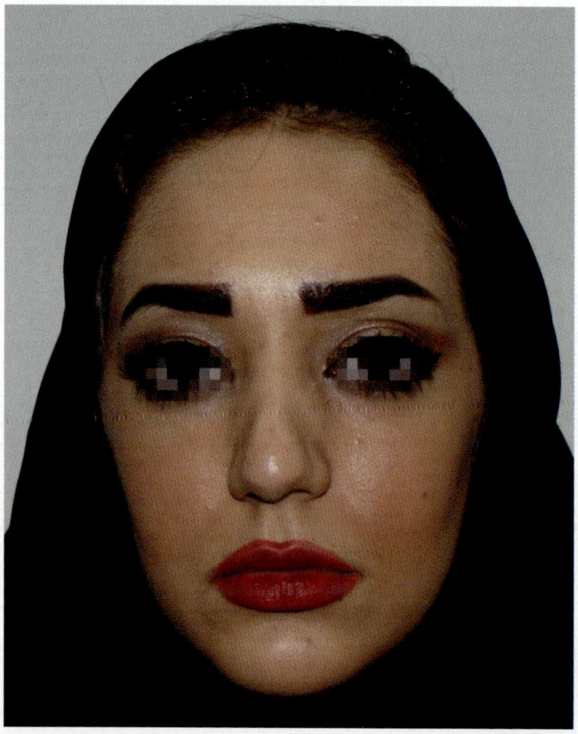

Fig. 28.30 Inverted-V deformity as a result of hump removal without inserting spreader graft.

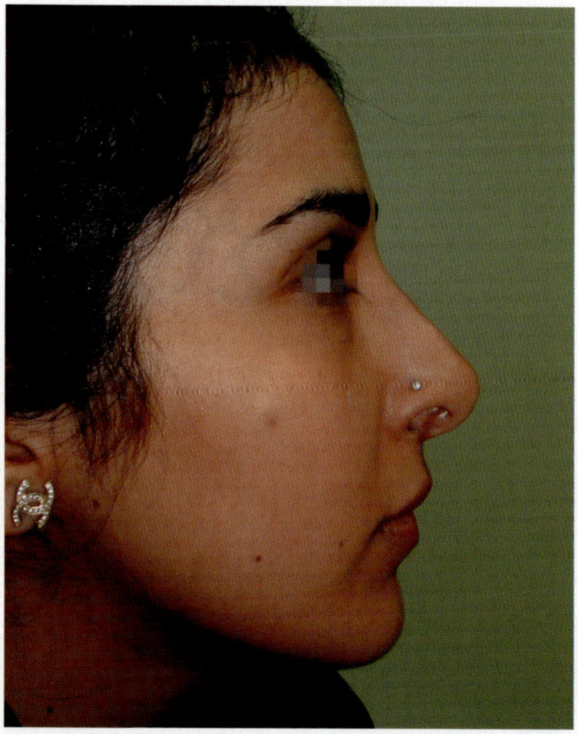

Fig. 28.31 Alar rim retraction as a result of tight domal and spanning sutures.

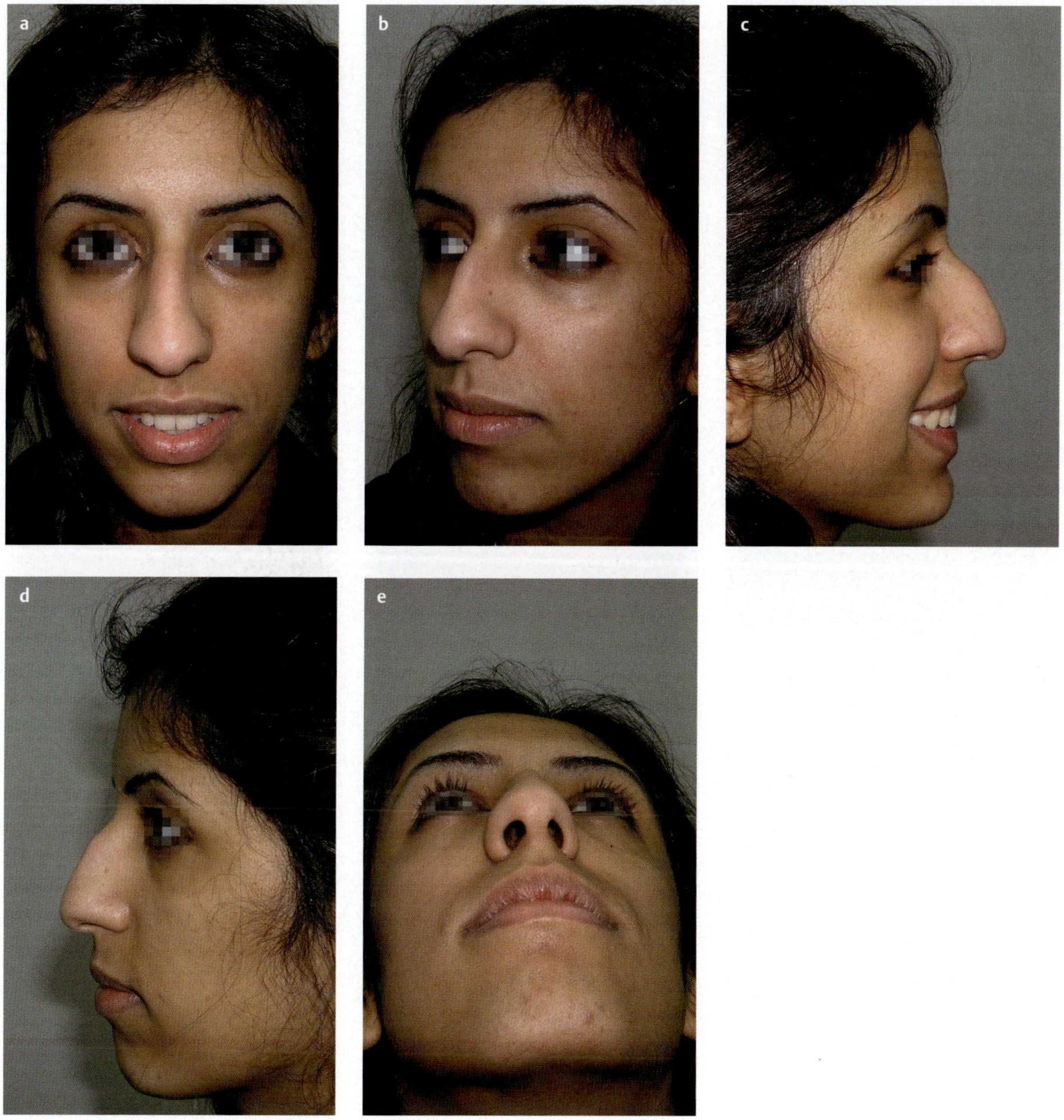

Fig. 28.32 (a–e) Preoperative views of 17-year-old patient.

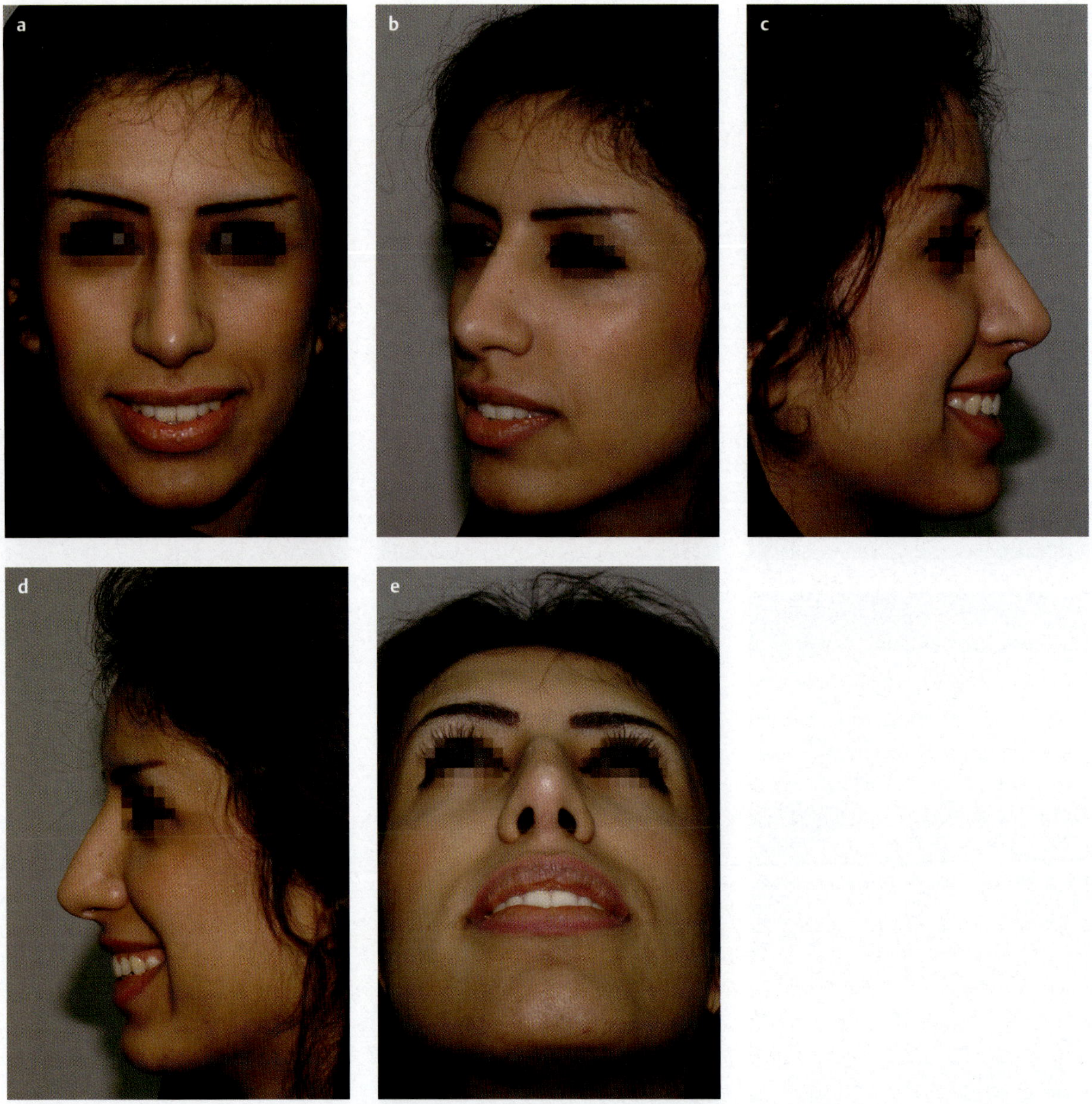

Fig. 28.33 (a–e) Postoperative views of same patient as in **Fig. 28.32.**

References

1. Bizrah MB. Rhinoplasty for Middle Eastern patients. Facial Plast Surg Clin North Am 2002;10(4):381–396
2. Al-Qattan MM, Alsaeed AA, Al-Madani OK, Al-Amri NA, Al-Dahian NA. Anthropometry of the Saudi Arabian nose. J Craniofac Surg 2012;23(3):821–824
3. Foda HM. External rhinoplasty for the Arabian nose: a columellar scar analysis. Aesthetic Plast Surg 2004;28(5): 312–316
4. Bafaqeeh SA, Al-Qattan MM. Open rhinoplasty: columellar scar analysis in an Arabian population. Plast Reconstr Surg 1998;102(4):1226–1228, discussion 1229
5. Alharethy S, Aldaghri F, Mesallam TA, Farahat M, Bukhari MA. Nasal bone length in Saudi rhinoplasty: a clinical-radiological study. Ann Saudi Med 2014;34(1):65–67
6. Elshahat A. Triple plane dissection in open primary rhinoplasty in middle eastern noses. Eplasty 2013;13:e40
7. Daniel RK. Middle Eastern rhinoplasty: anatomy, aesthetics, and surgical planning. Facial Plast Surg 2010; 26(2):110–118
8. Azizzadeh B, Mashkevich G. Middle Eastern rhinoplasty. Facial Plast Surg Clin North Am 2010;18(1):201–206
9. Rohrich RJ, Ghavami A. The Middle Eastern nose. In: Gunter JP, Rohrich RJ, Adams WP, eds. Dallas Rhinoplasty: Nasal Surgery by the Masters. St Louis, MO: Quality Medical Publishing; 2007:1139–1165
10. Foda HMT, Kridel RWH. Lateral crural steal and lateral crural overlay: an objective evaluation. Arch Otolaryngol Head Neck Surg 1999;125(12):1365–1370
11. Bafaqeeh SA. Open rhinoplasty: effectiveness of different tripplasty techniques to increase nasal tip projection. Am J Otolaryngol 2000;21(4):231–237
12. Silver WE, Zuliani GF. Management of the overprojected nose and ptotic nasal tip. Aesthet Surg J 2009;29(3): 253–258
13. Rohrich RJ, Muzaffar AR. Rhinoplasty in the African-American Patient. Plast Reconstr Surg 2003;111:1322

29 Midface Lift: Our Current Approaches

Giovanni Botti and Chiara Botti

29.1 Introduction

A misguided idea has spread among plastic surgeons all over the world. Some researchers have claimed that facial aging changes are essentially related to fat atrophy, and they propose to treat every defect with fat grafts or fillers alone. This is simply wrong. In fact, aging generally entails alterations in the skin texture (atrophy, elastosis, etc.), which give rise to its relaxation and "enlargement," as well as modifications of the inner tissues (fat and bone atrophy, fat ptosis, loss of muscular and fascial tone, etc.), with a consequent reduction of their volume and loss of projection and support to the midface structures and overlying lower lid. This gap between the container and its contents is one of the most important causes of the aging-related facial aesthetic problems.[1] Any experienced surgeon knows that, in the vast majority of cases, it is impossible to obtain natural and long-lasting results without removing excess skin. This is the main reason why the so-called thread-based treatments (insertion in the fat of barbed sutures, which are supposed to lift the soft tissues without any skin removal) fail to correct aging problems in the face. The same unnatural and ineffective outcomes often can be observed after the injection of excessive quantities of various substances (fat, hyaluronic acid, etc.) in an attempt not only to correct the soft and hard tissue atrophy, but also to fill out the enlarged skin, which instead should have been partially removed.

Facial plastic surgeons confront two main problems, skin "expansion" and fat/bone atrophy; consequently, to obtain the best outcomes, we should try to solve or, at least, to improve both problems. These considerations are particularly valid for the midface area, where quite often the simple use of fillers that nowadays seems to be so much in fashion gives a funny appearance or, in the worst cases, a monstrous look to the unlucky patient. Only in cases where internal atrophy is prevalent should one resort to "filling" by itself. Fat grafting, implants, and hyaluronic acid injections alone can be quite effective when dealing with only a well-delimited local defect, like a deep tear trough or lack of cheekbone projection, but if relevant excess skin is detected, the surgeon also should consider a midface lift procedure, to be performed at the same time as augmentation or by itself (**Fig. 29.1**).

Over the past 30 years, many new treatments have been proposed to improve the midface area. Some of them were greeted with a lot of enthusiasm, but, unfortunately, with time their use and overuse resulted in terrible complications. Among them, for example, are the so-called permanent fillers. At the beginning, they were proposed and used by several eminent plastic surgeons (in Italy, they were supported by almost all plastic surgery program directors), but quite shortly they gave rise to very bad problems, often almost impossible to correct completely. In the 1990s, removal of the Bichat fat pad through an intraoral approach was introduced as the best option to enhance cheekbone projection and was performed by many "advanced" surgeons. Ten to 15 years later, many of those poor patients had to return to the operating room in order have hollowed cheeks filled by fat grafting. Extended lower blepharoplasties with sub-orbicularis dissection and muscular suspension[2,3] seemed to be the best solution for malar festoons, but in many cases they had very annoying complications (scleral show, ectropion, etc.), until a better comprehension of the lid suspension system was reached. Nowadays, the latest fashion is to treat midface defects with fat grafting alone, based on some debatable pathophysiological findings that have led some to think that no sagging and downward shifting of soft tissues would actually take place. We completely disagree and are deeply convinced that to correctly solve the aging-related aesthetic defects of the midface area with natural and harmonious results, a more comprehensive and complete approach should be considered. First, a proper and unbiased diagnosis should be made, and then

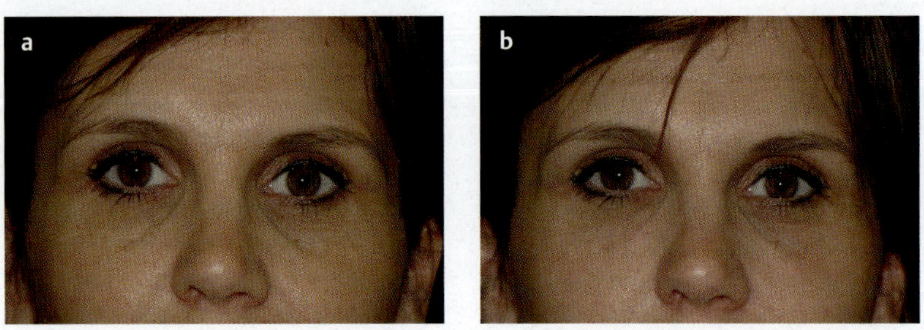

Fig. 29.1 (a,b) Hyaluronic acid injections. When the aesthetic defect is limited to the tear trough without any soft tissue laxity, one can resort to hyaluronic acid injection with acceptable but short-lasting results. In this case, a nonhydrophilic hyaluronic acid is preferable to prevent excessive swelling of the treated area.

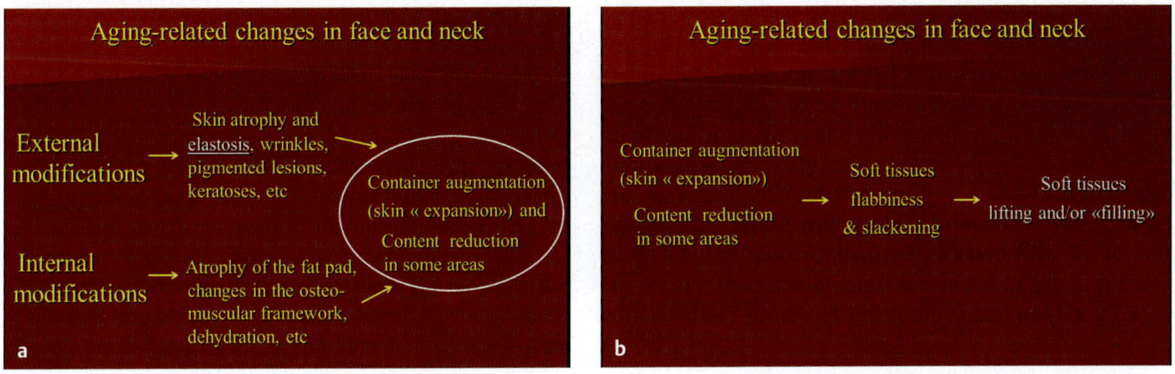

Fig. 29.2 **(a,b)** Flowchart for the treatment of midfacial aging-related changes. If the problems are related to both ptosis and deflation, we should try to both lift and fill the soft tissues. Quite often, though, repositioning of lax soft tissue alone is sufficient to give excellent, stable results. That is the "pure" midface lift.

the consequent logical treatment should be performed. In only a few patients should midface defects be corrected by fat grafting or midface lift alone, while in the majority of cases both procedures should be used in varying degrees (**Fig. 29.2**).

29.2 History

In the 1980s, plastic surgeons were already capable of consistently improving aging-related defects in the lower part of the face and the neck, but they could not obtain any concrete improvement in midface problems. In fact, at that time it was quite common to find in scientific publications postoperative pictures with inharmonious outcomes: well-treated lower face, neck, and even forehead, and undertreated infrapalpebral and malar areas. Realizing that midface enhancement techniques were still lacking, a few surgeons around the world tried to focus on malar bags, the tear trough, flatness under the eyes, etc.—in other words, midface defects.[4]

The authors' personal crusade began in the late 1980s. Disappointed with the outcomes of many inferior blepharoplasties performed to treat lower lid and extraorbital defects, following De La Plaza, Hinderer, and Faivre,[5] we first tried extending the usual palpebral undermining downward outside the orbital rim, to lift that specific area. The widened dissection was performed between the fat pad behind the orbicularis muscle (the so-called SOOF) and the periosteum, at a level that many years later B. Mendelson called the prezygomatic space. Sometimes, the wide, deep dissection and sagging soft tissue reposition gave good results, but in the majority of cases the results were not long-lasting, and a few surgeries were followed by complications like ectropion and scleral show. The main problem was the instability of the fixation. In fact, even if any incidental hypotony was corrected by deep and superficial canthopexy, sometimes the lower lid border still had a tendency to move downward. Moreover, that technique didn't allow filling of any deep palpebrojugal grooves with a thick layer of soft tissue, as was often required. However, in selected cases, it proved to be an effective operation: for example, in treating festoons due to skin and/or muscle laxity. When both festoons and deep tear troughs were present, we used to couple the extended blepharoplasty (superficial midface lift) with dermal-fat grafts or with Flowers implants placed over the orbital rim. When the problem was just deep tear troughs without any skin-muscle sagging, our preferred treatment was fat grafting alone, with no undermining, which in many cases provided good results, although not always predictably. At that time, exactly like today, the major drawback of the approach lay in its uncertain results (**Fig. 29.3** and **Fig. 29.4**).

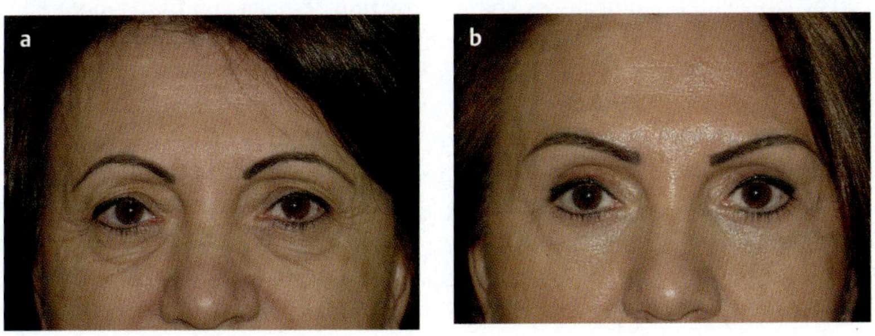

Fig. 29.3 **(a,b)** Extended lower blepharoplasty. If the patient's request is limited to excess skin removal and the soft tissues are still in their correct position, an extended blepharoplasty with deep and superficial canthoplasty is often sufficient to repair the situation. The patient must be aware that no change in the shape of midface area will be obtained.

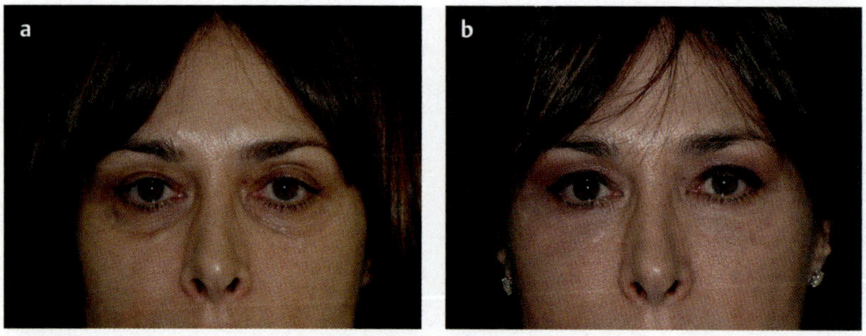

Fig. 29.4 (a,b) Fat grafting. When the patient complains of empty lower lids with deep palpebrojugal grooves, the surgeon should consider fat grafting. The main drawback of this procedure is its lack of longevity. In fact, even if some cases have long-lasting results, in other cases the fat take rate is quite low and the operation needs to be performed many times to get a permanent outcome.

In the late 1990s, we began carrying out the midface lift with a subperiosteal dissection, as was proposed by Tessier and Krastinova and was popularized by Psillakis et al, and we immediately realized that the operation had many more potential advantages than the midface lift with more superficial undermining.[2] The subperiosteal dissection, followed by the release of the midfacial "mask" and its fixation to solid anchoring points, ensures a more secure and stable reposition of the sagging midface soft tissues.[3] In fact, the periosteum underneath the flap strongly adheres in the new position to the local nondissected periosteum. Furthermore, the thicker layer of soft tissue can be lifted and can be used to fill deep palpebrojugal grooves. This deep undermining is still the basis of our midface lift,[6] even if with time we realized that only individualized treatment, based on very meticulous attention to all details, allows the surgeon to obtain consistent major improvements of the main defects of this area. Among the most common ancillary procedures that we add to midface lifting are fat grafting and lateral canthopexy (**Fig. 29.5**).

29.3 The Main Midface Problems

The majority of midface defects are age-related, even if sometimes we have to deal with congenital problems, like the negative vector (when the eyes are more prominent than the inferior orbital rim and the malar soft tissues) or deep tear troughs. The latter deformities can be congenital or acquired, but in both cases a midface lift can generally help to improve the situation.[7,8,9] Additional defects in the area are festoons, too high and/or too sunken lower lids, too evident lid–cheek transition area, wrinkles, discoloration, and some midface-related problems in the lower lids, like scleral show and ectropion. With reference to the latter defects, the skin gathered in the lid with lifting the midface is quite helpful for skin deficiencies, even if additional procedures are necessary.

29.4 Basic Techniques of Midface Lifting

Subperiosteal dissection is relatively easy to perform, is almost bloodless, avoids injury to facial nerve branches, and guarantees much longer-lasting results than a supraperiosteal approach. To carry out complete subperiosteal undermining of the midface area, the easiest access to the deep plane is undoubtedly a paracanthal stab incision, prolonged with a subciliary extension when it is evident that it will be also necessary to remove a strip of excess skin from the lower lid. Another useful approach is the transoral incision, performed perpendicular in the vestibular fornix. One could pass through a temporal scalp incision as well, or even through the usual preauricular facelift approach, deepening the dissection at the lateral border of the malar bone.[10,11] Resorting to two simultaneous approaches often provides a more precise undermining and an easier and faster operation. The dissection should be performed both in the malar and maxillary subpalpebral areas and should be extended above and below the infraorbital bundle. It is important to completely release the periosteum, which is rigid and inextensible, at the periphery of the dissected zone: at the base of the malar area, along the oral upper fornix, and at the level of the orbital rim. This will allow easy movement of the midface flap upward. In this area, soft tissues can be lifted along different vectors, the main ones being superolateral and superomedial. Pulling in these two directions has different effects. A superolateral vector of pull allows better correction of malar soft tissue mounding and festoons. Furthermore, improved cheekbone projection can be obtained thanks to a deep periosteal plication. A superomedial vector of pull is more effective when the main issue is the correction of a deep tear trough. The midface flap can be fixed to the periosteum of the periorbital rim or, better yet, directly to the bone at the same level through drill holes. Another solid anchoring tissue is the deep temporal fascia (the muscular aponeurosis), but this can be reached only by means of long "suspender" sutures.

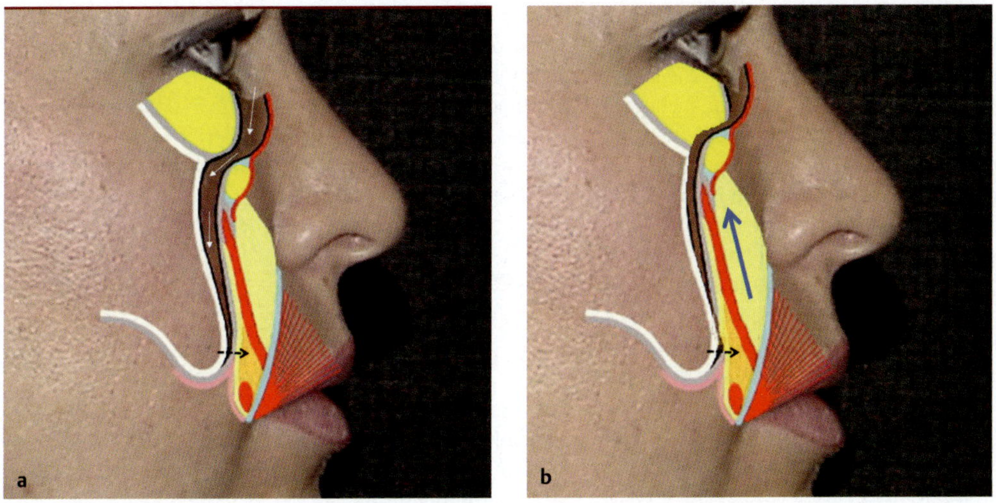

Fig. 29.5 Subperiosteal dissection. **(a)** The downward extension of subperiosteal dissection is illustrated, which, together with the lower section of the periosteum, will allow lifting the flap. **(b)** The soft tissues have been moved upward, thus filling the nasojugal groove, correcting any festoons that may be present, and adding volume to the cheekbone area.

29.5 Analyzing Different Operations to Treat Midface Aesthetic Defects

As already mentioned, several operations have been proposed to correct midface problems.[12,13,14] The two main procedures are based on different levels of dissection: a more superficial and a deeper one.

The technique based on *superficial dissection* usually starts with a subciliary incision, followed by a subcutaneous dissection and by the incision of the orbicularis oculi muscle below the lower tarsal margin. Then a palpebral myocutaneous flap is elevated, reaching the lower orbital rim. At this point the undermining is extended caudally, passing between the SOOF (sub-orbicularis oculi fat) and the periosteum, and then further downward behind the lower extension of the orbicularis muscle and the anterior cheek fat pad, but in front of the lip elevator muscles. This dissection can reach medially the nasolabial fold, but it should be interrupted laterally halfway across the malar bone, to avoid severing a branch of the facial nerve directed to the orbicularis oculi muscle,[15,16] which runs above the zygomaticus major muscle. The flap thus obtained is lifted and fixed with a few sutures to the periosteum of the lower orbital rim. When necessary, i.e., in case of lower lid hypotony, a deep and/or superficial canthopexy is also performed. Finally, excess skin is removed and the wound is sutured.

The deep (subperiosteal) dissection is used in three main different procedures.[17,18] Two are based on a superolateral vector of pull, one on a superomedial vector of pull.

The midface lift with subperiosteal dissection is a "closed approach" procedure, actually performed through only three small stab incisions. The first incision is in the scalp of the temporal area, ~ 1.5 cm behind the hairline. Through this incision, a tunnel is created between the superficial and the deep temporal fascia. The dissection is extended subperiosteally in the forehead and both the insertions of the frontal periosteum and of the superficial temporal fascia along the superolateral orbital rim are disrupted and completely released. The second incision is made lateral to the lateral canthus (as the usual extension of the lower blepharoplasty incision). Through it, subperiosteal undermining of the malar and maxillary areas is performed. Care should be taken to avoid any damage to the infraorbital bundle,[19] even if the dissection has to be extended below and above it to move soft tissues from the midface area to the lid. The zygomaticofacial bundle is usually sectioned without any detectable change in local sensitivity. A third incision is made in the mouth, perpendicular to the vestibular fornix. This last incision will allow a complete and verified midface dissection and the insertion of a Reverdin needle, used to anchor the wide flap. The needle is passed through the buccal incision and the dissected midface area and exits the paracanthal incision. Then a suture is mounted on its eye, and the needle repierces the flap and exits again from the paracanthal incision. Now, the suture is withdrawn from the needle and its two extremities are passed through the temporal tunnel and are pulled and fixed to the deep temporal fascia (muscular aponeurosis) under appropriate tension. A second, similar fixation, with a suture pulled along a slightly different vector, is often performed. The operation is completed with a couple of sutures between the superficial and deep temporal fasciae, with the aim of lifting the paracanthal soft tissues and the eyebrow tail.

The second operation based on a subperiosteal dissection is substantially similar to the first one, but in this case the paracanthal incision is extended underneath the lashes to the medial canthus. Through this approach, anchorage is easily performed with no need for any supplementary oral incision. After the scalp incision and temporal undermining are performed, the subciliary incision is made, and through it the malar/maxillary undermining is done. Then, through the same incision, the midface flap is directly anchored (with no need of a Reverdin needle) with a long "suspender" suture that is fixed to the deep temporal fascia. The upper margin of the orbicularis oculi muscle flap is also fixed to the periosteum of the superolateral orbital rim through the paracanthal tunnel. The most important difference between the first and the second type of midface lift with subperiosteal dissection is that the latter allows the removal of potential excess skin at the level of the subciliary incision. If the lower lid suspension system (canthal tendon–canthal ligament–orbicularis muscle) is not adequately strong and tight, then a "deep" canthopexy must also be performed. In that case, the surgeon should take care to anchor the orbicularis oculi muscle outside the orbital rim and the canthal ligament and/or tendon inside, to avoid any pulling away of the lower lid from the ocular globe **(Fig. 29.6)**.

The third operation based on subperiosteal dissection has a different vector of traction. While the first two procedures rely on a superolateral pull, the last one has a superomedial vector. With this technique there is no need of buccal or temporal incisions, because it is completely performed through the lid. The operation starts with a small incision in the lateral part of the upper lid groove extended for a few mm externally to the orbital rim or, instead, when needed, with the usual upper blepharoplasty skin removal. Then a paracanthal incision with a subciliary extension (as in any lower blepharoplasty) is performed. Subperiosteal dissection is performed in the malar/maxillary area, as in the other techniques, but in this case it is extended to the internal side of the inferior and superolateral orbital rims. Then, two or three drill holes are created in the bone along the inferior orbital rim and one on its superolateral part. The midface flap is grasped with a suture under direct vision ~ 1 cm inferiorly and laterally to each drill hole and then the same suture is passed through the respective hole. By the sutures, the midface flap is lifted and fixed in its new position. An orbicularis flap is taken from the subcanthal portion of the muscle (Adamson flap) and is passed through the paracanthal tunnel and is anchored to the upper drill hole. In the majority of cases, canthopexy is also performed, taking care to pass the retaining suture from inside to outside the orbital rim. This last maneuver is facilitated if two drill holes are also created along the superolateral orbital rim. Frequently, large quantities of skin can be removed at the end of the operation but, as in any procedure involving lower lid dissection, care should be taken to leave at least 3 mm of apparent excess skin to prevent lid margin displacement due to inner scar retraction.[20] The usual suture completes the operation. We prefer 5–0 silk interrupted sutures. Because silk is a soft material, we avoid having the suture ends inadvertently scratch the cornea in the postoperative period **(Fig. 29.7)**.

29.6 Indication for Midface Lift Procedures with Subperiosteal Dissection

The "closed approach" without subciliary incision should be used when there is no extra skin to resect in the lower lid. The best candidates are younger patients who desire just a better definition and shape of the midface area.

The second technique, with complete subciliary incision, orbicularis oculi flap, and temporal fixation, should be chosen when there is excess skin to be removed from the lower lid, if a superolateral traction vector is needed (to be discussed with the patient in front of a mirror), and when cheekbone projection needs to be improved.

The third technique, with a purely trans-palpebral approach and orbital rim drill holes, should be preferred when a superomedial traction vector is needed, if a temporal incision should be avoided (bald men), and when the main issue is the correction of a deep tear trough. In fact, this procedure allows better elevation of the most medial midface soft tissues, thus covering the exposed lower orbital rim caused by anterior cheek fat pad and SOOF ptosis **(Fig. 29.8, Fig. 29.9, Fig. 29.10)**.

29.7 Other Techniques Used to Correct Midface Aesthetic Defects

In some cases, fat grafting can be considered a valid alternative to midface lift. The best candidates for lipofilling or lipostructure (in contemporary surgical language, these two words are considered synonyms) are patients who show mainly lack of soft and/or hard tissue thickness. Very often, aging entails atrophy of both fat and bone and, although less frequently, this atrophy can occur congenitally. Very rarely, the laxity that develops with the aging process is totally due to fat depletion and/or bone atrophy, because a very important role is played by skin thinning and enlargement.[21] Beyond face and neck, this same phenomenon is easily detectable in almost every other area of the body, even if it is more evident in specific zones, such as the inner and anterior/posterior sides of the thighs, the arms, the abdomen, and the breasts. In other words, as already mentioned, two different phenomena take place: on the one hand, the extension of the skin surface (the

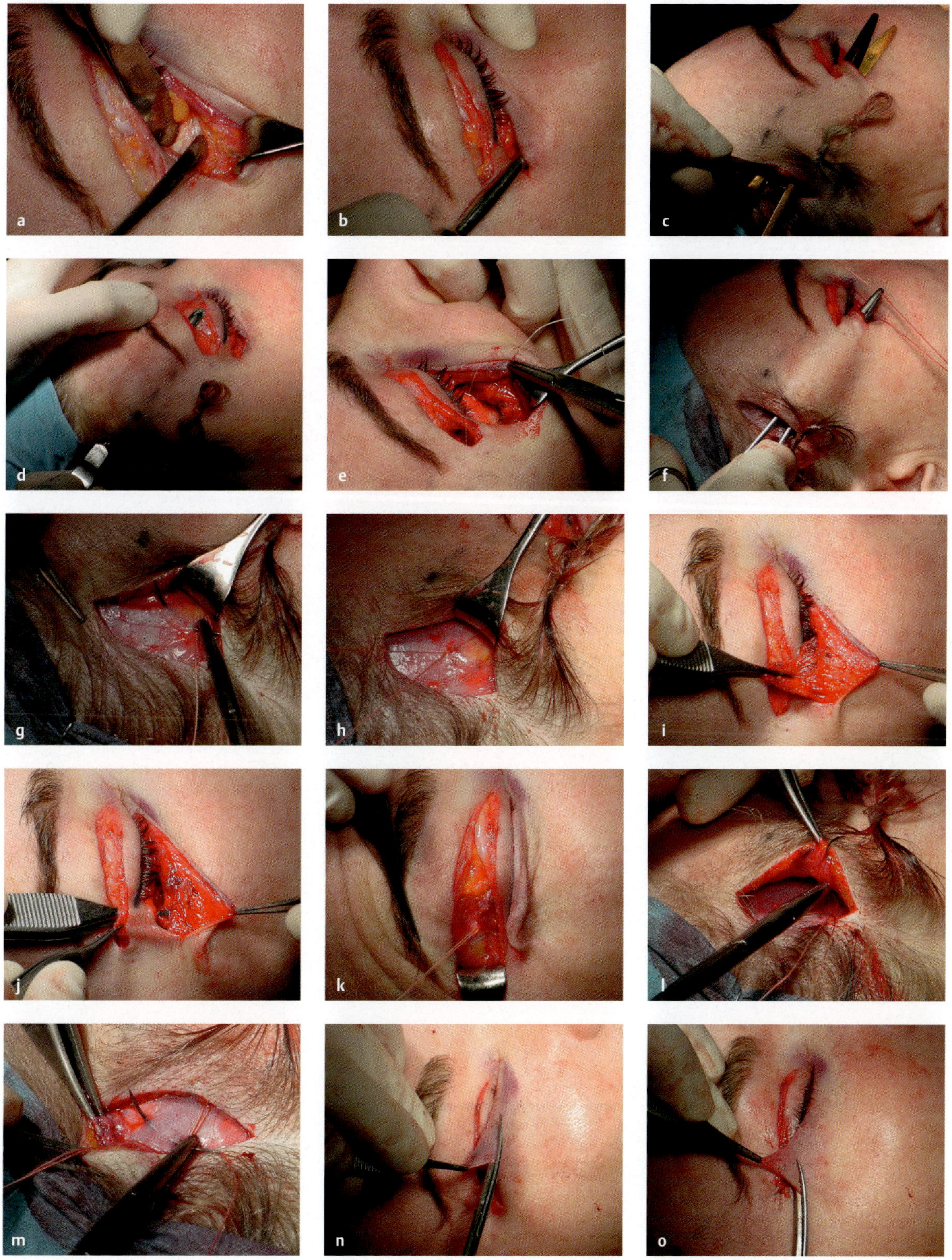

Fig. 29.6 "Suspender" midface lift: surgical technique. **(a)** On the left, the orbital rim periosteum is accessed and the subperiosteal dissection is begun. **(b)** Dissection is extended to the malar and maxillary areas, where a fingertip protects the infraorbital bundle. **(c)** A subfascial tunnel is created, connecting the temporal scalp incision to the midface. **(d)** The temporal undermining is extended subperiosteally to the forehead; the surgeon must take care to avoid damage to the supraorbital bundle. **(e)** On the left, the flap is passed through with a 3–0 Vicryl suture. **(f)** The suture is grasped with a needle holder and is driven through the temporal tunnel. **(g)** The upper extremity of the long suture ("suspender") pierces the deep temporal fascia and **(h)** it is tightened. **(i)** The creation of an orbicularis oculi flap, which is passed through a paracanthal tunnel and **(j)** is fixed to the periosteum of the lateral orbital rim and **(k)** to the deep temporal fascia. **(l)** The temporal flap is grasped by a Vicryl 3–0 suture. **(m)** The same suture also pierces the deep temporal fascia and, when pulled and tightened, lifts the eyebrow tail. **(n,o)** A strip of excess skin is conservatively removed along the subciliary incision.

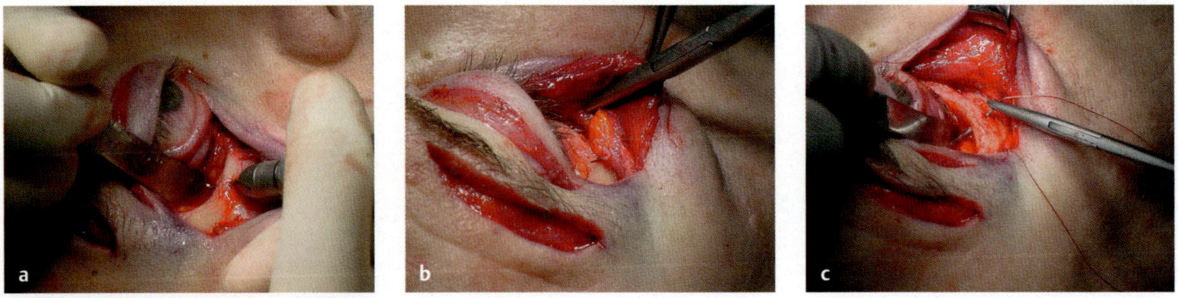

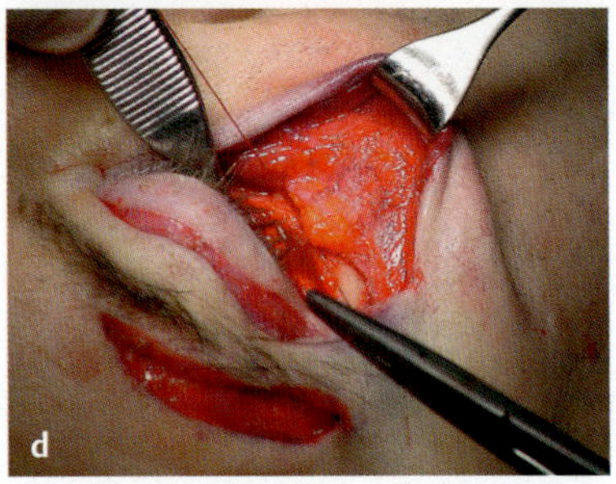

Fig. 29.7 "Belt" midface lift: surgical technique. **(a)** A drill hole is created in the orbital rim. **(b)** Then the flap is pierced with a suture needle that afterward **(c)** passes through the hole in the bone. **(d)** Finally, the suture is tied. This lifting maneuver allows the repositioning of the SOOF (suborbicularis oculi fat) on the orbital rim (as is clearly seen in the illustrations), thus filling the palpebrojugal groove.

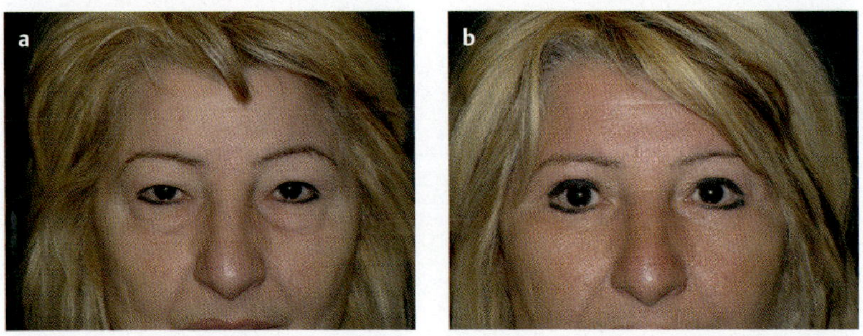

Fig. 29.8 **(a,b)** Basic midface lift. Upper lid dermatochalasis and lower lid fat bags are evident in this patient, as well as soft tissue ptosis in the midface. A good correction cannot be obtained with fat grafting, which would cause only more heaviness in the orbital/periorbital area. Instead, soft tissue repositioning addressed the patient's problems with a very natural result. Notice that no fat was removed from the lower lid because fat herniations (fat bags) were pushed back into their original position by midface and orbicularis oculi tightening.

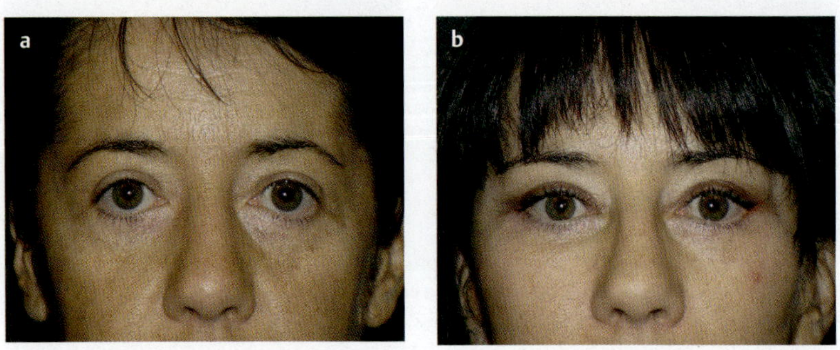

Fig. 29.9 Scleral show corrected by midface lift and canthoplasty. **(a)** An overzealous blepharoplasty produced round eyes. **(b)** The great quantity of skin moved upward from the midface area allowed the surgeon to fill the gap (scleral show) between the lower limbus (inferior margin of the pupil) and the lower lid margin.

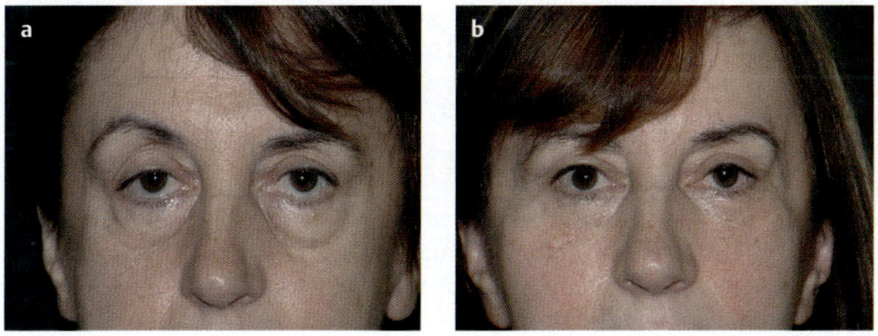

Fig. 29.10 (a,b) Senile soft tissue ptosis and scleral show. This case was treated with a midface lift along with canthopexy, fat grafting in both upper eyelids, and ptosis correction in the right upper eyelid. No fat was injected in the lower eyelid or in the cheekbone area.

container) increases, and, on the other hand, fat and bone volume (the contents) decreases.[22] But in selected cases fat grafting (or HA injections/implants) alone provides very good outcomes, while in other cases these procedures should be coupled with a midface lift or, at least, with a regular lower face and neck lift[23,24] (better, in that case, if resorting to the high-SMAS technique) (**Fig. 29.11**).

29.8 Drawbacks of Various Procedures

The main complication of midface lifting is lower lid displacement, which seems odd, because this operation is frequently performed with the aim of correcting scleral show and ectropion, thanks to the large quantity of skin that can be recruited. Nevertheless, if not correctly performed, it can be the cause of such defects.[25] At the beginning, there is a steep learning curve,[26] and a very important rule the surgeon should bear in mind from the outset is to leave, at the end of the operation, at least 3 mm of extra skin. This is very important to compensate for postoperative scar retraction, which always takes place, especially if a skin flap was lifted. To avoid lower lid displacement, it is also fundamental to detect and correct any hypotony of the suspension system during the operation and to avoid any hematomas.[27,28] Another possible complication of a subperiosteal midface lift is in an unnatural outcome, which is more frequent if canthopexy is also done,[29] but this is surgeon-dependent, and certainly experience helps the surgeon appreciate the different vectors and strengths of pull and to obtain a well-balanced and natural result.[30]

With fat grafting, the most frequent complication is reabsorption, but the opposite can occur as well, meaning

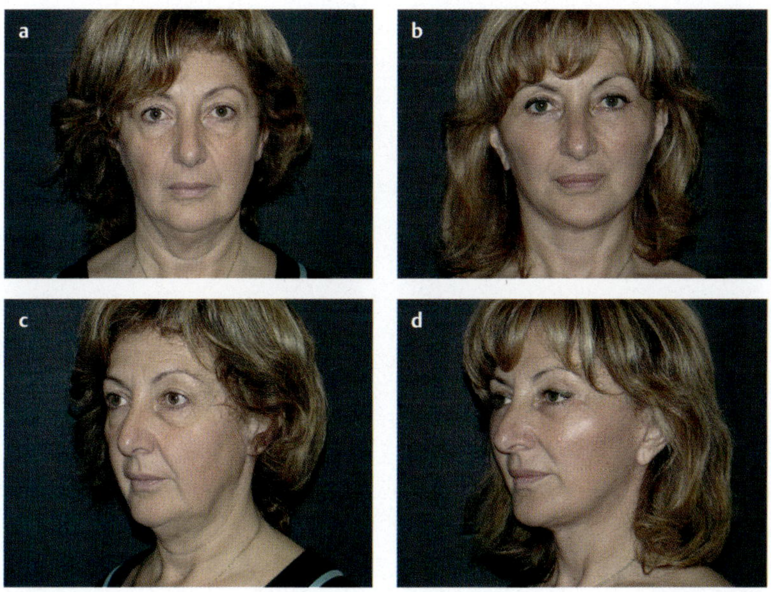

Fig. 29.11 (a–d) Midface, lower face, and neck lifts. This patient had soft tissue ptosis of both face and neck. Fat grafting would have "overloaded" her general appearance; instead, we performed a regular cervicofacial lift coupled with a midface lift. This latter provided correction of the deep palpebrojugal groove and enhancement of the cheekbone projection.

too much fat taking. Generally it is common practice to slightly overcorrect defects because some adipose tissue will certainly atrophy and will be eliminated by the body. Nevertheless, not infrequently excess fat is found postoperatively in the tear through (and sometimes even on the zygoma) and needs to be removed. To prevent this annoying complication, fat should always be injected deeply along the orbital rim, beneath the orbicularis oculi muscle, while only very tiny quantities (drops) could be put directly under the skin. Unfortunately, there is no special technique that can always guarantee fat taking. One can choose different harvest areas, one can use various preparation treatments (such as filtration, decantation, centrifugation), and one can use special devices or even follow particular procedures (fat condensation, ADSC enrichment, etc.), but even in the best hands the percentage of fat taking is still unpredictable. We noticed that fat has a tendency to survive more in some areas than in others, and fortunately the midface is a favorable environment. Perhaps the use of cannulas with small holes for harvest and injection of fat helps get more stable results, but, even following any general rule, fat can still partially diminish or completely disappear, and the patient should be warned about it.

Hyaluronic acid (HA) has a specific complication: its reabsorption. The midface is relatively immobile, and perhaps HA lasts a bit longer in the midface than in more mobile areas. Nevertheless, it would be wrong to guarantee that the correction obtained will last more than 1 year. Another possible complication is the Tyndall effect, which is a bluish discoloration due to localized swelling when hydrophilic HA is injected at the level of the tear trough. To correct this particular problem, hyaluronidase should be infiltrated in the affected area. Finally, all facial implants are subject to dislocation, but this complication is relatively rare if the pocket is created with precision and if the prosthesis is anchored to the bone (**Fig. 29.12** and **Fig. 29.13**).

29.9 Conclusion

The midface lift consists of repositioning malar and maxillary (infrapalpebral) sagging soft tissues. It is indicated when the major defect is soft tissue laxity. If the main problem is atrophy, instead, it is better to resort to filler. In many cases, it is convenient to reposition soft tissues with a midface lift and to correct their atrophy with fat grafting, filler, or implants in the same operation.[31] Fat and fillers can be injected superficially, while implants should be fixed at the bone, eventually through the same drill holes as the midface lift, otherwise the wide recipient pocket would allow unwanted movements. We prefer to carry out the midface lift with a subperiosteal dissection because it provides long-lasting outcomes.[32,33] Our clinical observations allow us to state that the durability of the results is not due to a readherence of periosteum to bone in the new uplifted position, but instead to the fact that nonextensible dissected periosteum adheres to nonundermined, unchanged bone. Midface lift allows one to truly recreate the youthful characteristics lost with aging, returning the soft tissues to their original position, volume, and shape.[34] Furthermore, the operation can be very helpful in treating scleral show and ectropion, along with canthoplasties, because it generates a great amount of skin with the same texture and color that the lower lid is lacking.[35] Generally, midface lifts give excellent, natural, and stable results when used for aesthetic or functional purposes.[36] But the midface lift is not an easy procedure and there is a steep learning curve before mastering it.

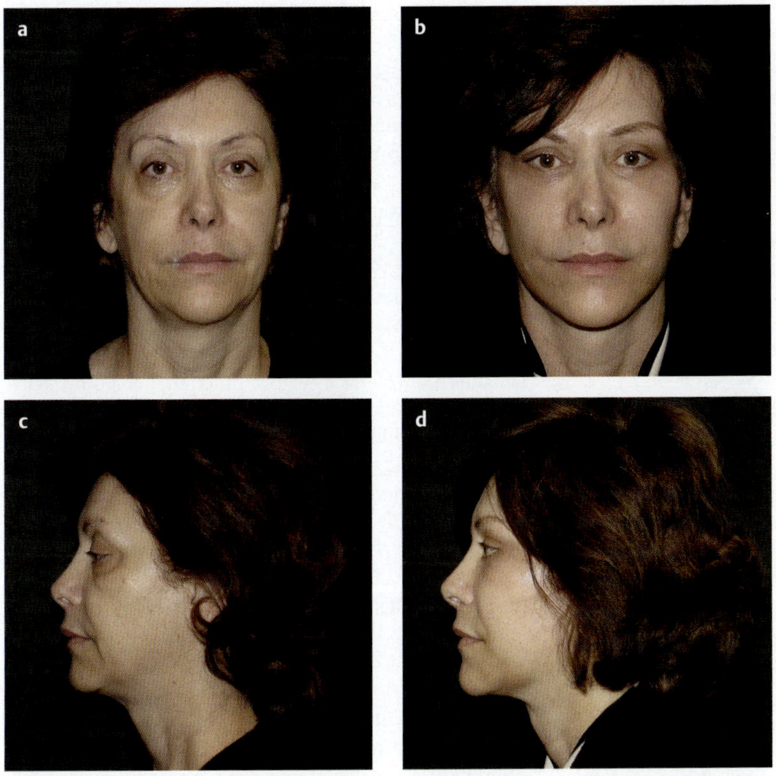

Fig. 29.12 **(a,c)** Midface lift and cervicofacial lift preoperative views. **(b,d)** Postoperative views. To obtain a more harmonious outcome, a complete lift was performed, treating the midface, lower face, and neck. Due to weakness of the lower lid suspension system, it was necessary to resort to a canthopexy, which gave this patient a slightly unnatural look.

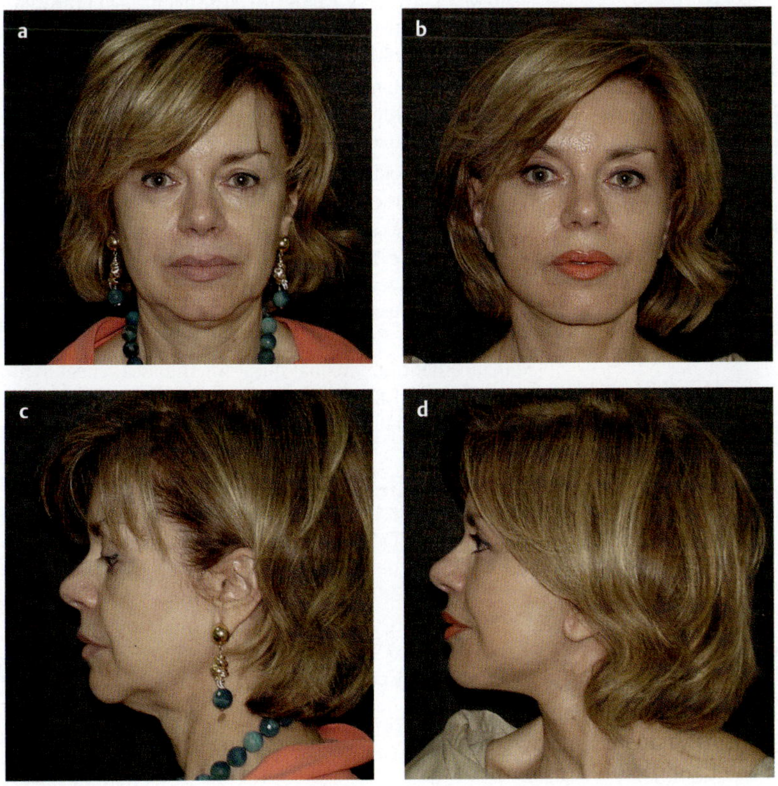

Fig. 29.13 **(a,c)** Midface, lower face, and neck lift preoperative views. **(b,d)** Postoperative views. This 58-year-old woman complained of an aged facial appearance. In cases like this, it is very important to correct all the aesthetic defects with a harmonious reposition of the ptotic soft tissues in both the face and the neck. Therefore, to obtain a natural result, a combined midface lift–lower face lift–neck lift should be performed. Thanks to this complete operation, the patient's sagging cheeks, tear troughs, jowls, and cervical bands were corrected.

References

1. Little JW. Volumetric perceptions in midfacial aging with altered priorities for rejuvenation. Plast Reconstr Surg 2000;105(1):252–266, discussion 286–289
2. Adamson JE, McCraw JB, Carraway JH. Use of a muscle flap in lower blepharoplasty. Plast Reconstr Surg 1979; 63(3):359–363
3. Adamson PA, Dahiya R, Litner J. Midface effects of the deep-plane vs the superficial musculoaponeurotic system plication face-lift. Arch Facial Plast Surg 2007;9(1):9–11
4. Paul MD, Calvert JW, Evans GR. The evolution of the mid-face lift in aesthetic plastic surgery. Plast Reconstr Surg 2006;117(6):1809–1827
5. De La Plaza R, Valiente E, Arroyo JM. Supraperiosteal lifting of the upper two-thirds of the face. Br J Plast Surg 1991;44(5):325–332
6. Alsarraf R, To WC, Johnson CM Jr. The deep plane facelift. Facial Plast Surg 2003;19(1):95–106
7. Barton FE Jr. The SMAS and the nasolabial fold. Plast Reconstr Surg 1992;89(6):1054–1057, discussion 1058–1059
8. Besins T. The "R.A.R.E." technique (reverse and repositioning effect): the renaissance of the aging face and neck. Aesthetic Plast Surg 2004;28(3):127–142
9. Binder WJ, Schoenrock LD, Terino EO. Augmentation of the malar-submalar/midface. Facial Plast Surg Clin North Am 1994;2:265–283
10. Botti G, Pelle Ceravolo M. Midface and Neck Aesthetic Plastic Surgery, Vol. I/II. Parma, Italy: Acta Medica Edizioni; 2012
11. Connell BF, Semlacher RA. Contemporary deep layer facial rejuvenation. Plast Reconstr Surg 1997;100(6): 1513–1523
12. Cornette de Saint-Cyr B, Garey LJ, Maillard GF, Aharoni C. The vertical midface lift. An improved procedure. J Plast Reconstr Aesthet Surg 2007;60(12):1277–1286
13. Dempsey PD, Oneal RM, Izenberg PH. Subperiosteal brow and midface lifts. Aesthetic Plast Surg 1995;19(1): 59–68
14. Fuente del Campo A. Cirugia reparadora del envejecimiento facial sin cicatrices visables. Cir Cir 1993;60:123–132
15. Hamra ST. Composite rhytidectomy. Plast Reconstr Surg 1992;90(1):1–13
16. Hamra ST. The zygorbicular dissection in composite rhytidectomy: an ideal midface plane. Plast Reconstr Surg 1998;102(5):1646–1657
17. Hinderer UT. The sub-SMAS and subperiosteal rhytidectomy of the forehead and middle third of the face: a new approach to the aging face. Facial Plast Surg 1992;8(1): 18–32
18. Krastinova-Lolov D. Le lifting facial sous-périosté. Ann Chir Plast Esthet 1989;34(3):199–211
19. LaFerriere KA, Kilpatrick JK. Transblepharoplasty: subperiosteal approach to rejuvenation of the aging midface. Facial Plast Surg 2003;19(2):157–170
20. Isse NG. Endoscopic facial rejuvenation. Clin Plast Surg 1997;24(2):213–231
21. Ivy EJ, Lorenc ZP, Aston SJ. Is there a difference? A prospective study comparing lateral and standard SMAS face lifts with extended SMAS and composite rhytidectomies. Plast Reconstr Surg 1996;98(7):1135–1143, discussion 1144–1147
22. Kamer FM, Mingrone MD. Deep plane rhytidectomy: a personal evolution. Facial Plast Surg Clin North Am 2002;10(1):63–75, viii
23. Le Louarn C, Buthiau D, Buis J. The face recurve concept: medical and surgical applications. Aesthetic Plast Surg 2007;31(3):219–231, discussion 232
24. Le Louarn C. [Midface region: functional anatomy, aging process, indications and concentric malar lift]. Ann Chir Plast Esthet 2009;54(5):411–420
25. McCollough EG, Scurry WC Jr, Shirazi MA. The "midface-lift" as a misnomer for correctly identifying procedures designed to lift and rejuvenate the cheeks and malar regions of the face. Arch Facial Plast Surg 2009;11(4): 257–262
26. Newman J. Safety and efficacy of midface-lifts with an absorbable soft tissue suspension device. Arch Facial Plast Surg 2006;8(4):245–251
27. Ortiz Monasterio F. Aesthetic surgery of the facial skeleton: the forehead. Clin Plast Surg 1991;18(1):19–27
28. Owsley JQ. Lifting the malar fat pad for correction of prominent nasolabial folds. Plast Reconstr Surg 1993; 91(3):463–474, discussion 475–476
29. Paul MD, Calvert JW, Evans GRD. The evolution of the mid-face lift in aesthetic plastic surgery. Plast Reconstr Surg 2006;117(6):1809–1827
30. Psillakis JM, Rumley TO, Camargos A. Subperiosteal approach as an improved concept for correction of the aging face. Plast Reconstr Surg 1988;82(3):383–394
31. Quatela VC, Jacono AA. The extended centrolateral endoscopic midface lift. Facial Plast Surg 2003;19(2):199–208
32. Ramirez OM, Maillard GF, Musolas A. The extended subperiosteal face lift: a definitive soft-tissue remodeling for facial rejuvenation. Plast Reconstr Surg 1991;88(2): 227–236, discussion 237–238
33. Ramirez OM. Three-dimensional endoscopic midface enhancement: a personal quest for the ideal cheek rejuvenation. Plast Reconstr Surg 2002;109(1):329–340, discussion 341–349
34. Tapia A, Ferreria B, Blanch A. Subperiostic lifting. Aesthetic Plast Surg 1991;15(2):155–160
35. Williams EF III, Vargas H, Dahiya R, Hove CR, Rodgers BJ, Lam SM. Midfacial rejuvenation via a minimal-incision brow-lift approach: critical evaluation of a 5-year experience. Arch Facial Plast Surg 2003;5(6):470–478
36. Williams JV. Transblepharoplasty endoscopic subperiosteal midface lift. Plast Reconstr Surg 2002;110(7): 1769–1775, discussion 1776–1777

Section VI

Special Topics

30 Nuances of Fat Grafting in the Face of the Mixed-Race Patient

Samuel M. Lam

30.1 Introduction

Volume restoration for the aging face has emerged as a cornerstone of the treatment strategy of many facial aesthetic practitioners over the past 10 to 15 years.[1,2,3] No longer is the gravitational model for aging the dominant paradigm for how the face changes over time. In the author's opinion, gravitational effects are secondary to the volumetric collapse that occurs over the patient's lifetime. Understanding how best to achieve aesthetically pleasing, technically proficient outcomes that are universal in scope regardless of the ethnicity of the patient, is a major goal of this chapter. Furthermore, points for superior fat grafting that relate to the varied mixed-ethnicity face are also elaborated.[4] Finally, it is imperative that the surgeon have meticulous dialogue with every prospective patient to minimize patient dissatisfaction, which can occur even with the greatest surgical outcomes due to poor communication.[5] The saying "The difference between an education and an excuse is that an education is given before a procedure, and an excuse is given afterward" is a maxim that the author lives by on a daily basis. It is preferable never to give an excuse if at all possible.

30.2 Aesthetic Philosophy, the Aging Process, and the Limitations of Fat Grafting

Fat grafting can be a technically straightforward procedure, but before the procedure is undertaken, the artistic underpinnings must be firmly grasped to avoid the overfilled, unbalanced results that have given the procedure an undeserved poor reputation in many circles. Fat grafting does not provide perfect volumetric results; instead, it provides shades of improvement that the surgeon must comprehend in order to master safe and reproducible work.

First, it is important to recognize the nature of the aging process so that the surgeon can understand how to rejuvenate the patient's face. If weight is held consistent over a lifetime, i.e., one does not gain or lose weight except for the growth associated with reaching adulthood, then one will notice a very distinct evolution of the face: it consistently and ineluctably deflates from birth until death. There is significantly more fat in the face of a 1-year-old child than in a 10-year-old's face, in a 10-year-old's face than in a 20-year-old's, in a 20-year-old's than in a 30-year-old's, etc. In fact, many women in particular are not very fond of how their faces appear in their twenties because there is almost too much fat, colloquially termed "baby fat," that they wish to shed, which magically occurs by their early thirties. Many women actually prefer this transformation, and the male-dominated world of surgery should understand this aesthetic value before endeavoring to plump up a face, because the result may be far in excess of what a woman wants and may even look unnatural. In particular, dark-skinned ethnic faces may age more slowly than the faces of fair-skinned races, which are more prone to sun damage and consequently cutaneous photodamage, volume loss, and gravitational forces. Accordingly, darker-skinned ethnic faces may show only signs of volume loss, since higher Fitzpatrick skin types resist cutaneous solar elastosis and facial gravity better than their lighter-skinned counterparts. This is why fat transfer can be so important for ethnic individuals (**Fig. 30.1, Fig. 30.2, Fig. 30.3,** and **Fig. 30.4**). Some words of caution should be offered about working on ethnic individuals. Some ethnic faces, like Asian faces, some Mestizo faces, and faces of patients who have Asian ancestry, may remain very round and fuller even into the patient's fourth decade, so fat transfer should be more conservative. In addition, owing to the flatter and wider aspect of Asian faces, fat should be conservatively and judiciously placed in the lateral portion of the face so as not to widen the face unduly and unaesthetically. These concepts are discussed further in detail below.

The concept of "blink," written about by Malcolm Gladwell in his book of the same title, is important to convey to the patient desiring cosmetic facial rejuvenation. Too often, women in particular are very focused on the minutiae of the face, such as fine lines around the mouth, that contribute little to the aging-related appearance. Instead, the surgeon should help the patient to understand that a major, if not the principal, goal of rejuvenation is to change the onlooker's "blink," i.e., the immediate perception of the beauty and youthfulness of the face that is determined in a nanosecond. To get a better "blink" outcome, the surgeon should focus on the light and shadow of the face that can indicate either youth or senescence. The progressive exposure of the bony landmarks of the face is a sign of aging and should be corrected by fat transfer. In addition, hollowing and narrowing occur in every subcomponent of the face, and the primary focus of a fat transfer procedure is to reestablish favorable highlights, to diminish unfavorable shadows, and to minimize transitions between the shadow points. Many times, surgeons are only interested in augmenting obvious deficits, like those in the cheek and the lower eyelid area, but doing so can lead to a disjointed rejuvenation where the size of the cheek, for example, does not match the rest of the face or to a face that simply appears inadequately rejuvenated. Instead, the goal should be to

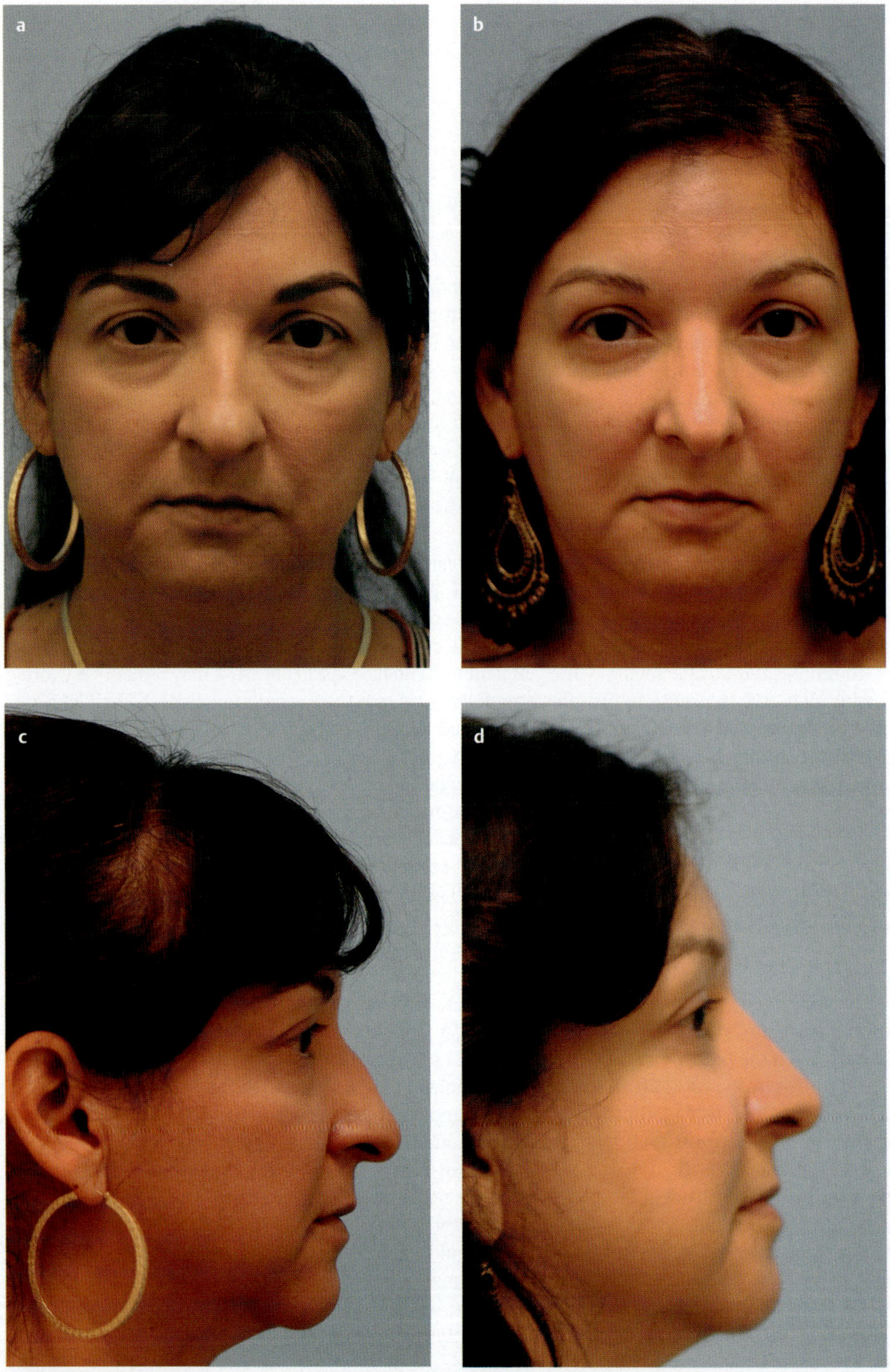

Fig. 30.1 This 47-year-old Hispanic woman is shown **(a,c)** before and **(b,d)** 1 year after a combined full facial fat transfer and cosmetic rhinoplasty.

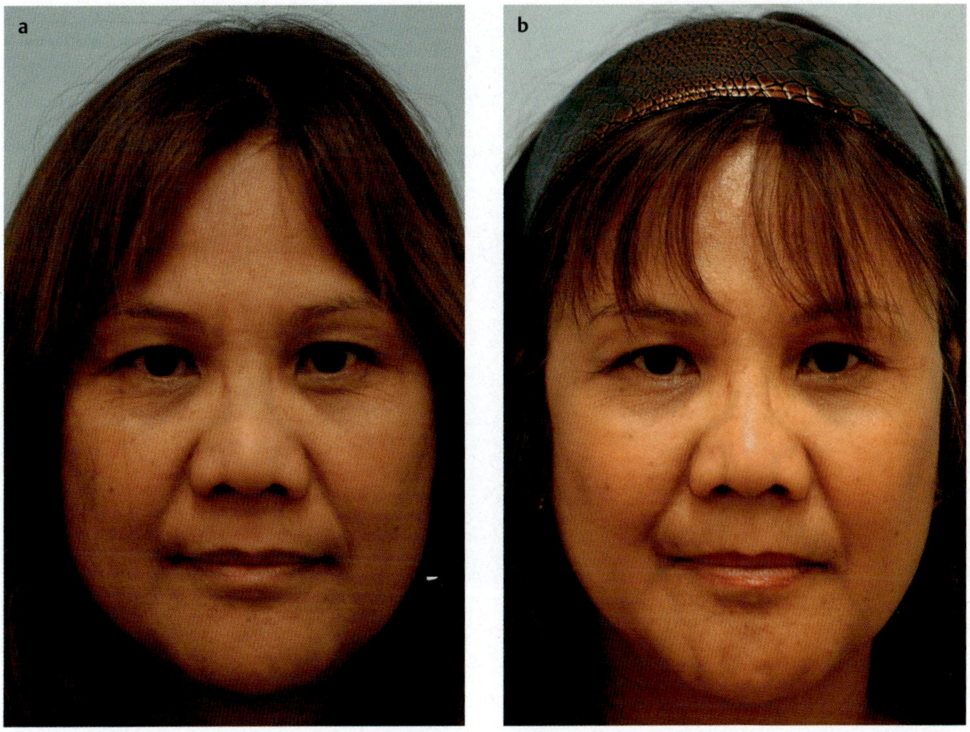

Fig. 30.2 This 51-year-old Filipina woman is shown **(a)** before and **(b)** 1 year after a full facial fat transfer procedure. The wide appearance of the face can be reduced by sculpting the anterior cheek and chin area to balance the outer facial shape.

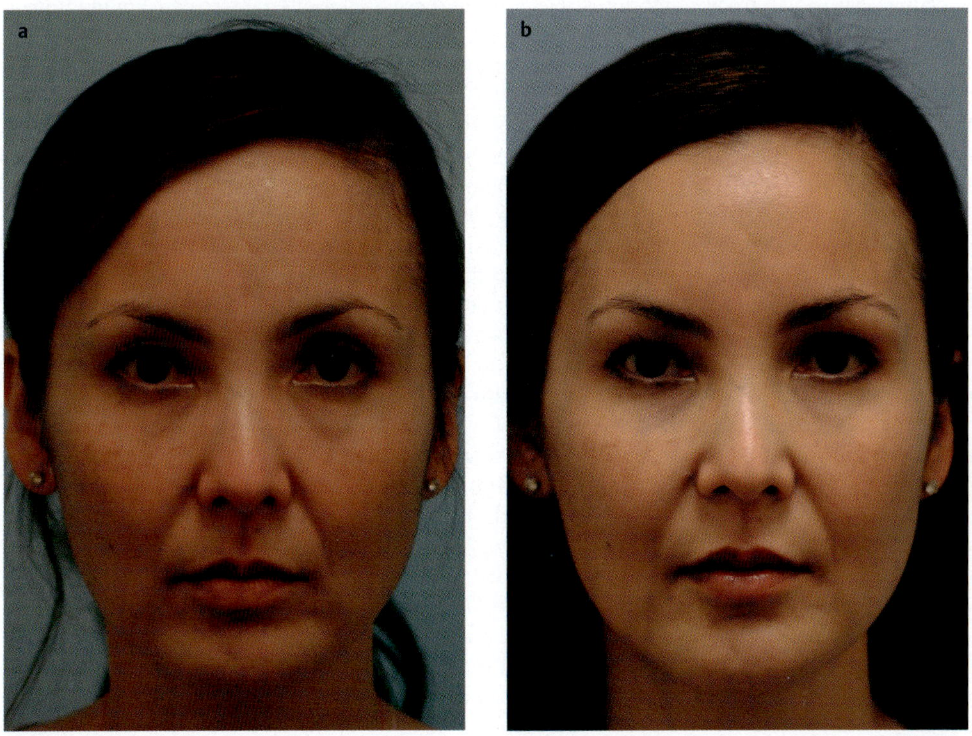

Fig. 30.3 This 41-year-old half-Asian, half-Caucasian woman is shown **(a)** before and **(b)** 1 year after a full facial fat transfer.

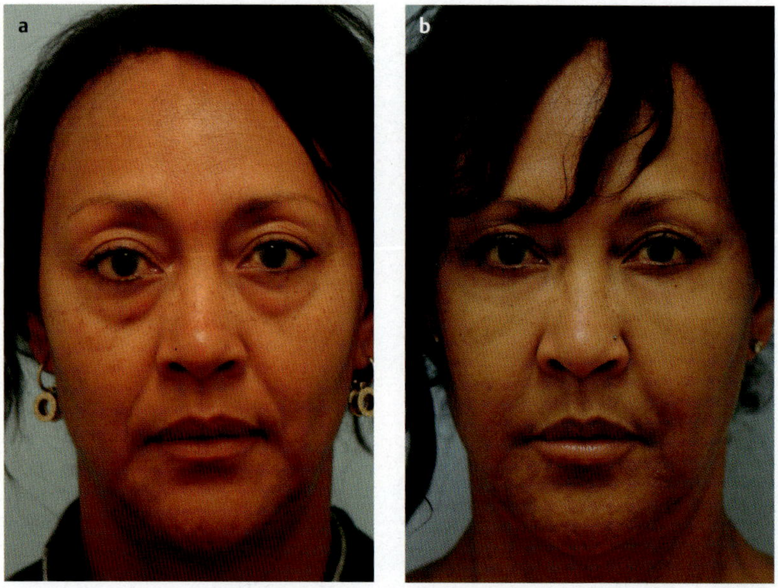

Fig. 30.4 This 51-year-old African woman is shown (a) before and (b) 5 years after a full facial fat transfer and lower transconjunctival blepharoplasty.

improve as many shadows and deficiencies of the face as possible by including all areas of volume loss—the temple, brow, upper eyelid, lower eyelid, outer canthus, nasojugal groove, anterior cheek, lateral cheek, subzygomatic region, central buccal region, canine, nasolabial groove, anterior chin, prejowl sulcus, and, as needed, the lateral mandible or entire mandibular expanse. In addition, by providing volume in the lateral face, particularly the temple, lateral cheek, and subzygomatic regions, the surgeon can reinflate the face so that the oval shape of the face is improved. Part of the blink effect is contributed by the overall shape of the face: an oval face has a more youthful effect than one that is starting to narrow in the lateral expanse. Identifying these deficits and understanding how to fill them properly are prerequisites to performing fat transfer in an aesthetic and effective way.

Many surgeons are frustrated with the outcome of the fat transfer procedure, largely because they do not understand the benefits, limitations, and risks of the procedure, which are very important to grasp. The benefits of fat transfer are outlined in the previous paragraph, i.e., to improve overall highlights, to diminish shadows, to diminish transitions of the face, and to create a better face shape, while providing a lasting result. The limitations of fat transfer are that it doesn't allow absolute precision. Why? First, the fat graft must have a blood supply to survive. If harvested gently, processed correctly, and injected appropriately, then fat should have very good viability (these technical aspects are discussed in the following section on technique). However, fat is still a graft, and it has variable resorption. Second, fat is a very soft filler compared to commercial injectable products, so it does not eliminate facial flaws as well as injectable fillers do. Last, fat should be placed relatively deep so that it is not visible. Despite these limitations, fat transfer should improve one's blink effect, especially if the procedure is performed as prescribed, with a little fat placed in a lot of areas, rather than a lot of fat placed in a few areas of the face. However, injectable fillers may be required in many cases to improve the fat grafting result. If this is the case, questions arise: When should you inject the fillers to touch up the fat grafting result? Should you instead perform multiple sessions of fat transfer or, better yet, skip fat transfer and just perform filler injection? Here are the answers. First, the fat graft takes time to mature and to achieve blood supply. The time required is very similar to that required for a hair graft after a hair transplant, which can take 6 to 12 months to achieve complete blood supply. Fat grafts can shrink in the first few months after a transplant and then start to evolve slowly over time to an improved condition after 9 months to a year. Therefore, a fat transfer should not be touched up with fillers until at least 9 months to a year after the fat grafting procedure.

If fat transfer is less precise than filler injection, why perform fat transfer at all? The reason is that fat is less expensive and gives more durable results for the entire face when it is performed in the prescribed manner, i.e., a little bit placed everywhere. Injectable filler procedures can use as many as 10 to 20 syringes, if not more, which can be quite costly to the patient; and if the filler is a hyaluronic acid–based product, the results begin to diminish as the patient leaves the office. That is not the case with a fat graft. Conversely, if a single session of fat transfer may be insufficient, why not perform multiple sessions of fat transfer to achieve an outcome? The reason is that fat transfer to the face incurs considerable morbidity and therefore has a protracted recovery time. In addition, the limitations of fat transfer already mentioned (viability of the graft, softer product, and deeper placement) make accuracy problematic. Therefore, patients are counseled that their fat graft should provide a very good "blink" improvement for their face but cannot completely manage all of the volumetric loss: approximately a year after the fat transfer, the patient will require a supplemental procedure with facial fillers targeted to the areas where fat did not perfectly survive or did not effectively correct the facial defect.

Another question that patients are concerned about is the longevity of a fat graft. Fat grafts have been characterized as strictly temporary, and, alternatively, it has been proposed that fat grafts last 2 to 4 years or some other particular stated time. However, these characterizations are made in ignorance of the nature of a fat graft. Since a fat graft is truly a graft, the proportion of the graft that survives will remain throughout the patient's remaining life. (Would a skin graft die suddenly 2 years after it was placed? Of course not. Neither would a fat graft.) In performing revision surgery 8 years after a fat graft into the lips, the author found the fat graft still present as discrete lobules of fat. Furthermore, Lambros has seen a patient who had a fat transfer years before start to have areas of the face enlarge unnaturally with weight gain, a risk that is further discussed below. In summary, a fat transfer is a graft that survives, and it must be treated as permanent because it is unequivocally permanent if performed correctly.

How, then, does a patient continue to lose facial volume as he or she ages? The answer is simple. The grafted fat remains, but the remainder of the native, untransplanted fat begins to dissipate over time. The author has seen in his patients that, many years after a fat transfer, the areas where less fat was transplanted begin to look unbalanced, not significantly so, but still enough to cause alarm, and they require either additional fat transfer or fillers to adjust the result. (Using the hair transplant analogy, it is like a hair transplant in which the transplanted hair survives but the original, untransplanted hair disappears.) It is very important that patients (as well as surgeons) understand this limitation so that there is no misunderstanding of the permanence of the fat graft.

The final point of discussion is the risk of poor results of a fat graft. Clearly, an overfilled result can look terrible, and it is critical that the surgeon be conservative, only gradually adding volume to the patient's face. Because it is nearly impossible to correct an overfilled face, it is imperative not to create one in the first place. However, even with the surgeon's best efforts, the patient can gain weight over time and make a previously excellent result appear overfilled and/or disjointed. Unlike off-the-shelf fillers, fat is truly a viable graft and behaves like the fat from the donor source, which is typically the abdomen and thighs, i.e., it is very resistant to loss but easily can expand with weight gain. For this reason, the author does not like to use fat transfer in three circumstances: (1) The patient's weight is unstable or the patient has had recent significant weight loss. (2) The patient is young and future weight gain is uncertain. (3) The patient requires a reconstructive procedure in which fat will be placed in the face asymmetrically. An individual who recently lost weight and who is now interested in a fat graft is a very high-risk surgical candidate, because if he or she regains the weight, the face can look disastrously overfilled and unnatural. A younger patient is defined as one under the age of 35 years, when metabolic slowdown starts to affect the waistline, and thus the younger patient has the risk of weight gain over time. Finally, asymmetrical injection is also problematic because the injected area can change as the person's weight profile fluctuates. For these reasons, in patients in these risk categories, injectable off-the-shelf fillers are preferable, and the risks of fat transfer must always be discussed with the high-risk patient before the procedure.

30.3 Special Considerations for Fat Grafting in the Ethnic Face

As discussed above, the universal elements of volume loss affect all ethnicities. However, some differences that have been briefly mentioned in the previous section also apply to ethnic faces.

In many cases, darker-skinned ethnic faces have an inherent resistance to solar damage, allowing for the persistence of more youthful countenances. The reason for most of the aging-related facial changes in different ethnicities is volume loss, whereas rhytids, cutaneous damage, and neck descent are largely delayed and occur to a lesser extent than in fairer-skinned races. This is why fat grafting and other procedures to restore volume loss can be so important for the ethnic face.

Many Asian faces are wider and flatter than Caucasian faces. African faces, too, can have a broader, wider nose and a flatter facial appearance. Mestizo patients who have a high proportion of indigenous Indian blood can also have a broader countenance, owing to descent from the distant lineage of Asiatic tribes who crossed the Bering Strait over to the New World. Therefore, it is important not to overfill the broad face, especially laterally, causing the face to appear too wide. The author uses fat grafting as a sculpting tool to subtly reshape the face (without changing identity) so that the face has overall better harmony. For example, if the chin is weak, additional fat can be placed there in lieu of a chin implant (but not too much, or the chin will look simply fat and not solidly projected). Or, for example, some Koreans have a very broad outer cheekbone. Fat can be placed more anteriorly and immediately below the large malar prominence to soften its appearance. Conversely, if an Asian patient has a very full anterior cheek, fat can then be placed in the lateral cheek to offset the dominant anterior cheek. While the surgeon is learning the subtle elements of aesthetic volume restoration, they can be practiced more safely using off-the-shelf fillers that are temporary and reversible.

Another issue is the complicated status of the aging Asian upper eyelid.[6,7,8] Many Asians experience age-related sagging of the upper eyelid but simply want a browlift and/or upper eyelid surgery to improve the situation. However, the real problem is that the upper eyelid crease should be relatively lower in the Asian patient than in any other race. Removal of skin from the upper eyelid and/or browlift can lead to a high upper eyelid crease that appears unnatural. Another difficulty is the patient who does not have a discernible crease in the upper eyelid and who would like to simply have skin removed. Simply removing upper eyelid skin in an Asian patient without a crease can cause unpredictable, visible scarring and a limited result, because the problem is not excess skin but a narrowed palpebral fissure caused by postseptal fat descending toward the ciliary margin. There are only two ways to solve this problem: fat transfer to fill out the eyelid and/or a formal Asian blepharoplasty to create a distinct supratarsal crease. Accordingly, fat transfer is a very important method for improving the aging Asian eyelid without risking an unnatural result or a visible scar with no discernible benefit.

30.4 Preoperative Considerations

All of the limitations, benefits, and risks should be fully grasped by the surgeon and should be accurately and fully discussed with the prospective patient. In addition, the surgical plan should be based on the key design strategies espoused in the previous section. If these elements are all well understood, communicated, and documented, the only other issues to be addressed are safety of anesthesia and the nature of the recovery time. Typically, the author tells the patient that, at 1 week, nobody will like the surgical result; at 2 weeks the patient may not like the result but others will think you look good; and it may take up to 3 weeks for the patient to like the result. The average patient takes ~ 7 to 10 days off from work but may take up to 2 weeks off if one's appearance is critical to the job description, e.g., a sales position. (More details of the recovery process are discussed under "Postoperative Considerations" below.)

30.5 Operative Considerations

The author prefers to perform fat transfer procedures with the patient under general anesthesia if at all possible, chiefly because there is significantly less patient discomfort. In addition, general anesthesia entirely eliminates the need for local anesthesia, which otherwise is associated with postoperative edema and ecchymosis. However, the procedure can be performed under twilight anesthesia, but the patient discomfort level is too high if the procedure is performed without any sedation at all.

30.5.1 Marking the Patient

For marking the regions of the face that will receive fat transfer, the patient should sit upright, because the shadows cast in the upright position allow the surgeon to have a much better appreciation of how much volume is needed in each region of the face. The author uses a black permanent marker to outline the areas in question and a red marker to circle the areas of proposed needle entries, where typically a small wheal is raised with lidocaine, as is explained below (**Fig. 30.5**). Before the marking begins, the author already has calculated how many milliliters of filler will be placed, and where, and that plan is rarely altered intraoperatively. Preoperative visualization of what is needed is much more effective, because once the patient is supine and with edema (especially if local anesthesia is used), it becomes progressively harder to determine what is needed. Furthermore, the patient's preoperative frontal and oblique photographs are always on display in the operating room to remind the surgeon of what needs to be accomplished with the fat transfer.

30.5.2 Infiltration of Local Anesthetic

The discussion here covers how to perform the procedure with the patient receiving twilight anesthesia, because under general anesthesia no local anesthetic is needed except at the entry sites.

After the patient is marked and brought into the operating theater, the donor and recipient sites are prepared with povidone-iodine and are draped with sterile towels per standard routine. With the patient properly sedated, anesthesia is first infiltrated into the donor areas to permit adequate time for anesthesia and vasoconstriction. A 20 mL syringe is filled with 10 mL of 1% lidocaine with 1:100,000 epinephrine and 10 mL of plain sterile saline and is outfitted with a 5 inch 22 gauge spinal needle. With the spinal needle, half of the syringe is infiltrated below the perceived fat plane and half of the syringe is infiltrated above the fat plane near the dermis.

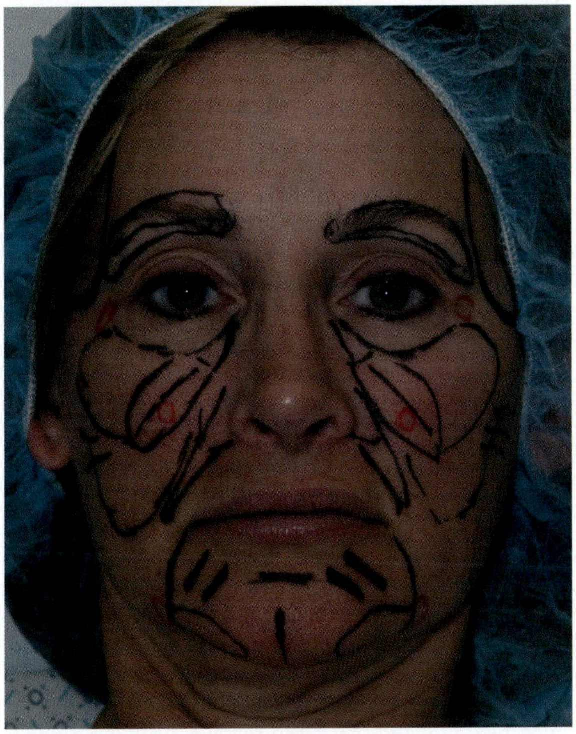

Fig. 30.5 A black marker is used to delineate all of the areas for fat augmentation, and a red marker is used to aid the surgeon in locating the proposed entry points.

A single 20 mL syringe can be used for the entire expanse of the abdomen. For the thighs, a single 20 mL syringe per thigh is preferred to attain adequate anesthesia. If the lateral thigh is also included, an additional syringe will be required for each side. Fortunately, dilute lidocaine that is infiltrated into adipose tissue (which readily absorbs the anesthetic) and is then suctioned out of the body rarely achieves toxic levels even if recommended textbook ranges are exceeded. However, the reader is advised to use caution with the amount of lidocaine in a given patient. The recipient area is then infiltrated with anesthetic. A 10 mL syringe with pure 1% lidocaine with 1:100,000 epinephrine is used for facial anesthesia. With a 30 gauge needle, the six entry sites are anesthetized with an aliquot of anesthetic to improve patient comfort and to facilitate vasoconstriction prior to creating the actual entry site with a standard 18 gauge needle. After a few minutes, the 18 gauge needle is used to create each entry site. An infiltration cannula is then fitted on the 10 mL syringe containing the remaining lidocaine and is used to infiltrate all of the recipient areas via the entry sites. To minimize distortion, generally speaking, a total of 10 mL of lidocaine should be sufficient to attain adequate anesthesia in the face so long as the patient is also supported with a comfortable level of intravenous sedation. If the patient is under only light sedation or oral medication, then a regional nerve block should precede blunt cannula injection of anesthetic to make cannula injection more tolerable. The reason for using a blunt cannula for local anesthetic injection is to minimize postoperative bruising by avoiding all sharp needle injections.

30.5.3 Harvesting the Fat

First, the donor site should be entered through a discrete entry point, e.g., the inferior aspect of the umbilicus for abdominal harvesting and the inguinal line for thigh harvesting. The entry site is made with a 16 gauge Nokor needle (Becton Dickinson), through which the harvesting cannula (Tulip Medical Products) can be easily inserted. The harvesting cannula is attached to an empty 10 mL syringe for hand harvesting. The Johnnie Lok (Tulip Medical Products) facilitates locking the syringe plunger to a degree of negative pressure and minimizes hand fatigue during harvesting. After insertion of the cannula through the entry site into the donor area, the Johnnie Lok is used to establish ~ 2 to 3 mL of negative pressure before harvesting is initiated. Of course, the syringe plunger can be manually retracted if the physician decides against the purchase of a Johnnie Lok device.

During harvesting, the surgeon should visualize where the tip of the cannula is at all times during passage through the donor area, for two reasons. First, the cannula tip is the site where fat enters the cannula so it must pass through the entire donor site evenly and deliberately. Second, if the cannula tip is passed too aggressively it can cause unnecessary trauma and related discomfort: if it is passed too deeply, it will abrade the fascia; too superficially, it will irritate the dermis; and too far past the donor area, it will disturb adjacent territories for no reason. With experience, the surgeon will be able to sense the position of the cannula tip at all times, and will be able to minimize discomfort and to maximize a uniform yield.

With that in mind, the next consideration is that the cannula tip pass across the intended donor area uniformly. It is important during fat harvesting that the cannula tip glide across the fat plane without distortion. To avoid uneven harvesting, the surgeon should not pinch or tent the skin upward with the nondominant hand during harvesting. Instead, the nondominant hand can brace the donor area gently so that the skin is held taut during fat harvest. It is also important that the cannula pass the entire expanse from entry site to the distal end of the donor site with each pass to avoid over- and under-harvesting the fat pad proximally or distally. That consideration also applies with the passage of the cannula from side to side. Accordingly, the cannula tip should be withdrawn all the way to the entry site before turning to harvest an adjacent area, because just turning the cannula tip while it is already fully inserted into the donor area will lead to over-harvesting of the same area, since the cannula tip has not truly advanced to the adjacent terrain. This technical error is revealed by the skin's kinking above where the cannula is merely torquing the tissue without actually being advanced.

When harvesting specific donor areas, all of the above guidelines should be followed plus the following recommendations related to the respective donor areas. In the lower abdomen, the harvesting should progress along the lower lateral quadrants, with feathering to include the regions just above superolaterally and toward the midline inferiorly. The midline generally is devoid of significant adipose tissue and is replete with more fibrous fascia. Nevertheless, the surgeon should feather across the transition zones, to ensure that the harvested area is uniformly blended to the adjacent nonharvested regions.

The inner thigh can be more technically difficult to harvest from and should be undertaken only by a more experienced surgeon. The cannula must pierce through an initial fascial layer so that the cannula tip is not observed tracking across under the skin, which would be too superficial and would most likely engender unfortunate contour deformities. To ensure more uniform harvesting, the patient's leg should also remain in a straightened position and should not be in the frog-leg position. In short, with the patient supine, no change in position is required for inner-thigh fat harvesting. As with abdominal harvesting, the surgeon should attempt to harvest not only in a discrete area but also to feather gently medially and laterally to provide a smooth transition to the unharvested zones.

30.5.4 Processing the Fat

The processing of fat involves separating and removing the blood, lysed fat cells, and lidocaine prior to infiltration—all of which is performed on a sterile table by the surgical assistant.

Once the fat has been collected, the syringes are centrifuged for distillation of impurities. Only centrifuges that can accommodate sterilizable sleeves (into which the syringes are placed) should be used, in order to maintain a sterile environment throughout the procedure.

The plungers are removed from the syringes and specially designed caps are secured to both ends of each syringe to avoid spillage during centrifugation. Of course, the prepared syringes of uncentrifuged fat are inserted into the sterile sleeves within the centrifuge so that they are across from one another, so as not to disrupt the balance of the machine. The syringes of fat are then centrifuged for 3 minutes at 3,000 rpm. They are removed from the centrifuge sterilely and are placed into a test-tube rack on the sterile field. The supranatant (yellowish oil that represents lysed fat cells) is first poured off from the plunger side into a waste bin. The screw cap on the other end can then be removed to drain the infranatant, consisting of blood and lidocaine. It is imperative that the supranatant always be poured off before the infranatant is drained, because proceeding in the reverse order will ensure that the column of fat will inadvertently fall out into the waste bin. After both supranatant and infranatant are decanted, the syringe is placed with the open plunger side up into the test-tube rack, and an uncut 4 × 4 gauze is inserted into the exposed plunger side to contact the column of fat. Allowing 5 to 10 minutes of contact time between the cotton gauze and the fat will help absorb any remaining supranatant before transfer. Of note, the cotton gauze should not be cut to avoid the risk that strands of gauze would splinter off and remain on the column of fat and in turn be injected into the face as a foreign body. When removing the gauze, any fat clinging to the gauze can be gently rubbed onto the side of the syringe so as to preserve it, but care should be taken not to work too vigorously and leave any cotton fibers behind on the fat.

To facilitate preparation, the 10 mL syringes can be emptied into a 20 mL syringe by pouring from open plunger side to open plunger side. Another reason to transfer from the 10 mL syringe into a 20 mL syringe before transferring the fat into the 1 mL infiltration syringes is to remove the small plug of blood that often remains behind even after decanting. Typically, since only ~ 5 mL of fat are collected from every 10 mL syringe (the remainder being unusable supranatant and infranatant), two to three 10 mL syringes of fat can be transferred into a single empty 20 mL transfer syringe. The plunger is then replaced into the backside of the 20 mL syringe, taking care not to eject the fat across the room during insertion of the plunger. All air is carefully removed from the 20 mL transfer syringe at this point.

A two-sided Luer-Lock transfer hub is used to attach the 20 mL syringe to a 1 mL syringe, which will be used to infiltrate the fat. Of note, if not already explicitly stated, all syringes used during fat transfer employ Luer-Locks. During transfer from the 20 mL to the 1 mL syringe, it is important to remove the plunger entirely from the 1 mL syringe so that the air bubble is taken out. The plunger is then reinserted back to the 1 mL mark.

As mentioned, typically only about half of the 10 mL syringe that is harvested contains usable fat. Therefore, as the surgeon is deciding the amount of fat necessary for transfer, he or she should plan according to this anticipated loss. At times, the fat harvested can be bloodier or oilier, and a greater percentage of waste then occupies each collected syringe and a greater number of syringes will need to be collected to attain the same volume of fat.

30.5.5 Fat Infiltration

Before giving a detailed description of fat transfer in each facial zone, some basic guidelines must be elaborated. As described, all fat transfer is undertaken with a blunt cannula on a 1 mL Luer-Lock syringe, and a 1.2 mm Tulip cannula serves as the workhorse for the majority of fat infiltration. There are two principal considerations in the basic fat transfer injection technique: the amount of fat transferred per cannula pass and the depth of injection (**Table 30.1**).

The amount of fat transferred per pass of the cannula can be divided into two standard injection amounts: 0.02 mL per pass or 0.1 mL per pass, depending on how sensitive the area in question is. For example, in the inferior orbital rim, it is very important that only tiny aliquots of fat be transferred per cannula pass, because of the risk that visible lumps of fat could become apparent over time. In the anterior cheek, a highly forgiving area, a more generous 0.1 mL per pass of the cannula is acceptable. A pass of the cannula is defined as the movement of the cannula in a single direction so that the fat in question is deposited as a discrete bolus. To transfer only 0.02 mL, the surgeon must depress the syringe plunger with an absolute feather-light touch. Furthermore, occasionally the plunger becomes occluded, and it is very important that the surgeon remove the syringe entirely from the injection site and clear the obstruction ex vivo before continuing. A sudden bolus of 0.1 mL or greater could be disastrous in highly sensitive areas like the inferior orbital rim. Injections are performed both in the push and pull directions (insertion and withdrawal phase) during cannula passage.

In addition to the amount of fat injected per pass, the other major consideration is the depth of injection. The depth of injection obviously cannot be immediately visualized but is based on tactile sensation of the cannula tip. When injecting in the deep plane, the cannula tip contacts the periosteum of the bone (but does not need to abrade or remove the periosteum). The index finger of the nondominant hand can be used to provide additional feedback about the proper depth and location of injection, as is elaborated in the pertinent sections below. The intermediate plane is truly an arbitrary plane of injection that corresponds with the plane of least resistance, i.e., the cannula is simply passed into the soft tissue so that it glides approximately somewhere between the deep bone and the

Table 30.1 Systematic fat infiltration, by facial region

Facial region	Entry site	Amount of fat per cannula pass (mL)	Depth	Amount of fat (mL)
Medial inferior orbital rim	A	0.02	Deep	1.0–1.5
Lateral inferior orbital rim	A	0.02	Deep	1.0–1.5
Lateral canthus	a	0.02	Deep	0.1–0.5
Nasojugal groove/tear trough	A	0.1	Intermediate to deep	0.5–1.0
Brow/upper eyelid complex	B	0.1	Intermediate	1.0–2.0
Temple	B	0.02	Intermediate	0.5–1.5
Anterior cheek	B	0.1	All planes	1.0–2.0
Lateral cheek	A	0.1	All planes	0.5–2.0
Medial buccal hollow	A	0.1	Intermediate	0.0–2.0
Central buccal area	A	0.1	Intermediate	0.0–6.0
Lateral buccal hollow (backfill)	A	0.1	Intermediate	0.0–4.0
Prejowl	C	0.1	Intermediate	2.0–4.0
Anterior chin	C	0.1	Intermediate	2.0–3.0
Lateral mandible	b, c, d	0.1	Intermediate	0.5–1.5 (per each of the three entry sites)
Canine (or precanine) fossa	A	0.1	Intermediate to deep	1.0–3.0
Nasolabial groove	A	0.1	Intermediate	1.0–3.0

superficial dermis. The superficial plane lies in continuity with the intermediate plane so that the cannula passes closer to the dermis. Again, the cutoff of what constitutes the intermediate and the superficial planes is arbitrary and continuous. With a basic understanding of these two parameters (amount per cannula pass and depth of injection), the surgeon can then apply these precepts to injection into each facial zone. Almost the entire procedure can be undertaken through three separate entry sites: entry site A (midcheek) **(Fig. 30.6)**, entry site B (near the lateral canthus) **(Fig. 30.7)**, and entry site C (lateral to the prejowl) **(Fig. 30.8)**. Additional entry sites can be used for areas like the lateral canthus and lateral mandible.

Medial Inferior Orbital Rim

The most sensitive area for injection is unequivocally the inferior orbital rim. In the past, it has been the source of most contention about why fat transfer should not be undertaken due to the high morbidity experienced in this region. However, with refinement in technique that focuses on depth, amount injected, and the direction of entry, the complications have been so reduced as to have become negligible. The inferior orbital rim should be approached perpendicularly from an inferior entry site rather than parallel from a lateral entry site. The lateral entry site has

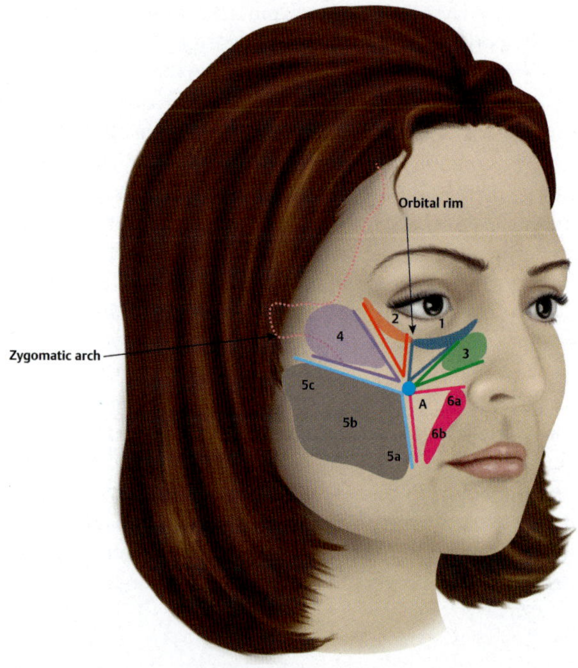

Fig. 30.6 This schematic illustration shows the facial regions that can be infiltrated with fat transfer from entry point A, including (1) the medial inferior orbital rim, (2) the lateral inferior orbital rim, (3) the nasojugal groove/tear trough, (4) the lateral cheek, (5a) the medial buccal hollow, (5b) the central buccal area, (5c) the lateral buccal hollow (or "backfill"), (6a) the canine/precanine fossa, and (6b) the nasolabial groove.

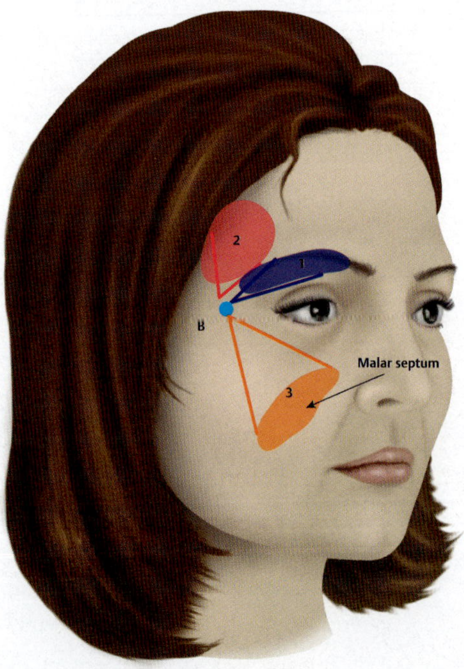

Fig. 30.7 This schematic illustration shows the facial regions that can be infiltrated with fat transfer from entry point B, including (1) the brow–upper eyelid complex, (2) the temple, and (3) the anterior cheek. The malar septum is the fibrous, linear fascia along which and through which the fat is infiltrated into the anterior cheek.

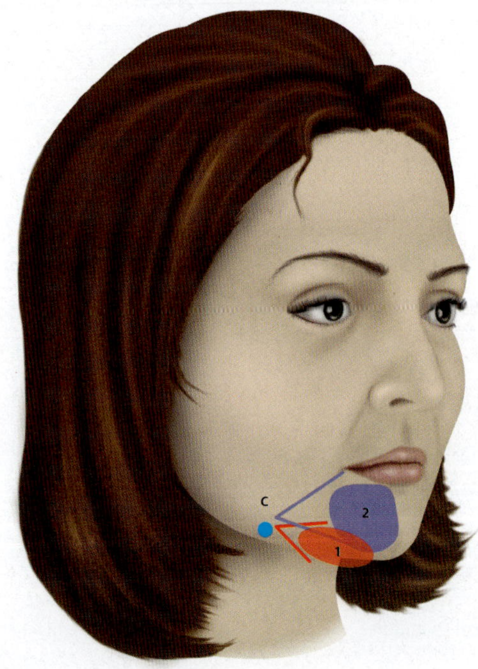

Fig. 30.8 This schematic illustration shows the facial regions that can be infiltrated with fat transfer from entry point C, including (1) the prejowl and (2) the anterior chin.

proven to be an unreliable method of placing fat along the inferior orbital rim that has led to significant contour problems, and it has been relegated to the past with the current perpendicular approach. From the midcheek entry site A, the cannula is inserted and passed superiorly to contact the inferior orbital rim. (This entry site can be divided into two entry sites [more lateral and more medial] to facilitate easier access to the medial and the lateral portions of the inferior orbital rim.) The index finger of the nondominant hand should already be positioned at the inferior orbital rim before insertion of the cannula to protect the globe and to guide injection. The cannula tip should pierce through a fascial layer to contact the orbital rim bone. Without the feeling of a puncture through a fascial tissue plane near the orbital rim, the cannula most likely is not deep enough to be in contact with the rim.

With the index finger of the nondominant hand guiding placement, the cannula tip is gently marched back and forth across the orbital rim, carefully depositing only 0.02 mL per pass across the medial half of the inferior orbital rim. The inferior orbital rim is divided arbitrarily in half medially and laterally to help ensure consistency of injection volumes.

Lateral Inferior Orbital Rim

The lateral half of the inferior orbital rim is approached identically to the method prescribed above for the medial inferior orbital rim. Another reason for dividing the inferior orbital rim into halves is that at times the medial half requires a different volume than the lateral half, based on perceived degrees of hollowness. Typically, the volumes are the same for the medial and lateral extents. However, less commonly, the lateral half may require less volume if the skin is very thin and has a shallow perceived depression.

Lateral Canthus

The cannula has a difficult time filling the very far lateral recess of the inferior orbital rim (referred to here as the lateral canthus) for two reasons. First, the curve of the inferior orbital rim upward makes it hard to deposit fat in this recess. Second, the lateral canthus possesses a greater extent of fibrous tissue. The separate entry site for the lateral canthus is not used for anything else other than placement of fat in the lateral canthus.

Brow/Upper Eyelid Complex

Some surgeons advocate filling principally the lateral extent of the brow, whereas others view the medial extent of the brow as the requisite focus of filling. The author believes that the entire extent of the brow should be filled, possibly with added emphasis to the lateral tail of the brow if need be, i.e., when the surgeon wants to create a brow highlight in this area. Besides creating fullness in the region of the brow proper, the bony step-off that corresponds with the exposed superior half of the orbital rim should be softened with fat transfer. The visibility of this bony landmark is a hallmark of aging and should be minimized if possible. Accordingly, fat is transferred on top of the bony rim (the region that corresponds with the brow) and just where the orbital rim edge is exposed, transitioning down to the upper eyelid region. The brow and upper eyelid complex are filled from entry site A by passing the cannula in an intermediate plane, i.e., the plane of least resistance, and fanning subtly to cover the above-described areas.

Temple

The temple should be considered an advanced area to fill. Technically, it is not very difficult, but the surgeon is advised to master the basic techniques of filling the remainder of the face before approaching the temple. From entry point B, the surgeon places very small aliquots (0.02 mL) per pass, fanning to encompass the entire temporal fossa from hairline laterally to the medial bony border. Generally, 0.5 to 1.5 mL are used to augment the temporal hollow. The plane of placement is in the subcutaneous plane along a plane of least resistance. The major adverse sequela is a hematoma arising from laceration of a superficial temporal vessel. With the appearance of an expanding hematoma, the surgeon should apply immediate sustained pressure, wait, and perhaps venture to the contralateral side until the bleeding ceases. Although some fibrous attachments may be encountered as the surgeon augments this area, the surgeon should be slower and more deliberate when breaking through these fibers to limit hematoma risk.

Anterior Cheek

The anterior cheek, as explained, can be one of the most important areas to fill aesthetically for the female patient. The luster of a bright anterior cheek can return a vibrant appearance to the eye. However, overfilling this area can also lead to an unnatural chipmunk appearance that is highly unfavorable. From entry point B, the surgeon passes the cannula in a fanning technique to break through the malar ligament. The malar ligament, or malar septum, is a fibrous entity that spans superomedially to inferolaterally across the anterior cheek, and its fibers run superficial to deep. It is important when filling the anterior cheek that the cannula pass through the malar ligament so that fat is deposited on either side of the ligament. The only way to accomplish this feat easily is to pass from a perpendicular orientation, i.e., from entry point B, which lies perpendicular to the malar depression. If the surgeon passes the cannula parallel to the malar ligament, there is a risk that the fat will be positioned on one side or the other of the ligament and create an unsightly bulge, thereby deepening, rather than effacing, the malar depression. Although the ligament is physically present in every individual, the surgeon may not feel a perceptible resistance as the cannula passes across it. Nevertheless, a perpendicular deposit of fat across the ligament is critical in every case. As the area is filled, the surgeon visualizes the cannula passing from a deep to a superficial orientation while fanning across the cheek. When starting deeply, it is not critical to hug the periosteum but just to start in a relatively deep subcutaneous plane and to march upward so that the fat is uniformly deposited across the entire expanse of the anterior cheek, focusing on the malar depression. By spreading the deposited fat over a wide area, the surgeon can increase the likelihood of fat survival, as the tiny microdroplets are suspended with greater contact to the surrounding native tissue and associated blood supply. Generally, for mild anterior cheek depression, 0.5 to 1 mL is sufficient to provide adequate augmentation, whereas 1 to 2 mL are preferred for someone with more notable anterior cheek hollowing. Placement of fat is performed with a more generous 0.1 mL per pass, as the area is very forgiving, with a negligible risk of lumpiness if the method prescribed is adhered to.

Lateral Cheek

The anterior cheek should be blended with the three surrounding adjacent facial territories: the lateral cheek, the inferior orbital rim, and the buccal region inferiorly (to be discussed). The lateral cheek is important to augment for three reasons: first, to cover the exposed bone of the malar eminence; second, to blend effectively with the anterior cheek; and third, to create a more vibrant light reflection over the augmented region that can be particularly attractive in the male patient. The lateral cheek is defined as the soft tissue region situated over the malar bony eminence. From entry point A, the surgeon fans the cannula superolaterally across the expanse of the malar bony eminence using the nondominant hand to guide tactile feedback by palpating the malar bone. The lateral cheek is also a very forgiving region, and 0.1 mL of fat can be transferred per cannula pass easily and quickly. Although the same deep-to-superficial passage of the cannula is ideal, it is very hard to accomplish this maneuver, as the soft tissue depth is relatively shallow. Therefore, the cannula can just be passed across this area subcutaneously along a plane of least resistance. Generally, ~ 1 to 2 mL are required to achieve a desirable augmentation. The author has become much more generous in the lateral cheek (at times using 4–5 mL) than in the anterior cheek, because the lateral cheek blends the face very well without contributing to the chipmunk appearance that can occur with on overfilled anterior cheek, especially observed during smiling.

Medial, Central, and Lateral Buccal Areas

The buccal area should be augmented in the gaunt patient and avoided or minimized in the heavier patient. In the very gaunt patient or the patient with significant volume loss, the buccal region can be one of the most important areas to fill to create a more youthful and balanced appearance of the face. From entry point A, the buccal area can be filled to soften the transition from the augmented anterior and lateral cheek. Recall that a youthful face exhibits very few transitions, so the buccal area can be viewed as an important area to fill to blend the augmented cheek region. The buccal area is filled from entry point A so that fanning of the cannula passes subcutaneously in a plane of least resistance. Because the buccal region is rather shallow, it is virtually impossible intentionally to pass the cannula from deep to superficial. Accordingly, the cannula simply traverses the plane of least resistance. The buccal area is a very forgiving area, and the cannula can be passed quickly and easily, depositing 0.1 mL per pass. Generally, in the heavy patient, the surgeon tries to avoid the buccal region but most likely will need to deposit a little fat there to soften the transition from the augmented cheek region. In this case, about 0.5 mL is sufficient. In mild cases of buccal hollowness, 1 to 2 mL are sufficient to accomplish the task, whereas significant buccal recession mandates 3 to 6 mL to camouflage the depression, especially in light of the greater disparity that arises between the augmented cheek and the yet-to-be-augmented buccal region.

Prejowl

The prejowl sulcus refers to the soft tissue depression that lies anterior to the jowl. The prejowl depression should be viewed as a three-dimensional cylinder that runs both along the inferior portion of the anterior face of the mandible and inferior to the mandible to capture the hanging portion of the jowl along with the transition zone between these two cylinders. Placement of fat occurs from the laterally based entry point C to fill the three aforementioned cylinders with 2 to 4 mL of fat along the plane of least resistance.

Anterior Chin

The anterior chin becomes progressively bonier with aging, and a chin implant fails to address this. The anterior chin deficiency resembles an upside down U, with the central limb of the U running across the mental sulcus toward the lateral mandibular hollow and downward toward the prejowl sulcus. From entry point C, the fat is transferred upward in an arc to address each limb of the inverted U, passing the cannula in a subcutaneous plane of least resistance while fanning across the deficient area and placing a generous 0.1 mL per pass, as this area is also very forgiving.

Generally, 2 to 3 mL are placed into each side of the anterior chin to create the desired aesthetic outcome.

Canine Fossa and Nasolabial Groove

Generally, the nasolabial groove and its superior aspect, the canine fossa, are filled with 1 to 3 mL of fat placed from entry point A so as to fan across the linear deficiency.

30.6 Postoperative Considerations

After a fat transfer procedure, very little aftercare is needed. There are no bandages, no drains, no use of oral antibiotics, and no other interventions. Icing of the transplanted areas can help reduce edema but the patient should be prepared for 2 weeks of potential facial distortion. The patient can resume light exercise without major consequence to the donor sites. However, the patient should minimize Valsalva-type maneuvers that could exacerbate facial edema. Listening to one's body to gauge workout intensity should be the universal dictum for all patients after cosmetic procedures.

30.7 Clinical Pearls

- Understanding that fat is a biologically active graft that can fluctuate with weight is very important. Because fat is a graft, it does not have perfect take, and fat grafting will often benefit from touch-up with an off-the-shelf filler.
- Volume loss occurs in all ethnicities as the principal process of aging, and in ethnicities with darker skin, it can be the only sign of aging for many decades.
- Artistic placement of fat is critical, and in the ethnic face, which tends to be wider and flatter, it is critical not to make the face appear wider or too full.
- Always be more conservative with quantities of fat transferred to the face, as removing transplanted fat is nearly impossible.

30.8 Conclusion

Fat grafting is a reliable and powerful way to rejuvenate the face so long as the surgeon and patient alike understand the benefits, risks, and limitations. Therefore, patient communication is critical as a first step in the process. Using off-the-shelf injectable fillers can be a good starting point for the physician who is in the early stage of acquiring the artistry to design and produce results that look balanced and natural. With the right technique and good aesthetic judgment, a physician can achieve remarkably durable and pleasing results for patients of all ethnicities.

References

1. Lam SM. A new paradigm for the aging face. Facial Plast Surg Clin North Am 2010;18(1):1–6
2. Glasgold MJ, Glasgold RA, Lam SM. Volume restoration and facial aesthetics. Facial Plast Surg Clin North Am 2008;16(4):435–442, vi
3. Lam SM, Glasgold MJ, Glasgold RA. Complementary Fat Grafting. Philadelphia, PA: Lippincott, Williams, & Wilkins; 2006
4. Shirakabe Y, Suzuki Y, Lam SM. A new paradigm for the aging Asian face. Aesthetic Plast Surg 2003;27(5): 397–402
5. Lam SM, Glasgold RA, Glasgold MJ. Limitations, complications, and long-term sequelae of fat transfer. Facial Plast Surg Clin North Am 2008;16(4):391–399, v
6. Lam SM, Karam AM. Management of the Asian upper eyelid. Facial Plast Surg Clin North Am 2010;18: 43–47
7. Lam SM. Aesthetic strategies for the aging Asian face. Facial Plast Surg Clin North Am 2007;15(3):283–291, v
8. Lam SM. Aesthetic facial surgery for the asian male. Facial Plast Surg 2005;21(4):317–323

31 Scar and Keloid Treatment in Patients with Dark Skin Types

J. Regan Thomas and Tatiana K. Dixon

31.1 Introduction

The goals of both keloid and scar revision surgery are to produce thin, flat scars that are level with, and have color matching, the surrounding skin.[1] To be able to consistently get this result in patients with dark complexions, there are a few special considerations the surgeon should be aware of.

First, hypo- and hyperpigmentation can be more pronounced and more noticeable in darker skin, and steps can be taken to avoid and treat dyspigmentation. As always, strict sun avoidance is observed during the healing phase for prevention of permanent hyperpigmentation. It also is imperative that the surgeon be aware of the benefits and possible side effects of different therapies.

Compared with Caucasian patients, patients of African, Asian, and Hispanic descent have a higher predisposition for developing keloid scars.[2] The incidence of hypertrophic scars is thought to be relatively equal across different ethnicities.[3] While they have different pathologies, hypertrophic scars and keloids are both fibroproliferative disorders.[4] Hypertrophic scarring results in an enlarged, raised scar, which stays within the confines of the scar, whereas keloids extend beyond the borders of the scar and can replace normal structures and tissue. The increased risk of aberrant wound healing is especially important to keep in mind when revising scars in people with history of keloids or when performing surgery to remove keloids.

In this chapter we review the different modalities available for treatment of scars and keloids, and with each modality we discuss the special considerations for dark-skinned patients.

31.2 Excision

Excision is often the first line of therapy for unsightly scars and large, mature keloids. This is also the only modality that can change the orientation of a scar or make a wide scar thinner. Incisions should be planned so that the resulting scars fall within the junction of facial landmarks or are parallel to the relaxed skin tension lines.[1] It is important to remember, when excising a keloid, that it is a benign growth and therefore does not need to be completely excised. Anatomical structures like the helical rim or lobule should not be sacrificed for removal of keloids.

To increase the chance of producing a thin, flat scar, there are a few surgical pearls recommended by the primary author. First, the surgeon should attempt to minimize trauma to the skin edges after the keloid or scar is excised. Use of toothed forceps, or preferably skin hooks, to gently grasp the skin edges as needed during resection and closure is recommended. Limiting undermining of the surrounding skin is also important to prevent trauma and further keloid growth in the surrounding tissue.[5] Second, the wound should be closed without tension and the skin edges should be everted. This is to be balanced with keeping subcutaneous stitches to a minimum, as dissolvable stitches can induce inflammation and subsequent pathologic scarring.

Excision alone is not recommended for keloids, as the trauma to the reticular layer of the dermis is thought to stimulate further keloid growth.[5] Keloid recurrence rates can be as high as 55 to 100% in single-modality therapy, and therefore keloids mostly require multimodality therapy for successful removal.[5,6] After excision, adjuvant therapy, such as steroid injections, silicone sheeting, and radiotherapy, are advocated in the literature. There is no level I evidence to support any one modality or gold standard of treatment for keloids.[3]

31.3 Steroids

Intralesional steroid injections are commonly used to treat small keloids, or as an adjunct to surgery to prevent keloid regrowth or hypertrophic scarring after surgery. When used as a sole therapy, steroid injections can soften and flatten scars, but they do not make a thick scar thinner. When combined with surgery, steroid injections can reduce recurrence of keloids to 14 to 40%.[7]

Corticosteroids work by inhibiting fibroblast proliferation and decreasing collagen production.[8] The corticosteroid triamcinolone is widely used and, despite limited controlled studies, it is considered to be the first-line therapy for keloids.[9] There is also no consensus about optimal dosage or strength of steroid in the literature.[3] However, studies have shown that starting with 10 mg/mL triamcinolone injections and then increasing the strength to 40 mg/mL for subsequent injections was most cost effective and showed the lowest recurrence rate.[10]

It is important to note that corticosteroid therapy requires a considerable time commitment from the patient to come into the office multiple times for injections. Patients are often seen on a weekly, then biweekly, and then monthly, basis for ~ 6 months or until there is no further growth of the keloid. Throughout the treatment, it is important to assess whether the scar is responding to the therapy, as an estimated 30% of patients don't respond to steroid injection.[11]

The risks of steroid injections are injection pain, skin atrophy, wound dehiscence, telangiectasias, and changes in pigmentation.[5,7,12] There have also been case reports of Cushing disease occurring after intralesional steroid injections.[7] To minimize the risk of side effects, small doses of intralesional steroids are recommended. The primary author uses a tuberculin syringe to inject just enough triamcinolone to cause blanching of the scar. Specifically in dark-skinned patients, permanent hypopigmentation is of concern and injections should be stopped at the first sign of depigmentation.

31.4 Silicone Gel Sheeting

Silicone sheeting has been shown to prevent abnormal scarring after surgery as well as to improve the thickness and color of existing scars; however, the supporting evidence is at best class 3 evidence, and has been shown to have a high risk of bias.[13]

The mechanism of action of silicone sheeting is unknown. It has been postulated that the sheeting exerts constant pressure on the wound, preventing thickening of the scar. Other theories are that there is an increase in temperature, a change in oxygen tension, or an increase in hydration under the sheeting.[13,14]

Silicone sheets are to be used on intact skin only and can be begun 2 weeks after wound healing. The recommendation is that the patient wear the sheets for 12 to 24 hours for at least 2 months after surgery.[5] However, there is no strong evidence to support any particular treatment regimen. Due to the length of treatment, patient compliance can be a problem.

Silicone gel has been noted to produce results equivalent to those with silicone sheets, and due to the contours and constant movement of the face, some physicians prefer gel over sheeting due to ease of use.[14]

The risks of silicone sheeting are pruritus, skin rashes, folliculitis, and infection. Presently there are no known risks of using silicone sheets specific to patients of dark complexion. The low risk of silicon sheeting makes it an attractive adjunct therapy, even if the supporting evidence is weak.

31.5 Lasers

Lasers are used for the prevention of pathologic scarring after surgery, as well as for contouring of keloids and treatment of hypertrophic scars. The mechanism by which the scars are improved is disputed, but thermal injury to the dermal layers has been shown to cause collagen deposition and dermal remodeling as well as neovascularization.[15] Keloids have been shown to soften and flatten, but wide scars are not made thinner.

The goal is to select a laser that provides thermal destruction of the target tissue while minimizing conduction of heat to surrounding structures.[16] However, in patients with dark skin, melanin acts as a competing chromophore and increases the collateral damage to the treatment area.[17] If the incorrect laser or energy settings are chosen for a specific skin type, scarring may be exacerbated rather than ameliorated.[17]

The best candidates for laser therapy are patients with immature scars less than 6 months old and ideally with Fitzpatrick skin types I to IV.[18] Leaders in the field of laser treatment of facial scars recommend that patients with Fitzpatrick types IV to VI be treated only with nonablative lasers or nonablative fractional lasers.[16]

The pulsed dye laser (PDL) is the nonablative laser of choice for the treatment of hypertrophic scars and keloids.[16,19] PDL targets blood vessels and has been shown to reduce erythema and to reduce thickness of scars by rearranging collagen fibers.[19]

Postinflammatory hyperpigmentation (PIH) is the most common adverse effect of laser treatment in dark-skinned individuals. Other complications include posttreatment purpura, hypopigmentation, blistering, and rash.[20] To help avoid complications, decreasing energy densities and increasing treatment intervals are recommended in dark-skinned individuals.[5] With this in mind, extreme caution should be used when performing laser therapy on people with dark skin.

31.6 Radiation Therapy

Radiation therapy to treat keloids has been shown to be effective in decreasing recurrence rates, especially when performed as an adjunct to surgery.[21,22] A possible advantage of radiation therapy is that fewer return visits are required than with steroid injections, thus increasing the likelihood of patient compliance.[22] The mechanism of action is thought to be the elimination of abnormally activated fibroblasts through radiolysis, thus controlling collagen synthesis.[23] However, the mechanism is still poorly understood.[23]

Large-scale studies with long-term follow-up are currently lacking, and recommended doses of radiation vary between 10 and 30 Gy.[21,24,25] It is also disputed whether the radiation should be given in one dose or multiple fractions.[23,24] The interval between excision and commencement of radiation is also controversial, with some advocating that the treatment should be administered within 2 days of surgery.[23,25]

The risk of inducing malignancies for treatment of a benign condition is a large deterrent for many patients and surgeons. However, the risk of radiation-induced carcinogenesis is low, with only five cases of carcinogenesis reported in the literature in 2009.[26] Other, less dangerous, but still undesirable side effects of radiation therapy include desquamation, telangiectasias, and severe hyper- or hypopigmentation.[23]

31.7 5-Fluorouracil (5FU)

Intralesional injection of the chemotherapy agent 5FU has been shown to be effective in treating keloids and in decreasing recurrence rates. 5FU is used as a monotherapy and as an adjunct to other keloid treatments. Specifically, 5FU has been shown to increase the efficacy of intralesional steroid treatments while reducing the side effects.[8]

The mechanism of action is thought to be inhibition of fibroblast proliferation by blocking DNA synthesis.[8,27] In vitro experiments have shown a significant suppression of collagen 1 synthesis in keloid fibroblasts when treated with a triamcinolone and 5FU mixture.[8]

Side effects of 5FU include ulceration and hyperpigmentation.[3]

31.8 Cryotherapy

Intralesional cryosurgery is performed by passing a cryogen, typically liquid nitrogen, through the lumen of a needle, which is introduced into the keloid.[28] Cryotherapy has been shown to be effective in flattening smaller, early-onset keloids.[29]

The mechanism of action is thought to be cellular injury from intra- and extracellular ice formation, as well as ischemic necrosis from vascular stasis after thawing.[28,29]

The side effects of cryotherapy are procedural pain and lesion depigmentation. Hypopigmentation is pronounced and exceedingly common in patients with dark skin types because melanocytes are destroyed at much higher temperature (−4 to −8°C) than fibroblasts (−30 to −40°C).[28] Therefore, specifically in dark-skinned individuals, cryotherapy produces less than desirable outcomes.

31.9 Miscellaneous Therapies

Many other recommended therapies for keloids are found in the literature, although good supporting evidence for these therapies has yet to be generated. Injection of calcium channel antagonist, such as verapamil, into the keloid is thought to reduce extracellular matrix production and to inhibit proliferation of fibroblasts.[12] Botox injections are thought to help prevent keloid recurrence by decreasing scar tension.[12] Bleomycin, a chemotherapy agent, is thought to induce apoptosis and to decrease collagen synthesis. Injections are thought to be effective in treating older scars that are not responding to steroid injections.[9,5] Interferon injections have been shown to increase collagen breakdown, but the injections are painful and require regional anesthesia, and patients sometimes experience flu-like symptoms after injections.[5]

31.10 Case Examples

Fig. 31.1, **Fig. 31.2**, **Fig. 31.3**, **Fig. 31.4**, and **Fig. 31.5** show examples of scar and keloid treatment.

31.11 Recommendations and Conclusion

There are many different treatment modalities for scars and keloids. No one treatment has been deemed far superior to others, and surgeons often use several treatment modalities to treat a single patient. Specifically for keloids, the exact mechanisms of action of the different treatments are still unknown. No gold standard of treatment has been found, and recurrence rates are still high.

The lack of evidence to support the treatment methods also means that there are few data on side effects, both for the population in general and even less so for patients with dark skin.

The primary author uses a combination of surgery, serial steroid injections, and silicone sheeting for the treatment of keloids and has noted low recurrence and complication rates in his dark-skinned patients. However, further research will have to be performed, specifically in dark-skinned individuals, before any one treatment can be recommended.

31.12 Clinical Pearls

- Surgical excision is the only modality that can change the orientation of a scar or make a wide scar thinner.
- Although steroid injections have been effective in decreasing hypertrophic scarring and keloid recurrence, permanent hypopigmentation is of concern in dark-skinned patients, and injections should be stopped at the first sign of depigmentation.
- Radiation therapy has been shown to decrease keloid recurrence rates after surgery, and documented cases of induced malignancies are very low.
- Postinflammatory hyperpigmentation is the most common side effect of lasers in dark-skinned individuals.
- Melanin acts as a competing chromophore in laser therapy and can increase collateral damage.
- Cryotherapy causes hypopigmentation because melanocytes are destroyed at a much warmer temperature than fibroblasts.
- 5FU has been shown to increase the efficacy of intralesional steroid treatments while reducing the side effects.

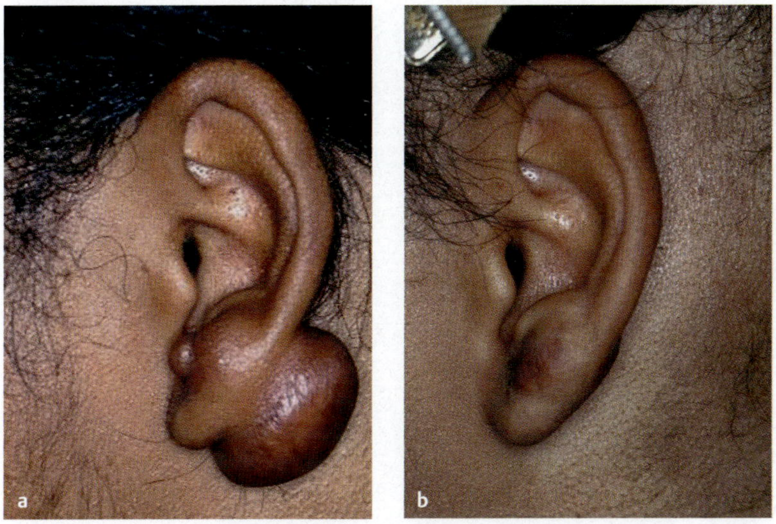

Fig. 31.1 **(a)** Small anterior and large posterior ear lobule keloid following ear piercing. **(b)** Appearance 1 year after treatment with excision and Kenalog injections of both anterior and posterior lobule keloids.

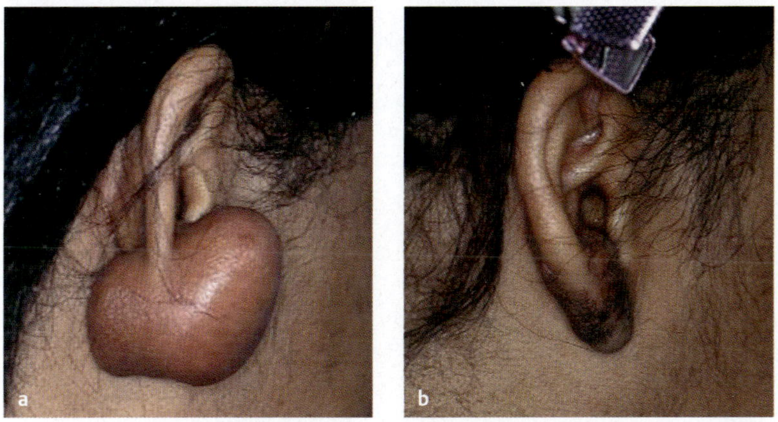

Fig. 31.2 **(a)** Large anterior and posterior ear lobule keloids following ear piercing. **(b)** Appearance 1 year after treatment with excision and serial Kenalog injections. The large keloid was carved to fashion a new lobule.

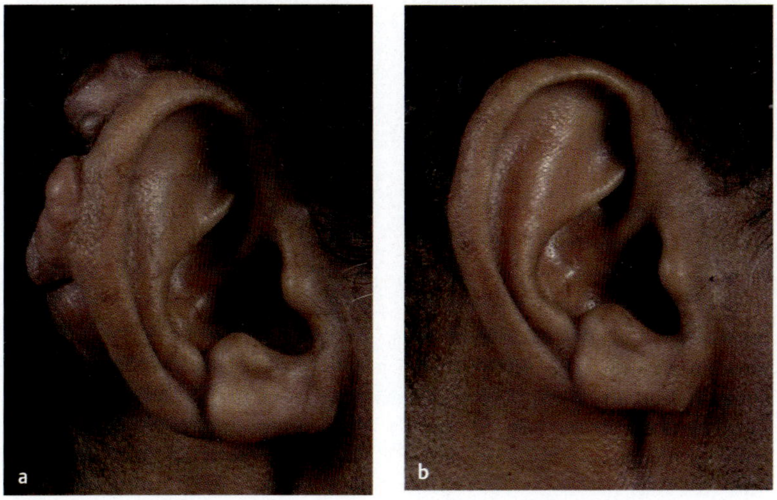

Fig. 31.3 **(a)** Preoperative anterior view. **(b)** Postoperative anterior view 1 year after excision and serial Kenalog injections.

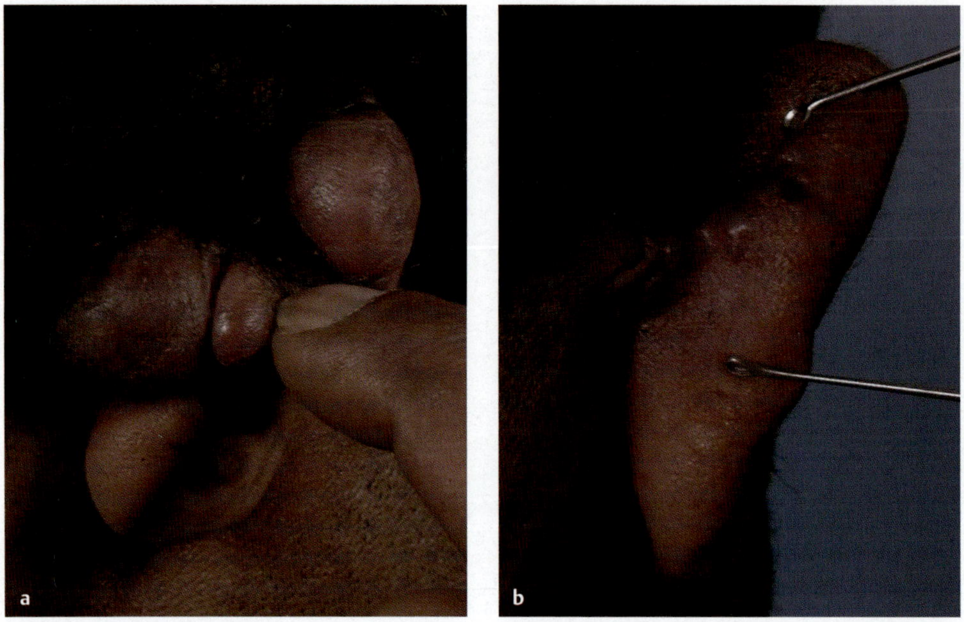

Fig. 31.4 **(a)** Preoperative posterior view. **(b)** Postoperative posterior view 1 year after excision and serial Kenalog injections. The incisions were hidden in the postauricular crease.

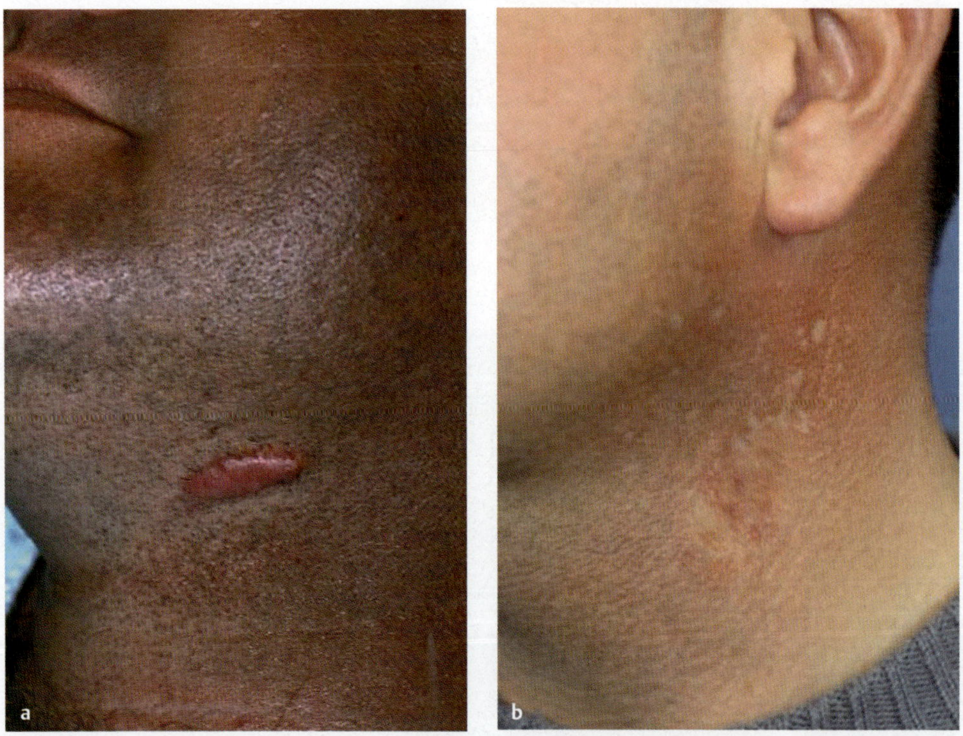

Fig. 31.5 **(a)** Preoperative view of Caucasian male with submandibular keloid after trauma. **(b)** Appearance 1 year after treatment with excision and serial Kenalog injections.

References

1. Thomas JR. Scar revision and camouflage surgery. In: Thomas JR, ed. Advanced Therapy in Facial Plastic and Reconstructive Surgery. Shelton, CT: PMPH-USA; 2010:687–693
2. Burchard AE, Lee AS. Treatment of keloid scars. In: Thomas JR, ed. Advanced Therapy in Facial Plastic and Reconstructive Surgery. Shelton, CT: PMPH-USA; 2010:695–701
3. Ud-Din S, Bayat A. Strategic management of keloid disease in ethnic skin: a structured approach supported by the emerging literature. Br J Dermatol 2013;169(Suppl 3): 71–81
4. Singer AJ, Clark RA. Cutaneous wound healing. N Engl J Med 1999;341(10):738–746
5. Arno AI, Gauglitz GG, Barret JP, Jeschke MG. Up-to-date approach to manage keloids and hypertrophic scars: a useful guide. Burns 2014;40(7):1255–1266
6. Butler PD, Longaker MT, Yang GP. Current progress in keloid research and treatment. J Am Coll Surg 2008;206(4): 731–741
7. Rosen DJ, Patel MK, Freeman K, Weiss PR. A primary protocol for the management of ear keloids: results of excision combined with intraoperative and postoperative steroid injections. Plast Reconstr Surg 2007;120(5):1395–1400
8. Huang L, Cai YJ, Lung I, Leung BC, Burd A. A study of the combination of triamcinolone and 5-fluorouracil in modulating keloid fibroblasts in vitro. J Plast Reconstr Aesthet Surg 2013;66(9):e251–e259
9. Mustoe TA, Cooter RD, Gold MH, et al; International Advisory Panel on Scar Management. International clinical recommendations on scar management. Plast Reconstr Surg 2002;110(2):560–571
10. Anthony ET, Lemonas P, Navsaria HA, Moir GC. The cost effectiveness of intralesional steroid therapy for keloids. Dermatol Surg 2010;36(10):1624–1626
11. Ud-Din S, Bowring A, Derbyshire B, Morris J, Bayat A. Identification of steroid sensitive responders versus non-responders in the treatment of keloid disease. Arch Dermatol Res 2013;305(5):423–432
12. Ledon JA, Savas J, Franca K, Chacon A, Nouri K. Intralesional treatment for keloids and hypertrophic scars: a review. Dermatol Surg 2013;39(12):1745–1757
13. O'Brien L, Jones DJ. Silicone gel sheeting for preventing and treating hypertrophic and keloid scars. Cochrane Database Syst Rev 2013;9:CD003826
14. Mustoe TA. Evolution of silicone therapy and mechanism of action in scar management. Aesthetic Plast Surg 2008;32(1):82–92
15. Nicoletti G, De Francesco F, Mele CM, et al. Clinical and histologic effects from CO_2 laser treatment of keloids. Lasers Med Sci 2013;28(3):957–964
16. Sobanko JF, Alster TS. Laser treatment for improvement and minimization of facial scars. Facial Plast Surg Clin North Am 2011;19(3):527–542
17. Jin R, Huang X, Li H, et al. Laser therapy for prevention and treatment of pathologic excessive scars. Plast Reconstr Surg 2013;132(6):1747–1758
18. Khatri KA, Mahoney DL, McCartney MJ. Laser scar revision: a review. J Cosmet Laser Ther 2011;13(2):54–62
19. Brown P, Miller ME, Bandino J, et al. Laser treatment of scars and keloids. Cosmet Dermatol 2012;25:318–325
20. Brewin MP, Lister TS. Prevention or treatment of hypertrophic burn scarring: a review of when and how to treat with the pulsed dye laser. Burns 2014;40(5):797–804
21. Ogawa R, Huang C, Akaishi S, et al. Analysis of surgical treatments for earlobe keloids: analysis of 174 lesions in 145 patients. Plast Reconstr Surg 2013;132(5):818e–825e
22. Sclafani AP, Gordon L, Chadha M, Romo T III. Prevention of earlobe keloid recurrence with postoperative corticosteroid injections versus radiation therapy: a randomized, prospective study and review of the literature. Dermatol Surg 1996;22(6):569–574
23. Sakamoto T, Oya N, Shibuya K, Nagata Y, Hiraoka M. Dose-response relationship and dose optimization in radiotherapy of postoperative keloids. Radiother Oncol 2009; 91(2):271–276
24. Song C, Wu HG, Chang H, Kim IH, Ha SW. Adjuvant single-fraction radiotherapy is safe and effective for intractable keloids. J Radiat Res (Tokyo) 2014;55(5):912–916 [Epub ahead of print]
25. Kal HB, Veen RE. Biologically effective doses of postoperative radiotherapy in the prevention of keloids. Dose-effect relationship. Strahlenther Onkol 2005;181(11): 717–723
26. Ogawa R, Yoshitatsu S, Yoshida K, Miyashita T. Is radiation therapy for keloids acceptable? The risk of radiation-induced carcinogenesis. Plast Reconstr Surg 2009; 124(4):1196–1201
27. Khare N, Patil SB. A novel approach for management of ear keloids: results of excision combined with 5-fluorouracil injection. J Plast Reconstr Aesthet Surg 2012;65(11): e315–e317
28. Zouboulis CC. Principles of cutaneous cryosurgery: an update. Dermatology 1999;198(2):111–117
29. Barara M, Mendiratta V, Chander R. Cryotherapy in treatment of keloids: evaluation of factors affecting treatment outcome. J Cutan Aesthet Surg 2012;5(3):185–189

32 Skin-Tightening Devices in Mixed-Race Patients

Rafael Espinosa Delgado, Miriam de la Torre Campos, and Rolando Hidalgo Moiron

32.1 Introduction

In 2013, the Associated Press reported that ethnic minorities composed half of the population in the United States under 5 years old, which means that in three decades, at least half of the population of the United States will be of non-Caucasian ethnicity.[1] Therefore, the number of mixed-race patients seen in aesthetic practices will grow at the same rate, and this is important because mixed-race skin reacts differently to light energy devices.

Safety has always been a concern in noninvasive rejuvenating procedures, especially for mixed-race patients, who have skin pigment disorders as their most common and important concern, and which can be seriously affected by energy-based treatments. Over the past 10 years, technology has developed at an accelerated pace in the aesthetic field, and a safe and effective noninvasive skin-tightening procedure has been a much-desired goal for the aesthetic industry.

It is said that the gold standard for skin tightening is the CO_2 laser.[1,2,3,4] The authors believe that CO_2 laser is great for improving overall skin quality (sun damage, sun spots, enlarged pores, acne scars), but after the swelling goes away, there is not as much tightening as with the radiofrequency (RF) devices.

Patients also are looking for skin-tightening procedures that are safe, have minimal to no downtime, and do not produce any pain.[5] Mixed-race patients are no exception. To meet these expectations, RF treatments are ideal because they have a high level of safety, they are non-ablative, and they incur almost no recovery time. Unlike laser energy, RF energy does not depend on selective photothermolysis of a chromophore; rather, RF depends on heating of water, and therefore any skin type may be treated.[3,4,5,6,7,8]

Radiofrequency was developed in the 1920s originally for electrocautery,[6] and in 2002 the Food and Drug Administration (FDA) approved the first RF device for facial wrinkle reduction, a monopolar RF device (ThermaCool; Thermage, Solta Medical, Hayward, CA), and in 2006 the device received FDA clearance for off-face use.[3,4,5,6] Today, RF is mostly used as a noninvasive procedure for skin tightening, circumferential reduction, and cellulite improvement.[7,8]

32.2 Radiofrequency Concepts

Radiofrequency produces electric current using electromagnetic radiation in the frequency of 3 kHz to 300 MHz.[6] Impedance is the resistance offered by a tissue as the RF current flows, and, as the RF meets resistance, it generates heat.[3,5] Radiofrequency can be monopolar, unipolar, bipolar, and fractional and it can be combined with light energy sources or vacuum.[3,5,6]

32.2.1 Monopolar RF

Monopolar RF uses one electrode in contact with the skin and a ground pad. It delivers electric current to the skin at the same time a cooling spray is applied to the epidermis, which protects it from heating. As the dermis heats uniformly and volumetrically, this causes partial collagen denaturation that leads to collagen contraction and thickening, which occurs immediately as the heat is applied. Some additional tightening occurs due to the natural inflammatory healing response in the form of neo-collagenesis.[3,4,5,6]

The depth of penetration of RF energy is inversely proportional to the frequency; in other words, lower frequencies of RF energy penetrate more deeply.[5]

Monopolar RF devices penetrate more deeply than unipolar or bipolar devices. The RF can be delivered in a static or a dynamic mode, by pulses or continuously, with constant movement of the handpiece. Pain during treatment depends on the duration of the pulse.[3,4,5,6,7,8]

An example of a monopolar device that delivers RF in a static mode with a short 1- to 2-second cycle is the Thermage device (Solta Medical, Hayward, CA),[3,4,5] and a monopolar device that delivers RF in a continuous pulse with the handpiece in constant movement is the Pellevé (Ellman International, Inc., Hicksville, NY).[9,10,11]

32.2.2 Bipolar RF

In bipolar RF devices, RF travels from a positive to a negative pole between two electrodes built into the handpiece; it is believed that the depth of penetration is half the distance between the electrodes. Bipolar RF is not as painful as monopolar RF because it has less penetration, so often bipolar RF devices are combined with other energies or have suction built into the handpiece.[5,8,12,13] An example of a bipolar RF device is the Viora Reaction (Viora, Jersey City, NJ).

32.2.3 Fractional RF

Fractional RF is a variation of the bipolar modality. The device uses mini bipolar electrodes or bipolar insulated needles, which can also be combined with a light-source device to potentiate treatment benefits.[5] Examples of fractional bipolar RF technology are the eMatrix (Syneron/Candela, Wayland, Massachusetts) and the ePrime (Syneron/Candela, Wayland, Massachusetts).

32.2.4 Unipolar RF

Unipolar RF delivers energy using one electrode with no grounding pad. This electrode produces a large, omnidirectional RF field. High-frequency electromagnetic radiation is produced by the device's quickly alternating the polarity of the electromagnetic field, producing rotation and oscillation in water molecules, which produce heat.[5,6,14,15] An example of a unipolar device is the Accent Rf (Alma Lasers, Caesarea, Israel).

Every year, new RF devices with various forms of delivery are inaugurated, and their manufacturers claim each one is the biggest breakthrough or the new gold standard in RF technology. To be fair, they all produce almost the same results. Some are better for facial skin tightening, some for cellulite treatment, and some for volumetric reduction. Each device has advantages and disadvantages, mainly because of their depth of penetration, their frequency, and the amount of effective heat they produce. We cannot write about all the RF devices, so here we review the three of them that we have experience with, which are also three of the most popular devices.

32.3 Monopolar RF Device—Thermage

Monopolar RF is an effective means of nonsurgical facial and body tightening. As mentioned above, it was the first nonsurgical technique developed for this purpose, and was cleared by the Food and Drug Administration for treatment of periorbital wrinkles and rhytids in November 2002.[3,4,5,6]

As also described above, monopolar RF uses a controlled RF pulse to selectively heat zones of the dermis and deeper tissues while using cryogen delivered to the tip membrane to cool the epidermis, preventing damage to the epidermis and upper dermis. The monopolar energy is delivered for ~ 1 to 2 seconds depending on the tip used. A pressure-sensitive tip prevents nonuniform application of the tip to the skin, and the cryogen spray applied to the tip keeps the epidermis cool, prevents blistering and crusting, and decreases the pain of the procedure.[3,4,16]

32.3.1 Procedure

Monopolar systems deliver the current through a single contact point with a corresponding grounding pad, which helps create a resistance path for the flow of current to complete the electrical circuit. The skin is cleansed and the grounding pad is placed in a naked area of the back, arm, or leg. A "calibration shot" is then made to establish treatment parameters.

For each patient, the initial impedance level setting is determined based on his or her heat sensation feedback. The amount of RF applied is configured to target specific tissues; therefore high-impedance tissues, such as subcutaneous fat, generate greater heat and account for the deeper thermal effects of RF devices.

Before treatment is started, pictures are taken. Patients may opt for treatment of the entire face, part of the face, or just the orbital area. With this information, the practitioner decides which tip is optimal for the treatment (for facial treatment, the two options are the Facial Tip, with 900 "shots" [passes] and the Total Tip, with 1,200 shots). With the chosen tip, the system divides the number of shots in half, so they are delivered equally on each side of the face or body.

The RF energy is delivered using a multiple, staggered pass technique (circle then square on the treatment grid), providing 50% overlap of each pulse on the body and a little more on the face. Three to four passes are applied over the gridded area and four to six passes are applied to vectors and problem areas until a visible and/or palpable clinical endpoint is achieved. Pulses are delivered distal to proximal and medial to lateral on the body, and from the forehead to the neck in facial treatment, avoiding treatment over the thyroid gland.[3,4,7,8] To ensure full tip-to-skin contact, the treatment tip is kept perpendicular to the skin and a generous amount of coupling fluid is applied throughout the procedure. The tip has a thermometer and is constantly measuring the temperature of the skin, so it has a low probability of damaging the skin by overheating.

After covering the area with individual passes, we then start a sweeping technique, applying energy through an area of two to three times the size of the tip, in the opposite direction of the aging descending vectors. This technique gives the practitioner the option of increasing the heat parameters, and it is well tolerated by the patient. We always leave 20 to 30 shots to retreat a special area chosen by the patient, and before finishing with the last one, we make cooling passes around the treated area to cool down the skin. When 50% of the shots have been delivered, the system stops automatically, so the patient may drink some water, and a picture is taken to compare the treated and untreated areas.

There are few contraindications to Thermage treatment. Typically, the technology should not be used on patients who have a pacemaker, patients who are pregnant or breast feeding, and patients who have skin cancer or lupus.[5,6] After Thermage, patients can also receive complementary treatments like botulinum toxin, hyaluronic acid injections, intense pulsed light (IPL), CO_2 laser, etc.[17]

32.4 Bipolar RF Device—Viora Reaction

The Viora Reaction device offers bipolar RF combined with suction and integrated cooling of the treated area. The Viora Reaction emits RF energy at three different frequencies: 2.45 MHz, 1.7 MHz, and 0.8 MHz, with a multimodal delivery that combines all three frequencies at the same time. This permits the energy to penetrate at three different depths, so that a specific layer of tissue can be targeted or combined energy can be delivered to a thicker layer of tissue.[5,12]

When the RF energy is applied to the skin, it generates an electromagnetic field, causing oscillation of molecules within the tissue. This molecular movement generates heat, causing two phenomena, the breakdown of collagen cross-links, which improves the elasticity of connective tissue for firmer skin, and gene expression of collagen types I and III, resulting in new collagen production and remodeling that goes on for 3 to 5 weeks after treatment.[4,5,8,12]

The Viora Reaction has two handpieces for use on the face: the skin tightening (ST) and the facial contouring (FC) device. They both have the capability of delivering the three RF frequencies, and the FC handpiece also incorporates suction in the applicator so that the energy can be delivered deeply to target the fat cells.[12]

32.4.1 ST Procedure

When using the ST applicator, cooling gel is applied on the area to be treated, the device is set in mode 1, and temperature is started at 52 J (joules), increasing from there until the patient feels the skin heating up at a comfortable temperature, which should be ~ 72 J. During treatment, the patient should not feel pain. Two passes are performed on the area to be treated, always proceeding from central to lateral. The machine is then set in mode 2, and four more passes are performed. Treatments can be personalized, targeting specific depths (this is done by changing the modes) and totaling four to six sessions, which should be performed 3 to 5 weeks apart to complete the treatment protocol. Thereafter, maintenance sessions can be done every 3 to 6 months (**Fig. 32.1**).[12]

32.4.2 FC Procedure

For the FC protocol, glycerin is used on the area to be treated so that the suction handpiece can seal completely for adequate suction and so that both electrodes are always in contact with the skin. This is very important because if one electrode fails to make contact, a burn will result. Half of the face is treated first with the following protocol: heat the skin in the combined mode (mode 4) and suction level 1 for ~ 6 minutes, while using an infrared thermometer to make sure the temperature is maintained between 38 and 42°C; then switch to mode 2 for 2 minutes, and then mode 3 for 2 minutes, repeating the procedure on the other side of the face and thus completing the session. A series of six to eight weekly treatments should be done to complete the protocol (**Fig. 32.2**).[12]

32.5 Monopolar RF Device—Pellevé

The Pellevé is a monopolar RF device in which the energy is applied to the skin by an electrode (GlideSafe handpiece) and a grounding pad receives the energy that goes

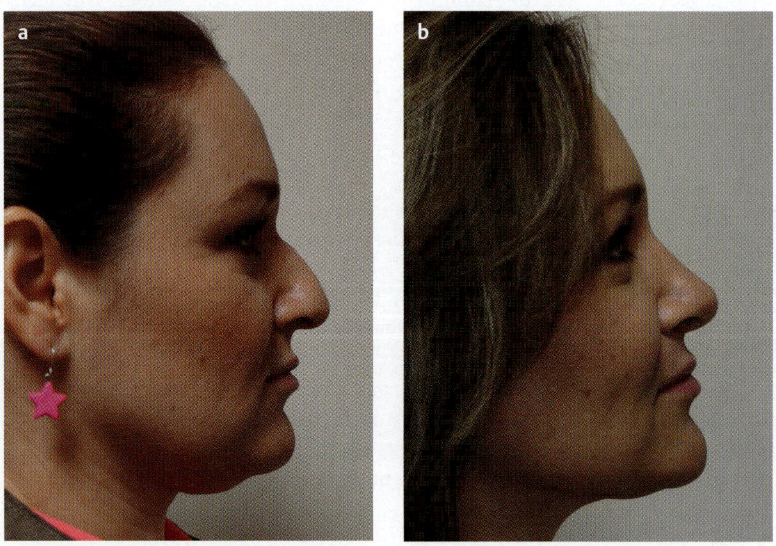

Fig. 32.1 **(a)** A 31-year-old female patient before treatment. Although she is thin, her genetically heavy chin and cheeks are evident. **(b)** Same patient after four Viora Reaction FC (facial contouring) lower face treatments and four ST (skin tightening) submental treatments combined with rhinoplasty and chin liposuction.

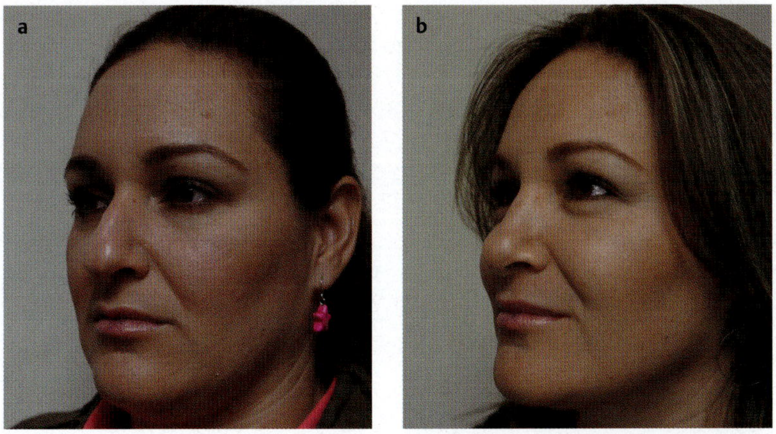

Fig. 32.2 Three-quarter views of same patient as in **Fig. 32.1** **(a)** before treatment and **(b)** after treatment.

through the body. When it is not in contact with the skin, the GlideSafe handpiece stops emitting RF to avoid electrical sparking and burning. As with the other devices mentioned previously, it works by delivering RF energy, causing heat that, at a superficial temperature of 39 to 42°C, induces collagen remodeling, new collagen formation, and elastin uniformity. The Pellevé is easy to use and has several handpieces that vary only in the size of the tip. The operator applies treatment gel before each pass, and the electrode is moved in a circular pattern, building up heat until it gets to 39 to 42°C, with that temperature maintained for ~ 8 passes. Like all the other RF devices, it produces skin contraction and contour remodeling as well.[9,10,11]

32.6 Patient Selection

The ideal patient for RF treatment is a patient between 30 and 60 years old, with modest to moderate laxity but relatively elastic skin and moderate to mild nasolabial and glabellar folds, and with realistic expectations. As with all medical procedures, patient education and informed consent are key elements.[7,8,18]

32.7 Complications of RF Treatment

Complications of RF treatment are often associated with overheating.[6] It is very important to monitor surface temperature during treatment and to keep it below 42°C, especially since the temperature below the skin is much higher. With pulse RF devices, be sure to avoid pulse stacking because it may lead to overheating and burns. With bipolar RF devices, a burn or sparking may occur when the handpiece is not fully in contact with the skin.[6,18]

With the first-generation monopolar devices, subcutaneous atrophy was reported as a result of a high-fluence treatment with the one-pass technique. To avoid this problem, a low-fluence protocol with a multiple-pass technique was introduced, lowering both the pain felt by patients and the risk of complications as well.[8] Avoid the use of RF in patients with pacemakers or patients who are pregnant, and avoid using monopolar devices when prosthetic devices are present in the patient.[5,6,18]

32.8 Conclusion

Ethnicity and culture play an important role in how people perceive beauty and how they take care of their skin. Mixed-race patients are an increasing percentage of aesthetic patients, and they require effective but safe procedures, so we as physicians have to invest a lot in training as well. The most common issue in mixed-race patients is post-inflammatory hyperpigmentation or hypopigmentation.[1]

Radiofrequency treatment is safe for all skin types because it does not depend on a target chromophore. Its mechanism of action is the production of heat, which induces collagen remodeling and new collagen formation, so skin color, melanin, and hemoglobin do not play any role in RF-based therapy.[3,4,5,6,7,8]

All RF devices produce mild to moderate results, so they should not be advertised as a nonsurgical facelift. They produce a refreshed look with some skin tightening. With some devices and proper patient selection, RF treatment can mildly reduce the fat under the chin and cheeks. RF treatment works better when combined with other noninvasive or minimally invasive procedures, such as botulinum toxin and filler injection. RF treatment is ideal after chin or face liposuction and as a post-rhytidectomy touch-up to tighten the skin **(Fig. 32.3)**.[7,8,16,17]

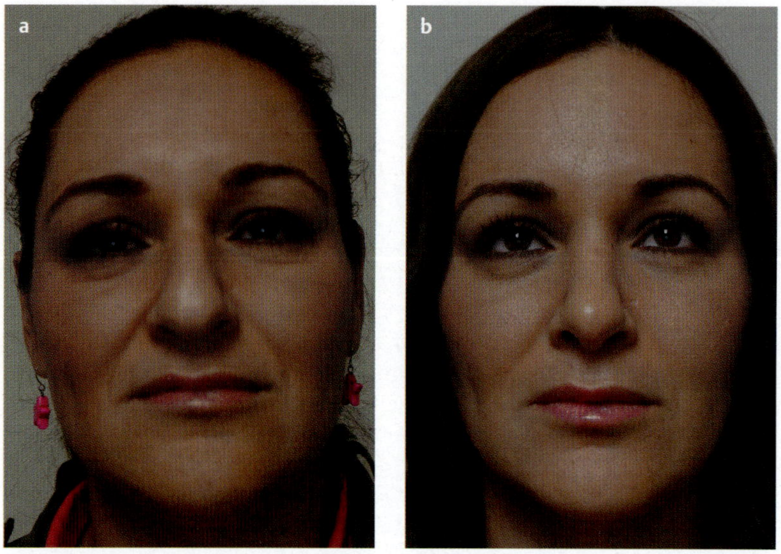

Fig. 32.3 Frontal views of same patient as in **Fig. 32.1 (a)** before treatment and **(b)** after treatment.

References

1. Delgado RE, Torre MdeL. Use of fractional laser in mixed-race patients. Facial Plast Surg 2013;29(3):161–166
2. Trelles MA, Shohat M, Urdiales F. Safe and effective one-session fractional skin resurfacing using a carbon dioxide laser device in super-pulse mode: a clinical and histologic study. Aesthetic Plast Surg 2011;35(1):31–42
3. Atiyeh BS, Dibo SA. Nonsurgical nonablative treatment of aging skin: radiofrequency technologies between aggressive marketing and evidence-based efficacy. Aesthetic Plast Surg 2009;33(3):283–294
4. el-Domyati M, el-Ammawi TS, Medhat W, et al. Radiofrequency facial rejuvenation: evidence-based effect. J Am Acad Dermatol 2011;64(3):524–535
5. Beasley KL, Weiss RA. Radiofrequency in cosmetic dermatology. Dermatol Clin 2014;32(1):79–90
6. Lolis MS, Goldberg DJ. Radiofrequency in cosmetic dermatology: a review. Dermatol Surg 2012;38(11): 1765–1776
7. Grimes PE. Aesthetics and Cosmetic Surgery for Darker Skin Types. Philadelphia, PA: Lippincott Williams & Wilkins; 2008:197–202, 207
8. Alam M, Bhatia AC, Kundu R, Yoo S, Chan HH. Cosmetic Dermatology for Skin of Color. Chicago, IL: McGraw-Hill; 2009:87–90
9. Stampar M. The Pellevé procedure: an effective method for facial wrinkle reduction and skin tightening. Facial Plast Surg Clin North Am 2011;19(2):335–345
10. Javate RM. Histopathological Analysis of Tissue Before and After Pellevé Treatment. Ellman International 2011:1–2
11. Taub AF, Tucker RD, Palange A. Facial tightening with an advanced 4.0 MHz monopolar radiofrequency device. J Drugs Dermatol 2012;11:1288–1294
12. Paun SD. Non ablative skin tightening and wrinkle reduction treatment with the Reaction system: a three month follow-up study and evaluation. Viora, Inc.:1–2
13. Adatto MA, Adatto-Neilson RM, Morren G. Reduction in adipose tissue volume using a new high-power radiofrequency technology combined with infrared light and mechanical manipulation for body contouring. Laser Med Sci 2014
14. Goldberg DJ, Fazeli A, Berlin AL. Clinical, laboratory, and MRI analysis of cellulite treatment with a unipolar radiofrequency device. Dermatol Surg 2008;34(2):204–209, discussion 209
15. Del Pino MA, Rosado Castro RH, Azuela A, Guzmán MG, Argüelles D, Rodríguez C. Efecto del calentamiento volumétrico controlado con radiofrecuencia en el tejido celular subcutáneo sobre la piel en muslos y glúteos, observado por medio de ultrasonido espacial en tiempo real. Alma lasers 2012; 1–10, http://www.accent.com.ar/files/ATT00035.pdf
16. Ruiz-Esparza J, Gomez JB. The medical face lift: a noninvasive, nonsurgical approach to tissue tightening in facial skin using nonablative radiofrequency. Dermatol Surg 2003;29(4):325–332, discussion 332
17. Fedok FG, Carniol PJ. Minimally Invasive and Office-Based Procedures in Facial Plastic Surgery. Hershey, PA: Thieme; 2014:147–157
18. Tosti A, Beer K, Pia de Padova M. Management of Complications of Cosmetic Procedures. Miami, FL: Springer; 2012:1–7, 23–33

Index

Note: Page numbers followed by f and t indicate figures and tables, respectively.

S

T

U

V

W

X

Y

Z